Sports and Soft Tissue Injuries

The fifth edition of the retitled *Sports and Soft Tissue Injuries* sharpens its focus on the treatment of sports injuries, providing the most complete evidence-based guide for physiotherapists, sports therapists and medical practitioners working with athletes.

Opening with chapters that examine the underlying science of tissue healing and principles of rehabilitation, the book employs a systematic approach, with chapters covering each area of the body, from facial through to ankle and foot injuries. Every chapter includes in-depth discussion and guidance on the treatment of common sports injuries through physiotherapeutic modalities, drawing on the author's wealth of personal experience and the latest peer-reviewed research.

A complete pedagogical resource, *Sports and Soft Tissue Injuries* is highly illustrated in full colour, and features a companion website with video examples of therapeutic techniques and a frequently updated blog on current issues in sports injury treatment. It is an important text for students of sports therapy, physiotherapy, sport medicine and athletic training, interesting further reading for sport and exercise science or kinesiology students with an interest in sports injury, and a crucial reference for practising physiotherapists and athletic trainers and the related disciplines.

Christopher M. Norris is a Chartered Physiotherapist (MCSP) and runs his own physiotherapy practice, Norris Health, in Cheshire, UK. He gained an MSc in Exercise Science from the University of Liverpool, UK, and a PhD on spinal rehabilitation from Staffordshire University, UK. He also holds postgraduate certification in Occupational Health, Orthopaedic Medicine and Medical Education.

Sports and Soft Tissue Injuries

A Guide for Students and Therapists

Fifth Edition

Christopher M. Norris

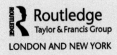
Routledge
Taylor & Francis Group

LONDON AND NEW YORK

Fifth edition published 2019
by Routledge
2 Park Square, Milton Park, Abingdon, Oxon, OX14 4RN

and by Routledge
711 Third Avenue, New York, NY 10017

Routledge is an imprint of the Taylor & Francis Group, an informa business

First edition published by Elsevier 1993
Fourth edition published by Elsevier 2011

British Library Cataloguing-in-Publication Data
A catalogue record for this book is available from the British Library

Library of Congress Cataloging-in-Publication Data
Names: Norris, Christopher M., author.
Title: Sports and soft tissue injuries : a guide for students and therapists / Christopher M. Norris.
Other titles: Managing sports injuries
Description: Fifth edition. | Milton Park, Abingdon, Oxon ; New York, NY : Routledge, 2018. | Revised edition of: Managing sports injuries : a guide for students and clinicians. 4th ed. Edinburgh : Churchill Livingstone/Elsevier, 2011. | Includes bibliographical references and index.
Identifiers: LCCN 2017058565 (print) | LCCN 2017059738 (ebook) | ISBN 9781315101521 (Master e-Book) | ISBN 9781351589321 (Adobe Reader) | ISBN 9781351589314 (ePub3) | ISBN 9781351589307 (Mobipocket) | ISBN 9781138106581 (hbk) | ISBN 9781138106598 (pbk) | ISBN 9781315101521 (ebk)
Subjects: LCSH: Sports injuries.
Classification: LCC RD97 (ebook) | LCC RD97 .N67 2018 (print) | DDC 617.1/027–dc23
LC record available at https://lccn.loc.gov/2017058565

ISBN: 978-1-138-10658-1 (hbk)
ISBN: 978-1-138-10659-8 (pbk)
ISBN: 978-1-315-10152-1 (ebk)

Typeset in Univers
by Servis Filmsetting Ltd, Stockport, Cheshire

Visit the companion website: www.routledge.com/cw/norris

Contents

List of figures

List of figures

List of figures

List of figures

List of figures

List of tables

List of tables

List of treatment notes

CHAPTER 1

Healing

Following injury, tissue which has been damaged must be replaced by living material. Two processes are possible, regeneration and repair. With *regeneration,* tissue is replaced by the proliferation of surrounding undamaged tissue. Therapy to produce this effect is currently in its infancy with stem cell therapy. With repair, however, lost material is replaced by granulation tissue which matures into a scar (Watson 2016), a process which most commonly reflects healing seen within the field of sports and soft tissue injury.

Therapists need to have knowledge of the processes which occur at each successive stage of healing to be able to select the treatment technique which is most appropriate for the stage the subject is presenting. A technique aimed at reducing the formation of swelling, for example, would be inappropriate when swelling had stopped forming and adhesions were the problem. Similarly, a manual treatment designed to mobilize soft tissue may not be helpful when inflammation is still forming and the tissues are highly irritable.

The stages of healing are, to a large extent, purely a convenience of description, since each stage runs into another in a continuum, the previous stage acting to initiate the next. The term *phasing* rather than separate stages may be more suitable. Traditionally, the initial tissue response has been described as *inflammation*, but some authors see inflammation as a response separate to the processes occurring at the time of injury. Both injury and inflammation may be viewed as a reactive phase of injury, with the classical inflammatory period preceded by a short (ten-minute) period before the inflammatory mechanism is activated. The reactive phase may also be viewed as a lag phase (Hunter 1998), before the strength of the healing tissues begins to change. In any traumatic injury the initial stage is *bleeding*, which is the precursor for the inflammatory cascade seen as both a vascular and cellular response.

The second stage of healing has been variously called repair, proliferation and regeneration. The tertiary stage is normally termed remodelling. The terms injury, inflammation, repair and remodelling will be used in this text

When describing the stages of healing, the terms acute, subacute and chronic are helpful. The acute stage (up to 48 hours following injury) is generally the stage of inflammation. The subacute stage, occurring between 14 and 21 days after injury, is the stage of repair. The chronic stage (after 21 days) may be viewed as the stage of remodelling. The term chronic is also sometimes used to describe self-perpetuating inflammation, where

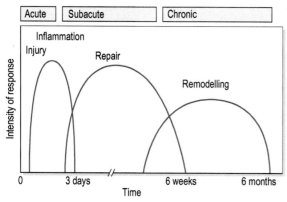

Figure 1.1 Timescale for healing. From Oakes, B.W. (1992) The classification of injuries and mechanisms of injury, repair and healing. In *Textbook of Science and Medicine in Sport* (eds J. Bloomfield, P.A. Fricker and K.D. Fitch). Blackwell Scientific Publications, Melbourne. With permission.

the inflammatory process has restarted due to disruption or persistent irritation of the healing tissues. The total healing process occurs over a continuum, shown in Fig. 1.1.

> **Keypoint**
>
> Treatment must be adapted to the stages of healing, which are injury, inflammation, repair and remodelling.

Injury

This stage represents the tissue effects at the time of injury, before the inflammatory process is activated. With tissue damage, chemical and mechanical changes are seen. Local blood vessels are disrupted causing a cessation in oxygen to the cells they perfused. These cells die and their lysosome membranes disintegrate, releasing the hydrolysing enzymes the lysosomes contained. The release of these enzymes has a twofold effect. First they begin to break down the dead cells themselves, and second, they release histamines and kinins which have an effect on both the live cells nearby and the local blood capillary network.

The disruption of the blood vessels which caused cell death also causes local bleeding (extravasated blood). More vascular tissue such as muscle will bleed more than less vascular tissue such as ligament. On average, bleeding following soft tissue injury stops within four to six hours (Watson 2016). The red blood cells break down, leaving cellular debris and free haemoglobin. The blood platelets release the enzyme thrombin, which changes fibrinogen into fibrin. The fibrin in turn is deposited as a meshwork around the area (a process known as walling off). The dead cells intertwine in the meshwork, forming a blood clot. This network contains the damaged area.

The changes occurring at injury are affected by age. Intramuscular bleeding, and therefore haemorrhage formation, is more profuse in individuals over 30 years of age. The amount of bleeding which occurs will be partially dependent on the vascularity of the injured tissues. A fitter individual is likely to have muscle tissue which is more highly vascularized, and therefore greater bleeding will occur with muscle injury. In addition, exercise itself will affect gross tissue responses. Muscle blood flow is greatly increased through dilatation of the capillary bed, and again bleeding subsequent to injury will be greater.

> **Keypoint**
>
> The tissues of an active individual are more highly vascularized than those of an inactive subject. The subject's tissues will therefore bleed more during injury, and bruising will be more noticeable.

Inflammation

The next phase in the healing sequence is that of inflammation, summarized in Fig. 1.2. This may last from ten minutes to several days, depending on the amount of tissue damage which has occurred, but generally reaches its peak by one to three days.

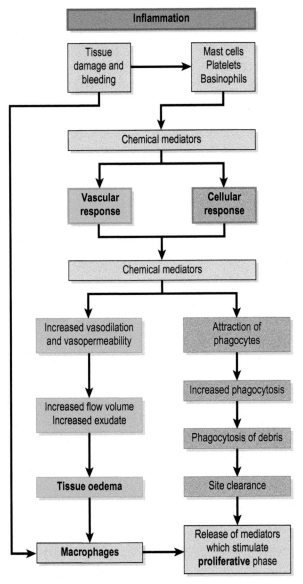

Figure 1.2 Inflammatory elements.

The inflammatory response to soft tissue injury is much the same regardless of the nature of the injuring agent or the location of the injury itself. Inflammation is not simply a feature of soft tissue injuries, but also occurs when the body is infected, in immune reactions and with infarction. Some of the characteristics of the inflammatory response seen with soft tissue injury may be viewed as excessive and better suited to dealing with infection than healing injury.

The cardinal signs of inflammation are heat (*calor*), redness (*rubor*), swelling (*tumor*) and pain (*dolor*). These in turn give rise to the so-called fifth sign of inflammation: disturbance of function of the affected tissues (*functio laesa*).

> **Keypoint**
> Inflammation is often seen as undesirable. However, inflammation is the first stage of healing and so is a vital step on the road to recovery. The aim should be to prevent excessive inflammation and move the subject on through the phases of healing towards eventual full function.

Heat and redness

Heat and redness take a number of hours to develop, and are due to the opening of local blood capillaries and the resultant increased blood flow. Chemical and mechanical changes, initiated by injury, are responsible for the changes in blood flow.

Chemically, a number of substances act as mediators in the inflammatory process. The amines, including histamine and 5-hydroxytryptamine (5-HT or serotonin) are released from mast cells, red blood cells and platelets in the damaged capillaries and cause vessel dilatation and increased permeability. Kinins (physiologically active polypeptides) cause an increase in vascular permeability and stimulate the contraction of smooth muscle. They are found normally in an inactive state as kininogens. These

Vascular and chemical cascades occur in parallel to drive the inflammatory process.

> **Definition:**
> A *chemical cascade* (signalling cascade) is a series of chemical reactions. As one reaches its completion, it triggers the next in a type of 'chain reaction'.

in turn are activated by the enzyme plasmin, and degraded by kininases.

The initial vasodilatation is maintained by prostaglandins. These are one of the arachidonic acid derivatives, formed from cell membrane phospholipids when cell damage occurs, and released when the kinin system is activated. The drugs aspirin and indometacin act to inhibit this change – hence their use as anti-inflammatory agents in sports and soft tissue injury treatment (see Treatment Note 1.1). The prostaglandins E1 and E2 will stimulate nociceptors and also promote vasodilatation, blood-vessel permeability and lymph flow.

The complement system, consisting of a number of serum proteins circulating in an inactive form, is activated and has a direct effect on the cell membrane as well as helping to maintain vasodilatation. Various complement products are involved, and these are activated in sequence. Finally, polymorphs produce leukotrienes, which are themselves derived from arachidonic acid, help the kinins maintain vessel permeability.

Treatment note 1.1 Medication used in soft tissue injury

Although inflammation is an essential part of the healing process, sometimes it can be excessive. Anti-inflammatory treatments are designed to limit inflammation and interfere with the chemical processes described above. Two groups of drugs are generally used in the treatment of soft tissue injuries in this respect: corticosteroids and non-steroidal anti-inflammatory drugs (NSAIDS). Analgesics are used to limit pain, and may be used in isolation or together with anti-inflammatories.

Non-steroidal anti-inflammatory drugs

NSAIDS have both anti-inflammatory and pain relieving (analgesic) properties, causing both local (peripheral) and mild central effects. They inhibit the cyclo-oxygenase (COX) system, which has an important function in the cascade of chemicals driving the inflammatory process (see above) and works to block the production of prostaglandin. Two types are generally used, COX-1 and COX-2. As COX-1 also has an important function on the gastric mucosa, COX-1 inhibitors can lead to gastritis, and with long-term usage ulceration. COX-2 inhibitors have fewer effects on the gastric mucosa and so are better tolerated, but can increase the risk of thrombosis. NSAIDS are also available as creams and patches which can be used for superficial injury such as muscle injuries, contusions, and knee arthritis. Drugs such as *aspirin*, *Volterol*, *Brufen* and *Naprosyn* are common oral NSAIDS.

NSAIDS can inhibit protein synthesis and affect satellite cell activity, detrimentally changing muscle repair (see Chapter 2). They may alter collagen formation and fibroblast proliferation, so long-term usage should generally be avoided. In addition, tenocyte action during tendon repair may be negatively affected, but pain reduced (Pollock 2017). The role of prostaglandins in bone repair is also a potential concern with NSAID usage, as osteoblast activity may be impaired, delaying callus maturation in bone (Wheeler and Batt 2005).

Targeting pain

Painkillers (analgesics) work on the peripheral or central nervous systems. Drugs such as *paracetamol* have painkilling (analgesic) and fever-reducing (antipyretic) effects, but do not generally reduce inflammation. This type of drug works by blocking a type of cell membrane receptor called a cannabinoid receptor, which drugs such as cannabis work on. *Codeine*, *morphine* and *ketamine* are more powerful painkillers and are opiates. They may be taken alone or combined with paracetamol. Opiate drugs are generally derived from the opium poppy or its synthetic equivalent (one of which is heroin) and are

Treatment note 1.1 *continued*

psychoactive compounds – ones which alter mood or consciousness. As such, one of their side effects is nausea and dizziness. Where pain is from a peripheral nociceptive stimulus, NSAIDS may be effective at targeting pain indirectly by reducing the inflammatory chemicals driving nociception. Their painkilling effect is generally non-addictive, unlike the narcotic group of painkilling drugs such as *morphine*, above.

Where neuropathic pain and central sensitization occurs, medications such as *Gabapentin* (an anti-epileptic) and *Pregabalin* may be chosen as these block the nociceptive signal by binding to the calcium channels on the nociceptor and reducing neurotransmitter release. These drugs can induce fatigue and have a sedative effect so subjects should be aware of this. Locally, counterirritant effects may be provided by massage or self-applied rubifacient rubs. These may reduce nociceptor transmission by depleting neurotransmitter activity.

Corticosteroids

Corticosteroids (such as *triamcinolone* and *hydrocortisone*) also reduce inflammation, but rather than targeting prostaglandin, they reduce activation of leucocytes and alter vascular permeability. These drugs tend to be injected to the site of a pathology and, although generally effective at reducing both pain and inflammation in the short term, can have a number of negative effects. Inhibition of collagen synthesis may occur, impacting on tendon healing, an effect most studied in the case of tendinopathy presenting as tennis elbow (Coombes et al. 2010). Injecting into a contained region such as a joint can reduce synovial inflammation. However, cartilage matrix degradation may occur with prolonged usage in weight-bearing joints. Combining a corticosteroid with a local anaesthetic followed by a quick return to running is said to be detrimental to articular cartilage (Pollock 2017). Fat atrophy and alteration of skin pigmentation can also occur as a result of corticosteroid injection.

References

Coombes, B.K., Bisset, L., Vicenzino, B. (2010) 'Efficacy and safety of corticosteroid injections and other injections for management of tendinopathy: a systematic review of randomised controlled trials'. *Lancet* 376(9754):1751–1767.

Pollock, N. (2017) 'Therapeutic medication in musculoskeletal injury'. In: Brukner, P., Clarsen, B., Cooks, J. et al. (eds) *Clinical Sports Medicine.*

Wheeler P., Batt, M.E. (2005) 'Do non-steroidal anti-inflammatory drugs adversely affect stress fracture healing? A short review'. *British Journal of Sports Medicine* 39(2):65–69.

Blood-flow changes also occur through mechanical alterations initiated by injury. Normally, the blood flow in the venules, in particular, is axial. The large blood proteins stay in the centre of the vessel, and the plasmatic stream, which has a lower viscosity, is on the outside in contact with the vessel walls. This configuration reduces peripheral resistance and aids blood flow.

In a damaged capillary, however, fluid is lost and so the axial flow slows. Marginalization occurs as the slower flow rate allows white blood cells to move into the plasmatic zone and adhere to the vessel walls. This, in turn, reduces the lubricating effect of this layer and slows blood flow. The walls themselves become covered with a gelatinous layer, as endothelium changes occur.

Definition

Marginalization is the build-up of white blood cells (leukocytes) on blood-vessel walls at the site of an injury.

Some four hours after injury, diapedesis occurs as the white cells pass through the vessel walls into the damaged tissue. The endothelial cells of the vessel contract, pulling away from each other and leaving gaps through which fluids and blood cells can escape (Fig. 1.3). Various substances, including histamine, kinins and complement factors, have been shown to produce this effect (Walter and Israel 1987).

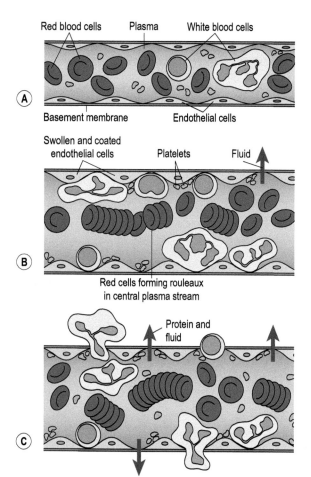

Figure 1.3 Vascular changes which occur in inflammation. (A) Blood vessel starts to dilate. (B) Dilated vessel showing marginalization. (C) White blood cells and fluid pass into tissue. From Evans, D.M.D. (1990a) Inflammation and healing. In *Cash's Textbook of General Medical and Surgical Conditions for Physiotherapists* (ed. P.A. Downie), 2nd edn. Faber and Faber, London. With permission.

Swelling

The normal pressure gradients inside and outside the capillary balance the flow of fluid leaving and entering the vessel (Fig. 1.4). The capillary membrane is permeable to water, and so water will be driven out into the interstitial fluid. However, because the tissue fluids usually contain a small amount of protein, and the blood contains a large amount, an osmotic pressure is created, which tends to suck water back from the tissue fluid and into the capillary once more. The magnitude of this osmotic pressure is roughly 25 mmHg. At the arteriole end of the capillary, the blood pressure (32 mmHg) exceeds the osmotic pressure and so tissue fluid is formed. At the venous end of the capillary, the blood pressure has reduced (12 mmHg) and so, because the osmotic pressure now exceeds this value, tissue fluid is reabsorbed back into the capillary.

During inflammation, the capillary bed opens and blood flow increases (heat and redness). The larger blood volume causes a parallel increase in blood pressure. Coupled with this, the tissue fluid now contains a large amount of protein, which has poured out from the more permeable blood vessels. This increased protein concentration causes a substantial rise in osmotic pressure, and this, together with the larger blood pressure in the capillary, forces fluid out into the interstitium, causing swelling.

Protein exudation in mild inflammation occurs from the venules only and is probably mediated by histamine. More severe inflammation, as a result of trauma, results in protein exudation from damaged capillaries as well.

During inflammation, lymphatic vessels open up and assist in the removal of excess fluid and protein. The lymph vessels are blind-ending capillaries which have gaps in their endothelial walls enabling protein molecules to move through easily. The lymph vessels lie within the tissue spaces, and have valves preventing the backward movement of fluid. Muscular contraction causes a pumping action on the lymph vessels and the

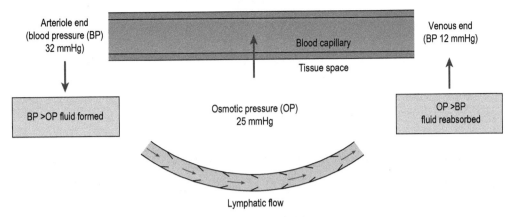

Figure 1.4 Formation and reabsorption of tissue fluid.

excess tissue fluid is removed to the subclavian veins in the neck.

Pain

Pain is the result of both sensory and emotional experiences, and is associated with tissue damage or the probability that damage will occur. It serves as a warning which may cause us to withdraw from a stimulus and so protect an injured body part. Unfortunately, pain often continues long after it has ceased to be a useful form of protection. Associated muscle spasm, atrophy, habitual postures, guarding and psychological factors all combine to make chronic pain a clinical state in itself.

Types of pain

Pain may be classified as somatogenic (acute or chronic), neurogenic or psychogenic. Chronic pain is traditionally said to last for more than six weeks, while acute pain is pain of sudden onset and lasts for less than six weeks. However, rather than distinct timescales, pain behavior is more appropriate as a classification.

> **Definition**
> Acute pain is traditionally said to have a sudden onset and lasts for less than six weeks, while chronic pain lasts for more than six weeks.

Musculoskeletal pain is not usually well localized – the surface site where the pain is felt rarely correlates directly to injured subcutaneous tissue. Generally, the closer an injured tissue is to the skin surface, the more accurate the patient can be at localizing it.

Deep pain is normally an aching, ill-defined sensation. It can radiate in a characteristic fashion, and may be associated with autonomic responses such as sweating, nausea, pallor and lowered blood pressure. Pain referral usually corresponds to segmental pathways, most often dermatomes. The extent of radiation largely depends on the intensity of the stimulus, with pain traditionally said to radiate distally, and rarely to cross the mid-line of the body (Cyriax 1982). In the clinic, however, these rules, while a useful guide, are often not adhered to rigidly.

Neurogenic pain is different again. Compression of a nerve root gives rise to ill-defined tingling, especially in the distal part of the dermatome supplied by the nerve. This is a pressure reaction, which quickly disappears when the nerve root is released. Greater pressure often causes the tingling to give way to numbness. Compression or tension to the dural sleeve covering the nerve root gives severe pain, generally over the whole dermatome. In contrast, pressure on a nerve trunk is conventionally said to cause little or no pain, but results in a shower of 'pins and needles' as the nerve compression is released. Pressure applied to a superficial nerve distally gives numbness and some tingling, with the edge of the affected region being well defined.

Irritability

Irritability may be defined as 'the vigour of activity which causes pain' (Maitland 1991). It is determined by the degree of pain which the patient experiences, and the time this takes to subside, in relation to the intensity of activity or mechanical stimulation. The purpose of assessing irritability is to determine how much activity (joint mobilization, exercise, and so on) may be prescribed without exacerbating the patient's symptoms.

An assessment of irritability may be made at the second treatment session. The amount of movement which the patient was subjected to in the previous session is known, as is the discomfort that he or she feels now. These subjective feelings are then used to determine the intensity of the second treatment session. Similarly, at the beginning of each subsequent treatment session the irritability is again assessed.

> **Keypoint**
>
> Irritability is a measure of the amount of pain a patient experiences as a result of movement (including that of treatment). Irritability can be used to guide the type and intensity of treatment to avoid excessive post-treatment soreness.

Treatment note 1.2 Pain description in examination

During both the subjective examination and the objective examination (see Treatment Note 1.8, p. 53) the patient will usually describe pain as part of their experience. In addition to psychosocial factors (see below), both the type (nature) of pain and its behaviour are important factors in making an accurate clinical diagnosis, and a number of factors should be considered:

▶ When pain is decreasing, the condition is generally resolving; increasing pain suggests a worsening condition.
▶ Constant pain which does not change with time, alteration of static posture or activities may suggest a non-mechanical condition such as chemical irritation, tumours or visceral lesions.
▶ Where pain changes (episodic pain), the therapist should try to determine what activities make the pain worse (exacerbation) and what make it better (remission).
▶ The therapist should try to determine if the pain is associated with particular events (e.g. movements, visceral function), or time of day.

▶ Pain with activity which reduces with rest in general suggests a mechanical problem, irritating pain-sensitive structures.
▶ Morning pain which eases with movement may indicate chronic inflammation which takes time to build up and reduces with movement.

The description of pain itself may indicate the structure causing it (see Table 1.1) and the

Table 1.1 Pain descriptions and related structures

Type of pain	
Cramping, dull, aching, worse with resisted movement	Muscle
Dull, aching, worse with passive movement	Ligament, joint capsule
Sharp, shooting	Nerve root
Sharp, lightning-like, travelling	Nerve
Burning, pressure-like, stinging, with skin changes	Sympathetic nerve
Deep, nagging, poorly localized	Bone
Sharp, severe, unable to take weight	Fracture
Throbbing, diffuse	Vasculature

Source: Magee (2002) and Petty and Moore (2001) with permission.

Treatment note 1.2 *continued*

behaviour of the pain on physical examination clarifies the picture.

Recording pain

The intensity of pain may be recorded on a visual analogue scale (VAS). The patient is asked to indicate the pain description or number which best represents their pain. Where a 10 cm line is used the distance from the left of the scale to the point marked by the patient may be measured in millimetres and used as a numerical value (Fig. 1.5).

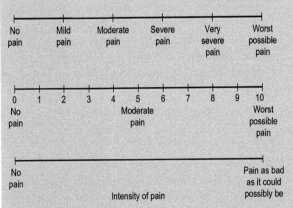

Figure 1.5 Visual analogue scales (VAS) used in pain description. From Petty and Moore (2001) with permission.

Red flags

It is important for the therapist to appreciate when pain and other symptoms may suggest serious pathology which requires medical investigation – so-called 'red flags' (Table 1.2). Where the patient has persistent pain and is generally unwell, the indication is that a pathology other than a musculoskeletal condition may exist. In addition, changes in bladder and bowel habits, alteration in vision or gross changes in gait all require further investigation.

Table 1.2 Red flags in sport examination indicating medical investigation

System/ possible pathology	Pain behaviour
Cancer	Persistent night pain
	Constant (24 hour) pain
	Unexplained weight loss (e.g. 4–6 kg in 10 days)
	Loss of appetite
	Unusual lumps or growths
	Sudden persistent fatigue
	Past history of carcinoma
Cardiovascular	Shortness of breath
	Dizziness
	Pain or feeling of heaviness in the chest
	Pulsating sensations in the body
	Discoloration in the feet
	Persistent swelling with no history of injury
Gastrointestinal/ genitourinary	Frequent or severe abdominal pain
	Frequent heartburn or indigestion
	Frequent nausea or vomiting
	Change in bladder or bowel habits
	Unusual menstruation
Neurological	Changes in hearing
	Frequent or severe headache
	Problems in swallowing or changes in speech
	Gait disturbance, or problems with balance/coordination
	Drop attacks (fainting)
	Sudden weakness

Source: Magee et al. (2002) and Waddell, G., Feder, G. and Lewis, M. (1997) Systematic reviews of bed rest and advice to stay active for acute low back pain. *British Journal of General Practice*, **47**, 647–652. With permission.

Pain production

Free or 'bare' nerve endings (type IV) respond to noxious stimuli and are termed nociceptors. They are largely unresponsive to normal stimuli but have a low threshold to mechanical and thermal injury, anoxia and irritation from inflammatory products.

> **Definition:**
>
> Nociceptors are sensory receptors which respond to harmful (noxious) stimuli

Tissues vary in the intensity of nociception they will produce when stimulated, compared to skin. The joint capsule and periosteum are the most sensitive to noxious stimuli. Subchondral bone, tendons and ligaments are the next in line in terms of sensitivity, followed by muscle and cortical bone, the synovium and cartilage being largely insensitive.

Nociceptors are supplied by a variety of different nerve fibres. Skin receptors are supplied by thinly myelinated (A delta) fibres which carry 'fast' nociceptive signals and respond to strong mechanical stimuli and heat above 45°C. They give the initial sharp well-localized pain feeling (pinprick). The function of fast nociception is to help the body avoid tissue damage and it often provokes a flexor withdrawal reflex.

Impulses from free nerve endings found in deeper body tissues are carried by non-myelinated C fibres. This is 'slow' nociception, which tends to be aching and throbbing in nature, and poorly defined. Its onset is not immediate, and the sensation it produces persists after the stimulus has gone. The function of slow nociception seems to be to enforce inactivity and allow healing to occur, and it is therefore often associated with muscle spasm. The C fibres respond to many different types of stimuli and, as such, are said to be 'polymodal'. However, they are most sensitive to chemicals released as a result of tissue damage. Histamine, kinins, prostaglandins E1 and E2, and 5-HT have

all been implicated in this type of nociceptive production during inflammation.

Following a soft tissue injury, both mechanical and chemical stimuli may occur. Mechanical nociception is the result of forces which deform or damage the nociceptive nerve endings, and so may be caused by stretching contracted tissue or by fluid pressure. This type of sensation is influenced by movement. Chemical nociception, on the other hand, results from irritation of the nerve endings, and is less affected by movement or joint position, but will respond to rest.

> **Keypoint**
>
> Fast pain may help the body avoid tissue damage by provoking a flexor withdrawal reflex. Slow pain can enforce inactivity (through muscle spasm) to allow time for healing.

Articular neurology

In addition to nociceptive receptors (Type IV), three other sensory receptors are important. Type I receptors are located in the superficial layers of the joint capsule. They are slow adapting, low-threshold mechanoreceptors, which respond to both static and dynamic stimulation. These receptors provide information about the static position of a joint, and contribute to the regulation of muscle tone and movement (kinaesthetic) sense. The Type I receptors sense both the speed and direction of movement.

Type II receptors are found mainly in the deeper capsular layers and within fat pads. These are dynamic receptors with a high threshold, and they adapt quickly. They respond to rapid changes of direction of joint movement.

The Type III fibres are found in the joint ligaments, and are again high-threshold dynamic mechanoreceptors, but are slow adapting. These receptors monitor the direction of movement, and have a 'braking' effect on muscle tone if the joint is moving too quickly or through too great a range

Table 1.3 Sensory nerve fibre types

Fibre type	Group	Diameter (µm)	Conduction velocity (m/s)	Mylinated	Receptor type	Function
A α	I	15	95	Yes	Muscle spindle & GTO	Proprioception
A β	II	8	50	Yes	Muscle spinal & tissue receptors (various)*	Proprioception, Superficial & deep touch, Vibration
A δ	III	3	15	Yes	Bare (naked) nerve ending	Nociception, Temperature (cool)
C	IV	0.5	1	No	Bare (naked) nerve ending	Nociception, Temperature (warm), Itch

GTO – golgi tendon organ
*Tissue receptors - Meissner corpuscle, Merkel receptor, Paccinian corpuscle, Ruffini receptor, Hair receptor.

of motion. Table 1.3 provides a synopsis of the various categories of sensory nerve receptors and fibre types.

Alteration in the feedback provided by joint receptors is of great importance following sports and soft tissue injury, and is dealt with in the section on proprioceptive training.

Nociceptive pathways

Three categories or 'orders' of neurone make up the nociceptive pathways. First-order neurones travel from the sensory receptors to the spinal cord, second-order neurones within the cord to the brainstem, and third-order neurones travel from the brainstem to the cerebral cortex.

Seventy per cent of the C fibres enter the spine via the dorsal root, while 30 per cent of the fibres enter via the ventral root. The C fibres synapse with second-order neurones in the substantia gelatinosa (SG) of the cord and these neurones ascend in the anterolateral funiculus on the opposite side of the cord (Fig. 1.6). From here they travel via the reticular formation to the intralaminar nuclei of the thalamus. The neurones synapse here once more and travel to the prefrontal region of the cerebral cortex. Some of the C fibres travel to the limbic

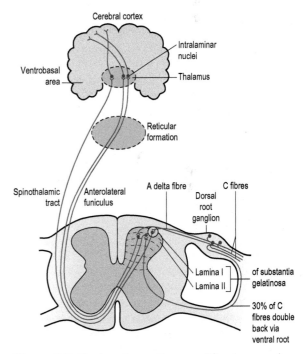

Figure 1.6 Nociceptive pathways. After Low and Reed (1990) with permission.

system (cingulate gyrus) and generate emotional responses to pain (described as anxiety, fear and dread). C fibre pain is therefore poorly localized with a large emotional effect (White 1999).

11

The A delta fibres (fast pain), on the other hand, synapse in the outer part of the posterior horn of the cord and cross to ascend in the spinothalamic tract to the ventrobasal nuclei in the thalamus, and then to the postcentral gyrus of the cortex.

Fast pain is registered in the parietal lobe and visceral pain in the insular cortex. With more major injuries both fibres will produce a nociceptive effect. The response to an ankle sprain, for example, will be an intense, well-defined stabbing sensation (A delta) followed by a dull ache accompanied by an emotional response (C fibre).

> **Keypoint**
> Acute soft tissue injuries often give a well-defined stabbing pain followed by a dull ache accompanied by an emotional response.

Managing pain

Essential aspects of neuroscience

When pain acts as an alarm, it signals that the body is under threat, or rather that the brain perceives that the body is under threat. In other words, rather than indicating actual tissue damage, pain indicates that the brain is of the opinion that damage exists – but it might not.

The traditional view of pain is that a stimulus occurs in the tissues which instigates an electronic signal that travels up a (sensory) nerve to the brain. Here, the sensation is felt as pain, in a 'pain centre'. However, a person who has had a limb amputated will sometimes feel pain in the leg which is no longer there (phantom limb pain). The tissues are no longer producing electric signals along the sensory nerve, but the brain is producing the illusion of pain. This example illustrates two directions involved in the production of pain: bottom up and top down. The bottom-up direction sees pain originating from the tissues and causing an input to the brain, whereas the top-down direction has pain originating as an output from the brain. Both bottom-up and top-down directions are important, as we will see.

> **Keypoint:**
> Pain may be viewed as an output of the brain rather than just an input from the tissues.

Nociception

Rather than pain receptors sending pain signals to the brain, we simply have danger sensors, which travel to the dorsal horn of the spinal cord. As we have seen, these sensors respond to noxious stimuli, hence their name – *nociceptors*. When stimulated, the nociceptor opens an ion channel, causing an electrical signal to build up and eventually fire off an action potential which travels to the dorsal horn of the spinal cord. The nociceptor signal travels to the dorsal horn via first-order neurons which synapse with second-order neurons in the dorsal horn. At this point the signal from the first-order neuron can be modulated (changed) by both local interneurons and descending (brain orchestrated) neurons so that the original nociceptor signal may not necessarily reach the brain. The brain itself is able to modulate the impulses in the dorsal horn and either increase (augment) or reduce (inhibit) nociceptive impulses coming from the periphery. Once on its way up the spinal cord, the signal enters the thalamus and from here is directed to several other brain regions – even at this point the action potential has still not been perceived at a conscious level. Only when the various brain areas (neuromatrix, see below) interpret the signal as threatening will it become what the patient traditionally knows as pain.

At the dorsal horn level, as the nociceptive impulse passes to the second-order neuron it may be further enhanced (a feature termed *wind-up*) if stimulation of the first-order neuron continues repeatedly. The second-order neuron is becoming hypersensitive due to neurotransmitter action on receptor sites which increase the post-synaptic response. Wind-up (part of the central sensitization process) describes an increased electrical discharge of the second-order neuron in response to repeated first order (C fibre) stimulation.

A further way that the nociceptive signal may be modified is due to changes within the tissue housing the nociceptive sensor. Significantly, as we have seen, local inflammation from a soft tissue injury may produce a variety of substances, including prostaglandins, pro-inflammatory cytokines, histamine, and substance P, within the tissues. These substances can lower the stimulus threshold of the nociceptors, making their activation more likely (Nils et al. 2015).

Descending nociceptive *facilitation* occurs when output from the brain enhances nociceptive signals reaching the dorsal horn. Catastrophizing (viewing a situation as worse than it actually is) and fear-avoidance behaviour (avoiding certain actions due to fear rather than pathology) are just two of the factors shown to activate this effect and give sustained arousal of the dorsal horn (Zusman 2002).

Descending nociceptive *inhibition* occurs from the periaqueductal grey matter (PAG) and medulla to the dorsal horn of the cord. This descending pain inhibitory pathway applies neurotransmitters (especially serotonin and noradrenaline) to suppress the primary afferent nociceptors. Interestingly the main focus of this effect is to target the state of excitation of the dorsal horn neurons by reducing the activity of the surrounding neurons (Nils et al. 2015). The process is known as diffuse noxious inhibitory control (DNIC) and it malfunctions in cases of chronic pain. A variety of therapy treatments have been shown to act as physical stressors to activate DNIC, including exercise, manual therapy and acupuncture/dry needling.

From the above description is should be apparent that tissue injury and pain are not directly related. As such, pain can be better viewed as a perception produced by the brain in response to perceived threat or danger. As we have seen, the sensation of touch can be intensified into a stronger danger signal (nociception) which indicates the possibility of harm. Defining whether the nociceptive signal is interpreted as pain is the job of the brain, and this decision is made on the basis of a number of elements. Several factors (stressors) can amplify the nociceptive signal, including poor sleep, anxiety and worry, stress, depression, negative expectations and negative beliefs about the injury. These types of factor can make the nervous system more sensitive to nociceptive signals, increasing the likelihood that these signals will be interpreted as pain. Pain itself acts as a stressor to activate the autonomic nervous system and the fight-or-flight system, which consists of the linkage between the hypothalamus, pituitary and adrenal glands (HPA axis). Normally, where the fight or flight response is seen, the natural result is a reduction in pain through the release of noradrenaline and cortisol, both of which inhibit pain. In chronic pain situations this seems to be reversed (Nils et al. 2015). The dorsomedial nucleus of the hypothalamus and ventromedial medulla are activated, triggering cells which promote nociception (ON-cells) and deactivating those which supress nociception (OFF-cells). The result is a lowering of sensory and pain thresholds, making stress management in cases of chronic pain especially useful.

Neuromatrix

Rather than a single location within the brain feeling a pain sensation, several regions interact to create a neuromatrix which interprets the pain experience. The neuromatrix consists of all the brain regions which are activated in the process of concluding that a subject's body is in danger – a conclusion which is highly individual (patient specific). The key point here is that the same amount of tissue damage can cause widely varying pain experiences between individuals.

> **Keypoint:**
> The same amount of tissue damage can create widely varying pain experiences between subjects.

Although the brain areas activated vary between individuals, and within individuals in different situations, imaging studies have consistently demonstrated several regions which typically form a pain neurosignature (neurotag) for a given situation (Fig. 1.7). Importantly, these regions do not just include neurones, but other neural cells including astrocytes, microglia and oligodendrocytes which have both immune functions and may communicate in both directions (bidirectional) with neurons. These cells play a part in learning and plasticity and may remain sensitized for many years (Austin and Moalem-Taylor 2010). In addition they may alter anti- and pro-inflammatory cytokine balance in the central nervous system (CNS). This connection may explain how psychosocial factors such as emotional stress can link to both immunological distress and pain.

Using pain to indicate tissue damage or to judge recovery is clearly an inaccurate measure if used to compare between individuals. Pain can be used with the same individual to measure between treatment sessions, but only with the knowledge that psychosocial factors will also be involved. For example, if someone states that their pain score (numerical rating score or NMS) is 5/10 on one

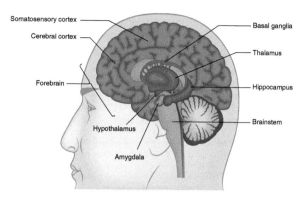

- ▶ Somatosensory cortex – identifies pain location
- ▶ Amygdala (with cingulate cortex and hippocampus) – memory of movement, fear
- ▶ Thalamus (with periaqueductal grey) – stress response
- ▶ Brainstem – descending inhibition

Figure 1.7 Pain neuromatrix.

occasion and 7/10 on another, it would seem that their pain is getting worse, perhaps implying a regression in tissue recovery. However, if prior to the second occasion an individual reports that they lost their job, or had an argument with their spouse, these changes may explain the alteration in pain score, not the tissue state. Allowing the patient to talk freely and tell 'their story' (patient narrative) rather than using a rigid questioning checklist, is more likely to reveal details which may impact on their pain experience.

Hypervigilance

Hypervigilance is a behaviour change where a patient places greater attention or awareness on a body part or tissue as a result of their belief. In sport this can distract from performance, and in general rehabilitation it may make the patient less compliant, when using exercise therapy, for example. Hypervigilance may be increased by focusing on localized tissue-based therapies rather than whole body actions such as exercise therapy. Even when tissue healing is complete, the neurosignature formed during injury will remain.

Hypervigilance sees the patient selectively focusing (attending) to sensations which he/she would normally ignore. It is as though they are in a room listening to someone's voice (foreground sound) but always hearing some background music which previously would have been ignored.

> **Definition:**
> Hypervigilance is a behaviour change where a patient places greater attention or awareness on a body part as a result of their belief.

One of the aims of rehabilitation is to increase adaptation and limit maladaptation. Traditionally this is seen as referring to the tissues, which is clearly appropriate in many cases – patients invariably have 'issues in the tissues' (Joyce and Butler 2016). However, as we have seen above, maladaptive beliefs about the threat of injury can often be limiting when tissue changes have typically resolved. Reassuring the patient that 'hurt does not mean harm' and that they can perform exercise and be 'sore but safe' is important, as patients will often believe that what they feel reflects the condition of their injured area. Using basic neuroscience education to explain the concepts of the neuromatrix and the nature of pain can be helpful, providing it is presented in a supportive and non-disparaging manner. The use of graded exposure (see Chapter 8) can also be helpful.

> **Keypoint:**
> Reassuring patients that 'hurt does not mean harm' and they can perform exercise and be 'sore but safe' is important during rehabilitation.

Central sensitization and wind-up

Sensitization may be either peripheral (within the tissues) or central (within the brain and spinal cord). Central sensitization (CS) is an increase in the responsiveness of central pain-signalling neurons to the input from mechanoreceptors. CS involves both altered processing of stimuli in the brain, resulting in signal amplification, and also a reduction of pain-inhibitory mechanisms. As we have seen, signals may be increased at the level of the dorsal horn as wind-up, while DNIC, the natural descending pain inhibitory mechanism, may be reduced. In addition, the neuromatrix may become overactive, and areas within the brain not normally associated with the pain experience (pain signature) may become activated, especially those associated with emotion and acute pain (insula, anterior cingulate and pre-frontal cortex). The synapses involved in the transmission of nociceptor signals become more efficient by firstly releasing more neurotransmitter and secondly enabling the neurotransmitter which is released to bind more effectively to post-synaptic sites. This process is called *long-term potentiation*.

> **Definition:**
> Long-term potentiation (LTP) is the persistent augmentation of a synapse, producing a lasting increase in signal transmission between two neurons.

Patients with CS often have the inhibitory neurotransmitter GABA (gamma-aminobutyric acid) reduced in quantity as a result of long-term stress leading to increased neural excitability. Table 1.4 highlights typical signs of CS seen in clinic by the therapist.

Table 1.4 Typical signs of central sensitization (CS)

▶ Perceived disability – demonstrating greater disability than functional tests suggest
▶ Self-reported pain distribution – larger region which is non-dermatomal and often varies
▶ Pain location – unrelated to source of nociception
▶ Allodynia – painful sensation to a normally non-painful stimulus (e.g. touch)
▶ Hyperalgesia – excessive sensitivity to a normally painful stimulus (e.g. pressure)
▶ Expansion of the receptive field – pain that extends beyond area of peripheral nerve supply
▶ Unusually prolonged pain after stimulus has been removed – usually burning / throbbing tingling / numbness

Treatment note 1.3   Dry needling

Dry needling (DN) uses a thin filiform needle which penetrates the soft tissues. Filiform needles are solid, flexible and have a pointed tip, in contrast to an injection needle, which is inflexible and has a bore through the centre for the passage of a fluid drug (Fig. 1.8). Injection needles have a cutting edge at their tip, whereas a filiform needle has a rounded tip. Needles typically used for DN are acupuncture type, and are described in terms of length and width (gauge) of the needle shaft in millimetres, with common needle sizes ranging from 15 x 0.22 mm for the head, face, hands and feet up to 60 x 0.32mm for the buttock. Needles used for DN are single use and disposable. The combination of needle tip shape, polishing and insertion technique has led to the term 'painless insertion' being applied to filiform needling, and although not strictly pain free, the sensation is usually that of a small local scratch on the skin surface followed by a diffuse dull ache.

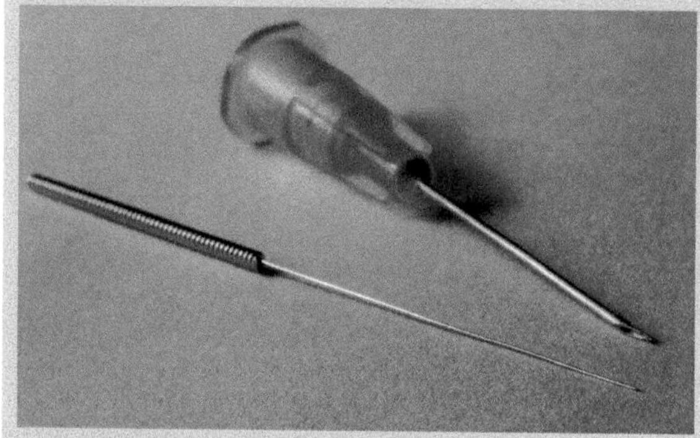

Needle depth

The depth of needle penetration into the soft tissues has led to the differentiation into superficial (SDN) and deep (DDN) dry needling types, with SDN typically less than 1 centimetre (< 1.0 cm) depth through the skin and into the subcutaneous tissue touching onto the muscle and DDN typically greater than 1 centimetre (> 1.0 cm) into the muscle bulk. Needles are inserted either perpendicular to the skin or at an angle, and once in place they may be stimulated manually or using an electrical impulse generated by a purpose-designed electro-stimulator (electroacupuncture or EAP) unit.

DN typically has effects on pain, healing and in the release of myofascial trigger points. The precise effect of DN depends on the target tissue penetrated, and the method used.

Dry needling effects

One of the primary reasons for applying DN is to release trigger points. These are hypersensitive local areas lying within a muscle. They are typically associated with muscle tightening and pain. Additional DN effects are seen on local tissue healing, and on general pain reduction, the latter response being similar to that of classical acupuncture. Needling into local soft tissue elicits a classic triple response (redness, heat, swelling and pain) demonstrating the beginning

Figure 1.8 Comparison between acupuncture (left) and injection (right) needles.

Treatment note 1.3 *continued*

of an inflammatory reaction. The response is due to the release of pro-inflammatory mediators including prostaglandin, calcitonin gene-related peptide (CGRP) and nitric oxide (NO) (see above). In studies of DN, blood flow assessed using near infra-red reflectance spectroscopy has been shown to improve, and oxygen saturation to increase, the changes remaining for some time following needle removal. DN treatment of a burn skin lesion in mice has been shown to decrease wound size and induce epidermal regeneration, with significantly increased levels of fibroblast growth factor and leukocyte infiltration (Lee et al. 2011).

The physical act of needling may also affect the soft tissue mechanically. As the needle is inserted through the skin it passes into the loose subcutaneous fascia. Stimulating the needle by twisting or thrusting (as is common practice) winds the fascial fibres to the needle shaft to create a whorl (Langevin 2006). Once the fascial fibres are attached to the needle, further movement pulls the fibre along the tissue plane from the periphery towards the needle. The loose connective tissue glides independently of the skin creating a localized tissue stretching effect (Langevin et al. 2004). Maintaining the fascial stretch by leaving the needles in place is claimed to cause visco-elastic relaxation, and change in the shape of the fibroblast cells. This process in turn gives rise to remodelling of the cellular cytoskeleton, and extracellular ATP signalling, also called purinergic signalling (Langevin 2013).

Effects on pain

The effects of DN on pain have been well researched with reference to acupuncture. Pain relief essentially occurs at four levels: local, spinal, brainstem, and higher centre. At a local level, the release of opioid chemicals (neuromodulators) has an effect on nociception. This effect builds to a peak within 20 minutes of needle retention and then subsides after the needles have been removed, and is reversed by the opioid antagonist naloxone.

At a spinal level, the sensory nerve synapses in the dorsal horn of the spinal cord, and at that point desensitization occurs, as a result of DN reducing nociception. Through interneurone effects at the dorsal horn, the sympathetic nervous system is also stimulated, creating the possibility for effects on internal organs, and changes in skin responses such as sweating. The nociceptive pathway from the dorsal horn ascends in the spinal cord to the brainstem, where nociceptive suppression occurs, not just to the injured body part but to the whole body. This type of 'top-down' pain inhibition occurs via several brainstem structures, including the periaqueductal grey matter (PAG) and the rostral ventromedial medulla (RVM). From these regions neurons ascend to higher centres in the brain to affect the pituitary gland and hypothalamus. Through action on these two centres, and by affecting the limbic system deep within the brain, neurohormonal effects are created which target not the pain sensation per se, but the emotional experience of pain. This latter effect is particularly important where a persistent pain state is part of the clinical picture.

Dry needling technique

Risks associated with DN can be minimized by good technique. First, prior to needle insertion a clean field should be established, ensuring that the immediate treatment area is clean and any potentially infectious material, such as dirty towels or clothing within a sporting environment, is removed. The patient is treated in a recumbent position (prone/supine/side-lying/long-sitting), supported by pillows or folded towels to discourage movement.

The risk of infection due to resident bacteria on the skin surface is low unless the patient's immune system in compromised, so disinfection of clean skin in not generally a requirement (Hoffman 2001). Infection with micro-organisms

Treatment note 1.3 *continued*

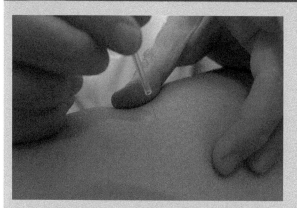

Figure 1.9 Needle insertion using plastic guide tube.

not normally resident on the skin (known as transient microflora) can pose a greater risk. The skin region to be needled should be clean and exposed, with the use of direct skin swabbing at the discretion of the practitioner. Gloves (single-use and disposable) may be used, especially on the palpating hand, and a hand sanitizing gel is generally applied to all surfaces of the hands and fingers. Single-use disposable needles are used, which are protected by a plastic guide tube. The insertion technique is to hold the guide tube and tap the needle into the skin (Fig. 1.9). Once the guide tube is removed, the portion of the needle

shaft (sterile) which will enter the patient's tissues is never touched by the therapist, to minimize the risk of infection. Where the needle is manipulated, the needle handle, rather than the shaft, is gripped. As the needle is withdrawn, pressure is applied over the needle area using a sterile cotton-wool ball until bleeding has stopped (haemostasis is established).

References

Hoffman, P. (2001) Skin disinfection and acupuncture. *Acupuncture in Medicine* 19(2):112–116.

Langevin, H. (2006) Connective tissue: a bodywide signalling network? *Medical Hypothesis* 66: 1074–1077.

Langevin, H.M. (2013) Effects of acupuncture needling on connective tissue. In: Dommerholt, J. and Fernandez, C. (eds) *Trigger point dry needling*. Churchill Livingstone.

Langevin, H.M., Konofagou, E.E., Badger, G.J. et al. (2004) Tissue displacements during acupuncture using ultrasound elastography techniques. *Ultrasound Med. Biol.* 30: 1173–1183.

Lee, J.A., Jeong, H., Park, H., et al. (2011) Acupuncture accelerates wound healing in burn injured mice. *Burns* 37(1): 117–125.

Management of inflammation

A number of outcomes are possible as a result of inflammation (Watson 2016). Complete resolution is possible only where there has been minimal disruption, often due to irritation rather than catastrophic cellular damage. Where microdamage occurs, failure to initiate repair mechanisms may result in further tissue damage. *Suppuration* may occur in open wounds where infection has occurred. Cell debris (dead and living cells) combines with inflammatory exudate to form pus, delaying wound healing. *Chronic inflammation* may occur in the presence of local irritants, inadequate circulation or immune disorders. Rather than swelling, more fibrous material is often produced as inflammation and proliferation may occur simultaneously (see below). *Resolution* of inflammation due to the progression to repair is the desirable outcome with the formation of granulation tissue which organizes into a scar.

Treatment note 1.4   Management of acute soft tissue injury

The early management of sports and soft tissue injuries has for many years been summarized in simple pneumonics. However, as scientific evidence has changed over time, so have the letters used in the pneumonics.

ICE

Initially, in the 1970s, the acronym ICE was used, standing for ice, compression and elevation. The original idea was to limit tissue damage by slowing the metabolic rate of the tissues, and reduce the spread of swelling into the surrounding area, which would eventually clot and potentially lead to adhesions. Studies showed decreased cell metabolism, changes in white blood cell activity and a reduction in both cell death due to trauma (necrosis) and ordered cell death (apoptosis) (Bleakley et al. 2012a). For every 10°C drop in temperature, chemical reactions are said to reduce by two or three times (Van't Hoff's law). The evidence for these changes in tissue, however, was based on early animal studies where cooling was much greater than that used in humans, and was applied for a greater time. Local temperature reduction to 10°C was reported using hamsters cooled for 60–180 minutes over a dorsal skinfold (Westermann et al. 1999). The effect of cold application is offset by the thickness of the subcutaneous fat layer, which is much thicker in humans than in the mammals used in the original studies. Using crushed ice application for 20 minutes on humans, intramuscular temperature, measured at 1 cm and 3 cm depth in the medial calf, has been shown to reduce to a maximum low of 21°C (Myer et al. 2001), considerably higher than that found in animal studies. In addition, the depth of the injury is of relevance. A 1 cm increase in tissue depth has been claimed to reduce the rate at which tissue cools from 0.72 to 0.45°C per minute (Myer et al. 2001), meaning that ice application would have to be left for far longer on deeper tissues. A deep tear of the quadriceps, for example, may be 3–4 cm

below the skin surface in an athlete, so a brief ice application is unlikely to record clinically significant tissue temperature reductions.

Ice is still useful, but nowadays its effects are more for the modulation of pain than to limit ongoing tissue degradation. Local cold-induced analgesia requires a reduction of temperature to 13°C, but of the skin surface, not the deep tissues. Temperature reduction to this level is achieved within 5–15 min of cooling and is more consistently applied using crushed ice or ice cubes in a bag which will adapt to the limb contour and remain at 0°C throughout treatment. Caution should be used with commercially available ice packs as the temperature applied may vary and sometimes cooling may be greater than 0°C.

Practically, ice, or cold application, should be applied using crushed ice in a wet cloth bag (wrapped in a tea cloth or thin towel, for example) to act as a protective barrier. If a commercial ice pack is used it should again be wrapped in a damp cloth to prevent ice burn to the skin. A damp cloth will conduct the cooling effect from the ice to the skin, but a dry cloth will reduce the cooling effect before it is saturated by melting ice. The pack should be left on for at least 10 minutes, but no more than 30 minutes, and symptoms should be monitored for pain relief. Ice can be reapplied every two hours to maximize the analgesic effect. If no ice is available, cold water is of use, but the tissue temperature changes are not as great as with ice, and so cold analgesia will be lessened.

As we have seen, following soft tissue injury, fluid (swelling/oedema) may accumulate as a result of changes to the pressure balance between the tissue in relation to that of the blood vessels (interstitial and osmotic pressure). These changes occur due to local blood vessel damage and the release of blood products into the surrounding tissues, which in turn changes

Treatment note 1.4 *continued*

blood viscosity (fluid stiffness). Elevating the lower limb decreases the effect of gravity and minimizes swelling and the pooling of fluid around the ankle after a sprain for example. The reduction in tissue pressure can result in a parallel reduction in pain, but when the limb is taken into a normal standing position a rebound effect may occur, increasing pain once more. This effect is reduced by allowing the subject to return the limb from elevated to dependent gradually. Applying compression may reduce this effect; however the amount of compression is unclear. A study applying 80 mmHg pressurse was unable to demonstrate a prevention of swelling, but lower pressures of 15 and 35 mmHg have been shown to at least lessen fluid pooling (ACSEM 2011). It is likely that the effect of compression will be dependent on a number of factors, including injury type, tissue depth, body part, stage of healing and body resting position. Rather than set time protocols, patient assessment (pain and swelling) should be made to monitor symptom modification and assess treatment outcome.

Compression is best applied contouring the limb (elastic tubular bandage for example). Intermittent compression through the application of electrically pumped garments (compression boot) is useful, as is graduated compression which applies a distal to proximal force. Limb circulation should be monitored while compression is on, with distal skin coloration and return of blood to the nail bed (squeeze the nail until it goes white and ensure normal pink coloration returns upon release) being practical forms of assessment.

Elevation should be above the level of the heart, so for lower-limb injuries the athlete should lie on the floor or bed with the leg up on a bench or stool. If this is not available, a kit bag may suffice. Symptoms should be monitored, with a greater angle of elevation and longer time period likely required for more distal (ankle) than proximal (knee or thigh) injuries.

RICE / PRICE / POLICE

The ICE mnemonic was replaced by RICE to emphasize the importance of using inactivity (Rest) to prevent further tissue damage. Unloading damaged tissue (by avoiding movements which replicate the injury force) in the acute phase of an injury to minimize bleeding and prevent re-injury is important. However, the advice on how this is achieved has changed over the years. Total immobilization (limb cast) will result in joint stiffness and change the morphological properties of the healing tissue and should be restricted to bone injury or complete rupture, where minimal movement would be a disadvantage. Protecting the area by using a support which allows some movement (functional bracing), or simply allowing the athlete to perform restricted activity, is likely to improve the quality of the healing tissue, and so the mnemonic PRICE came into usage. As an example, following acute ankle sprain mobilizing with an external support gives a superior result to cast immobilization. In a systematic review of nine RCTs, return to pre-injury fitness, re-injury rate and subjective ankle stability have all been shown to be superior with early immobilization (Jones and Amendola 2007).

Limited mechanical loading of tissue has been shown to upregulate gene expression of important proteins in tendon healing, for example, and mechanotransduction which results from movement may enhance the healing process. The transition from rest & protection must be closely monitored by assessment of patient symptoms. Loading damaged tissue may be both negative and positive. Further injury may result if loading is excessive, and few positive tissue changes may occur if loading is too light. The requirement for optimal loading has led to the use of the latest mnemonic, POLICE, standing for protection, optimal loading, ice, compression and elevation.

Treatment note 1.4 *continued*

Optimal loading has been defined as 'the load applied to structures that maximises physiological adaptation' (Glasgow et al. 2015). Some of the aims of applying optimal loading are to change collagen reorganization and improve tensile strength, increase stiffness of the muscle-tendon unit, or improve motor (neural) control. Variation in both load magnitude and timing of application can have significant effects on tissue recovery. Moderate loads (55% maximum voluntary contraction (MVC)) on tendons have failed to increase tissue stiffness, while near maximal loads (90% MVC) increase tendon stiffness and elasticity, and result in tendon hypertrophy. These results indicate that a threshold may exist for mechanical stimuli to produce mechanotransduction (Arampatzis et al. 2007). Similarly, high-impact actions produce a greater stimulus to increase bone mineral density (BMD) than slow actions, especially in the hip (Zhao et al. 2014).

Optimal loading must address both the mechanical properties of the affected tissues and the central nervous system (CNS), to challenge the complete neuromusculoskeletal system. Rather than simply increasing load on tissues we are seeking to increase variation in movement to encourage tissue adaptation in parallel with changes to motor control, and Glasgow et al. (2015) cite three categories in which load may be varied. To reduce repetitive loading, magnitude, direction and rate of loading should be varied. Secondly, stimulation of the mechanotransduction effect may be enhanced by varying loading to prevent accommodation to stimuli, where the body simply gets used to a stimulus and it no longer has an effect. Finally, variable tensile, compressive and torsional forces may build a stronger biological scaffold, which creates tissue resilience equipped to withstand a wider range of loading.

Chronic inflammation

Inflammation is the beginning phase in the healing process. Ordinarily, tissues progress through the healing process sequentially to restore full function. However, in certain cases injuries remain in the inflammatory period, like a computer program that has become stuck in a loop. This is then termed chronic inflammation and occurs because macrophages have been unable to completely clear (debride) the area of foreign substances. This material may be dead cells, extracellular blood, or sand or dirt in some cases. Either way, the material is surrounded by collagen to isolate it from the body. This mass of encapsulating scar is called a granuloma.

Definition

A granuloma is a mass of collagen which occurs in chronic inflammation. It surrounds and isolates foreign material in a wound.

Chronic inflammation has been shown to have a low concentration of growth factors and a high concentration of protease (Hom 1995). Adding growth factor to a chronic wound has been shown to improve healing in a number of soft tissues. Platelet-derived growth factor has been used to treat ligaments and tendons in general (Evans 1999), whilst insulin-like growth factor (IGF-1) has been used with the Achilles tendon (Kurtz, Loebig and Anderson 1999) and articular cartilage (Nixon, Fortier and Williams 1999).

Repair

Inflammation may continue for five days, but with minor trauma it is usually complete by the third day after injury. Following this, tissue repair can take place. Repair is by resolution, organization or regeneration, depending on the severity of the injury and the nature of the injured tissues. A minor injury will result in acute inflammation as described above, and the phagocytic cells will clear the area. If there is little tissue damage, the stage of resolution will result in a return to near normal conditions. True resolution rarely occurs with soft tissue injuries, but is more common with inflammatory tissue reactions such as pneumonia.

The proliferation of new tissue is by two processes, *fibroplasia* (the production of fibrous material) and *angiogenesis* (production of new blood vessels). This process is instigated by cytokines and growth factors released from macrophages during the inflammatory stage of healing, so limiting this stage may impair subsequent proliferation (Watson 2016)

Definition:

Fibroplasia is the production of fibrous material within healing tissue. *Angiogenesis* is the formation of new blood vessels.

On the periphery of an injured area, macrophages and polymorphs are active because they can tolerate the low oxygen levels present in the damaged tissue. Cellular division by mitosis (cells splitting to create two identical copies of themselves) is seen in the surrounding capillaries about 12 hours after injury. During the next three days, capillary buds form and grow towards the lower oxygen concentration of the injured area. These capillaries form loops and blood begins to flow through them. This new capillary-rich material is known as granulation tissue. Plasma proteins, cells and fluid pour out of these highly permeable vessels. The gradually increasing oxygen supply to the previously deoxygenated area means phagocytosis (ingestion of material by specialized white blood cells) can now begin.

New lymphatic vessels bud out from the existing lymphatics, linking to form a renewed lymphatic drainage system. As this process is occurring, fibroblast cells multiply and move towards the injured tissue. Myofibroblasts (specialized fibroblast cells similar to smooth muscle cells) are responsible for wound contraction, pulling the edges of the wound towards each other to reduce the size of the final scar.

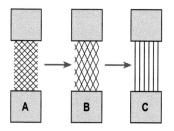 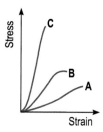

Figure 1.10 Relationship between fibre orientation and stress–strain response. From Oakes, B.W. (1992). The classification of injuries and mechanisms of injury, repair and healing. In *Textbook of Science and Medicine in Sport* (eds J. Bloomfield, P.A. Fricker and K.D. Fitch). Blackwell Scientific Publications, Melbourne. With permission.

By the fifth day after injury, fibrils of collagen begin to appear, a process requiring adequate amounts of vitamin C. The individual fibrils form into parallel bundles lying in the direction of stress imposed on the tissue. If no movement occurs to stress the collagen bundles, they may be laid down in a haphazard and weaker pattern. Controlled movement causes the fibrils to align lengthways along the line of stress of the injured structure. Variation in longitudinal fibre alignment will determine the stress–strain response of the tissue to loading (Fig. 1.10). Where fibre alignment is parallel to the tissue body, the steep stress–strain curve (C) indicates that less deformation will occur for a given tissue loading. The tissue is therefore 'stronger'.

It becomes clear that external mechanical factors, and not the previous organization of the tissue, dictate the eventual pattern of fibril arrangement. Total rest during this stage of healing is therefore contraindicated in most cases.

Keypoint:

External mechanical factors have a positive influence on tissue healing and can dictate the eventual strength of the healing tissues. Long periods of total rest are therefore rarely required when treating sports injuries.

In some tissue full regeneration occurs, damaged cells being replaced by functioning normal tissue. Fractured bone exhibits this property, as do torn ligaments and peripheral nerves providing conditions are suitable (Evans 1990b).

Remodelling

The remodelling stage overlaps repair, and may last from three weeks to twelve months, in some cases continuing for longer. During this stage, collagen is modified and refined to increase its functional capacity. Remodelling is characterized by a reduction in the wound size, an increase in scar strength, and an alteration in the direction of the collagen fibres.

Contraction of granulation tissue (see above) will occur for as long as the elasticity of the fibres will allow. Fibroblast cells transform into myofibroblasts, which then form intercellular bonds. These contain contractile proteins (actomyosin) and behave much like smooth muscle fibres.

Three weeks after injury, the quantity of collagen has stabilized but the strength of the fibres continues to increase. Strength increases are a result of an expansion in the number of cross-bonds between the cells, and the replacement collagen cells themselves. There is a continuous turnover of collagen, and several factors may delay this stage of the healing process (Table 1.5).

Table 1.5 Factors slowing healing rate

Age (slower with ageing)
Protein deficiency
Low vitamin C levels
Steroids and Non-steroidal anti-inflammatory drugs (NSAIDS)
Temperature (reduced rate when cold)
Poor local blood supply (ischaemia)
Adhesion to underlying tissue
Prolonged inflammation
Wound drying
Excessive mechanical stress (disrupts healing tissue and may restart inflammation)

Data from Watson 2016

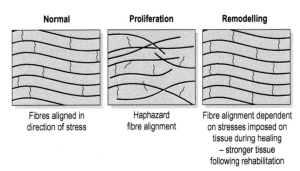

Normal	Proliferation	Remodelling
Fibres aligned in direction of stress	Haphazard fibre alignment	Fibre alignment dependent on stresses imposed on tissue during healing – stronger tissue following rehabilitation

Figure 1.11 Changing collagen fibre alignment during healing.

Final collagen fibre alignment should match the tissue function (Fig. 1.11). Fibres within a ligament will respond to a range of motion exercises which tense the ligament rhythmically. This may cause mild discomfort (VAS 2–3) but not pain (VAS 7–8). Excessive loading can hamper the healing process, causing it to revert back from the remodelling stage to the inflammatory stage. Fibres within muscle respond similarly, but to force transmission encountered by active and light resisted exercise during rehabilitation.

Keypoint:

▶ Tissue should be subjected to mild stress during rehabilitation but NOT severe loading.

▶ Mild discomfort indicates that tissue is stimulated to remodel, encouraging correct collagen fibre alignment.

▶ Excessive mechanical stress on the damaged area may cause tissue disruption, forcing the healing process to revert back to its inflammatory stage.

Matching treatment to the healing timescale

The tensile strength of injured soft tissue will reduce substantially after injury due to mechanical damage to the tissues. By the first post-injury day, tensile strength may have reduced by some 50 per cent. Although healing begins immediately, we have seen that collagen is not laid down until the fifth post-injury day. The period between injury and the beginning of collagen synthesis has been described as the 'lag phase' (Fig. 1.12). Therapy techniques applied in this period should be aimed at pain resolution and oedema reduction. Only when collagen synthesis begins should therapy aim to mobilize tissue and align collagen fibres in the direction of stress.

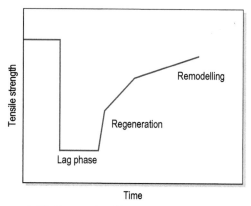

Figure 1.12 Strength of healing tissue following injury. From Hunter (1998) with permission.

Treatment note 1.5   Influencing the mechanical properties of healing tissue

Mechanotransduction

Stimulation of the healing tissue through mechanical loading such as exercise or manual therapy results in mechanotransduction (Khan and Scott 2009). This process has three interrelated components: mechanocoupling, cell-to-cell communication, and effector cell response.

▶ Mechanocoupling is the method through which forces created through manual therapy (or exercise), such as shear, compression and tension, deform the tissue cells and are transformed into chemical signals. The effect of cell deformation is not restricted to the local area of therapy, however, as cell-to-cell communication will also occur.

▶ Cell-to-cell communication involves signals being conducted from the treated area throughout the wider tissue region. At the points where cells touch each other, gap junctions are formed. Through these, charged particles (calcium and inositol triphosphate) pass so that cells can communicate with each other directly, to cause an effector cell response.

▶ Effector cell response. Integrins (receptors on the outside of the cell) form a bridge between the extracellular region (outside) and the intercellular region (inside). The cytoskeleton of the cell sends a direct physical stimulus to the cell nucleus, and biochemical signals (gene expression) are caused by the integrins. As a result, the cell nucleus gives a signal to begin protein synthesis and the new protein is secreted into the extracellular matrix, causing it to remodel.

Manual therapy and exercise therefore cause direct chemical changes which promote repair and remodelling of the injured tissues. Tissue overload from manual therapy or exercise leads to the increased release of mechano-growth factor (MGF), a member of the insulin-like growth factor (IGF) family. MGF has been shown to activate satellite cells within muscle (Goldspink 2003) and is important in both muscle injury and age-related muscle wasting or sacropenia (Kandalla et al. 2011).

Soft tissue manipulation

The use of deep transverse frictional massage (DTF) has been claimed to assist soft tissue healing. By applying shear and gliding movements to an injured tendon, ligament or muscle, tensile strength of the healing scar may be improved and adhesions potentially reduced. Gentle DTF applied in the acute phase of healing could increase the rate of phagocytosis by inducing agitation of tissue fluid. In the chronic stage of healing the therapeutic movement produced by DTF is said to soften and mobilize adhesions (Kesson and Atkins 1998), but there is little evidence to support this claim.

Specific soft tissue mobilization

Specific soft tissue mobilization (SSTM) is a technique pioneered by Hunter (1998). The procedure involves tensioning the tissue using physiological joint movement and accessory joint movement and adding a dynamic soft tissue mobilization. In the acute phase of healing, SSTM is claimed to influence the mechanical properties of healing tissue by altering collagen and ground substance synthesis.

A sustained load of five repetitions of a 30-second hold is used in a treatment session and the patient performs home exercise by self-stretching for three repetitions of a 30-second hold every three to four hours. Using the Achilles tendon as an example (Fig. 1.13), the mobility of the tendon is assessed by subjecting it to shearing forces, beginning distally and moving proximally. The aim is to fix the proximal segment of the tendon with the fingers and then move the tendon in the opposite direction with the fingers of the other hand. The shearing motion is moved up the tendon progressively, assessing range and quality of movement.

This same shearing action is used with the tendon on stretch (passive loading) or loaded by mild muscle contraction (dynamic loading). Pain modulation is a likely effect, rather than mechanical change.

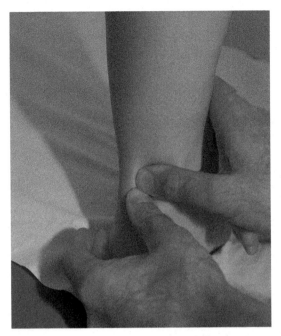

Figure 1.13 Specific soft tissue mobilization (SSTM) of the Achilles.

Individual tissue response to injury

In this section we will look at the responses of the individual tissues to injury, and the effects these have upon subsequent rehabilitation. Aspects of tissue structure relevant to sports injury are discussed.

Synovial membrane

The synovium consists of two layers, the intima, or synovial lining, and the subsynovial (subintimal) tissue. The intimal layer is made up of specialized cells known as synoviocytes, arranged in multiple layers. Two types of synoviocytes are present, type A cells, which are phagocytic, and type B cells, which synthesize the hyaluronoprotein of the synovial fluid. The two types are not distinct, however, and appear to be functional stages of the same basic cells.

The subsynovial tissue lies beneath the intima as a loose network of highly vascular connective tissue.

Cells are interspaced with collagen fibres and fatty tissue. The subsynovial tissue itself merges with the periosteum of bone lying within the synovial membrane of the joint. Similar merging occurs with the joint cartilage through a transitional layer of fibrocartilage.

The blood vessels of the joint divide into three branches, one travelling to the epiphysis, the second to the joint capsule and the third to the synovial membrane. From here the vessels of the subsynovium are of two types. The first is thin-walled and adapted for fluid exchange, and the second thick-walled and capable of gapping to allow particles, especially nutrients, to pass through.

Once free of the vessels, any material must pass through the synovial interstitium before entering the synovial fluid itself. The passage of this material is by diffusion on the whole, but by active transport for glucose molecules.

The synovium must adapt to movement with normal function of the joint. Rather than stretching, the synovium unfolds to facilitate flexion.
The synovium is well lubricated by the same hyaluronate molecules found within the synovial fluid itself, and so the various layers slide over each other. Since the synovium must alter shape within the confines of the joint capsule, the process of synovial adaptation is at its best when the fluid volume of the joint is at a minimum.

Synovial fluid plays a significant role in joint stability. The negative atmospheric pressure within the joint creates a suction effect, which, aided by the surface tension of the synovial fluid, draws the bony surfaces of the joint together.

Response to injury

With minor trauma the synovium is not microscopically disturbed, but will instead suffer a vasomotor reaction. The synovium will dilate and fluid filtration increases. Protein leaks into the interstitium, changing the osmotic pressure and causing local oedema and joint exudation. This process constitutes a post-traumatic synovitis.

Keypoint:
Post-traumatic synovitis initially involves a vasomotor reaction of the synovium rather than actual structural damage.

The slight hyperaemia gives way later to alterations of the intimal layer, the total number of layers increasing threefold. If the trauma does not continue, the protein molecules which were released are cleared by the lymphatics and the osmotic pressures return to normal. If mechanical irritation persists, the intimal layer will continue to thicken. The deep synovial cells now show increased activity and protein synthesis escalates.

Alterations occur in the number of type A and type B synoviocyte cells. The number of type A cells reduces as some of these move into the synovial fluid to become macrophages. The synovial lining becomes filled with fibroblasts, which in turn change into type B cells. Neutrophil cells die, releasing proteolytic enzymes which attack the near joint structures. This process can self-perpetuate the synovitis, even in the absence of further trauma, giving rise to a reactive synovitis.

Onset of symptoms following post-traumatic synovitis usually occurs between 12 and 24 hours after injury and can last for between one and two weeks. Patients complain mainly of joint tightness, with warmth, erythema and pain being encountered less often. The tightness is due to joint effusion, the increased fluid volume causing the normally negative intra-articular pressure to become positive.

The stability of the joint, no longer created by a negative intra-articular pressure, comes from joint distension instead. This places a traction force on the joint capsule and surrounding ligaments. Pressures are greatest in the effused joint in extremes of flexion and extension, and are reduced at about 30° flexion, this being the resting position taken up by the patient. Haemarthrosis is usually present if swelling occurs within two hours of injury, and pain is intense.

Surgical removal of the synovial membrane (synovectomy) may be performed in a number of inflammatory joint disorders. With time the synovium will regrow, and the use of continuous passive motion (CPM) may be used to assist this process. Without mechanical stimulation synovial membrane will degenerate through the loss of proteoglycan, so movement is vital to its effective healing.

Synovial fluid

Synovial fluid is similar in many ways to blood plasma. The main differences being that synovia does not contain fibrinogen or prothrombin and so is unable to clot. The mucopolysaccharide hyaluronate (hyaluronic acid) secreted by the synoviocytes is contained within the fluid.

The amount of synovial fluid present in a joint is very little – about 0.5–4 ml within large joints such as the knee – and this is spread throughout the joint by structures such as the cartilage, menisci and fat pads.

Synovial fluid is a highly viscous fluid, which becomes more elastic as the rate of joint movement increases. As weight is taken by the joint, synovial fluid is squeezed out from between the opposing joint surfaces. This is resisted by the tenacity of the fluid itself.

As the joint moves, the synovial fluid is pulled in the direction of movement and so a layer of fluid is maintained between the joint surfaces. Any friction produced by movement will therefore occur within the synovial fluid rather than between the joint surfaces. When the joint is statically loaded, however, fluid flows away from the point of maximal load and the joint relies on the articular cartilage to provide lubrication (see below). The synovial fluid provides nutrition for about two-thirds of the articular cartilage bordering the joint space

Following injury, fluid volume may increase as much as 10 or 20 times, with a decrease in hyaluronate and, with it, fluid viscosity. Pain due to the accumulation of synovial fluid is dependent not on the amount of fluid present, but on the speed with which it forms. As much as 100 ml may be extracted from a joint which caused little pain because it took a long time to form, while 15 ml may be painful if formed rapidly following trauma.

With injury in which bleeding is not present, the constituents of the synovial fluid remain basically the same. In reactive synovitis, the protein concentration is slightly elevated, and the number of white blood cells increases somewhat, from normal values of 100/ml to as much as 300/ml. With post-traumatic synovitis, however, the white cell count is further increased, to as much as 2000/ml.

Haemarthrosis (blood within the joint) causes rapidly developing fluid, which contains fibrinogen. If the synovial membrane is torn, fat can enter the joint from the extrasynovial adipose tissue and will show up in the synovial fluid. The blood from haemarthrosis will mostly stay fluid, and is quickly absorbed by the phagocytic cells to ultimately disappear after several days.

Bone

Types

Bone is essentially a fibrous matrix impregnated with mineral salts (mainly calcium phosphate), and it therefore combines the properties of both elasticity and rigidity. It is a living tissue, which is continually remodelled, and subject to hormonal control. Bone injury within sport is assessed using X-ray – see Treatment Note 1.6.

Treatment note 1.6   Diagnostic imaging

Diagnostic imaging is used to support a thorough examination and should not be relied upon as the only means of clinical diagnosis. In some cases physical examination will be superior to imaging, a situation recognized, for example, with ankle injury (see Ottawa ankle rules, Chapter 6).

Imaging types

There are several imaging types used within the management of sports injuries. Reflective imaging includes ultrasound (U/S) and magnetic resonance imaging (MRI).

With this type of imaging, energy is passed into the tissues and reflected back to form an image. Ionizing radiation imaging includes standard X-rays (plain films) and computed tomography (CT). X-rays use radiation which passes through the tissues onto film to cause an image, whereas CT again uses radiation but converts the radiation into digital units to create slices (3 mm minimum) through the body. Emission imaging (bone scan) uses a radiopharmaceutical agent injected into the blood. This is taken up by areas of the body with increased metabolic activity and these show up as images.

Standard X-rays

X-rays pass through the tissues at different rates depending on tissue density. Air is the least dense (radiolucent) and metal the most dense (radio-opaque). X-rays pass easily through air, creating the darkest image on X-ray film. The lungs, airways and colon therefore appear black. Fat is the next densest tissue and so appears as very dark grey and is found throughout the body. Fluid absorbs more of the X-rays than air or fat, giving a whiter image. Bone is the most dense naturally occurring tissue, appearing white on X-ray film. This may be either bone itself or where tissues have calcified, for example in myositis ossificans or calcific tendon pathology. Metal completely blocks X-rays and so metal implants are easily visualized on plain film as totally white.

Because X-rays pass through the body in a straight line, they create a planar image, that is one structure superimposed on another. Two images are therefore used, lying at 90 degrees to one another, most commonly anteroposterior (AP) and lateral (lat.). X-rays obey the laws of light, and so body positioning is important. The closer the body area to be imaged is to the X-ray film (further from the X-ray beam) the clearer the image will be.

X-ray analysis

A systematic analysis of X-rays may be made using the ABCs mnemonic, standing for alignment, bone density, cartilage and soft tissue (Table 1.6).

▶ Alignment is assessed by comparing the contour of one bone to that of the adjacent bone. This is normally assisted by drawing a mental line along the edge of the bones. Changed alignment suggests altered stability through soft tissue changes and/or fracture.

▶ Bone is assessed for changes in both density and dimension. In long bones the shaft should appear uniform, with increased density towards the edge and less density within the medullary canal. The periosteum should not be lifted and

Treatment note 1.6 *continued*

Table 1.6 A systematic analysis of X-rays, using the ABCs mnemonic. After Magee (2008)

		Overview	Normal	Abnormal
A	Alignment	Alignment to adjacent bone Bone contour	Normal size and number Smooth & continuous outline Normal spatial relationships	Deformity or extra bones Fracture/dislocation/subluxation Bone spur/osteophyte
B	Bone density	Density change Texture abnormality	Contrast between bone and soft tissue greyness Normal trabeculae Contrast between cortical and cancellous bone	Loss of bone density showing as poor contrast between bone and soft tissue Altered trabeculae Changed appearance within bone
C	Cartilage spaces	Normal joint space Epiphyseal plate	Well preserved joint space Normal size of epiphysis for age	Decreased joint space Cartilage erosion
s	Soft tissues	Muscle Fat pad Capsule Periosteum	Normal soft tissue size Capsule and fat pad indistinct	Swelling/wasting changing alignment Periosteal reaction Gas bubbles

the edge of the bone should be continuous. At the bone ends, the trabeculae of the cancellous bone should be uniform. Bone dimension is compared to neighbouring segments, for example within the spine to the vertebrae above and below, to identify wedging.

▶ Cartilage evaluation includes both hyaline cartilage across the joint surface and menisci or labral cartilage within a joint. An arthrogram is required to identify cartilage damage, but when cartilage is changed, bone alignment alteration and bone density change normally follow.

References

Magee, D.J., 2008. *Orthopedic Physical Assessment*, fifth ed. Saunders/Elsevier, St Louis, Missouri.

Two types of bone are generally described, *cancellous* (spongy) bone and *compact* (cortical) bone, and important differences exist in both their mechanical properties and methods of healing. Cancellous bone is found at a number of sites, including the bone ends, and is arranged in a system of trabeculae (bands or columns) aligned to resist imposed stresses. Compact bone is dense, with a solid matrix made from an organic ground substance and inorganic salts.

Keypoint:

Cancellous bone is made up of trabeculae, *compact* bone has a solid matrix.

The shaft of a long bone consists of a ring of compact bone surrounding a hollow cavity, containing marrow. In infants the bone marrow is red, but this is gradually replaced by yellow bone marrow until, by puberty, only the cancellous bone cavities at the ends of the long bones contain red marrow. With age, the bone marrow in these cavities too is replaced, but red bone marrow may still be found in the vertebrae, sternum and ribs, as well as the proximal ends of the femur and humerus.

The bone is enclosed in a dense membrane called the *periosteum*, which is absent in the region of the articular cartilage. The periosteum is highly vascular and responsible for the nutrition of the bone cortex which underlies it. The deep layers of periosteum contain bone-forming cells (osteoblasts). These lay down successive layers of bone during growth, and so the periosteum is responsible for alterations in the bone width; in addition, these cells play an important part in bone healing. In contrast, the bone cavity is lined by bone-destroying cells (osteoclasts) which erode the inner surface of the bone.

A direct blow to the bone may damage the periosteal blood vessels, giving rise to a periosteal haematoma. The blood formed beneath the periosteum can lift it, causing bone deposition by the osteoblasts. This is a common problem over the anterior tibia in footballers and hockey players and gives a pronounced lump.

Keypoint:

A direct blow to unprotected bone (with a hard ball or boot, for example) may cause bleeding beneath the bone periosteum. Ultimately this may lead to calcification (bone deposits) within the bruised area.

Bone may be further classified into four major types. The long bones are found within the limbs, and consist of a shaft and two enlarged ends. Short bones have a block-like appearance such as those of the carpals, and are mainly cancellous bone. Flat bones are thinner, and consist of two layers of compact bone sandwiching a thin layer of cancellous bone; examples are the skull vaults and the ribs. Finally, irregular bones consist of a thin layer of compact bone surrounded by cancellous bone; examples are the vertebrae.

Definition:

Bones may be classified as long (limbs), short (carpals), flat (scapula) and irregular (vertebrae).

Development

Skeletal development begins with loosely arranged mesodermal cells, which are mostly converted to hyaline cartilage. Between the seventh and twelfth intrauterine week, a primary ossification centre appears within the shaft of the long bone, and spreads towards the bone ends. The centre of the shaft is hollowed out and filled with red bone marrow, and the whole shaft is called a diaphysis. At the end of the bone, secondary centres of ossification appear, usually after birth. Gradually the main part of the cartilage is replaced, leaving only the articular cartilage, and a cartilage plate (growth plate, or physis) between the shaft and end of the bone.

The growth plate is of great importance in paediatric sports medicine. This cartilage layer is responsible for the increase in bone length. As the cartilage grows it becomes thicker, and its upper and lower surfaces are converted to bone. Eventually the cartilage stops growing, but its ossification continues so that the cartilage becomes thinner, until it eventually disappears. At this point the diaphysis and epiphysis are united, and growth in length of the bone is no longer possible. The point at which this occurs may be influenced by a number of factors, including impact stresses (see below).

Intramembranous ossification occurs in the mandible, clavicle and certain bones of the skull. Here, the intermediate stage of cartilage formation is omitted, and the bone ossifies directly from connective tissue.

Epiphyseal injury

Two types of epiphysis are found. Pressure epiphyses are found at the end of long bones, and are interarticular. They are subjected to compression stress with weight bearing, and are responsible for changes in bone length. Traction epiphyses (apophyses) occur at the insertion of major muscles. They experience tension stress as the muscles contract, and alter bone shape.

The growth plate itself forms a weak link in the immature skeleton, and shearing or avulsion stresses can cause it to be dislodged. Because the epiphyses are weaker than the major joint structures, injuries which in the adult would cause dislocation or tendon rupture may cause epiphyseal injury in a child.

Five types of injury are traditionally described, as shown in Fig. 1.14. The Type I lesion involves horizontal displacement of the growth plate, while with the Type II lesion the fracture line runs through to the adjacent metaphysis. In the Type III and IV fractures the joint surface is involved, so the complication rate is higher. Gentle manipulation under anaesthetic is normally used to realign the epiphysis in the first fracture types. Crush injuries and those through the growth plate may cause more severe problems of growth disturbance. When a fracture crosses the growth plate, bone may fill the gap formed, giving unequal growth. Crush injuries may lead to premature closure of the plate, with associated deformities of shortening and altered bony angulation.

> **Keypoint**
>
> If a fracture involves a bone growth plate, bone deformity such as angulation or shortening may result.

Osteochondrosis

Osteochondrosis affects the pressure epiphyses during their growth period, and are the most common overuse injuries seen in children. There is an interference with the epiphyseal blood supply, causing an avascular necrosis to the secondary ossification centre. The bone within the epiphysis softens, dies and is absorbed (Fig. 1.15). Because the cap of articular cartilage surrounding the epiphysis receives nutrition from the synovial fluid, it remains largely unaffected. The combination of softening bone contained within an intact articular cap leads to flattening of the epiphysis. Gradually the dead bone is replaced by new bone by a process of 'creeping substitution'. Trauma may be one factor which initiates the ischaemic process,

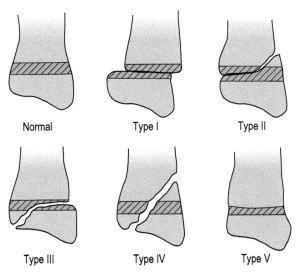

Figure 1.14 Epiphyseal injuries. After Salter and Harris (1963) with permission.

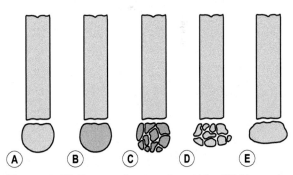

Figure 1.15 Stages of osteochondritis. (A) Normal epiphysis. (B) The bony nucleus undergoes necrosis, loses its normal texture and becomes granular. (C) The bony nucleus becomes fragmented during the process of removal of dead bone. (D) If subjected to pressure the softened epiphysis becomes flattened. (E) Re-ossification with restoration of normal bone texture, but deformity may persist. The whole process takes 2–3 years. From Gartland (1987) with permission.

either through direct injury or vascular occlusion as a result of traumatic synovitis.

The osteochondroses may be categorized into four groups:

1. Traction osteochondroses (apophysitis) affect the attachments of major tendons, particularly to the knee and heel.
2. Crushing osteochondroses occur in the hip, wrist and forefoot.
3. Articular chondral osteochondroses involve splitting of bone near an articular site, with resultant bone fragment formation.
4. Finally, physeal injuries affect the growth plate and result in irregular growth and/or angular deformity.

Any pressure epiphysis may be affected by osteochondrosis, the condition taking the name of the person who first described it in that region. The most common conditions are shown in Table 1.7, and details of these are given in the relevant clinical chapters in this book.

Table 1.7 The osteochondroses

Classification	Name	Site(s)
Non-articular traction (pulling)	Osgood–Schlatter's	Tibial tubercle
	Sinding–Larsen—Johannsson's disease	Interior pole of patella (quadriceps)
	Sever's disease	Calcaneous (gastrocnemius)
Articular subchondral (crushing)	Perthes' disease	Femoral head
	Kienböck's disease	Lunate (wrist)
	Köhler's disease	Navicular (mid-foot)
	Freiberg's disease	Second metatarsal head
Articular chondral (splitting)	Osteochondritis dissecans	Medical femoral
		Condyle (knee)
		Capitellum (elbow)
		Talar dome (ankle)
Physeal	Scheuermann's disease	Thoracic spine
	Blount's disease	Tibia (proximal)

Healing

Bone healing is governed by a number of factors, including the type of tissue which is damaged, the extent of the damage and position of the bony fragments, the amount of movement present at the fracture site as healing progresses, and the blood supply. In a long bone, healing may be divided into five stages, as shown in Fig. 1.16.

▶ Stage one is that of tissue destruction and haematoma formation. As local blood vessels

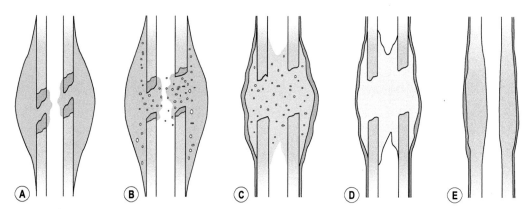

Figure 1.16 Stages of fracture healing. (A) Haematoma. Tissue damage and bleeding occur at the fracture site, the bone ends die back a few millimetres. (B) Inflammation. Inflammatory cells appear in the haematoma. (C) Callus. The cell population changes to osteoblasts and osteoclasts, dead bone is mopped up and woven bone appears in the fracture callus. (D) Consolidation. Woven bone is remodelled to resemble the normal structure (E). From Apley and Solomon (1988) with permission.

are torn at the time of injury, blood is released, forming a haematoma within and surrounding the fracture site. The bone periosteum and surrounding soft tissues contain the blood, and the periosteum itself is lifted from the bone surface. The deprivation of blood to the bone surfaces immediately adjacent to the fracture line causes these surfaces to die back for up to 2 mm. Some eight hours after fracture, inflammation and proliferation may be detected as stage two of healing.

▶ In stage two, the deep periosteal cells and those of the damaged medullary canal proliferate, and cellular tissue begins to grow forward to meet similar material from the other side of the fracture site and bridges the area. Capillary growth into the region allows the haematoma to be slowly reabsorbed, and the congealed blood itself takes little part in the repair process.

▶ Stage three is marked by the appearance of osteogenic and chondrogenic cells. New bone and, in some cases, cartilage are laid down, while osteoclastic cells remove remaining dead bone. The cellular mass which forms is called a callus, and becomes increasingly mineralized into woven bone, uniting the fracture. The callus is larger where there has been much periosteal stripping, when bone displacement is marked and if the haematoma has been large.

▶ During the fourth stage of healing, the woven bone is gradually transformed into lamellar bone by osteoblasts.

▶ The fifth and final stage of healing is remodelling, when the fracture site is bridged by solid bone. A combination of bone reabsorption and formation reshapes the callus, laying down thicker lamellae in areas of high stress and removing excessive bone. The medullary cavity is re-formed.

The rate of healing is dependent on a number of factors. The type of bone is important, cancellous bone healing far more quickly than cortical bone. Also, the fracture type will dictate the speed of healing, with a spiral fracture healing more quickly than a transverse type. If the blood supply has been compromised at the time of injury, or if the fracture has occurred in an area with a poor blood supply, the healing rate will be slower. The age and health of the patient are other determining factors, with fractures in children healing almost twice as fast as those in adults. In general terms, callus may be visible radiographically within two to three weeks of injury, with firm fracture union taking about four to six weeks for upper limb fractures and eight to twelve weeks for those in the lower limb. Full consolidation may take as much as eight and sixteen weeks for upper and lower limb fractures, respectively.

In contrast to long bone, cancellous bone remains fairly immobile when fractured, and heals by 'direct repair' with a minimum of callus formation. The main difference occurs because there is no medullary canal in cancellous bone, and the area of contact between the two injured bone fragments is much greater. Following haematoma formation, new blood vessels and osteogenic cells penetrate the area and meet similar tissue from the opposite bone fragment. The intercellular matrix which is laid down by osteoblasts is calcified into woven bone. This type of healing also occurs when internal fixation is used.

Mechanical properties

Bone responds to mechanical stress in similar ways to other connective tissue, but at a considerably slower rate. Its ability to adapt its structure, size and shape depends on the mechanical stresses placed upon it. When stress is reduced, by prolonged bed rest for example, mineral reabsorption occurs and the bone reduces in strength. Raising stress to an optimal level, by exercise, leads to an increase in bone strength.

In addition to changes in total mineral content, bone varies its strength according to the direction of the imposed stress. At bony attachment sites such as tubercles, alignment of collagen fibres is parallel to the direction of the imposed force. In the shaft of a long bone, fibre orientation is along the bone axis, indicating that this part of the bone is designed to resist tension and compression forces. In cancellous bone at the epiphysis, shear stresses are maximal and so fibre alignment is in the direction of the shearing forces.

> **Keypoint**
>
> As with other tissues in the body, bone responds to mechanical stress by adapting its structure. If stress is reduced (prolonged rest) bone reduces in strength. Raising stress to an optimal level (exercise) leads to an increase in bone strength.

Osteoporosis

Osteoporosis (bone mineral loss) has now reached epidemic proportions in the Western world (Carbon 1992). The condition involves a progressive decrease in bone mineral density (BMD), due to an imbalance between bone formation and bone reabsorption. Bone mass reaches its peak in the third and fourth decade, and loss occurs normally in both sexes with ageing, but this rate is increased markedly with osteoporosis. Normal bone loss of 3 per cent per decade may increase to as much as 10 per cent per decade for trabecular bone. This leads to a reduction per decade in ultimate stress of 5 per cent, ultimate strain of 9 per cent and energy absorption of 12 per cent (Behiri and Vashishth 2000).

Osteoporosis may be either *primary*, governed by age and sex, or *secondary* as a result of disease. The most common primary types are postmenopausal osteoporosis and senile osteoporosis

> **Definition**
>
> Osteoporosis may be either primary, governed by sex (postmenopausal) or age (senile), or secondary, resulting from disease.

The loss of mass makes the bone susceptible to fracture, particularly as a result of microtrauma. Common fracture sites include the distal radius and vertebrae for postmenopausal osteoporosis,

and the proximal femur for senile osteoporosis. Fracture of the distal radius presents as a Colles' fracture, while vertebral wedging gives rise to an increased thoracic kyphosis or 'dowager's hump'.

There is a marked increase in the risk of fracture once bone density reduces below a certain level (known as the fracture threshold, Fig. 1.17). The incidence of hip and vertebral fractures rises with age (Fig. 1.18), but the rise in hip fracture incidence

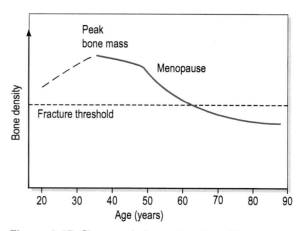

Figure 1.17 Changes in bone density with age. From Wolman, R.L. and Reeve, J. (1994) Exercise and the skeleton. In *Oxford Textbook of Sports Medicine* (eds M. Harries et al.). Reprinted with permission of Oxford University Press, Oxford.

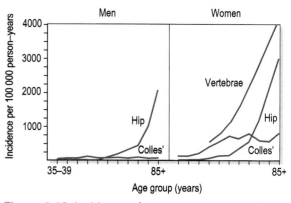

Figure 1.18 Incidence of common osteoporotic fractures. From Wolman, R.L. and Reeve, J. (1994) Exercise and the skeleton. In *Oxford Textbook of Sports Medicine* (eds M. Harries et al.). Reprinted with permission of Oxford University Press, Oxford.

in men occurs some five years later than in women (Wolman and Reeve 1994), an indication of the effect of postmenopausal osteoporosis.

Assessment of osteoporosis

Change in BMD is the standard objective measure for osteoporosis, but low bone density in itself is asymptomatic. It is only when a fracture occurs or an individual develops pain or substantial postural changes that they seek help. Assessment of BMD may be made by direct examination of X-rays, normally taken where a patient has a separate pathology or bone injury. *Cortical index* measures the thickness of the bone cortex in comparison to the bone shaft. The combined width of the two cortices should be 50 per cent of the total width of the bone at mid-shaft (Apley and Solomon 1993). *Trabecular index* is a method of assessing bone mass from the radiographic pattern of bone trabeculae in the proximal femur or calcaneus. A more accurate measure of BMD is obtained by *dual energy X-ray absorptiometry* (DEXA or DXA scan). Measurement is taken yearly, and only changes greater than 2 to 3 per cent are significant (Bennell, Khan and McKay 2000). Results are expressed as BMD in g/cm^2, as a Z score which compares the value to an age-matched group, or as a T score which compares the obtained value to a young healthy population. The World Health Organization has classified degrees of BMD loss as shown in Table 1.8.

Subjective assessment includes elements such as family history, fracture status, history of falls, menstrual history, smoking and dietary habits, and exercise status. Objective examination is of posture, pain and functional limitation (CSP 1999; Bennell, Khan and McKay 2000).

Three main factors are important in the development of osteoporosis: diet, oestrogen level and physical activity.

Diet

Modern diet can fail to provide an adequate daily intake of calcium. Recommended requirements as high as 1500 mg of calcium and 400 IU of vitamin D have been made for postmenopausal women, but many women may consume as little as 300 mg of calcium, placing themselves in negative calcium balance. Excess salt or caffeine, and a large intake of meat, promote calcium loss in the urine, and an excessive intake of fibre and alcohol can bind calcium in the gut, preventing its absorption.

Calcium deficiency in animals has been shown to produce osteoporosis (Martin and Houston 1987), but effects in humans are less clear. Studying early postmenopausal women, Nilas, Christiansen and Rodbro (1984) gave a 500 mg calcium supplement over a two-year period and assessed bone density in the distal radius, while Ettinger, Genant and Cann (1987) gave a 1000 mg supplement and assessed the lumbar vertebrae. Both of these studies failed to show any significant differences between the treatment and non-treatment groups. However, in late postmenopausal women calcium supplementation may be more beneficial (MacKinnon 1988).

However, the effect of calcium supplementation on the incidence of fractures remains unproven (Evans 1990b).

Adequate calcium is clearly necessary for health, and those individuals who show a deficiency in their calcium intake may need dietary supplementation. Others should receive advice on good diet to enable them to maintain an adequate intake of calcium and vitamin D, remembering that excessive vitamin D intake can be toxic.

Table 1.8 Classification of osteoporosis

Classification	DXA reading
Normal	>−1
Osteopenia	−1 to −2.5
Osteoporosis	<−2.5
Severe osteoporosis	<−2.5 plus history of fragility fracture

BMD expressed as standard deviations (SD) below the mean of a young adult (T score). World Health Organization (1994) Assessment of Fracture Risk and its Application to Screening for Osteoporosis. Report of WHO study group. World Health Organization, Geneva. With permission.

Exercise

Weight-bearing exercise creates bone stress and acts as a stimulus for maintaining bone mass (osteogenic stimulus).

> **Definition:**
>
> An osteogenic stimulus is one which stimulates new bone formation

Loss of bone mass has been reported both as a result of prolonged bed rest (Donaldson, Hulley and Vogel 1970) and following weightlessness (Mazess and Whedon 1983). Similarly, athletes have been shown to have greater bone density than non-athletes (Nilsson and Westlin 1977), and tennis players have been shown to have a greater bone density in their dominant arm (Huddleston, Rockwell and Kuland 1980).

A number of authors have demonstrated the beneficial effects of weight-bearing exercise in slowing bone loss. Smith, Smith and Ensign (1984) assessed the effects of exercise (45 minutes, 3 days per week) on bone loss in postmenopausal women and showed a 1.4 per cent increase in bone mass during the second and third years of their study. Krolner, Toft and Nielsen (1983) studied the effects of exercise (1 hour, twice per week) on postmenopausal women. They showed a 3.5 per cent increase in bone mineral content of the lumbar spine for the exercising group compared to 2.7 per cent for their control.

High-impact exercise which generates a ground reaction force greater than twice body weight is likely to create bone remineralization (Heinonen, Kannus and Sievanen 1996). Exercise should be performed at least three times per week at intensities beginning with 40 to 60 per cent maximal oxygen uptake (VO2 max) and progressing to as much as 80 per cent VO2 max, even in the elderly (ACSM, 1998). Strength (weight) training at 70 per cent 1 RM has been shown to maintain hip and spine BMD, but programmes must be given progressively, taking clinical history into account. High-intensity progressive resistance training has been used successfully to treat osteoporotic seniors (mean age 66.1 years). An eight-month programme of twice weekly 30-minute weight training exercise was shown to improve femoral neck and lumbar spine bone mineral density (0.3 and 1.6 per cent respectively) compared to a control group of low-intensity exercise of the same duration (Watson et al. 2015). A flowchart to guide exercise prescription is shown in Fig. 1.19.

Clearly, regular weight-bearing exercise is important for the prevention and management of osteoporosis. However, the increased risk of fracture in this group means that caution must be shown. Repeated spinal rotation or flexion should be avoided, and high-impact activities should be limited at the early stages of treatment, especially where osteoporosis already exists.

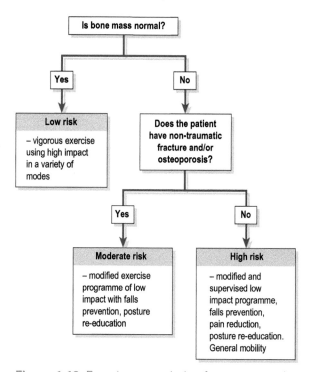

Figure 1.19 Exercise prescription for osteoporosis. Adapted from Bennell, Khan and McKay (2000), with permission.

Keypoint

Regular weight-bearing exercise slows, and can reverse, bone mineral loss seen in osteoporosis.

Definition

Core decompression is a surgical procedure which involves taking a plug of bone out of the centre of a bone to reduce pressure.

Transient osteoporosis

Transient osteoporosis most commonly affects the hip, where it is termed idiopathic transient osteoporosis of the hip (ITOH) (Harrington et al. 2000). It is a relatively rare condition which must be differentiated from both stress fracture and avascular necrosis. The condition was first described in women during late pregnancy. However, the main group to suffer from this condition are middle-aged (40–70 years) men, who represent over 70 per cent of cases (Lakhanpal, Ginsburg and Luthra 1987). ITOH is a self-limiting condition which demonstrates bone marrow oedema and slight bone cortex thinning. There is no evidence of the focal subchondral bone defect of the femoral head seen in avascular necrosis (Harrington et al. 2000). Joint fluid is sterile (non-infected) and only mild synovial thickening is present (McCarthy 1998).

Subjective examination reveals progressive unilateral hip pain referred into the groin and anterior thigh. Pain is exacerbated with weight bearing and eased with rest (contrast with malignancy, which gives pain at rest). Typically, pain is worse four to eight weeks after onset, and enforced rest may show disuse atrophy of the quadriceps and gluteal muscles. The joint and greater trochanter may be tender to palpation and the FABRE test positive.

Management is by protected weight-bearing (crutches) and non-weight-bearing or partial weight-bearing exercise to pain tolerance (pool/walking/jogging). Non-steroidal anti-inflammatory drugs (NSAIDs) may be of use, and protracted cases have responded to core decompression of the femur (Apel, Vince and Kingston 1994).

Articular cartilage

Cartilage is essentially a connective tissue consisting of cells embedded in a matrix permeated by fibres. Two major types are recognized, hyaline cartilage and fibrocartilage. Hyaline cartilage is found over bone ends and is described in more detail below. Fibrocartilage may be either white or yellow. White fibrocartilage is found in areas such as the intervertebral discs and glenoid labrum. Yellow fibrocartilage is found in structures such as the ears and larynx.

Definition

Hyaline cartilage is found in synovial joints, white fibrocartilage in the vertebrae and yellow fibrocartilage in the ear and larynx.

Articular (hyaline) cartilage is made up of collagen fibres, a protein–polysaccharide complex, and water. Fibres of collagen are embedded in a ground substance of gel-like material. The water content of cartilage is high, between 70 and 80 per cent of its total weight.

Cartilage has no blood vessels, lymphatics or nerve fibres. Nutrition is supplied directly from the synovial fluid, and by diffusion of blood products from the subchondral bone. The tangled structure of cartilage causes it to behave in some ways like a microscopic sieve, filtering out large molecules such as plasma proteins. Fluid movement through the cartilage is by osmosis and diffusion. Movement of the joint increases the rate of diffusion, but in the mature joint there is no transfer across the bone–cartilage interface.

Intermittent loading creates a pumping effect, squeezing fluid from the cartilage and allowing fresh fluid to be taken up as the load is released. Prolonged loading will gradually press fluid out of the cartilage, without allowing new fluid to be taken up. As much as a 40 per cent reduction in cartilage depth can occur by compression (Hettinga 1990).

Keypoint

Because cartilage has no direct blood supply, regular movement is vital to supply it with nutrients from the synovial fluid.

The cartilage is arranged in four layers (Fig. 1.20). The collagen fibres of the calcified zone bind the cartilage to the subchondral bone, resisting shear stresses. Within the mid-zone the fibres are randomly oriented. With joint compression, these

fibres stretch and will resist the tension forces created within them (Fig. 1.21). This property of elastic deformation (spring) occurs instantly. However, the fluid within the matrix of the cartilage will be compressed. As it does so, proteoglycans within the cartilage will tend to retain water and control its movement through the cartilage matrix. The cartilage will slowly flow away from the compression force, demonstrating the property of creep. When the load is removed, the fluid lost at the time of compression is reabsorbed. These two properties of instant spring and slower creep make cartilage a viscoelastic material.

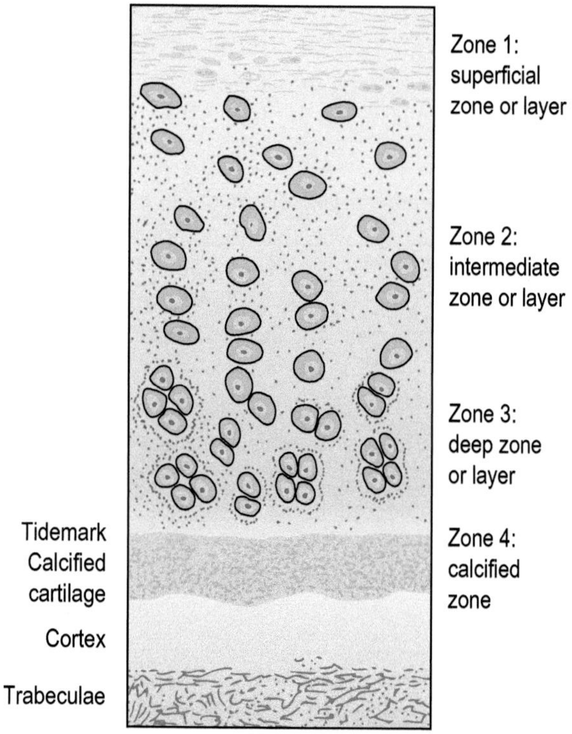

Keypoint

Cartilage assists joint lubrication by boundary lubrication and weeping lubrication.

Injury

Articular cartilage is to a great extent protected from injury by the elasticity of other joint structures, and the neuromuscular reflexes. Reflex muscular contraction and soft tissue 'give' will largely dampen shock before it reaches the cartilage. However, unexpected loading (such as trauma) which occurs too rapidly to invoke reflex protection will cause injury, but this is more frequently bony fracture rather than damage to the cartilage itself.

If cartilage injury does occur, it is most likely due to slip or shear. Three injury stages are generally described: first, splitting of the cartilage layer at the tidemark between the calcified and uncalcified tissue; second, cartilage depression into the subchondral bone; and third, fissuring of the cartilage and underlying bone.

Partial thickness injuries, limited to the articular cartilage alone, heal poorly. The healing which does take place is by proliferation and invasion from soft tissue, and the further away from this tissue the injured area is, the poorer the healing. Full thickness defects, extending through the subchondral bone, heal by superficial tissue

Zone 1: superficial zone or layer

Zone 2: intermediate zone or layer

Zone 3: deep zone or layer

Zone 4: calcified zone

Tidemark
Calcified cartilage

Cortex

Trabeculae

Figure 1.20 Zones in articular cartilage. From Gould (1990) with permission.

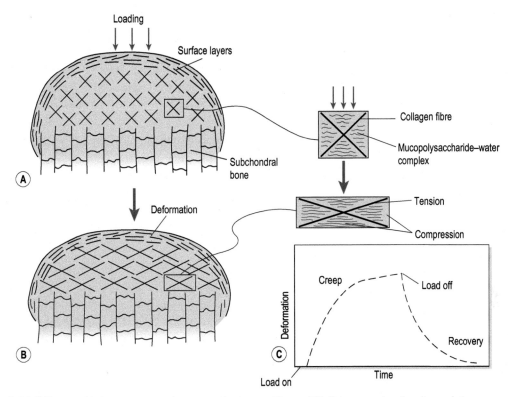

Figure 1.21 Effects of joint compression on articular cartilage. (A) Compressive loading of the cartilage results in (B) tension stress to the collagenous elements and compression stress to the mucopolysaccharide–water complex. (C) The total response is viscoelastic. The viscous creep with sustained loading is largely the result of a time-dependent squeezing out of fluid. From Hertling, D. and Kessler, R.M. (1990) *Management of Common Musculoskeletal Disorders*. JB Lippincott, Philadelphia. With permission.

bridging the break. Blood vessels grow into the uncalcified cartilage. Osteogenic cells and granulation tissue from the base of the break invade the area, resulting in the formation of fibrous tissue, bony trabeculae and fibrocartilage. There is obvious demarcation of the region into zones, a chondrin-free ring surrounding the uninjured tissue. The healed defect appears as a slightly discoloured roughened area of fibrous tissue.

Cartilage repair

Several surgical techniques may be used to aid repair of injury to articular cartilage (Table 1.9). The joint surface may be debrided (scraped) and the joint itself washed out (lavaged) to remove fragments of cartilage or subchondral bone. Damaging enzymes produced through cartilage degeneration are also removed. New cartilage cells may be introduced into the damaged area to stimulate healing. Osteochondral grafts of this type may be taken from the patient (autografts) or from cadaveric donors (allografts). A number of tissues have been used for autografts including rib perichondrial cells, periosteum and chondrocytes themselves. The technique involves two surgical procedures. First the cells must be removed, then allowed to grow in a laboratory, and finally the cells must be replanted into the damaged cartilage. Allograft techniques can result in high degrees of

Table 1.9 Management of articular cartilage degeneration

Method	Technique
Debridement	Cartilage layer is removed down to subchondral bone. Results may be poor
Arthroscopic washing	Washing out loose fragments of cartilage/subchondral bone and joint fluid containing degradative enzymes
Drilling, abrasion and microfracture	Work by penetrating the subchondral bone and stimulating cell regrowth. Fibrocartilage rather than renewed hyaline cartilage is produced
Autologous implantation	Transplanting cells of various types into chondral defects. Cells used include rib perichondrial cells, periosteum and chondrocytes
Allograft	Implanting cadaveric cartilage. Rejection is possible

rejection as a complication (Wroble 2000) but only involve a single surgical procedure.

> **Definition**
>
> Autografts involve implanting cells or tissue taken from the patient. Allografts are taken from a cadaver (dead person).

Drilling, abrasion and microfracture all work by penetrating the subchondral bone and stimulating cell regrowth. The aim is to allow a conduit for clot formation containing mesenchymal stem cells capable of forming repair tissue (Steadman, Rodkey and Singleton 1997). Unfortunately, fibrocartilage rather than renewed hyaline cartilage, is produced by these procedures.

Arthritis

The term arthritis tends to be used to describe any chronic inflammatory reaction affecting a joint. However, the term simply means 'joint inflammation', and as such must be qualified by a description of the cause of inflammation. Acute joint injury which causes intracapsular swelling may be termed 'traumatic arthritis'. True osteoarthritis involves cartilage degeneration, initially with little inflammation, so the term osteoarthrosis would seem more appropriate. This condition must be differentiated from inflammatory states affecting multiple joints such as rheumatoid arthritis. The following description is concerned with osteoarthritis (OA) and its connection to sport and exercise.

The initial changes in OA are usually painless and show no gross joint swelling. The tissue affected first appears to be the joint cartilage. As we have seen above, joint cartilage is under a process of continual remodelling. Degradation (breaking down) and synthesis (building up) are balanced, so that the total volume of cartilage remains the same. In OA, however, this balance is disrupted and the enzymes which break down the cartilage are overexpressed, resulting in a net loss of collagen and proteoglycans from the cartilage matrix. This shows as an increased water content resulting from proteolysis of the cartilage macromolecules.

> **Definition**
>
> Proteolysis is the degradation (digestion) of protein molecules by protease enzymes.

In a normal joint, proteases (breakdown enzymes) are secreted by synovial cells and chondrocytes in an inactive form. When activated they are counteracted (balanced) by protease inhibitors secreted by the same cells. In OA the proteases are greatly increased so the protease inhibitors become overwhelmed, leading to overall cartilage degradation.

Mild fraying or flaking of superficial collagen fibres within the hyaline cartilage occurs. This happens first at the periphery of the joint in the non-weight-bearing region. Later, damage (fibrillation) is to the deeper cartilage layers in the weight-bearing areas of the joint, extending down to one third of the cartilage thickness. Small cavities form (blistering) between the cartilage fibres, which gradually extend to become vertical clefts. If cartilage fragments break off, they may float free in the joint fluid as loose bodies, giving rise to joint locking and sudden twinges of pain. The presence of a loose body and the by-products of cartilage destruction causes the synovium to inflame, and it is only now that many patients become aware that a problem exists.

> **Keypoint**
>
> Patients usually only become aware that they have arthritis when a joint becomes inflamed and painful. Treatment aimed at reducing pain/inflammation and restoring function will often alleviate the problem, but the structure of the bone remains the same.

Turnover of proteoglycan and collagen within the cartilage ground substance is increased, and the proteoglycan molecules near the fibrillated cartilage are smaller than normal. Mechanically, this altered cartilage is weaker to both compression and tension stresses, but it is still resistant to gliding, and its coefficient of friction remains low (Threlkeld and Currier 1988). As the cartilage thins the joint space is reduced.

The subchondral bone beneath the fibrillated cartilage becomes shiny and smooth (eburnated). Below the eburnated region the area becomes osteoporotic and local avascular necrosis causes cyst formation where there is complete bone loss. Osteophytes covered with fibrocartilage form at the periphery of the joint, and may protrude into the joint space or more frequently into surrounding soft tissue.

> **Definition**
>
> Two classic signs of osteoarthritis are eburnation, where the joint cartilage becomes shiny and smooth, and osteophytes, which are bony spurs forming at the edge of the joint.

The synovial membrane becomes thickened and its vascularity increases in line with an inflammatory response (see above). The joint capsule demonstrates small tears filled with fibrous tissue, causing thickening. Contracture usually alters both physiological and accessory movements. For example, when OA affects the knee joint, flexion is often limited and mediolateral stability reduced. It is important to appreciate that many tissues are affected by arthritis, and bone itself is often not the most important tissue clinically. The synovial proliferation alters the consistency of the synovial fluid. There is an increased production of synovial fluid which has a lower viscosity. Injections of hyaluronic acid are designed to slow this process. Increased growth of blood vessels (angiogenesis or neovascularization) occurs in OA in bone, synovial membrane and joint capsule. In addition, new vessels may also grow across the subchondral barrier, dragging nerve fibres with them (Jones 2007). Table 1.10 summarizes the common tissue changes seen in arthritis, and further details of arthritis with respect to the knee are given in Chapter 4.

Table 1.10 Tissue changes in knee arthritis (Adapted from Jones and Amendola, 2007)

Tissue	Effect
Cartilage	▶ Initially increased hydration & softening ▶ Fibrillation & thinning ▶ Healing through fibrocartilage
Bone	▶ Adaptive thickening ▶ Early subchondral osteoporosis
Blood vessels	▶ Hypervascularity ▶ Ingrowth into cartilage ▶ Associated pain fibres
Fibrocartilage	▶ Early fibrocartilage degeneration
Synovium	▶ Degrading enzymes found ▶ Increased number of proinflammatory cells ▶ Decreased fluid viscosity
Tendons & ligaments	▶ Early adaptive changes
Muscles & nerves	▶ Pain inhibition ▶ Weakness ▶ Wasting

The joint capsule

The joint capsule is in two parts. The outer part (stratum fibrosum) is fibrous and thickened in areas to form ligaments. The inner layer (stratum synoviale) is loose and highly vascular and blends with the synovial membrane. The capsule consists of parallel fascicles of collagen and some fibrocytes. Blood vessels enter the subchondral bone at the line of capsular attachment and small vessels are found between the individual cartilage fascicles. The nerve supply is very rich, with large fibres giving proprioceptive feedback and small fibres terminating in pain endings.

The capsular response to trauma is an increase in vascularity and eventually the development of fibrous tissue. Cross-linking of collagen fibres occurs, causing a palpable thickening of the capsule. Capsular shrinkage combined with fibrous adhesions will cause loss of movement and occurs particularly after immobilization.

> **Keypoint**
>
> The joint capsule will become thickened and less elastic following trauma and prolonged rest. Ultimately, capsular shrinkage will significantly limit movement.

Accumulation of joint fluid through swelling will stretch the capsule and capsular ligaments. The nerve endings situated between the collagen fascicles of the capsule will be stretched, giving rise to mechanical pain. Should the fluid accumulation exceed the elastic limit of the joint capsule, rupture may result.

Joint effusion will stretch portions of the capsule which are normally lax, to facilitate movement. The patient will tend to rest the joint in a position where the joint cavity is of maximum volume; in addition, passive movements will be limited in characteristic 'capsular patterns' (Table 1.11).

Ligaments

When a ligament is put under stress, it responds by getting progressively stiffer before later deforming

Table 1.11 The capsular patterns

Shoulder—so much limitation of abduction, more than that of lateral rotation, less than that of medial rotation
Elbow—flexion usually more limited than extension, rotations full and painless except in advanced cases
Wrist—equal limitation of flexion and extension, little limitation of deviations
Trapezio-first metacarpal joint—only abduction limited
Sign of the buttock—passive hip flexion more limited and more painful than straight leg raise
Hip—marked limitation of flexion and medial rotation, some limitation of abduction, little or no limitation of adduction and lateral rotation
Knee—gross limitation of flexion, slight limitation of extension
Ankle—more limitation of plantiflexion than of dorsiflexion
Talocalcanean joint—increasing limitations of varus until fixation in valgus
Mid-tarsal joint—limitations of adduction and internal rotation, other movements full
Big toe—gross limitations of extension, slight limitation of flexion
Cervical spine—equal limitation in all directions except for flexion which is usually full
Thoracic spine—limitation of extension, side flexion and rotations, less limitation of flexion
Lumbar spine—marked and equal limitation of side flexions, limitation of flexion and extension

in a regular manner. There are two reasons for this. First, the collagen fibres within the ligament are not in line, and so the initial tensile stress is used up by pulling the fibres straight. Second, the fibres are not attached to a single point but to an area of bone, and so are of slightly different lengths. When the fibres are stretched, there will be a progressive tightening of the ligament, with some fibres becoming taut sooner than others.

> **Keypoint:**
>
> When a ligament is loaded it gets stiffer in a progressive manner, as its fibres take up slack, and different lengths of fibre become tight at different points.

Ligaments demonstrate viscoelastic properties. Rapid stretch has been shown to increase stiffness by as much as 20 per cent, and sustained stretch to cause ligament tension to reduce significantly after just two minutes. The mode of failure also changes with speed, avulsion occurring at slower speeds and ligamentous rupture at higher speeds.

Clinically, three grades of ligament injuries are generally described. Grade I sprains involve minimal tissue damage with some local tenderness. Swelling is only slight, and function is almost normal. With the Grade II sprain, more ligament fibres are injured or the ligament may become partially detached from its bony attachment. Local pain is more intense and movement more limited. Grade III injuries constitute a complete loss of function, often with rupture. There is a rapid onset of effusion with considerable pain, and the joint is unstable with marked loss of function (Table 1.12).

With Grades I and II, pain is increased by placing the ligament on stretch. With a Grade II injury, some instability may be present, but with a Grade III injury (rupture) instability is always present.

Table 1.12 Ligament injuries (Adapted from Reid (1992) with permission)

Grade	Signs and symptoms
(I) Mild	Minimal loss of structural integrity
	No abnormal motion
	Little or no swelling
	Localized tenderness
	Minimal or no bruising
(II) Moderate	Significant structural weakening
	Some abnormal motion
	Marked bruising and swelling
	Often associated with haemarthrosis and joint effusion
(III) Severe	Loss of structural integrity
	Marked abnormal motion
	Significant bruising which may track away from area
	Definite haemarthrosis if capsule remains intact

However, clinically this may be difficult to assess in instances of severe pain and muscle spasm.

Definition

Grade I ligament injuries are mild, Grade II moderate and Grade III severe.

Grade I and II injuries normally require pain relief (modalities or medication) and progressive joint mobilization and limb re-strengthening governed by the severity of tissue damage and the amount of joint instability. Grade III injuries will often require protective bracing, and in some cases surgical repair or reconstruction. As recovery progresses with all ligament injuries, rehabilitation is aimed at progressive limb strengthening and proprioceptive training to enhance joint stability.

Ligamentous viscosity changes with age. The collagen fibres within the ligament enlarge, reducing the water content in the ground substance. Noyes and Grood (1976) showed marked reductions in tensile strength of ligament in the 48–83-year age group when compared with the 16–26-year age group. Noyes et al. (1984) showed threefold decreases in maximum stress, elastic modulus and strain energy between the ligaments from donors aged 50 years compared to those aged 20 years. The older ligaments failed by bony avulsion rather than ligamentous failure as occurred in the younger tissues. They claimed that ageing produced changes in the ligament/bone systems similar to those found through disuse.

Immobility also has marked effects on ligaments. Laros, Tipton and Cooper (1971) showed strength reductions of 39 per cent after nine weeks' immobilization, full strength not being regained for thirty weeks. Exercise has been shown to have a beneficial effect on ligament tensile strength, as it seems to act as a 'mechanical stimulant' (see mechanotransduction above), causing increased collagen turnover within the ligament (Weisman, Pope and Johnson 1980).

This has important implications for rehabilitation following ligament injury. Wherever possible, complete immobilization should be avoided. While an injured ligament should be protected against excessive external forces which could cause further damage, gentle exercise within the pain-free range should still be encouraged.

The effect of corticosteroids on ligament failure is important. Decreases in maximum load of 21 per cent and 39 per cent have been shown six and fifteen weeks after large dosage cortisone injection (methylprednisolone acetate), with a load reduction remaining for one year. In addition, fibrocyte death was seen within the ligament, with delay in reappearance of new fibrocytes for fifteen weeks (Noyes et al. 1984).

Muscle injury

Common terminology for soft tissue injuries includes 'sprain' for a ligament and 'strain' for a muscle. Athletes often refer to muscle injuries as a 'pull' or 'spasm'. Terminology for muscle injuries has been defined by the Munich consensus statement (Mueller-Wohlfahrt et al. 2013). Injuries may be classified as direct where the force is externally applied or indirect where internal forces are involved (Table 1.13). Direct muscle injury includes contusion (bruising) and laceration (cutting). With contusion the muscle is frequently compressed between the externally applied force and the bone beneath. The injury may be mild to severe, with compressed muscle fibres causing pain and loss of motion. If fibres are torn at the time of impact some structural damage may occur, with bruising either restricted locally or tracking through the muscle compartment, this type of injury in the thigh is often termed a 'dead leg' or 'charley horse'.

Table 1.13 Munich classification of muscle injuries in sport

Indirect	Functional	Type 1 – overexertion related	1A – fatigue induced
			1B – DOMS
		Type 2 – neuromuscular	2A – spine related
			2B – muscle related
	Structural	Type 3 – partial tear	3A – minor
			3B – moderate
		Type 4 – (sub) total	Subtotal or complete tear
			Tendinous avulsion
Direct		Contusion	
		Laceration	

(Modified from Mueller-Wohlfahrt et al 2012)

The blood released into the muscle with a direct injury may be contained within the muscle sheath (intramuscular haematoma) or rupture through the sheath to track down the limb within the interstitial space, appearing in the periphery (intermuscular haematoma). Intramuscular haematoma will normally present as a firm localized mass, with the interstitial pressure limiting further blood release. Myositis ossificans should always be considered as a complication. Intermuscular haematoma is less firm as blood has spread.

Indirect injuries

Indirect injuries can be both *functional* and *structural*. Functional injuries do not include structural damage but may be either the result of overexertion (Type 1) or changes to the neuromuscular control of a muscle (Type 2). Overexertion is subdivided into those disorders associated with fatigue and those linked to delayed onset muscle soreness (DOMS). Muscle fatigue has been related to injury, with fatigued muscles absorbing less energy than their non-fatigued counterparts. Fatigued muscle also shows increased stiffness and tightness predisposing to injury (Mueller-Wohlfahrt et al. 2013). Timing is also important. Delayed onset muscle soreness occurs some time after training, whilst fatigue is seen at the same time as a training bout. DOMS is often characterized by inflammation to the muscle area, especially following prolonged use or eccentric loading. Tenderness is to the whole muscle rather than a focal area. See Chapter 2 for more details on DOMS.

Functional muscle injuries with a neuromuscular background may be due to peripheral or central dysfunction. Changes to muscle tone and/or pain within the muscle region can alter muscle function. For example, nerve root impingement within the lumbosacral spine may alter hamstring function, often shown on a positive slump test. These neuromuscular changes will show the muscle as MRI negative or with very minimal local muscle oedema. Peripheral neuromuscular changes of this type can result from increasing fatigue, as described above. Typically, functional muscle disorders show increased tone to palpation and muscle guarding to stretch. Return to graded training can be expected within less than seven days unless lumbosacral pathology coexists.

> **Keypoint**
>
> Functional muscle injuries do not generally show structural tissue damage on MRI or U/S scanning.

Structural muscle changes include both partial and full muscle tearing. Muscle is typically stretched over its normal limits, whilst undergoing a powerful contraction which generates significant internal force. There is macroscopic structural damage, which can be visualized on an ultrasound or MRI scan. Partial tears are the most common type of

Table 1.14 Common sites for avulsion injuries

Site	Muscle
Anterior superior iliac spine (ASIS)	Sartorius
Anterior inferior iliac spine (AIIS)	Rectus femoris
Iliac crest	External oblique
Ischial tuberosity	Hamstrings
Olecranon process	Triceps
Patella	Quadriceps tendon
Lesser trochanter	Iliopsoas

muscle injury and normally show minor to moderate damage. In terms of general definition, the Munich consensus defined minor partial tears as having a maximum diameter less than a muscle fascicle or bundle, and moderate tears being greater than this. Parallel injury to the muscle perimysium can cause interstitial bleeding, and larger injuries may result in impaired healing with scar tissue formation. Partial (Type 3) tears of this type can take from two to six weeks to show full recovery.

The most severe structural muscle injuries are those which show complete muscle tearing or musculotendinous avulsion (Type 4). Injuries of this type generally involve 50 per cent of the muscle diameter, while avulsions involve total tearing to the origin or insertion of muscle. Common sites for avulsion injuries are shown in Table 1.14.

Muscle healing following injury

Following structural injury, muscle fibres and blood vessels are ruptured, a haematoma formed and inflammation begins (see above). Repair involves removal of dead material and the development of a scar, which begins to shrink. Remodelling sees tissue maturation and the progressive recovery of muscle function.

At the time of injury, blood vessels have ruptured and released blood into the local area to form a haematoma. Reduced oxygenation of local tissue (hypoxia) and cell death (necrosis) drives the inflammatory process, and phagocytes (white blood cells) gradually destroy the clot. Fibrin (a blood protein) from the clotting blood begins to form granulation tissue, in turn trapping fibroblast cells. This process increases the density and strength of the clot structure to help it withstand the forces created by muscle contraction. These early proteins are followed by the formation of type III collagen around day one after injury and type I collagen two days post injury (Jarvinen et al. 2008).

The increasingly dense granulation tissue forms into a scar, marking the beginning of the repair phase of healing, with two principal processes, scar development and myofibre regeneration.

Individual myofibres are torn, and as they are long, necrosis could travel their whole cell length, spreading out from the injury site. To limit this, a *contraction band* is formed as the muscle cytoskeleton shrinks. Local blood vessel damage has caused the release of histamine and prostaglandins (both inflammatory products), and satellite cells (normally dormant) are activated within the dying muscle fibres. Macrophages and fibroblasts begin to release chemicals to attract other circulating inflammatory cells and bring them to the injured region, a process called *chemotaxis*. Growth factors, cytokines, and tumour necrosis factor (TNF-α) have all been identified as having this role in skeletal muscle regeneration.

Definition:

Satellite cells are undeveloped cells which act as precursors to muscle cell formation

The *satellite cells* lying at the end of the myofibres provide a source of undifferentiated cells (not yet developed) as a reserve which may be activated through injury. Two types exist, committed satellite cells (CSC) and stem satellite cells (SSC). Activation during the initial phases of injury causes the satellite cells to proliferate and then to differentiate into myofibres. The CSC react immediately post injury while the SSC divide first to increase their number before differentiation. The ability of the SSC to divide means that the satellite cells are not all used up, stocks being replenished to await future injury.

The regenerating myofibres on each side of the injured area grow towards each other. The cylinder which contained the old (now necrotic) myofibre forms the casing for the regenerating fibre. The stumps of this new fibre grow outward, forming several branches which pierce the scar as they approach each other. The ends of the stumps actually adhere to the scar, a process which requires mechanical stimulation and does not occur as effectively with total immobilization.

Keypoint:

Regenerating myofibre stumps grow towards each other, a process stimulated by movement.

Ultimately, the two approaching myofibres from each side of the injury interlace and contract synchronously (at the same time) but may never completely unite (Jarvinen et al. 2002).

The young myofibres have very few mitochondria and largely rely on anaerobic (without oxygen) metabolism. As they grow, their need for aerobic (with oxygen) metabolism increases. This need is fulfilled by the ingrowth of blood capillaries into the scar. Capillary sprouts form from the ends of the old ruptured vessels and grow into the scar. Where fibrosis is excessive and capillary ingrowth is limited, myofibre regeneration will in turn be limited. Re-innervation is also required if myofibre development is to continue. In cases of nerve axon damage (axonotmesis), muscle wasting remains until nerve regeneration is complete.

Myositis ossificans traumatica

Myositis ossificans traumatica (MOT) is soft tissue ossification of muscle resulting in the formation of non-neoplasmic bone. It usually occurs in the proximal limb muscles, and is seen most commonly following contusion of the quadriceps femoris musculature, although other regions include the elbow flexors and hip abductors.

Several aetiological theories have been suggested. Calcification of a muscle haematoma can occur following fibrosis, or intramuscular bone formation may result from periosteal detachment. Rupture of the periosteum may lead to the proliferation of osteoblasts and their escape into the surrounding muscle. Intramuscular connective tissue may undergo metaplasia into bone, and Urist et al. (1978) demonstrated that certain skeletal muscle cells, known as inducible osteogenic precursor cells (IOPC), have the capability of differentiating into osteoblasts.

Clinically, the patient presents with severe post-traumatic pain and limitation of movement. Typically, knee flexion is greatly limited (45–90°) in the case of a thigh haematoma. There is local swelling and erythema, with the area being warm and tender to palpation, with a characteristic firm 'woody' tissue feel. Tenderness usually becomes more pronounced with time, and tissue signs do not respond to conservative management. The factor which should alert the practitioner to the possibility of MOT is a reduction in movement range over time. Normally, an increasing range would be expected as a condition resolves. Radiological evidence of ossification is usually seen within two months following injury, and other investigations, including computed tomography and ultrasound scanning, can be used. In addition, MRI may show inflammatory oedema, which precedes tissue calcification.

> ### Keypoint
> Myositis is most common after quadriceps haematoma (dead leg). The classic sign is reduction in movement range over time.

Management of MOT is aimed at lessening any disability rather than affecting the bone mass. Initially, the soft tissue response to trauma, especially bleeding, is limited by the use of such regimens as protection, optimal loading, ice, compression and elevation (POLICE). Rehabilitation is slower than with a normal muscle haematoma, isometric exercises being used for seven to fourteen days following injury, but active exercises (within the pain-free range) are not used until two to four weeks after injury.

Tendons

Tendons are fibre-composites – that is, they are made by combining several differing materials, each with individual characteristics (Screen 2015). In the case of tendons, the two materials are mainly type I collagen (up to 90 per cent of volume), forming an extracellular matrix (ECM), and tenocyte cells (10 per cent). Small amounts of proteoglycans (2–5 per cent) and elastin (0.5–3 per cent) are also present, providing lubrication/resistance to compression, and elasticity, respectively. The ratio of collagen to elastic differs depending on tendon type (see below).

Tendons form a junction between solid bone and elastic muscle, and so offer a graded transformation from stiffness to compliance. The positioning of a tendon allows the muscle to be placed away from the moving joint, and transmit contraction force from the muscle to the point of application some distance away. In the case of the long finger tendons, for example, the advantage becomes obvious as the bulk of muscle is held away from the fine joint movements.

The length and shape of some tendons can be used to create a mechanical advantage, as is the case of the patella tendon. By positioning force away from the centre of rotation of a joint, tendons can act as levers to increase the effect of forces generated by muscle contraction.

The long finger tendons have to be able to transmit the subtle changes in muscle contraction to position the fingers accurately. The finger tendons are called *positional tendons* and are stiff (non-elastic), a feature suitable to their low loading. Tendons of the lower limb (Achilles and patellar) are subjected to the high forces of locomotion, and so need to absorb force and act a little like springs, having greater elasticity than stiffness. They are therefore termed *energy-storing tendons*, as they can store and release mechanical energy efficiently.

Definition:

An *energy-storing tendon* is one which can store and release mechanical energy with great efficiency

Tendon sheath injury

Injuries to a tendon sheath (paratenonitis) includes tenosynovitis, and tenovaginitis. Tenosynovitis is a lesion to the gliding surfaces of the outside of the tendon and the inside of its sheath, but not the sheath itself. The lesion is usually as a result of overuse or compression. Pathological features include an increase in the number of lining cells of the sheath, together with proliferation of local blood vessels, oedema and cellular changes. As the roughened surfaces of the sheath move against each other pain and crepitus occur, most commonly within the wrist tendons. The same condition occurring to tendons which do not have a true sheath is termed peritendonitis. Here, the paratenon thickens, and shows fibrinoid degeneration and dense fibrous adhesions. Local oedema is evident, sometimes with palpable crepitus, and pain which may disappear with activity.

Tenovaginitis occurs when the tendon sheath is chronically inflamed and thickens. It is the fibrous wall of the tendon sheath rather than the synovial lining which is affected. Common sites include the flexor sheaths of the fingers or thumb. When the sheaths of extensor *pollicis brevis* and abductor *pollicis longus* are affected, De Quervain's syndrome is present.

Keypoint

Tenosynovitis is a lesion of the gliding surfaces of the tendon and its sheath; *tenovaginitis* is a chronic inflammation and thickening of the tendon sheath

Tendinopathy

Tendinopathy is pain and swelling (thickening) of tendon, and although it can occur in any tendon,

Table 1.15 Phases of tendinopathy

Reactive tendinopathy	Tendon dysrepair	Degenerative tendinopathy
▶ Tenocyte activation	▶ Greater ECM breakdown	▶ Areas of tendon cell death
▶ Proteoglycan increase	▶ Tendon cells take on a more rounded appearance.	▶ Large regions of disordered ECM
▶ Increased bound water concentration	▶ Collagen & proteoglycan increase	▶ ECM filled with cells, vessels, & disorganized collagen
▶ Increased tendon volume	▶ Collagen separation	▶ Focal nodular regions interspaced with normal tendon
▶ Little significant collagen fibre disruption	▶ ECM disorganized	▶ Increased risk of tendon rupture
▶ Little significant inflammation	▶ Possible ingrowth of small nerve fibres & blood vessels.	▶ Significant blood vessel ingrowth
	▶ Hypoechoic areas on U/S.	▶ Large focal hypoechoic regions.

ECM – extracellular matrix, U/S – ultrasound, (Cook and Purdam 2009, Warden, Cook and Purdam 2017)

particular focus is placed in this publication on the Achilles (Chapter 5), patellar tendon (Chapter 4), and supraspinatus tendon (Chapter 12) in the relevant chapters referring to these regions. Details of the pathology of tendinopathy are given in Chapter 5, with tendinopathy healing stages illustrated in Table 1.15

Nerves

The nervous system can be affected by injury through both internal (intraneural) and external (extraneural) means. Intraneural pathology can have an effect on the elasticity of the neural system. When tension is taken up at one point in the nervous system, this is transferred further along, a little like pulling on a rope. Altered mechanics may be accompanied by changes in physiology. Altered microcirculation and axonal transport may occur through compression, with nerve swelling occurring both proximally and distally to a compression force.

The nervous system consumes 20 per cent of the oxygen used by the body, so it is highly metabolically active. The blood flow to a neuron comes from branches of the vessels running parallel to the nerve, which form epineural vessels passing into the nerve. A pressure gradient is required to maintain the neural microcirculation, which may be disrupted during entrapment neuropathy.

Nerve compression changes the pressure gradient in the nerve microcirculation leading to ischaemia and local oedema. An alteration in pressure to the blood vessels supplying the nerves of as little as 20 mmHg will affect the nerve, and at pressures of 80 mmHg the nerve blood flow may be cut off completely. When mild or short-lived, ischaemia may exist in isolation, but where the pressure change is higher or longer, lasting metabolic activity may be disrupted, causing ectopic firing (Schmid 2015). In prolonged cases, oedema may lead to fibrotic changes, reducing neural gliding, and ischaemia to focal demyelination, slowing nerve conduction. Demyelination may occur as a result of ischaemia leading to Schwann cell changes, but also due to mechanical compression and subsequent inflammatory changes, and may extend beyond the entrapment site.

Following injury or entrapment, axon debris causes activation of immune cells, including phagocytes and macrophages. This in turn leads to activation of pro-inflammatory mediators (see above), which lower the firing threshold of neurons, altering nerve conduction. Anti-inflammatory medication may therefore be helpful in cases of radiculopathy.

Normally a nerve action potential travels from the periphery towards the central nervous system (CNS), a directional movement termed *orthodromic*. However, when sensitized, nociceptive fibres especially can cause action potentials to travel towards the periphery (*antidromic* movement). Antidromic impulses of this type lead to the release of inflammatory mediators (especially CGRP, mentioned above), a process termed *neurogenic inflammation*. The resulting skin changes on objective examination are trophic changes, skin reddening and increased temperature to palpation.

Nerve injury which arises through repeated movement (overuse) may occur at a number of sites, especially where nerve movement is restricted (Fig. 1.22). Typically, pathology is through friction, compression or stretch, which cause changes in neural tension or gliding demonstrated on neurodynamic testing. Whilst mild pressure or friction can lead to oedema of the epineurium, tearing of the epineurium may occur with a traumatic soft tissue injury such as an ankle sprain, with rupture of the epineural vessels. Examples of neurodynamic treatment for the upper limb is given in Chapters 10 and 12, and for the lower limb in Chapter 8.

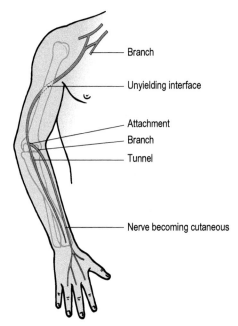

Branch

Unyielding interface

Attachment
Branch
Tunnel

Nerve becoming cutaneous

Figure 1.22 Sites of restricted movement in a nerve. From Butler (1991) with permission.

Fascia

What is fascia?

Fascia is connective tissue which envelops organs, providing support and shape, and surrounds muscles, creating and transmitting force. Fascia links parts of the body together, providing a continuous tract covering several bones and muscles leading to a 'line of pull' that is not restricted to a single muscle or body region.

Connective tissue in general is made up of fat used for storage, and fibrous tissue used for structure. It is the fibrous tissue we are interested in when describing fascia. It contains collagen (white), a strong tough substance giving the tissue its strength, and elastin (yellow), giving fascial tissue recoil. The ratio of collagen to elastin makes the particular connective tissue type either tough or pliable. Tendons, ligaments and the membranes covering bones and certain portions of the fascia contain mainly white fibres and are tougher, whereas specific fascia such as the ligamentum flavum in the neck, and the walls of blood vessels

are mainly yellow elastic tissue, giving them a more malleable nature.

Types of fascia

Fascia is subdivided into two types, *superficial* and *deep*. The superficial fascia lies just beneath the skin, acting as a base to enable the skin to move freely over the underlying structures. A loosely arranged, folded meshwork with the folds filled with fat, the superficial fascia dictates the body contours and gives each of us our unique look. This portion of the fascia is the main place where fat is deposited in obesity, hence the use of skin-fold measurements to assess body-fat percentage. The fat within the superficial fascia provides us with insulation and is important in preventing heat loss. On its under-surface, the superficial fascia becomes more fibrous and forms a distinct layer, which normally connects to the deep fascia.

The deep fascia is tougher and more fibrous than the superficial and surrounds almost every structure in the body. The deep fascia tends to be laid down in the direction of stress and attaches itself to bony projections as it passes over them. The under-surface of the deep fascia travels between muscle layers as the *inter muscular septa*, separating the groups of muscles from each other and forming muscle compartments. In the case of the arms, these are the flexor and extensor compartments, and in the thigh they are the flexor, extensor and adductor compartments.

The fascial membrane takes on a variety of names depending on its anatomical position. Around the brain and spinal cord it is the *meninges*, around the heart it is the *pericardium*, within the abdomen it is called the *peritoneum* and around the bones it is known as the *periosteal*. Even within the musculo-skeletal system fascia may be specialized. At the side of the leg we have the ilio-tibial band (ITB) and in the back the thoraco-lumbar fascia (TLF). The important feature, however, is that all of the layers of fascia are connected to each other. Fascia is really a 'soft tissue skeleton', as it supports the body, forms boundaries and moulds the shape of the body tissues. It is not really possible to exercise one muscle in isolation; when we stretch, for example, one muscle may receive the greater stretching effect, but both the muscle and the fascia will change tension. For this reason, we can talk of muscle and fascia as a single inseparable unit called *myofascia*.

Fascial response to injury and therapy

Fascia contains both myelinated and non-myelinated nerve fibres, together with a variety of mechanoreceptors. Many nerves are oriented perpendicularly to the collagen fibres and may act as stretch receptors (Simmonds et al. 2012). In addition to fibrocytes, myofibroblasts are also present (and the former may change into the latter). These cells have a contractile nature, enabling them to alter tissue tension (Nekouzadeh et al. 2008).

The ground substance within the fascia consists of fibrocytes, which regulate interstitial fluid volume and respond to mechanical deformation through mechanotransduction (Eagan et al. 2007). Although mechanical stress can induce a change in cell morphology, this change has been shown to take roughly two hours to occur (Langevin et al. 2005). In addition, the low forces used within manual therapy are unlikely to cause collagen microfracture (Simmonds et al. 2012). Any therapeutic change occurring at the time of treatment is therefore likely to be due to neurophysiological modulation, such as alteration in pain tolerance, changes in vagal tone, and mechanical hyperalgesia.

Fascial pathways

Four main fascial pathways have been described (Myers 2014). The superficial back line (SBL) supports the body in full extension, preventing it from collapsing into flexion. It is therefore important in forward bending and lifting tasks. The superficial front line (SFL) transmits muscle force to create powerful flexion of the legs and trunk. The lateral line (LL) is important for single-leg actions during walking and running, as well as for lateral bending activities of the trunk. Finally, the spiral line (SL) creates rotational movements of the body, which are important during functional activities such as walking and running, as well as during sport (Table 1.16).

Table 1.16 Fascial pathways

Pathway	Position
Superficial back line	Connects posterior surface of body from toes to knees and then knees to brow
Superficial front line	Anterior body surface from top of feet to the sides of the skull.
Lateral line	Foot and outside of ankle along the lateral aspect of the leg and trunk to the ear.
Spiral line (takes portions from the other three)	From one side of the skull, across the back to the opposite shoulder and then back across the chest and down the side of the body. From the foot up the back to rejoin the skull fascia.

Treatment note 1.7   Training the fascia

As with any other tissue, training requires overload. Fascia demonstrates great adaptability, remodelling effectively through fibroblast activity. While muscle strength increases relatively quickly, fascial adaptation takes longer, with 30 per cent of collagen fibres replaced within a six-month period and 75 per cent within twenty-four

months (Schleip and Muller 2013). One of the traditional images of a fascial component in the human body is the muscle-tendon unit (MTU). The traditional view of muscle action is that a muscle contracts to create force and a tendon applies the force but does not create it. Elements of this model are certainly true, in that muscle contracts

Treatment note 1.7 *continued*

to create force and tendon does not. However, muscle ultrastructure shows us that fascia occurs in parallel with the muscle as tendon, and in series with the muscle as the muscle framework (epimysium, perimysium). Fascia is elastic and can create force (elastic strength) through recoil. The recoil combines with active muscle contraction to create both active and passive force, through the *stretch–shortening cycle* (SSC). When training performance athletes, the SSC consists of an eccentric action (controlled lengthening) immediately followed by a rapid concentric action.

Maintaining the elasticity of fascia is an important aim of stretching. It has been shown that fascia is more elastic in the young due to its two-dimensional lattice structure, an architecture which changes to a more haphazard multidirectional alignment with age (Schleip and Muller 2013). Lack of movement results in a loss of fascial tissue elasticity and reduced tissue gliding. Eventually, non-use may cause adhesions and fibre matting (Jarvinen et al. 2002).

In addition to alteration in fibre direction, reduced fascia tissue usage can change tissue hydration. Fascia is 70 per cent water in volume, and mechanical loading squeezes the water from the fascia, release of the tension causing rehydration and refreshment of the tissue fluid. Training which is repetitive and rhythmical rather than

high load and reduced volume would seem more appropriate to achieve fascia hydration.

Proprioception may also be important to fascia training. Proprioceptive receptors are located in several structures, including joint tissues, muscle and fascia. It is known that proprioception may be impaired through both injury and lack of use, and that exercise is key to its enhancement. However, proprioceptors located within joint structures have been shown to be stimulated at end-range motion and those in fascia more within mid-range, so fascial proprioception may be more important for functional day-to-day activity. Static stretching does overload the proprioceptive system, but focuses on range of motion (movement quantity). Dynamic stretching, especially that involving more complex motion in several planes, is more challenging. In addition, focusing on refining a complex action (movement quality) requires a greater amount of motor skill, demanding more input from the proprioceptive system.

Fascial stretching, then, is ultimately dynamic, with rhythmic changes in direction using an interplay between muscle contraction and connective tissue elasticity. At the end of an action, movement slows down as tissue is stretched and speeds up as the tissue recoils followed by muscle contraction to create active force forming a ballistic action.

Skin

Skin wounds may be divided into two categories: open and closed. Closed wounds occur when there is no penetration of the epidermis, and open wounds are those where the epidermis has been pierced. Closed wounds encompass contusions, abrasions and friction burns, such as those caused by gravel. Open wounds in sport include cuts such as lacerations and puncture wounds.

Keypoint:

With *open* wounds the epidermis in pierced, with *closed* wounds it remains intact.

A contusion or bruise involves a direct blow to the skin surface. Bleeding occurs from torn blood vessels into the skin and subcutaneous tissues, forming a bruise or ecchymosis. The size of the bruise is dependent on the vascularity of the affected tissue, as well as the size of the blood vessels damaged and the laxity of the surrounding tissues. Normally, bruising requires conservative management, but conditions such as retrobulbar haemorrhage (behind the eyeball) and scrotal haematoma may require surgical evacuation. Following contusion, released blood will clot and degrade, producing superficial colour changes.

An abrasion or graze occurs through a glancing injury or repeated microtrauma to the skin surface. The skin surface breaks through, but the damage is not full thickness. The condition may be complicated by ingrained tattooing, where embedded particles remain beneath the surface. The material may become covered by epithelium, giving a visible and hypertrophic scar. An abrasion of this type should be treated as early as possible after the injury by vigorous scrubbing with a stiff nail brush and an antiseptic wash to remove the embedded dirt.

Keypoint:

An abrasion from a fall onto a grit surface runs the risk of ingrained tattooing. The wound must be thoroughly scrubbed with an antiseptic wash to remove all dirt, before being dressed.

Extensive areas of skin may be affected during an abrasion, and intense pain usually occurs as raw nerve endings are exposed. Bleeding may be widespread, but healing is rapid unless infection ensues. Extensive debriding injuries involving large areas of skin loss (for example from a motor-cycle accident) may require grafting.

A laceration is a full-thickness skin injury which exposes the subcutaneous tissue. A force sufficient to break the skin in this way will also give considerable associated deep tissue damage. In addition, the edge of the skin break will be uneven and surrounded by a contusion. Clean lacerations may require stitching but heal well; jagged injuries involving skin tearing may leave more scarring.

Pressure or friction may cause an abrasion where the skin surface is removed, or a blister where the epidermal surface skin layer is detached from the underlying tissue. The gap between the two layers is filled with lymph, exposing nerve endings to fluid pressure, so causing pain. When pressure or friction is applied progressively, the epidermal skin layer may adapt to form a thickened callus.

Healing of an incised wound such as a cut, where the wound edges are in apposition, occurs by *first intention*. If the wound edges are separated and more major skin damage has occurred (or if infection has intervened), then healing is by *second intention*.

With healing by first intention, slight haemorrhage occurs and the cut is filled with a blood clot on the first day. By the second and third day the clot has become organized and epithelial cells from the two sides of the cut have joined. This single layer of covering multiplies to form stratified squamous epithelium – normal epidermis. Fibroblasts lay down collagen in the granulation tissue and a band of scar tissue is formed by two weeks after the injury.

Healing by second intention takes longer as the spread of epithelial cells over the larger area takes time. The large amount of granulation tissue results in more extensive scarring and likely contracture.

Treatment note 1.8   Principles of physical examination

Physical examination is conducted after a full subjective examination (see Treatment note 1.1), and aims to determine the structure(s) which are responsible for producing the patient's symptoms.

The examination consists of a number of stages within the whole framework of clinical diagnosis (Table 1.17) and some or all of the elements will be used on each patient.

Treatment note 1.8 *continued*

Table 1.17 Clinical examination

Element	Detail
Observation	Face
	Gait
	Posture
History (subjective examination)	Age, occupation, activities
	Site and spread
	Onset and duration
	Symptoms and behaviour
	Past medial history (PMH)
	Other joint involvement
	Drug history (medication) (DH)
Inspection	Deformity (bony?)
	Colour changes
	Muscle wasting
	Swelling
Palpation	Temperature
	Swelling
	Synovial thickening
Active movements	Range/movement pattern
	Pain/symptoms
	Power
	Willingness
Resisted movements	Pain/symptoms
	Power
Passive movements	Pain/symptoms
	Range and quality
	End-feel

After Kesson and Atkins (1998).

Observation and inspection

1. The patient should be observed in general before the individual body part is focused on more closely. Postural characteristics, gait and facial expression can be important pointers in both static and dynamic situations. Simple tasks such as walking into the treatment room and undressing can hold valuable clues.

2. Inspection of the affected body part must identify any deformity, such as alteration in joint or spinal alignment, as well as skin colour changes, including redness (indicating inflammation), and any rashes or skin injury. Swelling indicates an inflammatory response, and the speed with which it formed is important. Other abnormalities such as soft/hard bumps, ganglia and nodules should also be noted and may require medical investigation. Muscle contour is important as it may indicate wasting, spasm or imbalance.

Palpation

1. General palpation of the area looks at temperature, swelling and synovial thickening before individual structures are identified through examination of surface anatomy. Increased temperature (heat) indicates inflammation as before, and a cold clammy skin feeling suggests autonomic disturbance. The firmness (condition) and mobility of the soft tissues should be determined, as well as the general presence of swelling. The production of muscle spasm suggests pain and/or trigger point activation.

2. The unaffected side of the body should be palpated first to establish a baseline for comparison with the affected body part. Superficial palpation should precede deep palpation so that important findings are not obliterated – in general, 'harder pressure feels less'.

Movements

1. Active movements may be used to assess willingness to move, and then resisted movements to look at the production of pain (or symptoms) and power graded to normal values and assessed in comparison to the uninjured side.

Treatment note 1.8 *continued*

Table 1.18 End-feel

Type	Example
Normal	
Hard	Bone to bone approximation—elbow extension
Soft	Soft tissue approximation—elbow flexion
Elastic	Tissue stretch—lateral rotation of the shoulder joint
Abnormal	
Hard	Bony degeneration—osteoarthritis (OA)
Springy	Mechanical joint displacement—loose body, meniscal tear
Spasm	Involuntary muscle spasm—irritable joint
Empty	Patient stops movement—anticipation of pain/instability

Kesson and Atkins (1998) with permission

2. Passive movements determine pain, range, and end-feel (Table 1.18) as well as the presence of a capsular pattern (see Table 1.11). They are used to examine non-contractile (inert) structures.

References

ACSEM, 2011. Guidelines on the management of acute soft tissue injury using Protection Rest Ice Compression and Elevation. ACPSM London 15–21.

American College of Sports Medicine (ACSM), 1998. Position stand on exercise and physical activity for older adults. *Medicine and Science for Sports and Exercise* **30**, 992–1008.

Apel, D.M., Vince, K.G., Kingston, S., 1994. Transient osteoporosis of the hip: a role for core decompression? *Orthopedics* **17** (7), 629–632.

Apley, A.G., Solomon, L., 1993. *Apley's System of Orthopaedics and Fractures*, 7th ed. Butterworth Heinemann, Oxford.

Arampatzis A., Karamanidis K., Albracht K., 2007. Adaptational responses of the human Achilles tendon by modulation of the applied cyclic strain magnitude. *Journal of Experimental Biology* **210**: 2743–2753.

Austin, P.J., Moalem-Taylor, G., 2010. The neuro-immune balance in neuropathic pain: Involvement of inflammatory immune cells, immune like glial cells and cytokines. *Journal of Neuroimmunology* **229**, 23–60.

Behiri, J., Vashishth, D., 2000. Biomechanics of bone. In: Dvir, Z. (Ed.), *Clinical Biomechanics*. Churchill Livingstone, Edinburgh.

Bennell, K., Khan, K., McKay, H., 2000. The role of physiotherapy in the prevention and treatment of osteoporosis. *Manual Therapy* **5** (4), 198–213.

Bleakley, C.M., Glasgow, P., Webb, M.J., 2012a. Cooling an acute muscle injury: can basic scientific theory translate into the clinical setting? *British Journal of Sports Medicine* 2012. Mar; **46** (4): 296–298.

Carbon, R.J., 1992. The female athlete. In: Bloomfield, J., Fricker, P.A., Fitch, K.D. (eds), *Textbook of Science and Medicine in Sport*. Blackwell Scientific Publications, Melbourne.

Chartered Society of Physiotherapy (CSP), 1999. *Physiotherapy Guidelines for the Management of Osteoporosis*. Chartered Society of Physiotherapy, London.

Cyriax, J., 1982. *Textbook of Orthopaedic Medicine*, 8th ed. **Vol. 1**. Baillière Tindall, London.

Donaldson, C.L., Hulley, S.B., Vogel, J.M., 1970. Effects of prolonged bed rest on bone mineral. *Metabolism* **19**, 1071–1084.

Eagan, T.S., Meltzer, K.R., Standley, P.R., 2007. Importance of strain direction in regulating human fibroblast proliferation and cytokine secretion. *Journal of Manipulative and Physiological Therapeutics* **30**, 584–592.

Ettinger, B., Genant, H.K., Cann, C.E., 1987. Postmenopausal bone loss is prevented by low dosage estrogen with calcium. *Annals of Internal Medicine* **106**, 40–45.

Evans, C.H., 1999. Cytokines and the role they play in the healing of ligaments and tendons. Sports *Medicine* **28**, 71–76.

Evans, R.A., 1990b. Calcium and osteoporosis. *Medical Journal of America* **152**, 431–433.

Glasgow, P., Phillips, N., Bleakley, C. (2015) Optimal loading: key variables and mechanisms. *British Journal of Sports Medicine* **49**, 278–279.

Goldspink, G., 2003. Gene expression in muscle in response to exercise. *Journal of Muscle Research and Cell Motility* **24** (2), 121–126

Harrington, S., Smith, J., Thompson, J., Laskowski, E., 2000. Idiopathic transient osteoporosis. *Physician and Sports Medicine* **28** (4), 1–9.

Heinonen, A., Kannus, P., Sievanen, H., 1996. Randomised controlled trial of effect of high impact exercise on selected risk factors for osteoporotic fractures. *Lancet* **348**, 1343–1347.

Hettinga, D.L., 1990. Inflammatory response of synovial joint structures. In: Gould, J.A., (ed.), *Orthopaedic and Sports Physical Therapy*. second ed. C.V. Mosby, St Louis, pp. 87–117.

Hom, D.B., 1995. Growth factors in wound healing. *Otolaryngologic Clinics of North America* **28**, 933–953.

Huddleston, A.L., Rockwell, D., Kuland, D.N., 1980. Bone mass in lifetime tennis athletes. *Journal of the American Medical Association* **244**, 1107–1109.

Hunter, G., 1998. Specific soft tissue mobilization in the management of soft tissue dysfunction. *Manual Therapy* **3** (1), 2–11.

Jarvinen, T.A., Jozsa, L., Kannus, P. et al., 2002. Organisation and distribution of intramuscular connective tissue in normal and immobilized skeletal muscles. *Journal of Muscle Research and Cell Motility* **23**, 245–254.

Jones, M.H., Amendola, A.S., 2007. Acute treatment of inversion ankle sprains: immobilization versus functional treatment. *Clin Orthop Relat Res* **455** (9), 169–172.

Joyce, D. and Butler, D., 2016. Pain and Performance. In: Joyce, D. and Lewindon (eds) Sports *injury prevention and rehabilitation*. Routledge. London.

Kandalla, P.K., Goldspink, G., Butler-Browne, G. et al., 2011. Mechano Growth Factor E peptide (MGF-E) derived from an Isoform of IGF-1, activates human muscle progenitor cells and induces an increase in their fusion potential at different ages. *Mechanisms of Ageing and Development* **132** (4), 154–162.

Kesson, M., Atkins, E., 1998. *Orthopaedic Medicine*. Butterworth-Heinemann, Oxford.

Khan, K.M. and Scott, A., 2009. Mechanotherapy: how physical therapists' prescription of exercise promotes tissue repair. *British Journal of Sports Medicine* **43** (4), 247–251.

Krolner, B., Toft, B., Nielsen, S., 1983. Physical exercise as a prophylaxis against involutional bone loss: a controlled trial. *Clinical Science* **64**, 541–546.

Kurtz, C.A., Loebig, T.G., Anderson, D.D., 1999. Insulin like growth factor 1 accelerates functional recovery from Achilles tendon injury in a rat model. *American Journal of Sports Medicine* **27**, 363–369.

Lakhanpal, S., Ginsburg, W.W., Luthra, H.S., 1987. Transient regional osteoporosis: a study of 56 cases and review of the literature. *Annals of Internal Medicine* **106** (3), 444–450.

Langevin, H.M., Bouffard, N.A., Badger, G.J. et al., 2005. Dynamic fibroblast cytoskeletal response to subcutaneous tissue stretch ex vivo and in vivo. *American J Physiology and Cell Physiology* **288**, C747–756.

Laros, G.S., Tipton, C.M., Cooper, R.R., 1971. Influence of physical activity on ligament insertions in the knees of dogs. *Journal of Bone and Joint Surgery* **53A**, 275–286.

MacKinnon, J.L., 1988. Osteoporosis: a review. *Physical Therapy* **68** (10), 1533–1540.

Maitland, G.D., 1991. *Peripheral Manipulation*, third ed. Butterworth-Heinemann, Oxford.

Martin, A.D., Houston, C.S., 1987. Osteoporosis, calcium and physical activity. *Canadian Medical Association Journal* **136**, 587–593.

Mazess, R.B., Whedon, G.D., 1983. Immobilization and bone. *Calcified Tissue International* **35**, 265–267.

McCarthy, E.F., 1998. The pathology of transient regional osteoporosis. *Iowa Orthopedic Journal* **18**, 35–42.

Mueller-Wohlfahrt, H.W., Haensel, L., Mithoefer, K. et al., 2013. Terminology and classification of muscle injuries in sport: the Munich consensus statement. *British Journal of Sports Medicine* **47** (6), 342–350.

Myers, T.W., 2014. *Anatomy Trains.* (4th ed.) Churchill Livingstone.

Myrer, W.J., Myrer, K.A., Measom, G.J. et al., 2001. Muscle temperature is affected by overlying adipose when cryotherapy is administered. *Journal of Athletic Training* **36**: 32–6.

Nekouzadeh, A., Pryse, K.M., Elson, E.L. et al., 2008. Stretch activated force shedding, force recovery and cytoskeletal remodelling in contractile fibroblasts. *Journal of Biomechanics* **41**, 2964–2971.

Nilas, L., Christiansen, C., Rodbro, P., 1984. Calcium supplementation and post-menopausal bone loss. *British Medical Journal* **289**, 1103–1106.

Nils, J., De Kooning, M., Beckwee, D., and Vaes, P., 2015. The neurophysiology of pain and pain modulation: modern pain neuroscience for musculoskeletal physiotherapists. In: Jull, G. et al. (eds) *Grieve's Modern Musculoskeletal Physiotherapy.* 4th ed. Elsevier, London.

Nilsson, B.E., Westlin, N.E., 1977. Bone density in athletes. *Clinical Orthopaedics and Related Research* **77**, 179–182.

Nixon, A.J., Fortier, L.A., Williams, J., 1999. Enhanced repair of extensive articular defects by insulin like growth factor 1 laden fibrin composites. *Journal of Orthopaedic Research*, **17**, 475–487.

Noyes, F.R., Grood, M.J., 1976. The strength of the anterior cruciate ligament in humans and rhesus monkeys: age-related and species-related changes. *Journal of Bone and Joint Surgery*, **58A**, 1074–1082.

Noyes, F.R., Kelly, C.S., Grood, E.S., Butler, D.L., 1984. Advances in the understanding of knee ligament injury, repair and rehabilitation. *Medicine and Science in Sports and Exercise* **16** (5), 427–443.

Schleip, R., Muller, D.G., 2013. Training principles for fascial connective tissues: scientific foundation and suggested practical applications. Journal of Bodywork and Movement Therapies **17**, 103–115.

Schmid, A., 2015. The peripheral nervous system and its compromise in entrapment neuropathy. In: Jull, G., Moore, A., Falla, D. et al. (eds) *Grieve's Modern Manual Therapy* (4th ed.). Elsevier.

Screen, H., 2015. Tendon and tendinopathy. In: Jull, G., Moore, A., Falla, D. et al. (eds) *Grieve's Modern Manual Therapy* (4th ed.). Elsevier.

Simmonds, N., Miller, P., Gemmell, H. (2012) A theoretical framework for the role of fascia in manual therapy. *Journal Bodywork and Movement Therapies* **16**, 83–93.

Smith, E.L., Smith, P.E., Ensign, C.J., 1984. Bone involutional decrease in exercising middle-aged women. *Calcified Tissue International* **36**, 129–138.

Steadman, J., Rodkey, W., Singleton, S., 1997. Microfracture technique for full-thickness chondral defects. *Operative Techniques in Orthopaedics* **7** (4), 300–304.

Threlkeld, A.J., Currier, D.P., 1988. Osteoarthritis: effects on synovial joint tissues. *Physical Therapy* **68** (3), 364–370.

Urist, M.R., Nakagawa, M., Nakata, N., Nogami, H., 1978. Experimental myositis ossificans: cartilage and bone formation in muscle in response to a diffusible bone matrix derived morphogen. *Archives of Pathology and Laboratory Medicine* **102**, 312–316.

Walter, J.B., Israel, M.S., 1987. *General Pathology.* 6th ed. Churchill Livingstone, London.

Warden, S., Cook, J., and Purdam, C., 2017, Tendon overuse injury. In Brukner, P., Clarsen, B., Cook, J. et al. *Clinical Sports Medicine.* 5th ed. McGraw Hill, London.

Watson, S.L., Weeks, B.K., Weis, L.J. et al., 2015. Heavy resistance training is safe and improves bone, function, and stature in postmenopausal women with low to very low bone mass: novel early findings from the LIFTMOR trial. *Osteoporosis International* **26** (12), 2889–2894.

Watson, T., 2016. Soft tissue repair and healing review. www.electrotherapy.org. Accessed 22/02/2017.

Weisman, G., Pope, M.H., Johnson, R.J., 1980. Cyclic loading in knee ligament injuries. *American Journal of Sports Medicine* **8**, 24–30.

Westermann, S., Vollmar, B., Thorlacius, H. et al., 1999. Surface cooling inhibits tumor necrosis factor alpha induced microvascular perfusion failure, leukocyte adhesion and apoptosis in striated muscle. *Surgery* **126**, 881–889.

White, A., 1999. Neurophysiology of acupuncture analgesia. In: Ernst, E., White, A. (eds), *Acupuncture: A Scientific Appraisal*. Butterworth-Heinemann, Oxford.

Wolman, R.L., Reeve, J., 1994. Exercise and the skeleton. In: Harries, M., et al. (eds.), *Oxford Textbook of Sports Medicine*. Oxford University Press, Oxford.

Wroble, R.R., 2000. Articular cartilage injury and autologous chondrocyte implantation – which patients might benefit? *Physician and Sports Medicine* **28** (11), 43–49.

Zhao, R., Zhao, M., Zhang, L., 2014. Efficiency of jumping exercise in improving bone mineral density among premenopausal women: a meta-analysis. *Sports Medicine* **44**, 1393–1402.

Zusman, M., 2002. Forebrain mediated sensitization of central pain pathways. *Manual Therapy* **7** (2), 80–88.

CHAPTER 2

Rehabilitation science

Principles of training

When a subject exercises, the body changes in two important ways. The first is immediate and is called the exercise *response*. Increased heart and breathing rate, sweat response and blood flow change are all examples of an exercise response. When the exercise session stops, these processes gradually slow down and the body returns to its normal physiological level. If the exercise bout is repeated, the same changes occur, but over a period of time the subject's body becomes better at coping with the exercise. Sweat response is lessened, heart and breathing rates lower and exercise can be maintained for longer periods. The longer-term changes represent an exercise *adaptation*.

Definition

A *response* is the immediate effect of exercise on the body, while *adaptation* represents longer-term and more enduring body changes.

Supercompensation

To be effective, exercise must challenge the body tissues, and this challenge is called an *overload*.

To achieve a training effect, the body must be overloaded, that is, exposed to a physical stress which is greater than that encountered in everyday living. The response to this training stress is catabolism, the breakdown of metabolic fuels or tissues. When muscle is the tissue being studied, the phenomenon is called Exercise Induced Muscle Damage (EIMD). Following this catabolic response, the tissues react by adapting and becoming better suited to coping with the imposed stress; this adaptation is known as anabolism, and involves tissue growth. With training, the anabolic effect is excessive, causing the tissues to grow stronger, a process called *supercompensation*.

Adaptation to exercise (a physical stress) can be understood through the principles of the general adaptation syndrome (GAS) first described by the Hungarian endocrinologist Hans Selye in the 1930s with reference to psychological stress. Plotting time against resistance to stress (Fig. 2.1a), the GAS consists of three phases. The first is the *alarm* phase as the body reacts by preparing its 'fight or flight' mechanisms, releasing hormones such as adrenalin and cortisol. Phase two is the *resistance* phase, when the body tries to cope with the imposed stress. The final phase is *exhaustion*, when the body has depleted its coping mechanisms and may suffer from pathologies such as high blood pressure or ulcers, for example.

(a) General Adaption Syndrome (GAS)

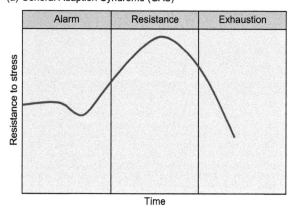

(b) Supercompensation

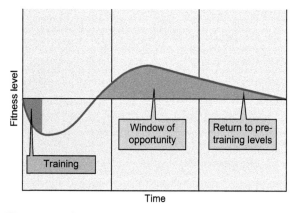

Figure 2.1 General Adaption Syndrome (GAS). From Norris, C.M. (2013). *The Complete Guide to Exercise Therapy.* Bloomsbury.

The key to the GAS is that the body can either positively adapt (called *eustress*), as when it becomes stronger through weight training, or negatively adapt (called *distress*), for example by overtraining.

The GAS is modified slightly when the imposed stress is exercise. The initial physical stress (exercise) is an overload which is at a higher level than that normally encountered. This stress causes body reactions which are physiological, biomechanical and psychological in nature. Immediately after training, fatigue in all three areas causes the body to be less able to react to an imposed stressor. For example, following

heavy weight training, muscles feel exhausted and the mind lacks motivation (Fig. 2.1b). The body gradually recovers, a process which may take one or two days, and even up to a week if the imposed stress is very great (running a marathon, for example). As the body adapts, pre-exercise levels are restored, but the adaptation continues (supercompensation) so that the body becomes better equipped to cope with the imposed stress. During this period, further exercise causes the whole cycle to be repeated, but this time, as the starting point (fitness level) is higher, the compensation is greater. For this reason, the period of supercompensation is often referred to as the *window of opportunity*. Two key points emerge from this process. The first is that the body has to be given the opportunity to adapt, with adequate rest and good nutrition, for example. The second is that the next training period must occur during the window of opportunity. Clearly, if the next training period occurs too soon the body will not have finished adapting, but if it occurs too late, the body will have returned to pre-training fitness levels.

> **Key point**
> Following training, the body must be given time to recovery for maximal tissue adaptation to occur.

The overload is made up of four factors, described by the simple mnemonic FITT, standing for *frequency, intensity, time* and *type*. Together, these variables make up the training volume, representing the total amount of exercise/work performed as shown in Table 2.1 For example, heavy weight training is clearly harder than light jogging (exercise type), while slow walking is easier than fast walking (intensity). Performing a trunk curl exercise every hour throughout the day is harder than performing it every other day (frequency), and performing 10 reps is easier than 100 reps (duration). Performing the trunk curl every day for 3 sets of 10 reps gives a larger training volume than

Table 2.1 Training variables using the FITT mnemonic

Variable	Meaning
Frequency	How often you practise an exercise, for example is it twice each day or three times each week
Intensity	How hard an exercise is. In strength training, this is normally measured in comparison to the maximum weight you can lift once (1 repetition maximum or 1 RM) or the maximum voluntary contraction (MVC) of a muscle. With stretching, it is how far you stretch as a proportion of your maximum range of movement (ROM), for example 60% max ROM or 80% max ROM.
Time	The duration of the exercise, for example running for 20 minutes or 1 hour. It also refers to the duration of a repetition, for example using a very slow action (superslow technique) in weight training to emphasize muscle contraction.
Type	The category of exercise, such as strength training, aerobics, stretching, plyometrics, and each of these can be subdivided depending on which of the 'S' factors of fitness are worked.

performing it 3 times each week for 2 sets of 12 reps.

> **Key point**
>
> *Training volume* is the total amount of work performed during an exercise by combining the training variables frequency, intensity, time and type.

As the body habituates (gets used) to the training stimulus, the stimulus must increase or *progress*. Failing to change the stimulus can lead to the subject's fitness gains plateauing.

> **Key point**
>
> To continue to gain benefits from training, the body must be subjected to a *progressive overload*.

As an example, a subject may be able to lift a 10 kg weight for 10 repetitions (reps) before fatigue. If they practise this action three times per week, after one or two weeks they will be able to perform a greater numbers of repetitions before fatigue sets in. If they are able to perform 15 or 16 reps, to continue to practise 10 reps with the same 10 kg weight will not stimulate continued adaptation. The overload needs to progress, and they may lift 12 kg for 10 reps, for example. As we will see later, increasing the resistance (weight in this case) is

only one way of progressing. Changing the action, altering the timing or rest period, changing the type of muscle work are all examples of progressing an overload.

Reversibility

Failure to overload tissue sufficiently will result in loss of the benefits gained as part of the training adaptation, a process called *detraining*. Training effects are not permanent. The motor system adapts to the level (overload) and type (specificity) of stress that is imposed on it. If the stress is removed, and training ceases, the motor system will again adapt to the new, now lower, level of stress, and detraining will occur. This transient nature of training adaptation is known as the *reversibility principle*.

> **Definition**
>
> The *reversibility principle* describes the gradual loss of training effects when the training overload is reduced, a process referred to as *detraining*.

However, athletes are often very anxious that even a single training session dropped or day lost will result in detraining, and this is far from the truth. Detraining must be differentiated from *tapering*. Tapering involves the gradual reduction in training volume prior to a competition to give a physical and psychological break from the rigours of continuous training. Tapering allows muscle to repair microdamage caused through intense training (eccentric actions especially) and to replenish the energy stores (muscle phosphocreatine and glycogen, and liver glycogen). Interestingly, the gains made by top-class training will remain for some time. Research has shown, for example, that swimmers who reduce their training by 60 per cent for up to 21 days show no loss of fitness (VO2 max), and actually improve muscle resistance to fatigue (lower blood lactate and increased arm power) (Costill et al. 1979). Similar findings occur in running, with a seven-day taper period in distance runners showing a significant reduction in 5k times.

Detraining sees the loss of the effects of training, but in a much slower way than injury or immobilization. The detrained athlete will show muscle wasting (atrophy) and this will be more noticeable in those who are highly trained because they obviously have more to lose. Atrophy is accompanied by reductions in muscle strength and endurance. Endurance begins to reduce after two weeks due to a reduction in oxygen usage capacity (fall in both oxidative enzyme activity and muscle glycogen storage). Loss of cardiorespiratory endurance is greater over a similar time period than strength, which requires only minimal stimulation to maintain it. Flexibility losses occur quite quickly. In a study looking at detraining in younger (<30) and older (>65) men, 8–13 per cent of strength gains were lost after 30 weeks to detraining (Lemmer et al. 2000). Power shows a more rapid reduction, however, with similar reductions occurring in just 4 weeks of detraining (Costill et al. 1985).

Individuality

Training responses are not equal between individuals, in the same way that treatment effects are largely patient-specific. Changes which relate to a specific person represent *individuality*. Each person reacts slightly differently to training stimuli due to differences in growth rate (genetically determined), and regulation of the cardiovasular and respiratory systems, for example. In studies using the same training programme, fitness levels (VO2 max) can vary from 0 to 50 per cent (Wilmore et al. 2008). The HERITAGE study in the late 1990s looked at family members' responses to training (Bouchard et al. 1998). Over 700 subjects completed a 20-week training programme and maximal oxygen uptake (VO2 max) was measured, together with risk factors for cardiovascular disease. Differences were shown to be related to genetics rather than age, sex or race.

Individuality explains why when two people begin a gym programme, for example, one may progress quite rapidly (*high responder*) while the other may struggle to make gains (*low responder*). The main reason for individuality is hereditary. A study of a 20-week endurance training programme using identical twins (Prud'homme et al. 1984) showed a similar training response for each twin pair, but a substantial variation across subjects of maximal aerobic power improvement (0–40 per cent). Assessing the difference in training response (VO2 max) using family members (Bouchard and Rankinen 2001) has shown that high or low responders tend to be clustered within families, again representing a genetic and/or familial tendency. The principle of individuality underlies successful exercise prescription. Variation in tissue adaptation, neural, cardiopulmonary and endocrine changes, and psychology dictate that subjects will often respond differently to similar exercise bouts.

Definition

Individuality is the familial and/or genetically determined aspect of an exercise response or adaptation.

Treatment note 2.1 Overtraining syndrome

Training involves stressing the body so that it overcompensates and gains a training effect. Some fatigue after exercise is therefore desirable, and this type of acute fatigue leads to an increase in performance. However, if the training volume is too great, or the recovery period between training bouts too brief, subjects will overreach, giving a temporary reduction in performance. Where overreaching (OR) is marked, stagnation will result in a brief performance reduction. This may occur, for example, after a hard training camp, and the effect would be positive providing recovery is adequate. Overreaching of this type is termed 'functional OR'. Continuing the increase in training intensity without allowing recovery will lead to a reduction in performance called non-functional OR. Generally, a short-term decrement in performance occurs which allows the subject to recover within a ten- to fourteen-day period. If recovery is not adequate and training continues, the progression is to overtraining. Recovery in this case may takes months, or in some cases even longer.

Overtraining syndrome (OTS) occurs when the body is subjected to stresses beyond its capacity to adapt. Typical triggers to OTS are shown in Table 2.2. Lack of adaptation to training leads in turn to a reduction in sports performance and a number of important potential health concerns. The symptoms of OTS are initially similar to those of hard training, such as muscle aching and fatigue. However, the experienced coach and subject can detect when these changes are greater than normal. Several physiological effects are thought to underlie OTS, including autonomic nervous system changes, alteration in endocrine response, suppression of immune function and variation in brain neurotransmitters. Alteration in sympathetic nervous system drive is seen in subjects who emphasize high-intensity resistance training, giving increased heart rate, blood pressure and basal metabolic rate, loss of appetite and decreased body mass.

Table 2.2 Common trigger of overtraining syndrome

Triggers to OTS
Increased training load without adequate recovery
Training monetary
Excessive number of competitions/games
Sleep disturbances
Personal stresses (partner, family, job)
Previous illness
Altitude or heat exposure
Severe glycogen depletion ('bonk')

(Data modified from Kreher & Schwarz 2012)

Symptoms of OTS

Common symptoms of OTS are shown in Table 2.3. One of the adaptations to normal training is a change in the hypothalamic pituitary axis (HPA), characterized by an increase in the ACTH/cortisol ratio during the post-workout recovery period. In OTS there is a change in the rise in ACTH following exercise and this has been used to identify non-functional OR and OTS. Using two exercise bout tests, Meeusen et al. (2004) were able to demonstrate large increases in hormonal release following the first exercise bout but suppression following the second. Time to fatigue tests, which are specific to a subject's sport, have also been used to detect OTS (Halson and Jeukendrup 2004). Typically, subjects suffering from OTS are able to begin an exercise session performing normally but then suffer from an unexplained performance drop. Fatigue tests are therefore more predictive than incremental tests (Meeusen et al. 2006).

Mood state questionnaires are very useful in the identification of OTS as negative affective states characterize the condition. Questionnaires such as the recovery-stress questionnaire (RestQ-Sport) may be used, but subjects should ideally be tracked throughout their training to identify a baseline to show deviation. This is

Treatment note 2.1 *continued*

Table 2.3 Symptoms of overtraining syndrome

Performance	Physiology	Psychology	Immunology	Biochemistry
▸ ↓ perfomance	▸ Altered resting HR & BR	▸ Apathy & depression	▸ Impaired immune function	▸ Altered cortisol & testosterone levels
▸ ↓ training tolerance	▸ Altered respiration	▸ ↓ self esteem	▸ ↓ rate of healing	▸ ↓ muscle glycogen
▸ ↑ recovery requirement	▸ Muscle soreness	▸ ↑ stress sensitivity	▸ ↑ respiratory infection	▸ ↓ blood haemoglobin and iron levels
▸ ↓ coordination	▸ Joint aching			
▸ ↑ faults	▸ Headaches			
	▸ Sleep disturbances			
	▸ Changed eating pattern			

↓ - decreased, ↑ - increased. Data from acsm.org

Table 2.4 Daily training log

Training details – FITT
Perceived exertion – RPE
Self-perception of training – worse/same/better than other days
Sleep quality (rating 1–5)
Muscle soreness (rating 1–5)
General fatigue (rating 1–5)
History of illness – UTI/MSK/menstruation

FITT: frequency, intensity, time, type; RPE: rating of perceived exertion; UTI: upper respiratory tract infection; MSK: musculoskeletal.

a 76-item questionnaire which assesses the physical and mental impact of training (Kellmann and Kallus 2001). Heart rate variability (HRV) has also been used as an assessment tool of OR. HRV increases with heightened parasympathetic tone and has been shown to be significantly elevated following chronic training (Meeusen et al. 2006).

Many subjects describe an increase in upper respiratory tract (URT) infections following hard training – the so-called open window effect. This effect seems to be more prevalent with OR and OTS. A two-week period of intense training has been shown to reduce bacterial defence response (bacterially stimulated neutrophil degradation) by 20 per cent (Robson et al. 1999) and a one-week intense programme to lower T-cell count (Lancaster et al. 2004).

The initial management of OTS is dependent on identifying OR. This is made easier by having the subject keep a training log (Table 2.4) so that changes in response to their baseline measure may be recognized early and appropriate action taken. Where OR is suspected, it is vital that training volume be reduced, and in more severe cases total rest may be called for over a period of many weeks. Prevention focuses on periodization of training to vary training variables including frequency, intensity, time and type (FITT). High-quality diet and adequate sleep play a pivotal role in exercise recovery and the prevention of OTS.

References

Halson, S., Jeukendrup, A., 2004. Does overtraining exist? An analysis of overreaching and overtraining research. *Sports Medicine* **34**, 967–981.

Kellmann, M., Kallus, K.W., 2001. *Recovery-Stress Questionnaire for Subjects: User Manual.* Human Kinetics Publishers, Champaign, IL.

Lancaster, G.I., Halson, S.L., Khan, Q., Drysdale, P., Jeukendrup, A., 2004. The effects of acute exhaustive exercise and intensified training on type 1/ type 2 T cell distribution and cytokine production. *Exercise Immunology Review* **10**, 91–106.

Lehmann, M., Foster, C., Gastmann, U., et al., 1999. *Overload, Performance Incompetence, and Regeneration in Sport.* Plenum, New York.

Meeusen, R., Duclos, M., Gleeson, M., Rietjens, G., 2006. Prevention, diagnosis and treatment of the

Treatment note 2.1 *continued*

Overtraining Syndrome. ECSS position statement. *European Journal of Sports Science* **6** (1), 1–14.

Meeusen, R., Piacentini, M.F., Busschaert, B., Buyse, L., 2004. Hormonal responses in subjects: the use of a two-bout exercise protocol to detect subtle differences in overtraining status. *European Journal of Applied Physiology* **91**, 140–146.

Robson, P.J., Blannin, A.K., Walsh, N.P., 1999. The effect of an acute period of intense interval training on human neutrophil function and plasma glutamine in endurance trained male runners. *Journal of Physiology* **515**, 84–85P.

Wilmore, J.H., Costill, D.L., Kenney, W.L., 2008. *Physiology of Sport and Exercise*, fifth ed. Human Kinetics Publishers, Champaign, IL.

Key point

Failure to allow sufficient recovery following a training session can lead to overtraining and exhaustion.

Recommended quality and quantity of exercise

When training for aerobic (cardiopulmonary) fitness or stamina, exercise intensity may be assessed by measuring heart rate or maximal oxygen uptake (VO2 max). The American College of Sports Medicine (1978) recommended the quantity and quality of exercise required to develop and maintain aerobic fitness and body composition. A training frequency of three to five days per week is required, at an intensity of 60 to 90 per cent of the maximum heart rate reserve, or 50 to 85 per cent VO2 max. This should be carried out for a duration of 15 to 60 minutes, and be continuous or rhythmical in nature. These recommendations were later updated to include the provision of resistance training, flexibility and weight loss (ACSM 1990, 2002) and neuromotor exercise (ACSM 2011). For strength gains, one set of 8–12 repetitions was recommended, with 8–10 exercises for the major muscle groups, for two days per week. A balanced flexibility programme should include both static and dynamic ranges of motion exercise to work the major muscle/tendon groups. Each stretch should be held for at least 10–30 seconds, and four repetitions should be used for each group two to three times per week. To achieve significant weight loss, 4.5 hours of moderate exercise, with an energy expenditure of at least 2,000 calories per week, is recommended.

To achieve this, either continuous or accumulative exercise may be used, at an exercise intensity of 55 to 69 per cent maximal heart rate. Accumulated daily duration should be 30 to 40 minutes per day. Neuromotor exercise should be practised two or three times each week for 20 to 30 minutes, using programmes which work on motor skills, proprioceptive exercise. Multifaceted activities such as yoga and tai chi are recommended for seniors to reduce the risk of falls (Table 2.5).

Components of fitness

Physical fitness can be viewed as a set of attributes that relate to the ability of a subject to perform physical activity. It is the ability of a person to function efficiently and effectively in demanding situation, and is closely related to health.

Fitness can be thought of as a continuum, from optimal fitness at one side, through average fitness, to complete lack of fitness and death (Fig. 2.2). The exact components of fitness required to make an individual optimally efficient and effective will be determined largely by the physical activity to be performed.

Fitness may be subdivided into two types: task (performance)-related fitness is that required for sport and within occupational activities; health-related fitness includes components which are associated with some aspect of health. Physical

Table 2.5 ACSM guidelines for maintaining fitness in apparently healthy individuals

Cardiovascular	
Frequency	3–5 times per week
Intensity	55–90% HRmax
Time	20–60 min
Type	Large muscle groups. Rhythmic and continuous activity
Muscular	
Frequency	2–3 times per week
Intensity	8–10 exercises 1 set of 8–12 repetitions to volitional fatigue 75% 1 RM resistance
Time	20 minutes
Type	Resistance training for major muscle groups
Flexibility	
Frequency	3 times per week
Intensity	3–5 repetitions for each exercise Maintain at point of mild discomfort
Time	10–30 second hold
Type	Static stretch for major muscle groups
Neuromotor exercise	
Frequency	2–3 times each week for using
Intensity	Varied
Time	20–30 minutes
Type	Work on motor skills, and proprioceptive exercise Multifaceted activities such as yoga and tai chi recommended for seniors to reduce the risk of falls

HR max: maximal heart rate; 1 RM: maximum resistance lifted for single repetition.
Source: ACSM (1990).

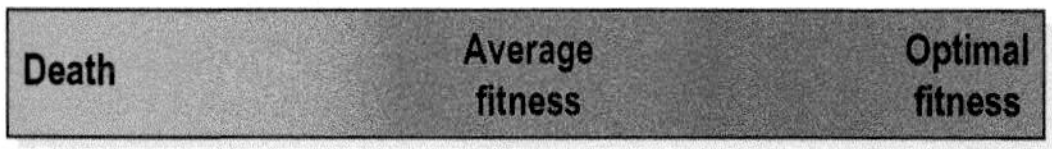

Figure 2.2 The fitness continuum.

training will improve fitness, but may not always enhance health. Extreme development of any one of the fitness components, in isolation, can upset the delicate balance between the components, and may actually be detrimental to health. For example, excessive development of

flexibility can lead to hyperflexibility and, when strength lags behind, may progress to instability. Excessive development of strength may reduce range of motion, leaving a subject 'muscle bound'. Favouring some muscles to the detriment of others could lead to a change in the equilibrium point (resting position) of a joint.

The benefits of exercise are numerous (Table 2.6). However, as we have seen (Treatment Note 2.1), there is a balance between training sufficiently hard to gain the effects of overload, but not so hard that the subject overreaches (OR) in the short term or eventually progresses to overtraining (OTS). Many subjects will be familiar with the symptom of staleness, and of an increased incidence of UTI.

Definition

Upper respiratory tract infection (UTI or URTI) is a condition affecting the nose, respiratory tract, sinuses, pharynx or larynx. Typical symptoms include nasal congestion, running nose, cough, sore throat and fever. Exposure to a virus, or less commonly a bacterium,

Table 2.6 Benefits of regular exercise

- ▶ Reduced risk of premature death
- ▶ Reduced risk of developing and/or dying from heart disease
- ▶ Reduced high blood pressure or the risk of developing high blood pressure
- ▶ Reduced high cholesterol or the risk of developing high cholesterol
- ▶ Reduced risk of developing colon cancer and breast cancer
- ▶ Reduced risk of developing diabetes
- ▶ Reduce or maintain body weight or body fat
- ▶ Build and maintain healthy muscles, bones and joints
- ▶ Reduce depression and anxiety
- ▶ Improve psychological well-being
- ▶ Enhance work, recreation and sport performance

Source: US Department of Health and Human Sciences (1999) Physical Activity and Health. Report of the Surgeon General. http://www.cdc.gov.

gives symptoms between one and three days later, which may last up to ten days. Common names for the condition include colds, sinusitis and laryngitis.

Infection of this type occurs because although training in general has been shown to enhance immune function, following intense training the immune system is depressed. This temporary depression leaves the subject susceptible to infection, and is called the 'open window'. It is thought that intense exercise changes adrenocorticotropic hormone (ACTH) and cortisol concentrations and has a knock-on effect on blood glucose concentration, negatively affecting the immune system (Nieman and Pedersen 1999). Moderate exercise does not have this effect, and the window remains closed, giving the long-term immune system the benefits of exercise without short-term immunosuppression.

Fitness components

The fitness components may be conveniently defined as 'S' factors (Table 2.7). The term 'stamina' is used to encompass both cardio-pulmonary and local muscle endurance. Cardiopulmonary endurance is associated with a reduced risk of coronary heart disease, and local muscle endurance is a factor in any sustained activity, especially joint stability. *Suppleness*

(flexibility) and *strength* (see below) are concerned with the health of the musculoskeletal system, to maintain both range of movement and joint integrity. *Speed* (rate of movement) and power (rate of doing work) are both needed in later-stage rehabilitation as part of proprioceptive training. *Skill* training is important, not just for sports specific actions, but for the skill of individual movement such as scapulohumeral rhythm or gait re-education, for example. *Structure* refers to body composition. Variance in body composition between subjects (for example, limb length) has an important bearing on exercise choice in strength and conditioning (S&C) especially. Body fat percentage and its relationship to obesity is an important health consideration for cardiopulmonary health and joint loading.

The term '*specificity*' refers to the SAID principle, that is 'specific adaptation to imposed demands'. The change taking place in the body of a subject (adaptation) as a result of training (the imposed demand) will be determined by the type of training which is used, and will be specific to it.

Specificity applies to strength and power development, but also to the energy systems used while exercising. A particular cardiopulmonary training programme will cause specific training adaptations. Aerobic fitness developed on a cycle ergometer, for example, will differ slightly from that obtained while running.

It is important, therefore, that training matches as accurately as possible the action which the subject will use in a sport in terms of joint range, muscle work, energy system and skill.

The term '*spirit*' covers the psychological effects of exercise as discussed below.

Table 2.7 Fitness component checklist

Factor	Interpretation
Stamina	Cardiovascular & local muscle endurance
Suppleness	Static & dynamic flexibility. Agility
Strength	Concentric/eccentric/isometric
Speed	Acceleration & deceleration/power
Skill	Movement quality/sensorimotor training
Structure	Body composition/anthropometry
Spirit	Psychological fitness/Psychological aspects of injury
Specificity	Task- & sport-related requirements

Key point

Specificity of training means that exercise must match, as accurately as possible, the actions which a subject will use in sport.

Treatment note 2.2   Tissue homeostasis

Homeostasis is the method by which the body actively maintains a constant state within its internal environment. To maintain tissue capacity there is a continuous process of physiological maintenance via adaptations in the body's metabolism (Dye 2005). Injury or overuse can disrupt homeostasis, leading to a cascade of biochemical changes. Excessive (supra-physiological) loading on tissue will cause adaptation, providing there is sufficient time for recovery. A sudden imposition of extreme force, however, may exceed the load capacity of tissue, leading to maladaptation. Similarly, repetitive small forces which occur too frequently may not allow sufficient time for the tissue to adapt to the new loading level. At the other extreme, too little (sub-physiological) loading, such as would occur with prolonged rest, also disrupts homeostasis, leading to changes such as muscle atrophy and bone mineral loss, reflecting deconditioning. Clearly it is a case of 'use it or lose it' with tissue function.

The region of loading between under and over usage has been described as an 'envelope of function' and represents the area of load acceptance (Dye 2005). Where loading exceeds the capacity of a body part, the action can be envisaged as occurring outside the envelope of function, and the tissues may be irritated, giving rise to symptoms such as pain and swelling. At this stage, reducing or changing loading may restore homeostasis, with a view to later increasing tissue capacity with progressive rehabilitation and elevating the upper limit of the functional envelope.

Poor load management can have effects both on the body as a whole and at a local tissue level. Repetitive loading without sufficient recovery can cause cumulative tissue fatigue, and increase susceptibility to injury. At whole-body level, inappropriate loading can impair a subject psychologically, for example with impaired decision-making ability, and physiologically, with compromised coordination and neuromuscular control. Fatigue of this type reduces both muscle force and muscle contraction velocity (Soligard et al. 2016). Joint kinematics and neural feedback can be compromised, with ongoing detriment to joint stability. Locally, excessive micro-damage may occur if the magnitude of loading is beyond the individual tissues' load-bearing capacity. Initially, when loaded, tissue changes are short term and reflect *reaction,* and include changes such as increased blood flow through muscle, and increased metabolic activity. When loading stops, these changes are reversed, homeostasis is restored, and the tissue resumes its resting state. Repeated loading causes the tissue to change more permanently, and *adaptation* occurs. Adaptation may include increased muscle strength, and increased bone mineral density, for example. Training loads which are too low may not stimulate sufficient adaptation and can impair the tissues' ability to cope with higher loads in the future. Adequate training stimulates biological adaptation to increase the subject's capacity to accept and withstand load, building resilience.

The aim of rehabilitation is to increase the capacity of the injured tissue, and to offload it by enhancing the strength of surrounding muscle. Tissue capacity may be built with progressive overload, which may be either simple or complex (Cook and Docking 2015). Simple loading targets the specific tissue (for example, the medial collateral ligament of the knee), while complex loading targets the tissue within the context of the whole limb or body region (for example, a squat action). The load chosen for rehabilitation must accurately reflect the type of load the tissue may be placed under during any functional action in daily living or sport. Training specificity of this kind is vital to increase tissue capacity relevant to the subject's actions (patient-centred) rather than increasing capacity to fulfil predetermined goals (therapist-centred).

Psychological effects of exercise

Exercise and self-concept

Several psychological characteristics have also been shown to change as a result of participation in a regular exercise programme. Enhancement of self-confidence, self-esteem, self-efficacy and body image are seen, and reductions in anxiety, depression, stress and tension have been demonstrated.

Definition

Self-esteem is the degree to which individuals feel good (positive) about themselves. *Body image* is the perception of one's own body and general physical dimensions. *Self-efficacy* is the strength of a subject's belief in their ability to complete tasks and reach goals.

Enhanced well-being

Subjects often claim that exercise makes them 'feel good', and the 'runner's high' is a widely reported phenomenon. Reductions in stress and anxiety have been reported following exercise, and decreased depression has been demonstrated. In addition, altered states of consciousness have been described following distance running, and weight-training programmes have been shown to enhance self-concept. Three theories exist to explain these phenomena: the distraction hypothesis, and the production of monoamines and endorphins.

How exercise makes a subject feel better

The *distraction hypothesis* proposes that participation in vigorous exercise distracts the subject from stress. Comparisons between exercise, meditation and distraction show similar reductions in state anxiety, but the effect resulting from exercise appears to last longer.

Depression is also affected by exercise. Reductions in noradrenaline (norepinephrine) and serotonin (5-HT) are associated with depressed states in humans, and these same chemicals have been shown to increase in rats subjected to chronic exercise. Increases in the release of endorphins and enkephalins, or slowing of the dissociation rates of these chemicals, has also been proposed. By measuring plasma levels of these chemicals, or using opiate antagonists to neutralize them, researchers have demonstrated some association between exercise and endorphins (Farrell et al. 1983).

Exercise addiction

Exercise addiction, or exercise dependence, is the physiological or psychological dependence on regular exercise, usually distance running, but other forms of exercise such as body-building may also show this trend. Subjects who are addicted to exercise show symptoms of withdrawal and uncontrollable craving for a particular exercise type at the expense of other training.

Definition

Exercise addiction is physical or psychological dependence on regular exercise of a single type. Subjects show uncontrollable craving and symptoms of withdrawal when the exercise is not practised.

The experience of exercise for a subject, and the way in which this fits into the rest of his or her life, is one factor which determines whether or not an exercise becomes addictive. An individual's need for exercise can be either positive or negative. *Positive addiction* exists when a subject receives some psychological or physical benefit from an activity, and is able to control the activity.

The *negatively addicted* subject is controlled by the activity and will experience severe negative effects (withdrawal) with a missed exercise bout. Such subjects often engage in an activity at the expense of their health or at the expense of other factors, such as relationships and career prospects. The negatively addicted subject may be failing

Table 2.8 Characteristics of exercise addiction

The athlete may:
1 Perform several bouts of exercise per week for up to an hour at a time
2 Experience a high degree of positive affect after exercising
3 Exercise alone or isolate themselves when in a group
4 Be highly satisfied and less self-critical when exercising than at any other time
5 Experience a state of euphoria when exercising
6 Be more depressed/anxious/angry after missing a workout
7 Tend to ignore physical discomfort/injury in order to complete exercise regime

Adapted from Glasser, W. (1976) *Positive Addiction*. Reprinted by permission of HarperCollins Publishers Inc. and Anshel, M.H. (1991) A psycho-behavioral analysis of addicted versus non-addicted male and female exercisers. *Journal of Sport Behavior*, 14 (2), 145–154.

to gain approval from significant others and may harbour feelings of inadequacy or unattractiveness. This type of subject often exercises alone or in isolation from the group. They experience feelings of enhanced self-concept and even euphoria during exercise. Importantly, such individuals are more likely to ignore pain or injury and work through this to complete a workout. In the same vein, they tend to be anxious if a workout is missed and almost appear to suffer 'withdrawal symptoms'. Table 2.8 illustrates some common features of exercise addition, and the *Exercise Addiction Inventory* (EAI) has been shown to be a valid and reliable tool to identify the at-risk individual (Griffiths et al. 2005).

Warm-up

Many subjects conscientiously warm up in the belief that they will protect themselves against injury, and enhance their sporting performance. While neither of these beliefs have been conclusively proven, there is mounting evidence in the literature to suggest that both may contain elements of truth. Wedderkopp, Kaltoft and Lundgaard (1999) found that warm-up significantly reduced both traumatic and overuse injury frequency. Players in the control group (non-warm-up) were found to be 4.9 times more likely to become injured than those who warmed up.

Looking at knee and ankle injury incidence in hard ball players, Olsen, Myklebust and Engebretsen (2005) studied 1,837 youth handball players in Norway and found a significantly lower incidence of injury in the warm-up group (0.5 injuries per 1,000 player hours) compared to the control group (0.9 injuries per 1,000 player hours). These same authors concluded that a warm-up programme reduced the incidence of injury by 50 per cent. Soccer-specific warm-up has been shown to reduce lower-limb injury rates in collegiate players (Grooms et al. 2013). The injury rate dropped from 8.1 injuries per 1,000 exposures, with 291 days lost, to 2.2 injuries per 1,000 exposures, and 52 days lost, with the inclusion of the specific warm-up. A systematic review and meta-analysis of 25 studies featuring neuromuscular training (NMT) as a warm-up has highlighted evidence for its effectiveness in the reduction of knee injuries within youth sport (Emery et al. 2015). In addition, NMT has been shown to significantly reduce injury risk rates in junior high school students (Richmond et al. 2017).

Definition

Neuromuscular training (NMT) is functional-based exercise involving multiple exercise types designed to reflect the demands of a sport or activity.

Table 2.9 gives examples of NMT which can be incorporated in an injury-prevention programme or warm-up.

Table 2.9 Example activities for neuromuscular training (NMT) as a warm-up

▶ Cardiovascular, strength & flexibility work
▶ Balance (balance board, single leg drills)
▶ Core training
▶ Agility (direction change)
▶ Acceleration/deceleration drills
▶ Plyometrics (jumps, bounds)
▶ Sport/activity specific exercise (throw, kick)

Warm-up types

Warm-up may be either *passive*, involving an external heat source, or *active*, involving body heat. An active warm-up, in turn, may be *general*, using the whole body, or *specific*, working only those body parts to be used in competition, and studies have shown physiological changes from each.

Many external heat sources are suitable for a passive warm-up. Common types used by subjects include hot baths or showers and saunas. Clinically, therapists use a number of modalities including hot packs, whirlpool baths and electrotherapy. Although benefits are often claimed to result from the increase in tissue temperature, pain modulation is also likely to be a significant mechanism.

With a passive warm-up, no significant active body movement is used, and little energy is expended. Subsequent physical work will not therefore be impaired due to depletion of energy stores. This type of warm-up can be useful clinically, when active movement is either not desirable or not possible.

Key point
Warming tissues passively may lead to pain modulation and can be useful therapeutically. Warm-water soaks and hot packs are simple home-use methods.

General warm-ups are the type most commonly used in sport. The overall body temperature is raised by active exercise, increasing the temperature of the deep muscles and body core. Specific warm-up involves movements which are to be used in actual competition, but at a reduced intensity. Rehearsal of body movement takes place, and the specific tissues directly involved in the activity are heated. This type of warm-up would seem especially appropriate for events requiring highly skilled and coordinated actions.

Definition
A *passive warm-up* increases tissue temperature by using an external heat source. An *active warm-up* uses body heat produced during exercise, and may be general, using the whole body, or specific, working body parts to be used in competition.

Effects of warm-up

A warm-up achieves its effect through physiological, psychological and biomechanical methods. Physiological effects are largely due to increases in tissue temperature and metabolic rate, while psychological effects are mainly due to practice. Biomechanical effects are achieved by alterations in the tissue response to mechanical strain.

Cardiovascular changes

The change from a relaxed resting state to a higher training level should be gradual, to avoid suddenly stressing the cardiovascular system. Equally, to stop training quickly, and reduce cardiac output too rapidly, can compromise venous return.

A warm-up of sufficient intensity will cause an alteration in regional blood flow. When resting, only 15–20 per cent of the total blood flow goes to the skeletal muscles, but after about ten minutes of general exercise this figure is increased to 70–75 per cent. During a warm-up, blood flow is increased to active muscles and reduced to visceral tissues earlier than would occur without a warm-up. Increased blood flow causes the delivery of nutrients and removal of metabolic wastes to be enhanced.

Classical studies from the early 1970s demonstrated the effects of sudden strenuous exercise on men with no symptoms of cardiac problems. Subjects ran vigorously on a treadmill for 10–15 seconds without a warm-up. In 70 per cent of these subjects, abnormal changes were seen on an ECG trace, indicative of subendocardial ischaemia.

These changes were reduced, or even abolished, when a warm-up was performed before activity. Similarly, the effect of sudden-onset exercise on blood pressure was improved. Average systolic blood pressures of 168 mmHg were seen without warm-up and these reduced to 140 mmHg when warm-up preceded exercise (Barnard et al. 1973).

One of the reasons for these changes is that the adaptation of the coronary blood flow to strenuous exercise is not instantaneous. The cardiac output is unable to increase quickly enough to meet the demands of sudden high-intensity work, and a warm-up gives the cardiovascular system time to respond.

Key point

A warm-up reduces the stress on the cardiovascular system by allowing the adaptation of coronary blood flow to occur more gradually.

Tissue temperature

The ability to perform physical work is improved by elevated temperature. Warm-up prior to maximal exercise will enable the adaptations necessary for these changes to occur sooner.

Oxygen dissociation from haemoglobin is more rapid and complete, and oxygen release from myoglobin is greater at higher temperatures. The critical level of various metabolic processes is lowered, causing an acceleration in metabolic rate and a more efficient usage of substrates. Muscle contraction is more rapid and forceful. The sensitivity of nerve receptors and speed of transmission of nervous impulses are both increased as temperature rises. This more rapid transmission of kinaesthetic signals is particularly important when complex highly skilled movements are used. These temperature-dependent changes are summarized in Table 2.10.

The increased tissue temperature created by a warm-up will alter the force–velocity curve

Table 2.10 Warm-up mechanisms

Improvement	Mechanism
Muscle work	Faster muscle contraction and relaxation speeds
Economy of movement	Lowered viscous resistance within muscle
Oxygen delivery and usage	Haemaglobin releases oxygen more easily as tissue temperature rises
Nerve conduction	Increased temperature accelerates metabolic rate within nerve.
Blood perfusion	Local vascular bed dilated
Psychological changes	Specific warm-up rehearses motor pattern increasing psychological preparedness for sport
	Enhanced motivation

(Data from McArdle, Katch and Katch 1996, Jeffreys 2016)

of a muscle. The effect is to shift the curve to the right by 12 per cent for each 1° C increase in temperature (Enoka 1994). The change in contraction velocity (maximal velocity of shortening) results in an increase in peak power output of the muscle (Fig. 2.3). Although laboratory studies are able to show increased metabolic activity, practically this may be difficult to achieve. The temperature change which the subject feels on the skin has to reach the depth of the muscle, and as the skin and subcutaneous tissue is an effective thermal insulator, this may not always be possible with passive warming.

Mobilization hypothesis

In the initial period of intense exercise, high amounts of energy are required immediately. The anaerobic reserves are quickly used up, and the aerobic system has not yet become fully functional. The difference between the energy needed and that which can be supplied is known as the *oxygen deficit*, and represents stored energy and the build-up of metabolic wastes (Fig. 2.4). When exercise stops, the body continues to provide energy aerobically to replenish the energy stores and metabolize waste products which have accumulated. This, in turn, creates the *oxygen debt*.

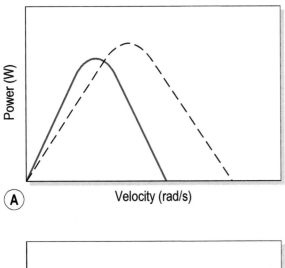

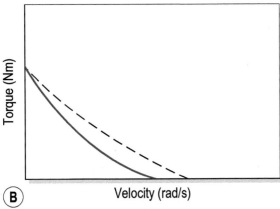

(B)

Figure 2.3 Effect of tissue temperature increase due to warm-up. (A) Peak power is increased demonstrated by increased height obtained on vertical jump test. (B) Maximum velocity of shortening increased and torque–velocity curve shifts to the right. Adapted from Enoka, R.M. (1994) *Neuromechanical Basis of Kinesiology*, 3rd ed. Human Kinetics, Illinois. With permission.

One of the functions of a warm-up can be viewed as mobilizing the body's cardiovascular system to reach a steady state. As warm-up is stopped, a brief rest period before competition should allow the oxygen debt to be repaid, without letting the cardiovascular system return to normal levels. When competition commences, the oxygen deficit would be smaller, and some anaerobic energy would be available to the subject at the end of

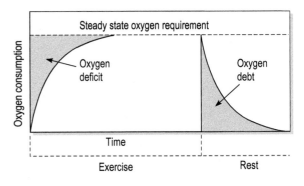

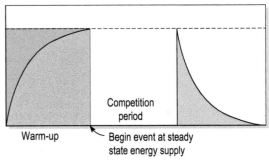

Figure 2.4 The effect of warm-up on oxygen deficit.

exercise. A rest period is essential after the warm-up, to allow the oxygen debt to be repaid. But, following rest, the body must be kept warm to maintain the warm-up effects until the subject competes. To achieve physiological changes of the type described above with a general warm-up, aerobic activity is required to increase heart rate, and blood flow with the aim of increasing deep muscle temperature. This is normally indicated by the development of light sweating.

Key point
A warm-up should be of sufficient intensity to induce mild sweating.

Biomechanical effects

Greater force and length of stretch is required to tear isometrically preconditioned muscles (Safran

73

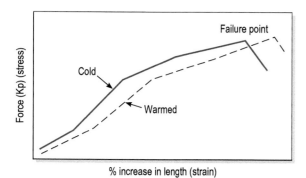

Figure 2.5 The effect of warm-up on tissue failure. The effect of warm-up on tissue failure. After Safran, M.R. et al. (1988) The role of warmup in muscular injury prevention. *American Journal of Sports Medicine*, 16 (2), 123–129. With permission.

et al.1988) (Fig. 2.5). The rise in temperature occurring during the warm-up period could alter the viscosity of the connective tissue within the muscle, and several early authors demonstrated an increase in the length of stretched tendon following temperature increase which mimicked warm-up (Warren, Lehmann and Koblanski 1971). Changes have also been noted in structural stiffness of muscle following warm-up and exercise. Immediately following activity, muscle stiffness is increased, but it can be significantly reduced by stretching. The increase in stiffness is thought to result from thixotropy, the property exhibited by materials whereby they become more fluid when disturbed (shaken). Within muscle, stable bonds are formed between actin and myosin filaments. The bonds are increased following activity, but disengaged by stretching. This has important implications for both warm-up and cool-down. Warm-up will help minimize general muscle stiffness, while cool-down will reduce the actin and myosin bonding which remains following exercise (see also DOMS).

Proprioception has been shown to improve as a result of warm-up (Bartlett and Warren 2002). Joint position appreciation is more sensitive in the knee after a warm-up, demonstrating that joints seem to accommodate to increased ligamentous laxity which results from a reduction in stiffness due to exercise. The method through which this occurs is thought to be an increase in the sensitivity of the proprioceptive mechanisms around the knee.

Psychological effects

Psychological aspects of warm-up fall broadly into two categories: first, there are psychological effects of a physical warm-up, and second, aspects of sports psychology, such as visualization and imagery, used in athlete preparation.

Two psychological factors are important in the context of warm-up; these are *rehearsal* and *arousal*.

Rehearsal

Rehearsal will only take place when a subject performs a specific warm-up, with actions relevant to the sport to be performed in competition. During the warm-up, the subject is re-familiarizing him- or herself with the skilled movements required by the sport. Confidence is improved, and the subject may be more relaxed following this practice.

When a subject is performing a skilled task, a period of rest followed by resumption of the same task may result in impaired performance. This phenomenon is called *warm-up decrement* (WUD) and is well documented (Schmidt and Lee 2011).

> **Definition**
> *Warm-up decrement* is the gradual loss of the effects of the warm-up in the period between the warm-up and competition.

A number of explanations have been suggested to account for WUD. At a basic level, it is seen as simply forgetting an aspect of the motor skill. WUD may result from a loss of 'activity set', comprising a number of variables, such as arousal level and attention, which have to be adjusted (tuned) to a specific task. With practice, the adjustments reach an optimal level, which is reduced with rest. WUD can be reduced if, during a rest period, a completely different movement is practised. The second movement does not contribute to the memory of the first task, but does require a similar activity set to the original skill.

So far, we have dealt with skills which were practised during the warm-up period to improve subsequent sporting performance. Where one type of training has a direct effect on another, a *transfer effect* is taking place.

Definition

A *transfer effect* is the interaction between two similar forms of training. An activity set is a group of variables which are adjusted or 'tuned' to a specific physical task.

When the practice of one task improves the performance of another, *positive transfer* is occurring. However, if, during a warm-up, skills are practised which are different to those needed for competition, they may interfere with the learning process and *negative transfer* can occur. Here, performance suffers because a slightly different skill, with a different activity set, is remembered. An example would be practising tennis strokes with a racquet of different weight and size to that of the one used in competition.

Arousal

The second psychological effect of warm-up is that of *arousal*. The relationship between level of arousal and performance is demonstrated by the inverted-U hypothesis (Fig. 2.6). In a plot of arousal level against performance, initially increased arousal correlates initially with improved performance. But, as arousal continues to increase, an optimal level is reached. Above this point, further arousal is detrimental to performance.

The point of optimum arousal is related to the psychological profile of the subject and the complexity of the task to be performed. Activities which require fine muscular control (such as archery) or involve important decision-making (such as wicket-keeping) generally require lower arousal levels. Where actions involve gross muscular actions without fine control and without complex

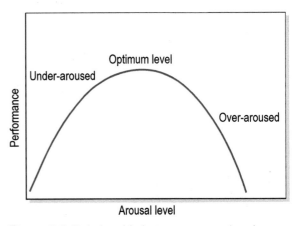

Figure 2.6 Relationship between arousal and performance.

decision-making (power-lifting, for example) a higher level of arousal is generally required.

The function of warm-up, therefore, must be to psychologically prepare the subject, and place him or her at the level of arousal appropriate to the task to be undertaken. A highly motivated (aroused) subject may need to be relaxed prior to a complex activity. Conversely, a poorly motivated subject due to compete in a strength event may need to be 'psyched up' to an increased arousal level.

Key point

A warm-up should psychologically prepare an subject, and place him or her at a level of arousal appropriate to the task to be performed.

Working with the RAMP method

A simple mnemonic to work with when planning a warm-up is RAMP, a three-phase programme standing for raise, activate and mobilize, and potentiate (Jeffrieys 2007). In Phase 1 (raise) the aim is to increase metabolic rate (as with a general warm-up above) but with the RAMP method actions to be used later in sports form the basis of the cardiopulmonary work, making the warm-up more functional from the outset.

Treatment note 2.3   Warm-up technique

The intensity and duration of the warm-up period will depend on both the type of activity to be undertaken and the subject's fitness. A fitter subject competing at a high level will take longer to warm up as the body's thermoregulatory system will be more efficient. In cold weather it will take longer for the body's core temperature to increase, and so the warm-up should be longer or more vigorous. Classically, a warm-up should be of sufficient intensity and duration to raise the body's core temperature by 1–2° C, recognized by the onset of mild sweating. Practically, the warm-up may be divided into three parts: *pulse raising*, *mobility* and *rehearsal*.

Pulse raising

The pulse raising (cardiovascular or 'CV') portion of a warm-up should induce mild sweating, and is best performed wearing a full tracksuit or other insulating clothing. This will retain body heat and maintain the benefits of the warm-up until competition. Gentle jogging, light aerobics or using CV machines in a gym are all pulse-raising activities.

Mobility

Mobility exercises should be performed that are sufficient to take the joints through their full range of motion, the exact range being determined by the movements to be used during sport or activity (activity-specific). The aim is to ensure that the movements used in sport will not overstretch the tissues. If stretching exercise is used in sports demanding a high degree of movement range, a distinction must be made here between *maintenance stretching* and *developmental stretching*. Maintenance stretches are used prior to a sport to take the tissues to their maximum likely to be encountered in the sport performance. For developmental stretching, exercises are used which aim to increase this range of motion, and so a thorough warm-up is performed first.

Maintenance stretches therefore form part of a warm-up, while developmental stretches are practised in a separate stretching session if required.

Rehearsal

To rehearse complex actions in a warm-up, sport-specific movements may either be performed at a lower intensity level or split up into their subcomponents. For example, in weight training, the first set of an exercise can be carried out with a light resistance, or even an unweighted bar or stick. In hurdling, the leg action may be practised slowly and to lower levels, gradually increasing in both speed and height until the normal hurdling action has been achieved.

Only when the individual can perform the movement correctly has the rehearsal portion of the warm-up achieved its aim.

Warm-down

On cessation of exercise it is important to reverse the processes which occurred during the warm-up. The heart is no longer helped by the rhythmic contraction and relaxation of the leg muscles. Consequently, to stop intense exercise immediately will increase the demand on the cardiovascular system, causing the heart rate to rise. Metabolic waste products formed during exercise, such as lactic acid, will no longer be carried away from the working area with so much vigour. Instead, they will remain in the area, causing ischaemic pain. Flushing the area with fresh blood by performing a gentle warm-down may reduce this effect.

Example NMT warm-up

The FIFA 11+ provides an example of a warm-up to prepare a subject for a particular sport, in this case soccer, using a variety of movements as part of a neuromuscular technique (NMT) warm-up. The programme begins with running drills at slow speed, combined with active (dynamic)

Treatment note 2.3 *continued*

stretching, working with a partner over an eight-minute period. Strength (core and leg), plyometrics and balance actions which target soccer-specific actions are practised for ten minutes with increasing difficulty in the second part of the programme. More intense running

at moderate to high speed, with soccer-specific planting and cutting actions, forms the third part for two minutes. The programme is available open source at

http://www.f-marc.com/downloads/workbook/11plus_workbook_e.pdf.

In Phase 2 (activate and mobilize) the aim is to increase range of motion using functional patterns likely to be used later in sports such as squat, lunge and press actions. The focus is on dynamic rather than static stretch to move through range of motion, and any weakness in movement patterns can be addressed at this stage prior to loading the body further. Phase 3 (potentiate) is similar to the specific warm-up detailed above, and includes sports-specific activities which gradually increase in intensity. This phase can be used to develop speed and agility relevant to the sport played.

Flexibility training

Flexibility is the range of motion possible at a specific joint or series of articulations, or the amount (amplitude) of joint movement and the general absence of stiffness.

Two types of flexibility are generally recognized, *static* and *dynamic*. Static (or extent) flexibility refers to the amount of movement obtained by passively moving a limb to a maximum degree. Dynamic flexibility is concerned with the amount of active movement possible as a result of muscle contraction. The concern here is not so much the degree of movement present as the ease with which it is obtained. This type of flexibility is more important in speed and power events in particular.

Definition

Static flexibility is the amount of movement obtained by passively moving a limb. *Dynamic flexibility* is the active movement possible as a result of muscle contraction.

Dynamic flexibility is contrasted with agility, which describes the ability to rapidly change the direction of either the whole body or individual body parts without loss of balance.

Effects of flexibility training

Flexibility training is generally thought to achieve effects in two broad areas, performance enhancement and injury prevention.

Improved performance

To achieve maximal performance, a limb must be able to move through a non-restricted range of motion. In sprinting, for example, lack of adequate dynamic flexibility could result in a reduced stride length, with possible reductions in sprinting speed. In addition, greater resistance to movement through increased joint inertia and muscle stiffness at the end of movement range is more energy consuming.

Good flexibility is associated with good sporting performance in activities where a maximal amplitude of movement is required to achieve the best technical effects. Similarly, a limited range of movement can reduce work efficiency in these situations. In addition, if flexibility is increased, force may be applied over an increased distance, thus facilitating acceleration of an implement. Static stretching may produce small performance enhancements in actions performed at long muscle lengths. However, small decrements to performance have also been shown immediately (3–5 min) after stretching due to a reduction in muscle activation (Behm et al. 2016).

Injury prevention

A variety of authors have argued that flexibility may condition tissues to have greater tensile strength and elasticity, leading to injury prevention and a reduction in soft tissue pain. This has led some to suggest that the type of training programmes undertaken could affect the number of injuries suffered (Ekstrand et al. 1983). Warm-ups which include stretching have been shown to be important factors in the prevention of hamstring injuries in Australian football (Seward and Patrick 1992). In a study of army recruits, Hartig and Henderson (1999) showed the effect of hamstring stretching over a thirteen-week period on overuse injuries. Using 298 subjects, they showed an incidence rate of 29.1 per cent for the control (non-stretching) group and 16.7 per cent for the stretching group.

Stretching to the glenohumeral (GH) internal rotators has been used as part of a shoulder injury prevention programme in elite handball players. A prevention programme including GH internal rotation stretching, GH external rotation strengthening and scapular muscle strengthening was used, together with kinetic chain actions and thoracic mobility, to reduce the injury risk by 28 per cent (Andersson et al. 2016).

Muscle stiffness has been shown to reduce as a result of stretching (McNair and Stanley 1996). Using five repetitions of a static stretch and holding each repetition for 30 seconds, stiffness was reduced to the same degree as with a warm-up for ten minutes at 60 per cent HR max. Static stretching has also been shown to improve muscle compliance and enhance muscle force development (Rosenbaum and Henning 1995) as well as reduce the passive resistance offered by a muscle. This latter effect has been shown to return to pre-stretching levels within one hour (Magnusson, Simonsen and Kjaer 1996). These biomechanical changes affecting muscle stiffness could lead to an injury-prevention effect of stretching.

Although individual studies indicate the possibility of an injury-prevention effect of stretching, taken as a whole the research does not support this.

Herbert and Gabriel (2002) summarized the information gained from five studies and concluded that there was no evidence that stretching either before or after exercise protects against muscle soreness or risk of injury. In a later study, Weldon and Hill (2003) conducted a review of seven papers and decided that no definitive conclusions could be made concerning the value of stretching, due to the poor quality of the available studies. Fradkin et al. (2006) conducted a systematic review of studies from 1966 to 2005 and concluded that, although there was insufficient statistical evidence to endorse or discontinue routine warm-up and stretching, 'the weight of evidence is in favour of decreased risk of injury'.

Tightness occurs in muscle groups in set patterns, with the biarticular muscles (mobilizers) showing a greater tendency to shorten. For example, of the hip extensors, it is the hamstrings (biarticular) rather than the gluteals (uniarticular) which commonly show tightness and injury through tearing, so muscle architecture may be an important determinant of stretching effect. The Canadian Society for Exercise Physiology (CSEP) position stand on the acute effects of stretching recommends the use of stretching within a warm-up to reduce muscle injury and increase joint range of motion (ROM), providing additional dynamic activity is practised after the stretching bout (Behm et al. 2016).

Flexibility training and muscle power output

Muscle power depends not just on muscle contraction, but on a combination of active contraction, muscle reflex activity and elastic recoil of the non-contractile elements associated with a muscle, within the stretch–shortening cycle (SSC). We have seen that one effect of flexibility training is to reduce muscle stiffness. This, in turn, could have a direct effect on power development by changing the elastic forces created by the rebounding muscle.

Kokkonen et al. (1998) tested subjects with a one repetition maximum (1 RM) lift, and found the subject's lifting ability to be reduced by 7–8 per cent following static stretching. Using a footplate to stretch and measure strength output from the soleus muscle, Fowles et al. (2000) used 13 maximal passive stretches over a half-hour period, holding each stretch for over two minutes. Again, they measured maximal muscle contraction and found that strength in the stretching group reduced by 28 per cent immediately after stretching, reducing to 12 per cent after 30 minutes and 9 per cent after 60 minutes. Using a leg-extension exercise, Behm et al. (2001) used 20 minutes of static stretching, with each repetition held for 45 seconds. These authors found a 12 per cent decline in maximal leg strength, confirming the results of the previous studies.

A number of mechanisms may be responsible for this stretch-induced decline in strength output. EMG measurement has revealed a 20 per cent decline in quadriceps activity after stretching (Behm et al. 2001). Muscle activation (using interpolated twitch) has also been shown to decrease by 13 per cent (Fowles et al. 2000).

In addition to alteration in muscle stiffness and electrical changes to the muscle, microscopic damage similar to that seen following eccentric activity also seems to occur. Creatine kinase (CK) levels have been shown to increase by over 60 per cent following intense stretching (Smith et al. 1993), confirming this.

Definition

Interpolated twitch (IT) is a method of electrically stimulating a muscle to create a muscle twitch which can then be measured. *Creatine kinase* (CK) is a chemical produced in a muscle following intense eccentric actions. It is created by the breakdown of damaged muscle cells.

Muscle reflexes

A number of structures can limit joint range of motion (Table 2.11) and the ability of muscle to

Table 2.11 Factors limiting range of motion at a joint

Osteological design of joint
Joint degeneration (osteophytes)
Cartilage and cartilaginous joint structures
Muscle tone (active)
Muscle elasticity (passive)
Ligament
Fascia
Tendon passing over the joint
Nerve length (passive)
Nerve activation (active)
Skin, scarring and subcutaneous tissue
Soft tissue contact
Joint fluid viscosity (ease of movement) and quantity (movement range)
Consolidated oedema, fibrous tissue

relax and allow a stretch to occur is one of the most important in sport. For this reason, three muscle reflexes are important when using flexibility training: the *stretch reflex, autogenic inhibition* and *reciprocal innervation* (Table 2.12).

When a muscle is stretched, elongation is detected by the muscle spindle afferent nerve fibres. These receptors send impulses to the dorsal roots of the spinal cord, and a reflex is caused which contracts the extrafusal fibres of the same muscle, in opposition to the original stretching force. The

Table 2.12 Muscle reflexes and stretching

Stretch reflex	
Responds to:	
— change in velocity (phasic) (e.g. knee jerk reflex)	Faciliatory (↑ tone)
— change in length (postural) (e.g. body sway)	
Autogenic inhibition	
(the reverse stretch reflex)	
— Golgi tendon organ (GTO) measures tension	Inhibitory (↓ tone)
Reciprocal innervation	
— Agonist contracts, antagonist relaxes to allow movement	Inhibitory (↓ tone)

reflex is therefore facilitatory. The stretch imposed may be either sudden (as in a knee-jerk reflex), where the muscle responds to a change in velocity, or prolonged (as with postural sway), where the muscle measures the change in length.

In addition to the muscle spindle, the Golgi tendon organ (GTO) in the muscle tendon will also register stretch. Both these receptors are affected by changes in muscle length, but the GTO is also receptive to changes in muscle tension.

When a muscle is stretched, there is a corresponding stretch of the muscle spindle. But, if the stretch lasts for longer than six seconds, the GTO registers not only the change of length of the muscle, but also the alteration in tension in the muscle tendon. The GTO will then cause a reflex relaxation of the muscle, a process known as autogenic inhibition or the reverse stretch reflex. This has a protective function, causing the muscle to relax and allowing it to stretch before it is damaged. It is therefore inhibitory.

Stretching which involves short jerking movements will tighten the muscle through the stretch reflex, while movements lasting for longer than six seconds will allow the muscle to relax again through stimulation of the GTO, which will override the stretch reflex. If the tension of the muscle to be stretched is increased through isometric contraction, once relaxed the muscle tone will reduce below normal resting levels, enabling a greater stretch to be applied. The stretch reflex (H reflex) has been shown to be suppressed for ten seconds following isometric contraction of this type (Moore and Kukulka 1991), giving a ten-second period during which stretching may be applied.

Definition

The H reflex (Hoffman reflex) is an artificially induced equivalent of the stretch reflex produced in a laboratory by stimulating a muscle with a single electric shock.

When a muscle is tensed, a reflex relaxation of the antagonist will occur, a process known as

reciprocal innervation. If, for example, the biceps muscle contracts to flex the elbow, its antagonist, the triceps, must relax to allow the movement to occur. This reflex is modified in co-contraction, where both the agonist and antagonist muscles contract simultaneously. Co-contraction functions to increase joint stiffness and contributes to stability and accuracy of rapid movements (Enoka 1994).

Most coaches, subjects and therapists would recognize that regular stretching can increase range of motion in many subjects. One of the methods by which this occurs may be neural plasticity at spinal level. Experiments with monkeys (Wolpaw, Lee and Carp 1991) have shown that the H reflex can be modified as a result of using EMG biofeedback. The magnitude of the H reflex can be increased, reduced or altered completely, and following surgical transection of the spinal cord these changes remain, indicating that the plasticity is occurring at spinal level rather than through brain influence. It may be possible that the threshold of the stretch reflex in man can be altered through a process of desensitization (habituation) so that the reflex threshold is higher (less likely to occur). This would modify the muscle's resistance to stretching and thereby increase available range of motion. Neuronal activity has been shown to reduce with both static and ballistic stretching (Vujnovich and Dawson 1994).

Definition

Habituation (desensitization) is a learning process which results in the reduction of a response or sensation. It occurs in the presence of continual stimulation with a constant stimulus.

Techniques of flexibility

Five methods of stretching are generally recognized: static, ballistic, active and two proprioceptive neuromuscular facilitation (PNF) techniques (Table 2.13).

Table 2.13 Summary of stretching techniques

1	Ballistic – rapid jerking actions at end of range to force the tissues to stretch
2	Static stretching (SS) – slowly and passively stretching the muscle to full range, and maintaining this stretched position with continual tension
3	Active stretch – contract the agonist muscle to full inner range to impart a stretch on the antagonist
4	Contract–relax (CR) – isometrically contracting the stretched muscle, and then relaxing and passively stretching the muscle still further. This action is usually performed by a partner
5	Contract–relax–agonist–contract (CRAC) – the same as CR except that during the final stages of the stretching phase, the muscle opposite the one being stretched is contracted

Static stretching

During static stretching, a muscle is stretched to the point of discomfort and held there for an extended period. As the muscle is held, the subject will feel a reduction in the pain stimulus, from sharp acute pain to a more dull diffuse sensation. If the static stretch is held by the therapist, the end-feel of the muscle resistance will change from a strong (firm) elastic feel to a more yielding feel. Static stretches should be held for a prolonged period. A thirty-second hold has been shown to be more effective than a fifteen-second hold, with no greater benefit seen when the holding time is extended to sixty seconds (Bandy and Irion 1994). Four or five repetitions should be performed, as no further benefit is seen when the number of repetitions is increased from this (Taylor et al. 1990).

Key point

Optimal static stretching is achieved by holding the stretch for thirty seconds and performing four to five repetitions of this movement.

Ballistic stretching

Ballistic stretching involves taking the limb to its end-of-movement range, and adding repetitive bouncing movements. There is a suggestion that injury may result from abrupt stretching of this type (Etnyre and Lee 1987) so the technique has become less popular. Although this may be true for vigorous ballistic stretches which are uncontrolled, adding small stretches to the end-of-range gained by static stretching (pulsing) has been shown to reduce neurone excitability further than static stretching alone (Vujnovich and Dawson 1994). To perform ballistic stretching more safely, first it should be given after static stretching, and second it should be given progressively in terms of both velocity of stretch and range of motion. Such a stretching session would begin with a warm-up and then move to static stretching (5 reps, each held for 30 seconds), which would then progress to 3–5 reps of end-range pulsing (high velocity, short range). This would then progress to longer range movements at slow velocity, and finally to long range movements at steadily increasing velocity.

Key point

Ballistic stretching must only be used as a progression on static stretching. Short-range high-velocity movements are used at end range (pulsing) to further increase flexibility. The movements must remain controlled throughout.

Active stretching

Active stretching involves pulling a limb into full inner range so that the antagonist muscle is stretched passively while the agonist is strengthened. This type of stretch can be important when targeting muscle imbalance around a joint. The inner-range contraction is used to shorten a lengthened (lax) muscle, while the shortened muscle is stretched using a functionally relevant movement.

When stretching a biarticular muscle, full inner-range contraction is not possible at both ends simultaneously and so the opposing muscle cannot be fully stretched. For example, the hamstrings

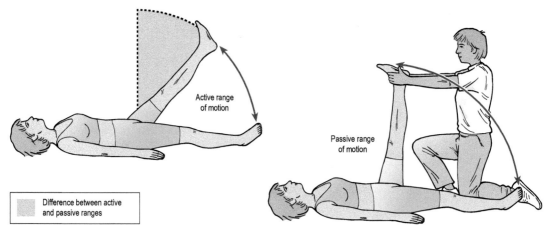

Figure 2.7 Difference between active and passive ranges of motion.

cannot pull the hip to full inner-range extension and the knee to full inner-range flexion at the same time, as they are activity insufficient. This means that the rectus femoris muscle will in turn not be fully stretched. Passive range of motion will therefore be greater than active range of motion for a biarticular muscle. One of the aims of stretching, however, should be to reduce this difference to a minimum, giving the subject active control over a greater range of motion (Fig. 2.7). In addition, although passive range of motion is greater than active, the active range normally more closely resembles the movements used in sport and so is more specific. Active stretching involving repeated eccentric lengthening followed by concentric action is often termed *dynamic* stretching, and when performed at speed to capitalize on the SSC, it forms the basis of *Plyometric* training.

> **Definition**
>
> *Active* stretching uses the strength of the agonist muscle to lengthen the antagonist, with the final stretch position held statically. *Dynamic* stretching uses repeated controlled full-range movement. *Plyometrics* uses faster muscle contraction following stretch.

One of the main advantages of active stretching in the early period of rehabilitation is the control that the subject has where pain is present. As one muscle is being tightened to stretch another, the subject is in control of the movement throughout. This may give the subject the confidence to stretch into ranges which they would not normally be prepared to enter in the presence of pain.

Treatment note 2.4   Passive stretching

There are several passive stretching techniques which are useful in the clinic situation. The therapist applies these on the subject, initially without the subject taking an active part in the procedure. Once full passive range has been obtained through a hold–relax technique, contract–relax and CRAC procedures may be used with the same exercise.

Hamstrings

Straight-leg raising may be performed with the subject's leg resting on the therapist's shoulder. The leg is held with one hand to stop it slipping and the other hand keeps the knee locked. The therapist takes up a walk standing position with the weight on the back leg to begin (Fig. 2.8); as the stretch is put on, the therapist shifts the

Treatment note 2.4 *continued*

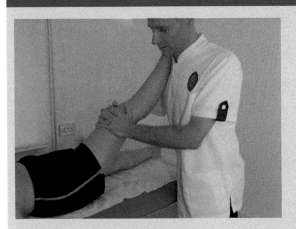

Figure 2.8 Hamstring stretch using straight-leg raise (SLR).

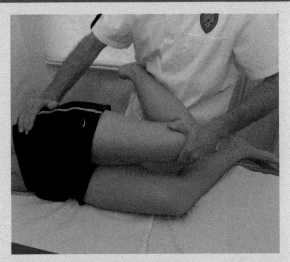

Figure 2.10 Rectus femoris stretch.

weight onto the front leg by lunging forward. In this way, the therapist protects his or her back and avoids moving into a flexed position of the trunk.

To emphasize the upper portion of the hamstrings (ischial origin), the subject's knee is flexed by 20 degrees by altering the hand position. The whole leg is pressed into hip flexion, maintaining the slightly flexed knee position (Fig. 2.9).

Rectus femoris

The rectus femoris is stretched in a side-lying position (Fig. 2.10). The affected leg is uppermost

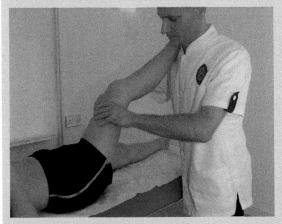

Figure 2.9 Emphasizing the upper portion of the hamstrings.

and the subject bends the underneath knee and holds onto this, to guard against anterior pelvic tilt and hyperextension of the lumbar spine as the stretch is put on. The therapist flexes the knee and holds this flexed position using pressure of his/her abdomen. The femur is then pulled back into extension using hand pressure over the knee and pelvis. Where the upper portion of the rectus is to be targeted, knee flexion is released slightly to allow for a greater extension stretch at the hip. It should be remembered that only 15 degrees of extension is available at the hip before anterior pelvic tilt begins. Further extension range will therefore affect the lumbar spine rather than impose a greater stretch on the rectus.

Upper trapezius

The upper trapezius is frequently overactive and may develop painful trigger points. The stretch is performed in supine lying, to allow the therapist to use massage techniques over the muscle belly if required.

For the right trapezius (Fig. 2.11), begin by elevating the right shoulder to relax the trapezius. Laterally flex the neck to the left and maintain this position using pressure with the right hand.

Treatment note 2.4 *continued*

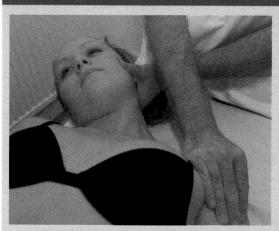

Figure 2.11 Upper trapezius stretch.

Impart the stretch by pressing down on the right shoulder with the left hand. An X grip of this type is easier for the therapist to apply, while pressing on the shoulder rather than the neck is more comfortable for the subject. The stretch may be varied by using neck flexion with the subject's head on a block or rolled towel.

When using massage techniques with the muscle on stretch, the neck and shoulder position may be maintained by using the left forearm as a 'strut' between the two structures. The right hand is then free to apply the massage technique.

> **Key point**
> With active stretching the aim is to match the range of motion available using a passive stretch.

PNF stretching

PNF (proprioceptive neuromuscular facilitation) techniques have been adopted by the sporting world from neurological physiotherapy treatments. These techniques use alternating contractions and relaxations of muscles and capitalize on the various muscle reflexes to achieve a greater level of relaxation during the stretch.

Two PNF techniques are used in sport: contract–relax (CR) and contract–relax–agonist–contract (CRAC). The CR technique involves lengthening a muscle until a comfortable stretch is felt. From this position, the muscle is isometrically contracted and held for a set period. The muscle is relaxed and then taken to a new lengthened position until the full stretch is again felt by the subject. The rationale behind the CR method is that the contracted muscle will relax as a result of autogenic inhibition, as the GTO fires to inhibit tension. The intensity of isometric contraction required to initiate post isometric relaxation may vary between patients. Initially, minimal contractions are used in the presence of pain, with intensity increasing if needed to increase movement range.

With the CRAC method, the muscle is stretched as above, but in the final stages of the stretch, the opposing muscle groups are isometrically contracted as the stretch is applied, to make use of reciprocal inhibition of the agonist and reduce its tension. PNF stretches have been shown to be more effective than static or ballistic movements (Etnyre and Abraham 1986), with CRAC methods generally being better than CR.

There are two major disadvantages to PNF techniques. First, the extra tension developed in the muscle may result in greater pain, and this in turn may reduce user compliance, an important consideration in early rehabilitation. Second, as PNF involves isometric contractions, the user must be discouraged from holding the breath and using a valsalva manoeuvre. The raised intra-abdominal and intra-thoracic pressure which occurs with this technique can lead initially to a reduction in venous blood flow to the heart and a decreased cardiac output. On expiration, increases in blood pressure in excess of 200 mmHg have been recorded (Alter 1996).

Factors affecting flexibility

The amount of movement present at a joint during a stretch (amplitude) is affected by internal (body) and external (environmental) factors (see Table 2.10). Internal factors include the bony contours of the joint, which may be affected by both morphology and pathology. Bone shape and proportion (morphology) will differ among individuals, and in certain disease states (pathologies) such as arthritis, movement will decrease as bone formation changes. These factors cannot readily be affected by flexibility training but must be taken into consideration when prescribing stretching programmes, especially with the elderly and during rehabilitation.

Definition

Morphology is the shape or form of a body structure, *Pathology* is the science of disease.

Other internal factors include volume of surrounding tissue, an obese individual frequently being less flexible than a lean one. Muscle tissue, tendons and joint capsules are other internal factors which may result in movement limitation. Jones and Wright (1982) indicated that 47 per cent of mid-range stiffness is due to the joint capsule, 41 per cent due to muscle fascial sheaths, 10 per cent due to the tendon and 2 per cent due to the skin. Other factors include cartilage and viscosity of joint fluid. Muscle tension will limit range of motion, providing *active resistance*. When a muscle is relaxed, the connective tissue framework of the muscle, rather than the myofibrillar elements, will provide a *passive resistance*.

Temperature is one external factor which affects flexibility. An increase in tissue temperature can result in both a reduction in synovial fluid viscosity and increased soft tissue extensibility. Elastic (recoverable) deformation of connective tissue is favoured by high-force, short-duration stretching, with tissue at normal body temperature or slightly cooled, while plastic deformation (permanent lengthening) is greater with lower-force, longer-duration stretching at elevated temperatures. If the tissue is then allowed to cool in this stretched position, results may be better (Sapega et al. 1981), but practically it is difficult to induce significant temperature changes to the tissues.

Individual variations in body structure can have apparent effects on flexibility. Individuals with long slender limbs are likely to be more flexible than shorter individuals with thicker musculature. However, good flexibility in one joint does not guarantee similar attributes in other joints, because flexibility is joint-specific.

In general, flexibility decreases with age, although among individuals this trend is very much dependent on activity levels and other lifestyle factors. A general belief is that girls are more flexible than boys, but it is not clear whether this is due to body structure or social and environmental influences (Goldberg, Saranitia and Witman 1980).

Therapeutic stretching

When stretching is used as a manual therapy to mobilize a joint after injury or surgery, various techniques will be combined. If muscle spasm is the limiting factor, ice may be used to limit the pain, and this may be combined with PNF stretching (cryostretch procedures). However, to change connective tissue effectively, higher than normal temperatures are required, so heat is the modality of choice, where muscle spasm does not limit movement.

The ability of the heat source to reach the tissue to be stretched must be considered, and this will largely depend on the tissue depth and vascularity. In superficial tissues and joints, superficial heat (heat lamp, hot pack, hot water soak) may have a beneficial effect on tissue extensibility. The deeper tissues will not be heated directly. However, muscle spasm may reduce as a result of pain modulation. Deeper heating (microwave, shortwave diathermy, ultrasound) may have a direct heating effect on deeper tissues, enabling some of the temperature-dependent effects on tissue to be achieved (Sapega et al. 1981), but the clinical usefulness of this may be questioned.

After heating, passive stretching may be applied by the therapist, or, where long-term stretch is to be used, pulley systems and weights can apply the passive stretch. This is especially useful for an immobile joint where adhesions limit movement.

Strength training

Strength is the ability to overcome a resistance, or the maximum tension which a muscle can produce. It is usually measured as the torque exerted in a single maximal isometric contraction of unrestricted duration. However, clinically it is important to define the type of strength by prefacing the term with the category of muscle contraction which was used. We should, therefore, talk of isometric or isotonic strength, rather than simply strength alone.

Adaptation to resistance training

Muscular contraction involves a combination of physiological and neurological processes, and consequently adaptations to resistance training are both *myogenic* (structural) and *neurogenic* (seen on EMG only) in nature (Table 2.14).

Key point

Adaptations to resistance training are from both myogenic (structural) and neurogenic (functional) sources.

Table 2.14 Adaptations to resistance training

Structural (myogenic)	Functional (neurogenic)
▶ Increased number of myofibrils ▶ Increased quantity of contractile and non-contractile muscle protein ▶ Increased muscle CSA ▶ Increased muscle energy stores and enzyme levels ▶ Alteration in capillary density	▶ Increased neural drive ▶ Increased MU recruitment ▶ Increased MU firing rate ▶ MU recruitment by size ▶ Increased neuronal firing rates ▶ MU synchronization ▶ Reduced muscle co-contraction ▶ Stretch reflex potentiation

CSA – cross-sectional area. MU – motor unit.

Myogenic changes

Hypertrophy

One of the most noticeable myogenic adaptations to resistance exercise is increased muscle size through muscle growth or *hypertrophy*. Increased cross-sectional area (CSA) has been found to result from an increase in size of individual muscle fibres. Hypertrophied muscle fibres may have 30 per cent greater diameter and 45 per cent more nuclei (McArdle, Katch and Katch 2001). The increase in size occurs in both Type I (slow-twitch) and Type II (fast-twitch) fibres. Selective hypertrophy can occur, causing just the Type I or just the Type II fibres to increase in size, the ratio between the two fibre types remaining the same. In normal adults, the ratio is about 1:1 or 2:1, but in competitive bodybuilders ratios as high as 6:1 have been found, compared to 0:1 in sprinters. In addition, heavy resistance training has been shown to increase the proportion of Type IIa (fast oxidative glycolytic) fibres, through transition from Type IIx and Type IIax intermediary fibres to Type IIa.

Hypertrophy involves the increase in the amount of actin and myosin proteins due to increased synthesis and reduced degradation. Further, the numbers of myofibrils within the muscle fibre increases, and there is an increase in the structural proteins *titin* (contractin) and *nebulin*. The additional material is added to the outside of the myofibril to increase diameter and ultimately CSA of the muscle itself.

Definition

Titin is the third most common form of muscle protein after actin and myosin. It is a folded protein which undergoes tension as the muscle is stretched, preventing overstretch and contributing to passive recoil and elastic strength. *Nebulin* is an anchoring protein for actin and has a regulatory role in actin-myosin coupling.

Hypertrophy occurs as a result of both mechanical and hormonal stimulation. Intense resistance training produces *exercise-induced muscle damage* (EIMD), which in turn influences gene expression to repair and remodel the muscle and prevent further damage. Both contractile and non-contractile protein increase occurs, together with increased water uptake.

Changes may also occur to the *pennation angle* within muscle. Long strap-like muscles such as the sartorius have fibres which run the full length of the muscle attaching to each end. Thicker muscles such as the quadriceps have a pennate structure, meaning that their fibres attach obliquely to a central tendon, giving a featherlike appearance. This arrangement reduces the speed of muscle contraction, but increases strength. The angle of pennation is normally around 15 degrees, but may increase with training, as can the length of each muscle fascicle.

In addition to the increase in fibre size, which occurs with hypertrophy, connective tissue proliferation is also seen. Thickening of the muscle's connective tissue support, and that of the musculotendinous junction, may reduce the risk of soft tissue trauma.

Key point

With resistance training, connective tissue as well as muscle is enhanced, providing the possibility for injury reduction.

Endurance training has long been known to increase the number of mitochondria and the capillary density (number per square millimetre of tissue). However, resistance training is thought to lead to hypertrophy without a significant increase in the number of capillaries. As the number of capillaries stays the same but the size of the muscle tissue increases, the capillary density is reduced. Each capillary must now supply a greater fibre area with oxygen and nutrients, a factor which may account for the relatively poor aerobic capacity of subjects who train solely for muscle size.

Alterations in muscle energy stores have been reported following resistance training programmes. Increased intramuscular stores of adenosine triphosphate (ATP) and creatine phosphate (CP) have been reported. Similarly, increases in two of the enzymes of anaerobic glycolysis (phosphofructokinase and lactate dehydrogenase) have been shown. Increases in phosphogen stores and the enzymes of anaerobic glycolysis could be expected to prolong the maintenance of a maximal muscle contraction.

Hypertrophy in seniors

With ageing, both body composition and functional ability frequently change. Loss of bone density and muscle mass decreases the ability to perform the activities of daily living (ADL) and increases the likelihood of injury, especially falls. Bone density changes as a result of *Osteopenia* are covered in Chapter 1, so here we will focus on muscle mass reduction, *Sarcopenia*.

Maximal strength decreases with age, due to both neurogenic and myogenic changes. Loss of muscle mass occurs, with a greater reduction in Type II fibres, switching the ratio of fibres to a higher percentage of Type I. Both the total number of muscle fibres and their CSA reduces with ageing, but resistance training seems to slow this loss. Motor neuron death in the spinal cord causes a reduction in Type II fibre innervation, with resulting fibre atrophy. Fibre reductions in the region of 10 per cent per decade after age 50 have been reported (Kenney et al. 2015). Motor unit (MU) activation is lowered with ageing, with older, inactive subjects demonstrating lower MU activation and longer twitch contraction duration. Loss of muscle strength independent of mass change is termed *Dynapenia*, and loss of muscle mass itself has been claimed to explain only approximately 10 per cent of strength reduction (Clark and Manini 2012).

Clinically, the important message is that many older subjects retain their ability to maximally recruit muscle, so many of the changes may represent de-training rather than ageing in isolation.

Definition

Sarcopenia is the age-related loss of muscle mass, strength and function. *Dynapenia* is a reduction in strength independent of structural muscle change.

While weight training was once thought of as the preserve of the young, research now shows that muscle training effects are significant in seniors as well. Increases of muscle volume of 26 per cent, peak torque of 46 per cent and 28.6 per cent in total work output have been reported following resistance training programmes for healthy men with an average age of 67 years (Sipala and Suominen 1995). In even older subjects, Fiatarone (1994) tested a ten-week resistance programme on 63 women and 37 men and showed average strength increases of 113 per cent and increase in cross-sectional area of 2.7 per cent. Perhaps of more importance were the improvements in functional ability which these physiological changes achieved, with significant improvements in gait velocity (11.8 per cent) and stair-climbing speed (28.4 per cent).

Key point

Muscle hypertrophy and functional improvements have consistently been demonstrated in seniors using resistance training.

Hyperplasia

The possibility of muscle fibre splitting (*hyperplasia*) in humans has always been a contentious subject. A greater number of muscle fibres is seen in competitive bodybuilders, but this is thought to be a congenital feature of the more successful subjects. New muscle fibres may develop from *satellite cells*. These cells lie between the sarcolemma and the basal lamina of the muscle fibre at the end of the muscle. They are normally dormant, but become active in the case of muscle injury, and when stimulated they proliferate. With high-intensity muscle training, satellite cell activation may occur to replace cells damaged by training. There may be no significant gain in fibre number, therefore. *Longitudinal splitting* may occur, where a large muscle fibre splits into two daughter cells (a process known as lateral budding). In mammals, hyperplasia through satellite cell proliferation and longitudinal splitting does occur, but only where hypertrophy is not the main system of muscle growth (McArdle, Katch and Katch 2001). In humans, most authors agree that the increase in cross-sectional area following resistance training is the result of hypertrophy rather than hyperplasia.

Neurogenic changes

Significant strength gains may be made at the beginning of a strength-training programme without noticeable changes in muscle size. The increase in strength is thought to be the result of more efficient activation of the motor units. As Sale (1988) stated, 'strength has been said to be determined not only by the quantity and quality of the involved muscle mass, but also by the extent to which the muscle mass has been activated'.

Increased EMG activity occurs during maximal muscle contraction following a resistance-training programme, indicating an increased recruitment of motor units and a greater firing rate (Bandy, Lovelace-Chandler and McKitrick-Bandy 1990). For a muscle to produce its greatest force, all of the motor units it contains must be recruited. Normally, high threshold motor units are only recruited in periods of extreme need, with the smaller motor units being recruited first, a feature known as the *size principle of motor unit recruitment*, originally described by Hennemann et al. (1965) following work on cat muscle.

Definition

The *size principle of motor unit recruitment* states that, under load, motor units are recruited from smallest to largest.

The small-diameter slow oxidative (SO) fibres are recruited at low force levels, while the larger fast glycolytic (FG) fibres may not be recruited until 90 per cent of maximum force production is reached. Between these two extremes, lower threshold FG and fast oxidative glycolytic (FOG) fibres are recruited (Fig. 2.12A).

Key point

Small-diameter motor units are recruited at lower resistances. The largest diameter fibres may not be recruited until 90 per cent of maximum voluntary contraction (MVC) is reached.

The size principle can be overridden, however. Where maximal contractions occur at very high speed (for example, during plyometric actions) *selective recruitment* can occur. Here, large diameter fibres are recruited first because the actions can be so rapid that graded recruitment of the entire motor unit pool, from small through to large fibres, would take too long (Nardone et al. 1989).

In addition to enhanced recruitment, an increase in firing rate (frequency) of motor units is also seen. A single nerve impulse will cause an isolated twitch response, while a number of impulses are required to produce a sustained contraction (Fig. 2.12B). The greater the excitation of a motoneurone, the greater the firing rate of the motor unit in impulses per second (Hz). Motor units fire at rates

of between 10 and 60 Hz, with large increases in force seen for small increases in frequency at the lower end of the spectrum. At the higher end (Fig. 2.12C), increasing the frequency of motor unit excitation has little effect on force production.

With strength training, a subject may gain the ability to recruit the large motor units more easily and so increase the muscle force production. In addition, the firing rate of the motor units utilized in a contraction may be enhanced with training.

In principle, both the rate (how many) and sequence (which size) of motor unit recruitment may change. However, clinically, small-diameter fibres increase their force production more through greater firing rate, while large-diameter fibres rely more on enhanced fibre recruitment (Gabriel et al. 2006).

Motor unit *synchronization* (groups of motor units being activated together) has been shown to be greater in strength subjects than control subjects, and is likely to increase as a result of a resistance training programme. This change is more likely to increase the rate of force development rather than peak force itself (Sale 1988).

Evidence for neural adaptation following strength training comes from EMG studies which show increased activation of prime movers, as a result of improved skill and coordination. For example, during plyometric exercise the high stretch load can result in a period of inhibition at the start of the eccentric phase, while the trained individual shows facilitation, possibly as an adaptation of reflex response.

Activation of the prime mover may be limited by insufficient motivation, or inhibition. During new strength tasks, excessive co-contraction may occur to stabilize and protect the moving joints. Simultaneous contraction of the antagonist will reduce the force output of the agonist through reciprocal inhibition. Training could reduce the co-contraction and allow greater activation of the agonist muscle group, resulting in a greater force output. Such inhibition may explain the phenomenon of *bilateral deficit* (Sale 1992). In a weight-training exercise which

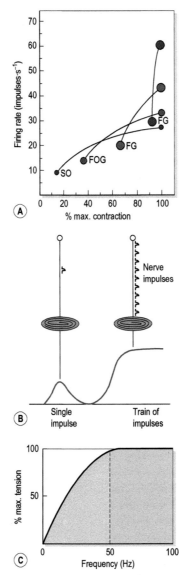

Figure 2.12 Neural adaptation to stretch training. (A) The size of motor unit recruitment. The small slow twitch oxidative (SO) motor units are recruited at low force levels. The largest high threshold fast twitch glycolytic (FG) are not recruited until 90 per cent maximal force is obtained. Between these two extremes are the lower threshold FG units and the fast twitch oxidative glycolytic (FOG). For each line, the low point shows the recruitment threshold and the high point shows the maximum firing rate obtained with maximum contraction force. (B) Effect of firing rate on muscle force. A single impulse from the axon to the muscle creates a twitch contraction, giving a low force output. A high-frequency train of impulses (high firing rate) creates a longer tetanic contraction, giving a force which is ten times greater. (C) Force–frequency curve. At low frequencies, small increases in frequency give very large increases in force. At high frequencies, the reverse is true, and doubling the frequency from 50 Hz to 100 Hz gives virtually no corresponding increase in force. From Sale, D.G. (1988) Neural Adaptation to Resistance Training, in *Medicine and Science in Sports and Exercise*, **20** (5), 135–145. With permission.

requires the simultaneous use of both limbs (for example, the squat, leg-press or arm-pressing movements), the total force which a subject can produce is often considerably less than the sum of the force of the individual limbs acting alone. The opposite effect may also occur, with bilateral facilitation showing an increase in voluntary recruitment of the muscle groups (French 2016).

In contrast to this inhibitory inter-limb effect, *cross-education* represents an overflow of chronic changes from the working muscle to the non-working muscle. This is commonly seen in rehabilitation, where an injured muscle may be enhanced by working its uninjured counterpart. Increases in strength in the range of 8 per cent may be expected with EMG activity rather than muscle structure changing (Carroll et al. 2006). Both bilateral deficit and cross-education represent neural adaptation as there are often no significant morphological changes.

Definition

Bilateral deficit represents a lower force produced when both limbs work simultaneously than the sum of the two individual limbs working unilaterally. *Cross-education* occurs when resistance training of a muscle on one side of the body (ipsilateral) produces increased strength and neural activation in the same muscle on the opposite side of the body (contralateral).

Changes to the stretch (myotactic) reflex occur when the protective nature of co-contraction is reduced, as described above. In addition, increased *stretch reflex potentiation* can occur to increase force output in high-speed (plyometric) actions, enhancing rate of force development (RFD). A fourteen-week programme of heavy resistance training has been shown to increase stretch reflex potentiation between 19 and 55 per cent (Aagaard et al. 2002).

Adaptation also occurs to the *neuromuscular junction* (NMJ), the interface between the nerve and the muscle fibre. Increased NMJ area, greater nerve terminal branching, and increased acetylcholine receptor spread have been described, which may enhance neural transmission (French 2016).

So, initial strength gains following a resistance training programme are largely through neural adaptation. Gains made later on are more likely to result from muscle hypertrophy. In addition, neural adaptation is likely to be one of the factors leading to specificity of strength training.

Specificity of strength training

Maximum force production from a muscle is, then, the result of a blend of myogenic and neurogenic adaptations which are specific to a particular movement pattern. Improvements in contractile properties such as maximum force, velocity of shortening and rate of tension development can vary with the type of contraction used in training. Training a muscle to perform in a particular movement is not simply a question of overloading it against a resistance. For example, strengthening the leg muscles with a squatting exercise will not increase the performance on a leg-extension movement to the same degree as training the same muscles on a leg-extension bench. To strengthen a muscle for a specific movement, an exercise must mimic the movement as closely as possible. Similarly, strength gains resulting from isometric training will be specific to the joint angle at which the training was carried out.

Training a muscle at a specific velocity will result in strength gains at speeds close to, or less than, the training velocity, a phenomenon known as *velocity specificity*. One explanation of this principle is that before training, subjects are unable to produce maximal contractions at all velocities, and through practice they learn to fully activate their prime movers only at the velocities used during training.

Another possibility is preferential hypertrophy of one fibre type. There is little evidence for transformation of one fibre type to another, except following electrical stimulation. Preferential hypertrophy of Type II fibres does occur, but at both fast and slow velocities, so the neural explanation seems more likely. *Joint angle specificity* refers to strength gains which are maximized to the joint angle at which isometric strength training is performed. The degree to which joint angle specificity occurs is influenced by a number of factors, including joint angle, training intensity and duration of isometric contraction. Joint angle specificity is most marked at inner-range positions, and lessened in outer range. Longer durations of isometric contraction result in less specificity, with greater carry-over to other joint angles. To minimize joint angle specificity, isometric training should be performed at multiple angles, or if this is not possible with the muscle in a lengthened position. Further, the contraction duration and number of repetitions should be larger.

Definition

With *velocity specificity*, strength gains are maximized to the velocity of dynamic (concentric or eccentric) training. With *joint angle specificity*, they are maximized to the joint angle of static (isometric) contractions.

Training principles for strength, conditioning and rehabilitation

Needs analysis

Just as a therapist would always assess a patient prior to treatment, before an exercise programme can be prescribed, a *needs analysis* should be performed (Table 2.15). The needs analysis looks at both the subject and the task or sport to be performed. Information gained about these two areas serves as a foundation for designing an individualized programme. Exercise history and current fitness level give a starting point in terms of skills which the subject possesses, and within this area we should consider injury history and any exercise adaptations required as a result of injury. Tests of neuromuscular skill level may

Table 2.15 Needs analysis in strength & conditioning

Subject/athlete	Task/sport
Exercise history	Movement analysis
Current fitness level	Physiological requirements
Neuromuscular skill level	Injury risk

Data from Baechle and Earle 2015

be relevant and can form part of a functional screen targeting the skill base of the task or sport to be performed. For example, a manual worker with a history of lower back pain may require screening for lifting and bending actions which mimic their working environment (height/weight/complexity), while a trail runner may need screening of lower-limb alignment in single-leg squat to reflect hill descent on uneven ground. Movement analysis forms an essential part of the preparation, and gives information on joint movements and muscle work especially. From this the physiological requirements of the task/sport can be implied, and a programme planned accordingly, with specific aims and objectives.

Definition

An *aim* is what is intended to be achieved (the 'what' of the programme). *Objectives* are the steps required to achieve them (the 'how' of the programme).

Exercise selection

Once the aims and objectives of the exercise programme have been established, the next step is exercise selection, which requires knowledge of several factors. Generally, exercises can be classified as multi-joint (whole-body) or single-joint (isolation) movements. In strength and conditioning (S&C) terms, multi-joint actions which involve large body areas (chest, shoulder, hip) are termed 'core' actions, and those targeting smaller body areas and fewer joints (upper arm, lower back, forearm) are termed 'assistance' exercises. However, these terms can sometimes be confusing for subjects, as the term core is often synonymous with core stability. Although many multi-joint actions (e.g. deadlift) do target core stability, isolation actions (e.g. abdominal hollowing) are also used as part of a progressive core-stability training programme.

Key point

Multi-joint actions target large muscle areas and involve movement of several joints at the same time. *Single-joint* actions target smaller body regions and fewer joints.

Single-joint actions are often more important in the early stages of rehabilitation as they can be used to target weak areas – for example, the quadriceps following a knee injury. Multi-joint actions will also often require whole-body balance and stabilizing the spine during their performance, and so may be less appropriate for the early stages of rehabilitation. In the early stages of rehabilitation, targeting muscle balance may be important to redress any imbalances determined in the needs analysis. In the later stages of rehabilitation, movements are generally progressed to become more functional, in that they mimic actions to be performed in a work task or sport (sport-specific). Finally, exercise technique obviously improves with practice, so in the early stages of training exercises should be simpler, or form components of a more complex task to be performed when training experience allows.

Exercise order

Once exercises have been selected, the order in which they are performed must be decided. In general, the aim is to ensure that the performance of one exercise does not interfere with (degrade) the performance of the subsequent movement. Usually, this is achieved by performing multi-joint actions (larger muscle-mass trained) before single-joint actions (smaller muscle-mass trained). This is because multi-joint actions generally require more skill, whole-body balance, and coordination. To degrade this type of action by performing several single-joint movements first may leave a subject more open to injury. Within the multi-joint ground, more complex actions (e.g. power clean) would be performed before simpler movements (e.g. rack squat).

Where actions are not complex, other orders such as alternating push (e.g. chest press) and pull (e.g. seated row) allow for recovery between exercises, and orders such as upper limb/lower limb/trunk are often used as part of circuit weight training.

Training frequency and volume

Volume is usually taken in S&C terms to mean the product of resistance and exercise number. In weight training terms it would be the weight lifted (kg) and the number of sets and reps performed, giving a volume which represents the total work done (joules). For example, 3 sets of 10 reps with a 5 kg weights gives a volume of 150, which is less than 2 sets of 15 reps with a weight of 10 kg, which gives a volume of 300.

Definition

Training *volume* is a measure of total work done. In weight training, it is reps multiplied by sets multiplied by weight.

Although many therapists work with the traditional '3 sets of 10' model originally developed by DeLorme and Watkins (1948), variations of training volume have been shown to work best for different outcome aims. When working to develop strength, repetition numbers of 6 or less are recommended for sets of 2–6, while power training sees fewer reps (1–4) and a mid-range number of sets (3–5). Hypertrophy is best achieved with 6–12 reps and 3–6 sets, while endurance is targeted with more reps (>12) and fewer sets (2–3).

Training frequency is the number of workouts completed in a given time, for weight training typically the number of gym sessions in a week. The aim is to allow sufficient recovery for adaptation to the training stimulus to occur. For less experienced subjects, this may involve a rest day between workouts – for example, training on Monday, Wednesday and Friday. For more experienced subjects, recovery from the muscles worked rather than total rest allows multiple-day training. Rather than training the whole body, only certain muscle groups are trained, using a *split routine*. This might mean working the lower body for two days (Monday/Thursday) and alternating this with upper-body workouts for two days (Tuesday/Friday), leaving a single recovery day (Wednesday).

Definition

A *split routine* separates body parts or muscle groups and trains them on different days.

Training frequency will also be changed when preparing for competition, with fewer training sessions used when in competition (in-season) and greater numbers when not competing (off-season). Variation of this type forms the basis of periodization (Treatment Note 2.5).

Treatment note 2.5   Periodization

Training in the same way all the time can lead to boredom and stagnation, with physical development reaching a plateau. Splitting training up, to coincide with a subject's individual goals, is a feature of *periodization*. Periodization enables a subject to concentrate on certain types of training at particular times in the year, allowing one stage of training to progress into another.

Four categories are generally used for periodization:

▶ Pre-season training
▶ Early season training
▶ Peak season training
▶ Off-season training

The aim is to cover all the components of fitness, and to build to a peak just before competition or a specific goal, with the overall periodization programme usually lasting a year. This year-long period is called a *macrocycle*.

The first phase is the preparatory phase, divided into *pre-season* and *early season* training. Within a yearly macrocycle, pre-season training lasts for about four months; early season training for about one month. As a subject approaches his/her peak season, more skill training and sport/task-specific work is included. During the peak or competitive season, training will be designed to maintain the particular fitness and skill needed for competition.

Off-season training acts as a recovery period, psychologically refreshing the subject and allowing the body to slow down after the intense demands of competition. The timing of this period will depend on the type of sport. During off-season training, moderate activity should be maintained so that the progress made in the other periods is not lost. Each of these four periods, being divisions of the year-long macrocycle, is known as a *mesocycle*.

Although this type of training was designed originally for competitive athletes, benefits can still be obtained by fitness enthusiasts. For example, the casual tennis player can concentrate on weight training in pre-season training, in order to build up a foundation of strength. Fitness training can be brought in during early training, and skill training introduced. Skill training comes to the fore during the peak season, while strength training is usually dropped.

Tennis should not be played during the off-season period so that the player has a psychological break. Instead, light weight training begins again in preparation for the heavy strength training of the pre-season cycle.

The four mesocycle periods can again be divided into typically week-long units called *microcycles*. The microcycle is used to plan individual workouts in the gym.

Training intensity

Training intensity is how hard a subject works during an exercise. Traditionally in resistance training, the weight lifted (load) is used as a measure of intensity. As load increases, the number of repetitions which can be performed reduces. The maximum weight which can be lifted is often used as an assessment of load and performing a single lift (one repetition maximum, or 1 RM) or a sequence of ten lifts (ten repetition maximum or 10 RM) are typical measures. Practically, there are a number of issues in determining 1 RM. Fatigue after each lift means that a rest period of one to five minutes has to be given after a single repetition before the test can be repeated to failure. Also, the relationship between the 1 RM and 10 RM changes with training: 7–10 RM has been shown to represent 68 per cent of the 1 RM for untrained subjects but 79 per cent of the 1 RM for trained subjects (McArdle, Katch and Katch 2001).

> **Key point**
>
> 1 RM is the maximum weight a subject can lift once. 10 RM is the maximum weight lifted for 10 repetitions, and will be a percentage of the 1 RM value. The percentage value is less for an untrained subject.

In rehabilitation, the load imposed on a tissue is often monitored using a variety of laboratory devices, such as dynamometry or EMG. This type of monitoring measures what happens to a subject from the outside (external load measurement) and may quantify training using sets and reps, poundage lifted, distance run, watts produced, for example. Measurement from within the subject (internal load measurement) assesses physiological and psychological responses to an activity – for example, heart rate, rating of perceived exertion, or psychological inventories. While external load gives an understanding of the work completed, internal load can be viewed as more patient-centred in that it determines whether training is creating an appropriate stimulus for optimal biological adaptation. Internal load monitoring is generally more sensitive than external measures in determining both acute and chronic changes to a subject's individual well-being (Soligard et al. 2016).

> **Key point**
>
> *External* load measurement quantifies training using performance. *Internal* load measurement assesses physiological and psychological response to an activity

There is a high correlation between the results of external measurement and the use of a rating of perceived exertion (RPE) scale focusing on each individual training bout. The RPE scale was originally developed in the 1970s by physiologist Gunnar Borg, and has been modified several times. It is currently a ten-point scale where the subject uses their body sensations to create a perception of how hard they are working. In statistical terms, this is described as a *category ratio* scale and hence the official title of the test is the Borg CR10 scale (Fig. 2.13). RPE is a measure of exercise intensity at a specific time point, and is extended to *sessional RPE* (sRPE) by multiplying the total time of an exercise session (minutes) by the exercise intensity (RPE score). For example, a 30-minute workout at an RPE intensity of 5/10 would give a sRPE value of 150 units, whereas a longer more intense workout of 40 minutes at 7/10 would give a sRPE of 280 units, clearly illustrating the difference between the two exercise sessions in terms of load.

Plyometrics

Rapid eccentric contraction used immediately before an explosive concentric action (stretch–shorten cycle, or SSC) forms the basis of plyometric training. This type of training was first used in Eastern Bloc countries in the development of speed (Verhoshanski and Chornonson 1967). The movements involve three phases. Phase I is a pre-stretch of a muscle which

0	Nothing at all	
1		How you feel sitting or simply standing
2	Weak	
3	Moderate	Exercise goal: How you feel when you exercise
4		
5	Strong	
6		
7	Very strong	How you feel when you really push yourself
8		
9		
10	Extremely strong	
•	All-out effort	You're unable to go on

Figure 2.13 The rating of perceived exertion (RPE) scale.

contracts eccentrically. At full stretch (Phase II), there is a transition between eccentric and concentric contraction. This is termed the amortization or coupling phase and should be keep brief to prevent dissipation of the energy stored within the eccentric phase. Phase III is a rapid concentric contraction, causing the subject to move in the opposite direction. Effects are achieved in both the contractile and inert structures of the muscle.

Key point

The *stretch–shortening cycle* (SSC) consists of three phases. An eccentric lengthening (Phase I), a transition phase (Phase II) and a rapid concentric contraction (Phase III).

The rapid stretch of the muscle stimulates a stretch reflex, which in turn generates greater tension within the lengthening muscle fibres. In addition to increased tension, the release of stored energy within the elastic components of the muscle makes the concentric contraction greater than it would be in isolation. Increased tension will in

turn stimulate Golgi tendon organ (GTO) activity, inhibiting excitation of the contracting muscle. Desensitization of the GTO has been suggested as a possible mechanism by which plyometrics allows greater force production.

The use of muscle contraction involving acceleration in the concentric phase and deceleration in the eccentric phase more closely matches the normal function seen in sport, and therefore has advantages in terms of training specificity. However, the rapid movements involved are not suitable in early-stage training as they can be relatively uncontrolled.

Several neuromuscular adaptations have been proposed for the effect of plyometric exercise (Table 2.16), and exercise of this type has been shown to significantly increase peak power output (Potteiger 1999). Comparing plyometric exercises with their non-power equivalents demonstrates the advantages of this training. A plyometric jump compared to a deep knee-bend action, used 22 per cent less energy, produced 9 per cent more work and was 40 per cent more efficient (Lees and Graham-Smith 1996), while a rebound bench press compared to a standard lift gives 30 per cent more work, allowing the subject to lift 5.4 per cent greater weight.

Practical considerations of plyometric training

Plyometric exercise is only effective when the concentric contraction occurs immediately following the pre-stretch cycle. If there is a pause in the transition phase, some of the benefits are lost as elastic energy is wasted, and the effect of the stretch reflex is altered. The ability to recover the stored elastic energy within the tissues depends on the time period between concentric and eccentric activity (coupling time). The stored elastic energy of the leg extensor muscles has a half-life of 4 seconds (Lees and Graham-Smith 1996), and the coupling time in plyometric exercise has been measured at average periods of 23 ms. Providing the coupling time remains at these levels, nearly all the stored elastic energy can be utilized.

Table 2.16 Proposed neuromuscular adaptations to plyometric training

Increased inhibition of antagonist muscles
Better co-contraction of synergistic muscles
Inhibition of neural protective mechanisms
Increased motor neuron excitability

Source: Potteiger, J.A. (1999) Muscle power and fiber characteristics following 8 weeks of plyometric training. *Journal of Strength and Conditioning Research*, 13 (3), 275–279. With permission.

Injury considerations in plyometrics

This type of training is intense, and should only be used after a thorough warm-up, and usually at the end of an exercise programme. To perform plyometrics, the subject needs a good strength base, and his proprioceptive activity should be tested using single-leg standing and single-leg half squats (eyes closed, position maintained for 30 seconds) before training commences. Any loss in proprioception may cause the subject to fall as fatigue sets in. Safety considerations, including proper clothing and footwear and a firm non-slip sports surface, are essential.

Compression forces present in plyometrics have the potential for injury. Spinal shrinkage has been measured at 1.75 mm after 25 repetitions of a drop jump from a height of 1.0 m so this type of exercise is not suitable for individuals with a history of lower back pain of discal origin. In normal walking, deceleration forces have been measured at 3 g

(three times earth's normal gravity), while in a drop jump from a height of 0.4 m the deceleration has been measured at 23 g (Lees and Graham-Smith 1996). This type of force acting on the lower limb makes plyometrics unsuitable for those with a history of arthritis in the joints of the lower limb or spine.

> **Key point**
> Plyometrics is an advanced, intense form of exercise, not suitable for the beginner. Safety considerations are essential throughout.

Three types of exercises are normally used: in-place, short response and long response (Table 2.17). In-place activities include such things as standing jumps, drop jumps and hopping. Short-response actions are those such as the standing broad jump, the standing triple jump and box jumps. Long-response movements include bounding, hopping and repeated hurdle jumps.

Although plyometric activity is primarily used for lower-limb training, is does have an important place for the upper limb and trunk. Overhead throwing actions using a medicine ball, and throwing and catching from a bent-knee sit-up position, are examples of this.

Resistance may be added to increase the overload on the working muscles as the plyometric activity is used. Vertical jumps may be performed using

Table 2.17 Plyometric exercises

Exercise type	Movement	Description
In-place	▶ Standing jumps	Jumping and landing on the same spot, to emphasize the vertical component of the jump
	▶ Drop jumps	Use gravity and body weight to increase resistance and emphasize eccentric component of movement
	▶ Hopping	Straight, zig-zag or rotatory hopping on the same spot
Short response	▶ Standing broad jump	Emphasizes horizontal component of jump
	▶ Standing triple jump	Combines several jumps and hops over a distance
	▶ Box jumps	Jump over an object to emphasize both vertical and horizontal component of jump
Long response	▶ Bounding	Greater horizontal range than others. Single/double/alternate legs
	▶ Hopping	Repeated combinations of straight/zig-zag/rotatory hopping
	▶ Repeated hurdle jumps	Horizontal and vertical jump component for endurance

light dumb-bells, or a squat/leg press machine, and horizontal movements (lateral jumps, side hops) can be overloaded using an elastic cord.

Plyometrics has its use in late-stage rehabilitation, and functional pre-competitive testing following injury. The adaptations produced by this type of activity within a previously injured muscle are likely to make it more capable of withstanding explosive effort, as encountered in sprinting and jumping activities, for example. This, in turn, may reduce the risk of re-injury. Using heavy-resistance exercise in late-stage rehabilitation of the injured subject may allow the limb to regain lost strength, but without plyometric activity it is likely that the limb could still break down in the competitive situation, because the strength activity does not match the speed and power of the action to be used on the field of play.

Exercise progression

As we have seen, training requires progressive overload. Increasing weight (resistance) is only one method of progression. Table 2.18 lists other methods of progressing overload during rehabilitation. Increasing the resistance, exercise duration and frequency will make the exercise harder, as will reducing the rest interval. Altering the effect of gravity, by inclining or declining a bench, will affect the point of maximal leverage. Changing the length of the lever arm will also alter the resistance, for example arm abduction performed in the standing position will be harder with a weight bag in the hand than with one fastened to the elbow.

Table 2.18 Methods of progressing overload

▶ Resistance	▶ Speed of movement
▶ Leverage	▶ Range of motion
▶ Isolation	▶ Duration of exercise
▶ Gravity	▶ Type of muscle work
▶ Sets/repetitions	▶ Group action of muscles
▶ Rest interval	▶ Starting length of muscle
▶ Frequency of training	▶ Momentum/inertia

The relationship between length–tension and force–velocity means that altering the starting length of a muscle or the speed of movement will change the overload. For example, when performing a sit-up exercise the hip flexors and abdominal flexors will work. By bending the hips, the work of the hip flexors will be reduced, increasing the overload of the abdominal flexors.

As the speed of movement increases, the force output from the muscle is reduced. In addition, more rapid actions have more momentum and are therefore harder to stop (a safety consideration) and are performed with ballistic muscle actions.

The type of muscle work (isometric or isotonic) and the function of the muscle (agonist/fixator, etc.) can be used to great effect, as can the range of movement. Initial rehabilitation exercises, where range of movement is limited, tend to be isometric in nature, progressing to isotonic and increasing the range of motion. The motor skill involved with group muscle action makes it vital that a muscle is not simply worked as a prime mover, but as a fixator and synergist as well.

The combination of repetitions (number of complete executions of an exercise) and sets (number of repetitions grouped together) in weight training is the subject of considerable debate. In general, low numbers of repetitions have been traditionally used to increase strength, while higher numbers have been favoured for endurance. Medium numbers of repetitions are usually referred to as 'power' training, although it is unlikely that this would be effective unless the speed of the movement were increased.

Kinetic chain exercise

Movement of the limbs occurs as a kinetic chain. Several joints arranged in sequence move together to produce a complex motor action. If the terminal joint in the kinetic chain can move freely, the chain is open. If this same joint is unable to move independently because it faces a significant

Treatment note 2.6   Historical resistance training methods

DeLorme and Watkins

One of the earliest combinations of sets and repetitions is that of DeLorme and Watkins (1948). This method requires the user to first discover the maximum weight which can be lifted for the 10-repetition maximum (10 RM). The programme then consists of three sets of 10 repetitions at percentages of this maximal value, as follows:

1. 1st set, 10 repetitions at 50 per cent of 10 RM
2. 2nd set, 10 repetitions at 75 per cent of 10 RM
3. 3rd set, 10 repetitions at 100 per cent of 10 RM

In the original programme, strength gains were assessed using a 1 RM (single repetition maximum) each week, and gains in strength from 20 lb lifted before the programme to 60 lb lifted after 36 days were seen. The DeLorme and Watkins programme enables the movement to be rehearsed before a maximal contraction is required, perhaps recognizing the importance of neurogenic factors in strength performance.

Pyramid system

In this routine, the number of repetitions performed with each set is reduced as the weight increases, the subject working on a 'light to heavy' system. This results in the subject performing a few repetitions to fatigue when the muscle is thoroughly warm. An example is given below:

1. 1st set, 12 repetitions at 50 per cent maximum
2. 2nd set, 8 repetitions at 65 per cent maximum
3. 3rd set, 6 repetitions at 75 per cent maximum, or to fatigue

Oxford technique (reverse pyramid)

This is the reverse of the pyramid system. Now the user adopts a 'heavy to light' system, starting by performing 10 repetitions at their 10 RM and reducing to 75 per cent and 50 per cent of this value:

1. 1st set, 10 repetitions at 100 per cent 10 RM
2. 2nd set, 10 repetitions at 75 per cent 10 RM
3. 3rd set, 10 repetitions at 50 per cent 10 RM

The Oxford technique (Zinovieff 1951) works on the principle that as the muscle fatigues, the weight should be reduced to take account of the reduction in force output.

---

resistance, the action constitutes a closed kinetic chain.

Definition

In a *closed-chain* action, both the proximal and distal ends of the chain of movement are fixed, and motion occurs between the two. In an *open-chain* action, the proximal segment is fixed but the distal segment moves freely.

Most functional activities involving the lower limb in sport are performed using a closed kinetic chain. Walking, running, jumping and rising from a sitting position are all examples of closed kinetic chain activities. One of the only open kinetic chain activities of the lower limb normally used in sport is kicking.

We have seen the importance of exercise specificity in terms of muscle work and energy system, but the exercise must also be specific to the type of kinetic chain action used. To exercise the quadriceps on a leg-extension bench (open-chain) does not accurately reflect the demands placed on the lower limb with running and jumping (closed-chain). As many of the adaptations produced during resistance training, particularly in the first four weeks of training, are neurogenic in nature, the mismatch in movement patterns could detrimentally affect the subject's performance (Palmitier et al. 1991).

A common open-chain movement used in knee training is the seated leg-extension exercise (Fig. 2.14a). The muscles primarily responsible for this action are the quadriceps. Contrast this to the closed-chain movement of the squat (Fig. 2.14b). When the leg extends to raise the body from the squatting position, the hamstrings extend the hip and assist in knee extension as the foot is stabilized. This co-contraction (co-activation) greatly reduces the anterior shear forces acting on the knee, and is of particular importance in the

rehabilitation of anterior cruciate ligament (ACL) repairs.

Several additional differences exist between open- (single joint or 'isolation') and closed-chain (multi-joint or 'general') exercises in resistance training. In an open-chain action, movement occurs mainly distal to the joint axis, whereas with a closed-chain action, motion is both proximal and distal to the joint. An open-chain action, when performed slowly, primarily emphasizes concentric work, but a closed-chain movement brings a more balanced action of concentric, eccentric and isometric contractions into play.

Open-chain actions, when performed rapidly (punching and kicking for example), are often *ballistic* in nature. Here, muscles begin the movement and end it, but the middle part of the action also uses momentum of the moving limb. The limb is literally thrown into the action. This requires large acceleration and deceleration forces at the beginning and end of the action, and the muscle work involved is very subtly coordinated. During the final stages of rehabilitation especially, the type of coordination required for ballistic actions is important to retrain. Ballistic actions are used functionally in sport, but less obviously in day-to-day actions. For example, a rhythmic gardening activity is ballistic in nature, as is swinging a child in her mother's arms.

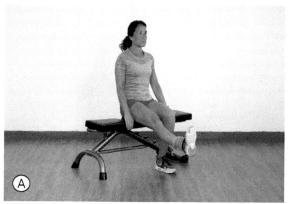

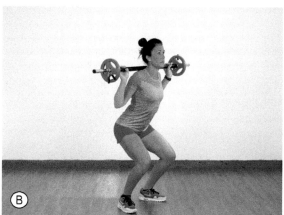

Figure 2.14 Open- and closed-chain movements.

Source: a) Leg extension – example of an open-chain movement b) Squat with barbell – example of a closed-chain movement.

Definition

A *Ballistic action* is high velocity, with rapid acceleration and deceleration. The EMG pattern is triphasic, showing activity in the agonist, then antagonist, and finally agonist muscles once more.

Implications for rehabilitation

The evidence on mixtures of sets, repetitions and types of muscle work indicates that no single combination yields optimal gains for everyone. In early rehabilitation, where range of motion is severely limited, isometric exercise is useful.

Performing this type of exercise in inner range will contribute to joint stability, and it is important that this be obtained before resisted movement is begun.

Because isometric gains are joint-angle specific, resistance training should progress rapidly to involve all types of muscle work. At the beginning of a weight-training programme we have seen that neurogenic changes predominate. Practising the skilled movement involved in the exercise is therefore important at this stage, so multi-set regimes are likely to be more successful. As rehabilitation progresses, all the fitness components must be worked. Power and speed are important and should be combined with rapid eccentric contractions in plyometric routines. Cardiopulmonary fitness may be maintained using circuit weight training, where lower-limb injury prevents activities such as running, cycling or swimming.

For pure strength gains, high-intensity programmes are more suitable for well-motivated individuals. Those who are poorly motivated may not be able to perform maximally in one set and so would be better to stay on more traditional multi-set programmes.

For a weight-training exercise to be maximal throughout the range of motion, the resistance offered to the muscle must change. Some form of accommodating resistance provided by an asymmetric cam or electronic braking system may be useful. Alternatively, free weights using body-building techniques such as 'forced repetitions' and 'cheating repetitions' can be used. Here, a training partner or body swing, respectively, is used to take the weight through the point of maximal leverage traditionally called the 'sticking point'.

Specificity of training makes it of paramount importance that exercise mimics as closely as possible the function which will be required of the subject. At this stage, sports-specific skills should be practised in preference to pure strength work.

Muscle pain

Muscle pain occurs under normal circumstances with exercise, and does not necessarily indicate injury. When training to maximum intensity, subjects will often be encouraged to continue an action until they reach *momentary muscular failure* (MMF), the point at which muscle strength fails to support a weight. The MMF point indicates that the muscle is exhausted, but, as we have seen with load measurement, above, there is a difference between performance (*external*) with a load and perception of that performance (*internal*), and muscle nociception can be a key component to this.

Two types of pain are generally recognized. First, pain which occurs during exercise but disappears when the activity stops (ischaemic pain). Second, with unaccustomed exercise, discomfort may not occur immediately afterwards, but pain comes on a number of days later (delayed-onset muscle soreness).

Key point

Ischaemic muscle pain occurs during exercise but disappears when activity stops. Delayed-onset muscle soreness (DOMS) does not occur immediately, but comes on a number of days later.

Ischaemic muscle pain

Pain of this type begins in the working muscle and increases in intensity as exercise continues. It disappears when exercise stops and generally leaves no after-effects. The rise in intramuscular pressure during exercise can compress the blood vessels running through a muscle, producing ischaemic pain.

The accumulation of metabolites is generally accepted to be the cause of the pain. Lactic acid is often cited as the culprit, but subjects who are unable to produce lactic acid (McArdle's syndrome) still suffer ischaemic pain. Histamine, acetylcholine, serotonin (5-HT), potassium and bradykinin are the most likely agents to cause the pain of ischaemia (Newham 1991).

Delayed onset muscle soreness

Delayed-onset muscle soreness (DOMS) is residual muscle pain which occurs 24 to 48 hours following unaccustomed bouts of intense exercise. Eccentric muscle work and exercise with a long muscle length have been shown to increase the intensity of the delayed-onset soreness (Jones, Newham and Torgan 1989). A number of possibilities exist for the cause of this pain, and it is probable that it is the result of a combination of factors, the contribution of each being related to activity type and individual differences (Table 2.19).

Mechanical trauma can develop as a result of the high tensions developed during eccentric contractions. More trauma is likely with eccentric work than with other muscle actions because the tensions created during eccentric contraction are usually greater. In a study of downhill running, increases in creatine kinase and myoglobin were seen, suggesting that structural damage was occurring within the muscle (Byrnes and Clarkson 1985).

Disruption seems to be to the connective tissue elements, rather than the contractile tissue within the active muscles. Hydroxyproline, a product of connective tissue breakdown, has been detected in the urine of subjects suffering from DOMS, suggesting connective tissue damage. The cytoskeleton of the muscle, when damaged, becomes more permeable, allowing excess leakage of muscle enzymes and an increased uptake of injected radioisotopes (Newham 1991). Further, changes in the sarcoplasmic reticulum of the muscle cell have been shown to depress calcium

muscle metabolism, altering muscle contraction and causing pain (McBride 1998).

Unaccustomed exercise can also produce a build-up of *metabolites* within the working muscle. This in turn will give rise to osmotic changes in the cellular environment of the muscle, resulting in fluid retention and subsequent pressure on sensory nerves. Similarly, ischaemia of the working muscle can occur, leading to an accumulation of pain (p) substance, bringing on reflex muscle spasm.

A number of methods have been suggested to relieve DOMS. Stretching has been shown to reduce pain in the anterior tibial muscles (DeVries 1961), and would certainly seem to be able to reduce muscle spasm. Increasing the blood flow to the muscle during the warm-down period is also helpful. This can be achieved by gentle exercise, hot showers or massage. In each case, a possible mechanism of relief is that of flushing fresh blood through the muscle to remove metabolic wastes, and pumping the lymphatic vessels to remove local oedema and reduce interstitial pressure.

Muscle fatigue

Muscle fatigue can present as a loss of force or power output, slowing of relaxation, changes in contractile characteristics and alterations in electrical properties, and represents the point of MMF detailed above. Two basic mechanisms of fatigue have been described, *central* and *peripheral*. Central fatigue refers to changes occurring proximal to the motor neurone, and involves neural and psychological changes such as motivation and recruitment. Peripheral fatigue involves the motor unit itself, and occurs chiefly through exhaustion of the muscle energy supplies. The type and intensity of activity being performed will decide whether central and peripheral fatigue occur separately or in combination.

Table 2.19 Factors associated with delayed-onset muscle soreness (DOMS)

- ▶ Micro-tearing of muscle contractile elements
- ▶ Resulting release of creatine kinase, myoglobin and troponin
- ▶ Damage to muscle connective tissue
- ▶ Local fluid retention due to osmotic pressure change
- ▶ Local inflammatory reaction
- ▶ Increased local muscle tone/spasm
- ▶ Change in calcium regulation within muscle cell

Key point

Changes in *central fatigue* are largely psychological in nature, those of *peripheral fatigue* are mainly physiological.

If a subject is told to push as hard as possible for as long as possible, without feedback, force output will fall due to fatigue. If central fatigue occurs, more force can only be generated when the muscle is stimulated electrically.

Traditionally, fatigue types have been studied by comparing forces generated by maximum stimulated contraction (MStC), with those of maximal voluntary contractions (MVC). In unfatigued muscle, the MVC is the same as the MStC. With central fatigue, the force produced during MVC is less than that from an MStC, while in peripheral fatigue there is no difference between force of MVC and MStC (Bigland-Ritchie 1981).

Peripheral fatigue can be further categorized into high- and low-frequency types. The natural firing frequencies of normal voluntary contractions are approximately 5–30 Hz. High-frequency fatigue occurs when a muscle is stimulated at high frequencies between 50 and 100 Hz, while low-frequency fatigue is the loss of force at low stimulation frequencies between 10 and 40 Hz.

Uncontrolled movement

The term uncontrolled movement (UCM) was proposed by Comerford and Mottram (2013) to build on a history of therapy based on movement change developed by a series of practitioners over the last 50 years. Within physiotherapy, classic work by Kendall et al. (1993), Janda (1993), Richardson (1992), Jull and Janda (1987) Sahrmann (1987), Hodges and Richardson (1995) and Norris (1995) have all outlined changes in movement which may be associated with a patient's symptoms. The key thrust to this concept is that rather than movement change simply being a result of pathology, it may be an important factor in its development.

Key point
Change in movement may be associated with pathology. Altered movement may precede or follow symptoms.

Basic concepts

Changes in muscle length or strength often occur in set patterns rather than at random. The relationship between the tone and length of muscles has been termed muscle imbalance (Janda and Schmid 1980). Muscles may be broadly classified into two types for convenience. Those whose actions are mainly to *stabilize* a joint and approximate the joint surfaces, and those responsible more for *movement*, which effectively develop angular rotation. The main differences between the two types of muscles are shown in Table 2.20. As we will see, this categorization helps to clarify exercise prescription but is not an exact science. Some muscles or portions of muscles fall into both camps, and importantly the classification does not infer pathology, so its clinical relevance must always be appraised.

Key point
Stability muscles hold a joint or body part firm and immobile. Movement muscles create body motion. Many muscles can act to achieve either function.

The stability muscles (stabilizers) tend to be more deeply placed, while the movement muscles (mobilizers) are superficial. In addition, mobilizers are often biarticular (two-joint) muscles (see Chapter 1). For example, in the leg, the rectus femoris is classified as a mobilizer, while the quadriceps are stabilizers. Stabilizer function is often more slow-twitch (Type I) or tonic in nature, while that of the mobilizers tends towards fast-twitch (Type II) phasic action. This physiology

Table 2.20 Muscle types (basic classification)

Stability	Movement
Deep	Superficial
Slow-twitch	Fast-twitch
One joint	Two joint
Weaken and lengthen	Tighten and shorten
Inhibited	Preferential recruitment

suits the functional requirements of the muscles, enabling mobilizers to contract and build maximal tension rapidly, but at the cost of fatiguing quickly. The stabilizers build tension slowly and perform well at lower tensions over longer periods, being more fatigue-resistant.

Classification of a muscle as a stabilizer with predominantly tonic functions refers to its most consistent response. Many muscles are able to exhibit both tonic and phasic contraction depending on requirement at the time. For example, transversus abdominis shows tonic activity during gait, when it contributes to spinal stability, but phasic activity associated with expiration during rapid breathing (Saunders, Rath and Hodges 2004). Both the diaphragm (Hodges and Gandevia 2000) and the pelvic floor muscles (Hodges, Pengel and Sapsford 2007) exhibit tonic activity during an active arm-lifting task and phasic activity during challenged breathing.

> **Key point**
>
> Muscles often exhibit both tonic (holding) and phasic (moving) responses, depending on the functional requirement at any one time.

In general, stabilizer muscles are better activated in closed-kinetic-chain actions, where movement occurs proximally on a distally stabilized segment. Mobilizer function is more effective in an open-chain situation, where free movement occurs without distal fixation. The structure and functional characteristics of the two muscle categories make the stabilizers better equipped for postural holding and anti-gravity function. The mobilizers are better set up for rapid ballistic movements.

> **Key point**
>
> Movement muscles (mobilizers) are better activated in open-chain actions. Stability muscles (stabilizers) are better activated in closed-chain actions.

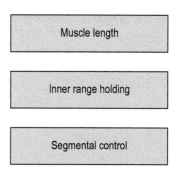

Figure 2.15 Assessing muscle imbalance.

Two of the fundamental changes seen in the muscle imbalance process include tightening of the mobilizer (two-joint) muscles and laxity/loss of endurance within the inner range for the stabilizer (single-joint) muscles. These two changes are often used as tests for the degree of muscle imbalance. The combination of length and tension changes can alter muscle pull around a joint and potentially pull the joint out of alignment. Changes in body-segment alignment and the ability to perform movements which dissociate one body segment from another form the bases of the third type of test used when assessing muscle imbalance (Fig. 2.15).

> **Key point**
>
> Through misuse or injury, stabilizing muscles tend to become lax (sagging) while movement muscles tend to tighten.

The mixture of tightness and weakness seen in the muscle imbalance process can alter body segment alignment and may change the equilibrium point of a joint. In addition, imbalance leads to lack of accurate segmental control. The combination of stiffness (hypoflexibility) in one body segment and laxity (hyperflexibility) in an adjacent body segment leads to the establishment of relative flexibility (White and Sahrmann 1994). In a chain of movement, the body seems to take the path of least resistance, with the more flexible segment moving first and furthest. We can take as an illustration two pieces of rubber tubing (Fig. 2.16) of unequal strengths. When the movement begins at

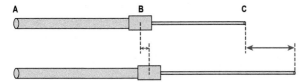

Figure 2.16 Relative stiffness. When the cord is stretched, the tighter segment (A–B) moves less than the looser segment (B–C).

C and A is fixed, the more flexible area B–C moves more. This will still be the case if C is held still and A moves.

Taking this example into the body, Figure 2.17 shows a toe-touching exercise. The two areas of interest with relation to relative stiffness are the hamstrings and lumbar spine tissues. As we flex forwards, movement should occur through a combination of anterior pelvic tilt and lumbar spine flexion. Subjects often have tight hamstrings and looser lumbar spine tissues due to excessive bending during everyday activities. During this flexion action, greater movement, and therefore greater tissue strain, will always occur at the lumbar spine. Excessive motion at this point can lead initially to pain, simply through overstretch of pain-sensitive structures. In the short to mid-term, the tissue insult creates an inflammatory response which both maintains the pain response and causes swelling. Longer term, the combination of altered movement and tissue stress may lead to overuse injury. It becomes apparent in the toe-

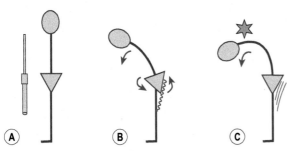

Figure 2.17 Relative stiffness in the body. (A) Tighter hamstrings, laxer spinal tissues. (B) Forward flexion should combine pelvis tilt and spinal flexion equally. (C) Tight hamstrings limit pelvic tilt, throwing stress on the laxer spinal tissues.

touching example that relative stiffness makes the toe-touching exercise ineffective as a hamstring stretch, unless the trunk muscles are tightened to stabilize the lumbar spine.

> **Definition**
>
> Relative flexibility (relative stiffness) occurs when the body takes the path of least resistance in a movement. Tighter tissues will allow less movement, while looser (lax) tissues allow more.

Muscle adaptation

Muscle adaptation to reduced usage has been extensively studied using immobilized limbs (Appell 1990). The greatest tissue changes occur within the first days of disuse. Strength loss has been shown to be as much as 6 per cent per day for the first eight days, with little further loss after this period. Greater reduction in size and loss of numbers is seen in Type I fibres, with a parallel increase in Type II fibres, demonstrating selective atrophy of Type I fibres (Templeton et al. 1984). However, not all muscles show an equal amount of Type I fibre atrophy. Atrophy is largely related to change in use relative to normal function, with the initial percentage of Type I fibres that a muscle contains being a good indicator of likely atrophy pattern. Those muscles with a predominantly anti-gravity function, which cross one joint and have a large proportion of Type I fibres, show greatest selective atrophy (e.g. soleus and vastus medialis). Selective wasting in the calf muscles illustrates this well, with the soleus wasting by 60 per cent and the plantaris by only 17 per cent (Thomason et al. 1987). Those predominantly slow anti-gravity muscles, which cross multiple joints, are next in order of atrophy (e.g. erector spinae); last are phasic, predominantly fast, Type II muscles, which can be immobilized with less loss of strength (e.g. biceps) (Lieber 1992). In addition to atrophy, apoptosis (programmed cell death) and infiltration of phagocytic cells has been shown to occur within

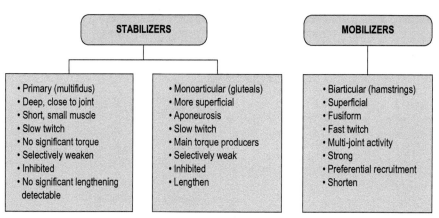

Figure 2.18 Muscle types (extended classification). After Jull (1994).

48 hours of immobilization in the soleus muscle (Ferreira et al. 2008).

> **Key point**
>
> Following immobilization, muscles with a large number of Type I (slow) fibres will show more marked atrophy. Muscles with predominantly Type II (fast) fibres show less loss of cross-sectional area (CSA) and strength.

These three categories of muscles have led to stabilizers being subdivided into *primary* and *secondary* types (Jull 1994), as shown in Figure 2.18. Examples of the three types include multifidus, transversus abdominis and vastus medialis oblique as primary stabilizers. The gluteals and oblique abdominals are classified as secondary stabilizers, while rectus femoris and the hamstrings are mobilizers, only acting as stabilizers in conditions of extreme need.

The primary stabilizers have very deep attachments, lying close to the axis of rotation of the joint. In this position they are unable to contribute any significant torque, but will approximate the joint. In addition, many of these smaller muscles have important proprioceptive functions (Bastide, Zadeh and Lefebvre 1989). The secondary stabilizers are the main torque producers, being large monoarticular muscles

attaching via extensive aponeuroses. Their multipennate fibre arrangement makes them powerful and able to absorb large amounts of force through eccentric action. The mobilizers are fusiform in shape, with a less powerful fibre arrangement, but one which is designed for producing large ranges of motion. In addition, the mobilizers are biarticular muscles, which have their own unique biomechanical characteristics.

Selective changes in muscle may also occur as a result of training (Richardson and Bullock 1986). In the knee, rapid flexion–extension actions have been shown to selectively increase activity in the rectus femoris and hamstrings (biarticular) but not in the vasti (monoarticular). In this study, comparing speeds of 75°/s and 195°/s, mean muscle activity for the rectus femoris increased from 23.0 uV to 69.9 uV. In contrast, muscle activity for the vastus medialis increased from 35.5 uV to only 42.3 uV (Fig. 2.19). The pattern of muscle activity was also noticeably different in this study after training. At the fastest speeds, the rectus femoris and hamstrings displayed phasic (on and off) activity, while the vastus medialis showed a tonic (continuous) pattern.

Even in the more functional closed-kinetic-chain position, similar changes have been found (Ng and Richardson 1990). A four-week training period of rapid plantarflexion in standing gave significant increases in jump height (gastrocnemius,

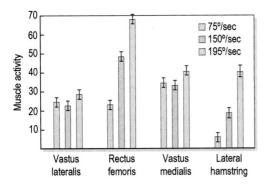

Figure 2.19 Changes in muscle activity with increases in speed. From Richardson, C.A. and Bullock, M.I. (1986) Changes in muscle activity during fast, alternating flexion–extension movements of the knee. *Scandinavian Journal of Rehabilitation Medicine*, **18**, 51–58. With permission.

biarticular) but also significant losses of static function of the soleus (monoarticular).

Changes in muscle length

Chronic muscle lengthening

Stabilizer muscles tend to 'weaken' (sag), whereas mobilizers tend to 'shorten' (tighten). Taking these responses further, primary stabilizers will react quickly to pain and swelling, by inhibition. Swelling has been shown to cause a reflex inhibition of muscles in the knee (Stokes and Young 1984). In addition, marked asymmetry of the multifidus has been shown using real-time ultrasound imaging. Adaptation of the primary stabilizers of the spine is covered in Chapter 8

Key point
Primary stabilizers adapt to reduced usage by (i) a shift in the recruitment patterns and timing of the synergistic muscle actions they are linked to, (ii) a reduction in cross-sectional area (CSA) and (iii) pathological changes to their muscle structure.

Adaptation of secondary stabilizers

The secondary stabilizer muscles show a tendency to *lengthen* and *weaken*. As postural muscles, they almost seem to give way to the pull of gravity and 'sag'. This reaction has been termed stretch weakness (Kendall, McCreary and Provance 1993). The muscle has remained in an elongated position, beyond its normal resting position, but within its normal range. This is differentiated from overstretch, where the muscle is simply elongated or stretched beyond its normal range.

The length–tension relationship of a muscle dictates that a stretched muscle, where the actin and myosin filaments are pulled apart, can exert less contractile force than a muscle at normal resting length. Where the stretch is maintained, however, this short-term response (reduced-force output) changes to a long-term adaptation. The muscle tries to move its actin and myosin filaments closer together, and to do this, it must add more sarcomeres to the ends of the muscle (Fig. 2.20). This adaptation, known as an increase in serial sarcomere number (SSN), changes the nature of the length–tension curve.

Definition
Serial sarcomere number (SSN) is the number of sarcomere units along an individual

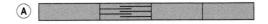
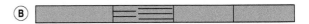
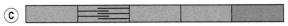

Figure 2.20 Muscle length adaptation. (A) Normal muscle length. (B) Stretched muscle—filaments move apart and muscle loses tension. (C) Adaptation by increase in serial sarcomere number (SSN), normal filament alignment restored, muscle length permanently increased.

> muscle fibre. Muscles held in a lengthened position for a prolonged period will adapt by increasing their SSN.

Long-term elongation of this type causes a muscle to lengthen by the addition of up to 20 per cent more sarcomeres (Gossman, Sahrmann and Rose 1982). The length–tension curve of an adaptively lengthened muscle moves to the right (Fig. 2.21). The peak tension that such a muscle can produce in the laboratory situation is up to 35 per cent greater than that of a normal length muscle (Williams and Goldspink 1978). However, this peak tension occurs at approximately the position where the muscle has been immobilized (point A, Fig. 2.21). If the strength of the lengthened muscle is tested with the joint in mid-range or inner-range (point B, Fig. 2.21), as is common clinical practice, the muscle cannot produce its peak tension, and so the muscle appears 'weak'. For this reason, manual muscle tests have been described as being more accurate indicators of positional (rather than total) strength (Sahrmann 1987).

In the laboratory situation, the lengthened muscle will return to its optimal length within approximately a week if once more placed in a shortened position (Goldspink 1992). Clinically, restoration of optimal length may be achieved by immobilizing the muscle in its physiological rest position (Kendall, McCreary and Provance 1993) and/or exercising it in its shortened (inner-range) position (Sahrmann 1990). Enhancement of strength is not the priority in this situation; indeed, the load on the muscle may need to be reduced to ensure correct alignment of the various body segments and correct performance of the relevant movement pattern.

Immobilization of cat hind limb in a lengthened position (four weeks) showed a 19 per cent increase in SSN of the soleus muscle but no change in individual sarcomere length. Immobilizing in a shortened position gave a 40 per cent decrease in SSN, again with no change in sarcomere length (Tabary 1972). It has been argued that this type of adaptation enables the muscle to develop maximum tension when movement of the muscle is limited (Jaspers, Fagan and Tischler 1985).

SSN may be partly responsible for changes in muscle strength without parallel changes in hypertrophy (Koh 1995). SSN exhibits marked plasticity and may be influenced by a number of factors. For example, immobilization of rabbit plantarflexors in a lengthened position showed an 8 per cent increase in SSN in only four days, while applying electrical stimulation to increase muscle force showed an even greater increase (Williams et al. 1986). Stretching a muscle appears to have a greater effect on SSN than does immobilization in a shortened position. Following immobilization in a shortened position for two weeks, the mouse soleus has been shown to decrease SSN by almost 20 per cent (Williams 1990). However, stretching for just one hour per day in this study not only

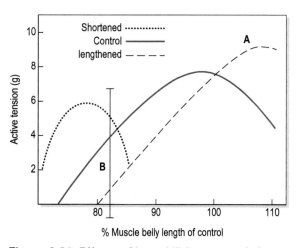

Figure 2.21 Effects of immobilizing a muscle in shortened and lengthened positions. The normal length–tension curve (control) moves to the right for a lengthened muscle, giving it a peak tension some 35 per cent greater than the control (point A). When tested in an inner-range position (point B), however, the muscle tests weaker than normal. Reprinted from Gossman, M.R., Sahrmann, S.A. and Rose, S.J. (1982) Review of length associated changes in muscle. *Physical Therapy*, **62** (12), 1799–1808. With permission.

eliminated the SSN reduction but actually produced nearly a 10 per cent increase in SSN. Static stretching, using a programme to mimic that used in sports (30 s hold, repeated for 25 reps with a 15 s rest, three times per week for four weeks), has been shown to increase SSN in rats, with corresponding changes to the biomechanical properties of the muscle-tendon unit (De Jaeger et al. 2015).

An *eccentric stimulus* may cause a greater adaptation of SSN than a concentric stimulus. Morgan and Lynn (1994) subjected rats to uphill or downhill running, and showed SSN in the vastus intermedius to be 12 per cent greater in the eccentric trained rats after one week. In contrast to this, however, Koh and Herzog (1998) used the dorsiflexor muscles of the rabbit to assess the effect of eccentric training on SSN. Using a two-week training session over a total of twelve weeks, they found little effect on SSN or fibre length, but the variation between the studies may well be related to species or training protocol differences.

Key point

Exercising at short muscle lengths reduces serial sarcomere number (SSN), while exercising at long muscle lengths increases SSN.

It has been suggested that if SSN adaptation occurs in humans, strength training might produce this type of change if it is performed at a joint angle different from that at which the maximal force is produced during normal activity (Koh 1995).

Rather than being weak, the lengthened muscle lacks the ability to maintain a full contraction within inner range. This shows up clinically as a difference between the active and passive inner ranges. If the joint is passively placed in full anatomical inner range, the subject is unable to hold the position. Sometimes the position cannot be held at all, but more usually the contraction cannot be sustained, indicating a lack in slow-twitch endurance capacity.

Key point

Clinically, lengthened muscles are identified by their inability to shorten completely and hold the joint they cross at full inner range.

Shortening posturally lengthened muscle

Clinically, reduction of muscle length is seen as the enhanced ability to hold this inner-range contraction. As the muscle is already strong, the focus is not on resistance but on *joint position* (alignment) and *holding time*. The muscle is passively positioned within its inner range and the patient is instructed to hold this position. Initially, this will not be possible and the limb will fall away from the inner-range joint position. The patient should be encouraged to slow the rate of limb fall to initiate an eccentric contraction. Once this is achieved, the eccentric action is emphasized, with the therapist placing the joint within its inner range and the patient using an eccentric action to guide the limb descent. Over time (sometimes within one treatment session, more normally within two to three sessions), the patient will be able to hold the inner-range position for a short period of time (seconds only). The next phase in the restoration of muscle balance is to emphasize the inner-range holding ability, building to 10–30 seconds holding. Finally, the patient uses a concentric action to pull the limb into its inner-range position, holds using an isometric action, and lowers under control (eccentric). At this point, muscle control through full range has been achieved.

Key point

Shortening a posturally lengthened muscle is achieved by working within inner-range only. The initial muscle work is eccentric, followed by isometric contractions with minimal loading.

Inner-range holding may or may not represent a reduction in SSN but is a required functional improvement in postural control. Muscle shortening may certainly be achieved through splinting. Muscles immobilized in a shortened position in this way show loss of sarcomeres in series within 14–28 days (Williams and Goldspink 1978). With training, there is less evidence for reduction in SSN in humans. Muscle shortening has been shown in the dorsiflexors of horse riders. Clearly, this position is not held permanently as with splinting, but rather shows a training response. Following pregnancy, SSN increases in the rectus abdominis in combination with diastasis. Again, the length of the muscle gradually reduces in the months following birth. It is generally thought that inner-range training is likely to shorten a lengthened muscle, although the precise method through which this adaptation is achieved in humans is not certain (Goldspink 1992). The treatment aim for a posturally lengthened muscle must ultimately be to change its resting length and therefore correct segmental alignment. In so doing, the joints within a body region will be able once more to move through an optimal movement range (Sahrmann 2002).

> **Key point**
>
> To restore the serial sarcomere number (SSN) and shorten a chronically lengthened muscle, it can be (i) splinted in a shortened position, (ii) worked within inner range, (iii) subjected to eccentric loading. A combination of these procedures will give the best clinical result.

Inner-range holding ability

The ability of a stabilizer muscle to maintain an isometric contraction at low load over a period of time is vital to its anti-gravity function. This may be assessed by using the classic muscle test position and asking the subject to maintain a contraction in full inner range. The important factor in the assessment is the length of time a static hold can be maintained without jerky (phasic) movements occurring. In each case, the limb is placed passively into full inner range. When released, if the limb drops, the passive range of motion differs from the active range, which is an important indicator of poor stabilizer function. Full stabilizing function is achieved when a subject can maintain the inner-range position for 10 repetitions, each of 10 seconds duration (Jull 1994). Often the first two or three repetitions are performed normally, and it is only with further repetitions that the deficit becomes apparent.

> **Key point**
>
> Inner-range holding ability is assessed by holding the test position for 10 seconds and repeating this action 10 times.

Segmental control

Segmental control is the ability to dissociate the movement of one body segment from that of a neighbouring segment. It is dependent on stabilization ability and adequate mobilizer length. Where imbalance exists, lengthened muscle will fail to act sufficiently and will be dominated by shortened overactive movement muscles. This imbalance leads to an alteration in the movement pattern controlled by the muscles, giving subtle changes seen on examination. The *quality* of the patient's movement changes, making movement less efficient. Subjectively, we can say that movement is suboptimal or incorrectly executed. The patient's action may be described as a *movement dysfunction*.

> **Definition**
>
> Segmental control is the ability to dissociate the movement of one body segment from another. It is dependent on stabilization ability and adequate mobilizer length.

The central features of segmental control require the pelvis to tilt independently of the lumbar spine in both frontal and sagittal planes, the shoulder girdle and thoracic spine to move in relation to each other, and the upper and lower portions of the cervical spine to move in a controlled fashion.

Restoration of muscle balance

Three elements combine to restore muscle balance: correction of *muscle length*, increasing *core stability* and correction of *segmental control*. The order in which these are used will depend on the patient's symptoms, and will often be governed by pain rather than alignment. For example, where a tight muscle is causing pain, this will be targeted first. If excess motion at the lumbar spine is causing overuse injury, stability may be chosen first to limit stress on inflamed tissue.

Muscle length

Tight muscles may inhibit their antagonists (Jull and Janda 1987) and often develop painful trigger points. This is especially the case in the upper limbs (Fig. 2.22). A trigger point (myofascial trigger point) is often located within a tight band of muscle. The point is painful to palpation and the muscle will often go into spasm if the trigger point is palpated briskly or flicked (the jump sign). For more information on trigger point pathology and treatment, see Norris (2001).

> ### Definition
> A trigger point (TrP) is a highly sensitive local area within a taut band of muscle fibres. TrPs are thought to result from: (i) muscle ischaemia, (ii) a hyperactive muscle spindle, (iii) excessive release of acetylcholine at the muscle motor end plate.

Furthermore, through relative flexibility, a tight muscle will throw stress onto a hyperflexible body segment, causing tissue stress and pain. Elimination of tightness and redevelopment of stability, coupled with correction of segmental movement, is therefore a key aim of treatment.

Where pain is a prominent factor, the elimination of this pain may be the primary aim of treatment.

Pain which occurs through muscle spasm, or through trigger points in tight muscle, may be relieved by treatment aimed at reducing muscle tone. This can be achieved by modalities or manual therapy, and will often involve the use of stretching (Table 2.21).

Stability

Where pain is the result of persistent overstress on a hypermobile segment, the initial treatment should be aimed at segmental control and stability. Stability may have to be applied passively at first (through taping or splinting) until sufficient control of the muscular stabilizing system has been gained. Core stability itself is divided into three overlapping phases: *muscle isolation*, *restoration of back fitness* and *functional actions*. For full details of back stability rehabilitation programmes see Norris (2015a).

Segmental control

Finally, where the tissues themselves are normal, but poor alignment has become habitual (particularly in adolescent athletes), coordination and alignment training may be all that is required. This will necessitate close inspection and regular feedback, and the use of a video in these cases is of great value.

Proprioceptive training
Background to proprioceptive training

Proprioception is a specialized variation of touch which encompasses both joint movement and joint position sense. Practically, it is the ability of the body to use position sense and respond either consciously or unconsciously to stresses imposed on the body by altering posture and movement. The conscious response to perception of limb or body position is sometimes referred to separately as kinaesthesia, leaving the term proprioception for unconscious perception. Some authors refer to kinaesthesia as motion sense and proprioception as position sense (Aman et al. 2014).

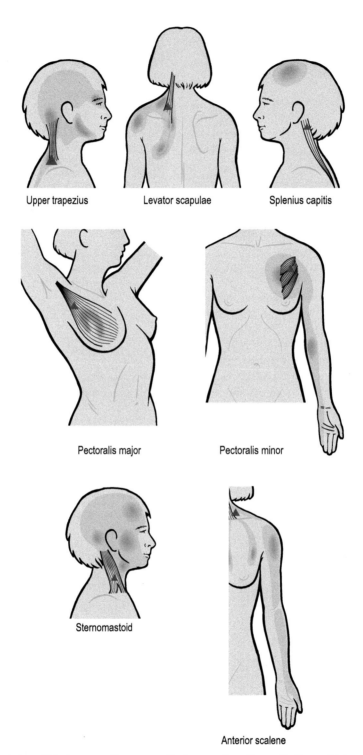

Upper trapezius

Levator scapulae

Splenius capitis

Pectoralis major

Pectoralis minor

Sternomastoid

Anterior scalene

Figure 2.22 Trigger points within hyperactive upper limb muscles. From Petty and Moore (2001), with permission.

Table 2.21 Methods of treating trigger points

Deep massage
Sustained local finger point pressure
Deep local circular massage (finger/probe)
Local and regional finger point pressure (acupressure)
Ice massage
Static stretching
PNF stretching
Muscle energy technique (MET)
Spray stretch (Vapocoolant spray)
Dry needling: shallow
Dry needling: deep (intramuscular stimulation, IMS)
Electrical point stimulation (non-invasive electroacupuncture)
Electrotherapy
Transcutaneous electrical nerve stimulation (TENS)
Interferential therapy (IF)
Low-level laser therapy (LLLT)
Ultrasound (U/S)
Vibration massage

Definition

Proprioception is the awareness of the body in space. It is the use of joint-position sense and joint-motion sense to respond to stresses placed upon the body by alteration of posture and movement.

Proprioceptive training uses exercises which challenge a joint to detect and react to afferent input about joint position (Schiftan et al. 2015). It aims to enhance sensorimotor function by using somatosensory signals such as touch or limb-position sense without information from other areas such as vision (Aman et al. 2014). In exercise terms, proprioception encompasses three aspects, known as the 'ABC of proprioception'. These are: agility, balance and coordination. *Agility* is the capacity to control the direction of the body or body part during rapid movements, while *balance* is the ability to maintain equilibrium by keeping the line of gravity of the body within the body's base of support. *Coordination* is the smoothness of an activity. This is produced by a combination of muscles acting together with appropriate intensity and timing.

Proprioceptive exercise is progressed in terms of skill and complexity rather than pure overload.

The aim is to perform gradually more challenging actions while maintaining movement accuracy. The emphasis therefore is on *quality* of motion rather than quantity (volume) of muscle work.

Proprioception and injury

Several factors may contribute to a reduction in proprioception following injury (Table 2.22).

Joint effusion contributes to a reduction in mechanoreceptor discharge, resulting in inhibition of muscular contraction. This is especially seen in the vastus medialis (VMO) of the knee, for example, where just 60 ml of intra-articular effusion may result in 30–50 per cent inhibition of quadriceps contraction (Kennedy, Alexander and Hayes 1982). Proprioceptive deficits have also been shown to parallel joint degeneration (Barrett, Cobb and Bentley 1991), but it is unclear whether this occurs as a result of degeneration, or is in fact part of its aetiology (Lephart and Fu 1995). Injury to mechanoreceptors at the time of injury reduces proprioceptive inflow, a situation which may continue for some time following resolution of gross tissue damage. In addition, fatigue will alter both muscle spindle discharge and spinal reflexes to impair the performance of fine motor skill performance (Röijezon et al. 2015).

Table 2.22 Factors contributing to reduced proprioception following injury

Joint swelling	▶ Inhibited skeletal muscle
	▶ Impaired proprioceptive inflow
Tissue injury	▶ Concurrent damage to mechanoreceptors at time of injury
Fatigue	▶ Altered muscle spindle discharge
	▶ Altered spinal reflexes
	▶ Clumsiness and difficulty performing fine motor tasks
Pain	▶ Altered reflex activity and sensitivity of muscle spindles
	▶ Altered body perception
	▶ Reorganization of somatosensory cortex

(Data from Röijezon et al. 2015)

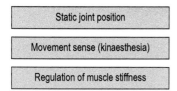

Figure 2.23 Components of proprioception.

> **Key point**
>
> Following injury, an athlete's proprioceptive ability will be impaired. Training to restore this is an important part of the rehabilitation of sports and soft tissue injuries.

From a clinical standpoint, proprioception may be seen to consist of three interrelating components (Fig. 2.23), representing activity at spinal, brainstem and higher-centre levels. Each component is assessed by a variety of different tests.

Static joint position sense

First, static joint position sense is used to maintain posture and balance at brainstem level. Input for these actions is from joint proprioception, the vestibular centres in the ears, and from the eyes. Balance and postural exercise with the eyes open and/or closed may be used to enhance static joint position sense. This component is commonly measured by tests which address reproduction of passive positioning (RPP) and reproduction of active positioning (RAP). The subject is required to return the joint to its start position after either an active or passive movement.

Movement sense

Second, kinaesthetic awareness, or 'movement awareness', is a result of higher-centre activity. This component encompasses the detection of both joint displacement and velocity change. It is commonly assessed by measuring the threshold to detection of passive motion (TTDPM), the subject simply stating when he or she feels movement has begun. Once movement has been detected through kinaesthetic awareness, motor

programmes may be performed automatically in many cases. Consciously performed joint-positioning activities, especially at end-range, will enhance the development of automatic control and cognitive awareness (Lephart and Fu 1995).

Regulation of muscle stiffness

Finally, closed-loop efferent activity is required for reflex (spinal) activity and regulation of muscle stiffness, leading to dynamic joint stability. This type of activity underlies all movements by supplying reflex splinting when a joint is stressed. Damage to joint receptors has been shown to affect co-contraction of muscles and reduce joint stability. This, in turn, can lead to an increase in the likelihood of injury.

Proprioception is enhanced at this level through the initiation of reflex joint stabilization, using activities which involve sudden alterations in joint position. Reflex stabilization is therefore assessed through measurement of the onset of muscle contraction in relation to joint displacement. The aim is to see if the muscles are able to limit joint displacement and effectively stabilize the joint.

> **Key point**
>
> Train static *joint position sense* using balance exercises with the eyes open/closed, *movement sense* with joint positioning activities at end-range, and *muscle stiffness* with sudden alteration of joint angle.

Proprioceptive research

Using TTDPM and RPP, Barrack and Skinner (1984) found decreased kinaesthesia with increasing age. In general, our highly mechanized Western society may fail to impose the variety of movements which an individual requires for optimal musculoskeletal health. This reduced movement 'vocabulary' decreases the proprioceptive stimulation needed for skilled motor action. After injury, proprioceptive input is further reduced due to prolonged inactivity and damage to proprioceptive nerve endings within the injured tissues. A number of authors have stressed the importance of proprioceptive training in rehabilitation following injury to the knee (Beard et al. 1994), ankle (Schiftan et al. 2015) and shoulder (Lephart et al. 1994). The functional importance of proprioceptive training has also been emphasized during rehabilitation of the spine (Norris 1995), although its use in spinal rehabilitation is less common than for other areas of the body.

Proprioception may be enhanced with training. Barrack and Skinner (1984) found enhanced kinaesthesia in trained dancers, and Lephart and Fu (1995) demonstrated the same in intercollegiate gymnasts. Both of these types of athletes practise free exercise using bodyweight as resistance, and use complex multi-joint activities. This type of training would seem appropriate for proprioceptive rehabilitation.

Training techniques

Proprioceptive training involves highly skilled actions, often performed at speed, with the aim of making the movement less attention-demanding (automatic). Proprioceptive exercises are progressed in terms of speed and complexity, aiming at quality of movement execution rather than simple overload. Multiple sensory inputs are used to improve the sense of both static position and movement. Once this has been achieved, dynamic stability exercises may be used.

Proprioceptive training may be performed by following the general stages by which an athlete actually learns any skilled action (Table 2.23).

Practical aspects of proprioceptive training

Localized proprioceptive training can involve reproduction of passive positioning (RPP), working with a partner, followed by active joint positioning, working alone. With a partner, the subject aims to reproduce the limb/joint position which was moved passively by their therapist or training partner.

Table 2.23 Proprioceptive training

Increase awareness of correct pattern
Split complex movement sequence into simple components
Increase awareness by passive movement using multisensory input
Gain voluntary control of movement pattern
Use multisensory stimulation during demonstration and performance of exercise
Start with slow precise movements Stop exercising when patient becomes fatigued Continually correct movement pattern passively Progress exercise only when movement pattern is correct Patient must perform independently before proceeding to more advanced actions Link simple tasks to form more complex actions
Gain automatic control of movement
Progress speed while maintaining accuracy of movement
Perform multiple repetitions of movement sequence
Perform actions with other body parts while maintaining accurate stability in the affected body part

From Norris, C.M. (1995) Spinal stabilisation, 2. Limiting factors to end range motion in the lumbar spine. *Physiotherapy*, 81, 4–12. Chartered Society of Physiotherapy. With permission.

Following practice, error is reduced and active position may be performed. Using a laser pointer, handheld for the upper limb, attached to a strap for the lower limb, or on a headband for the neck, is a useful method of self-monitoring.

General proprioceptive training begins by splitting complex movements into a number of simple component sequences, with the choice of exercise being determined by the functional requirements of the subject. Splitting the movement in this way enables the subject to focus their attention selectively on a single action, making learning far easier. Initially, actions must be slow and precise, with the emphasis on control of the correct body position. The rate of movement is progressed, while maintaining accuracy, and the simple movement components are linked together to form the total activity sequence. The subject must stop when they become fatigued; failure to do so will often lead to practice of incorrect exercise technique and negative transfer effects.

Treatment note 2.7   How subjects learn skilled movements

Proprioceptive exercises are highly skilled, and in order to effectively prescribe this type of training we need to understand the way that an athlete actually learns a skilled movement. There are three overlapping stages to motor skill (movement) learning (Fitts and Posner 1967, Schmidt and Lee 2011), as shown in Table 2.24.

Stage I (cognitive)

The first stage is *understanding*, where the athlete attempts to form an idea of the whole skill. The process is cognitive (thinking) rather than motor (doing) in nature, hence the title of this learning stage. The athlete is learning what to do (and, importantly, what not to do), and how to do it.

Environmental cues which later will go unnoticed are important to this early stage of learning. They provide an important frame of reference for building the new skill. For example, when learning a new dance step, a person will often focus attention on the foot position, which they later take for granted.

In this stage, movements will be poorly coordinated. The athlete must concentrate intensely and will therefore tire easily. The therapist can assist by providing clear instructions and feedback. Complex actions should be split up into more simple components. For example, a single-leg hop and twist would be learned as a single-leg balance first in Stage I. This would be followed by straight-line hopping, and, eventually, hopping and twisting on the spot, and finally hopping and twisting over a distance, in Stages II and III.

Demonstration of the movement is important, and the athlete will need constant coaching and correction of the skill to prevent them practising mistakes.

Table 2.24 Learning motor skills

Stage of learning		
Stage (I) – understanding	**Stage (II) – effective movement**	**Stage (III) – automatic action**
Understand what is required from action	Refine action	Less attention required
Environmental cues important	Able to recognize own mistakes	Movement seems to 'run by itself'
Movements poorly coordinated	Movements more consistent and efficient	Speed of movement increased
Demonstration and movement cueing important	Energy expenditure lower	
Practical implication		
Split complex movement sequences into simple components	Correct movement pattern when/if it erodes	Distract athlete to ensure less attention is used
Increase movement awareness by cueing	Stop if athlete becomes fatigued	Progress speed of movement while maintaining accuracy
Use palpation and passive movement to facilitate learning	Link simple actions together into sequences	Increase repetitions
Slow precise actions	Reduce environmental cues	Alter environmental cues
Progress only when athlete can perform action independently of therapist	Increase repetitions as endurance improves	Perform multiple actions
	Require athlete to recognize their own mistakes (self-monitoring)	

Treatment note 2.7 *continued*

One of the ways we can help learning in this stage is to use *cueing*, to paint a mental picture of an action in terms which an athlete can easily understand. For example, an abdominal hollowing action may be cued by asking the athlete to pull the tummy button in (visual), or use the fingers to feel the abdomen tightening (tactile). The instructor may use voice intonation (auditory) to indicate the intensity of the movement.

Definition

A cue is a signal which facilitates a particular action, and may be verbal, visual or tactile in nature. When a number of cues facilitate an action, multisensory cueing is being used.

Stage II (motor)

This is the stage of *effective movement*, when the athlete will try to make the motor programme more precise and refine the action. It is as though the original clumsy action is 'whittled down' to a smoother defined movement. Through practice, the athlete is now able to recognize mistakes, and so self-practice (unsupervised) can now be allowed.

The dependence on visual and verbal cues (Stage I) now gradually gives way to the reliance on proprioceptive information. Movements become more consistent and the athlete is able to work on the finer details of an action. As the action becomes more efficient, energy expenditure is reduced because the athlete does not have to work as hard to produce the action. Environmental cues are used for timing and, as anticipation develops, movements become smoother and less rushed.

Key point

As a motor skill becomes more efficient, energy expenditure is reduced and movements become smoother.

The individual movement sequences used in Stage I are now linked together to give a longer skill sequence. The actions must still be slow and precise, with progression made only when the movement sequence is correct.

Stage III (automatic)

In this stage, the action 'runs by itself' or becomes *automatic* (grooved). Movements in this stage demand less attention to perform, so the athlete can now perform other actions at the same time. The speed of the movement may be increased, and functions such as muscle reaction time become important. Here, the body is challenged (for example, knocking it off balance) and the athlete must react quickly, with appropriate changes in posture and movements. This type of final training is used with balance balls and gym balls, for example.

Definition

A negative transfer effect occurs when an activity in training is learned to such a degree that it actually interferes with a skilled movement in sport performance.

Movement of other body parts draws the athlete's attention away from the conscious control of the core action, and assists in the development of automatic actions. Rather than practising isolated exercises to repetition, functional activities should be built into an athlete's activities of daily living (ADL).

Using proprioceptive training of the ankle as an example, single-leg standing may begin, followed by single-leg standing with quarter-squat activities, and finally, the same base activity with throwing and catching. This could be built into a subject's daily activities (ADL) by performing simple home exercises, such as cleaning the teeth while standing on one leg!

Once an action can be performed correctly on a stable surface, the subject may use a moving base of support such as a balance cushion, balance board or vibration plate. The subject must now use not just joint position and movement sense, but anticipation of body displacement, requiring reflex stabilization. Initially, the mobile surface should involve uniaxial movements, for example a rocker board. Placing the pivot of this type of board in the frontal plane will work the flexion and extension reaction, while placing the pivot in the sagittal plane will work abduction and adduction. If the pivot is then placed diagonally, movements will be biaxial in nature. Progression is made to the balance board, where the pivot point is dome-shaped to allow triaxial motion. Other apparatus useful for balance work and muscle reaction includes the large-diameter (65 cm) gymnastic ball and the mini-trampette, or simply a cushion placed on the floor.

Examples of proprioceptive training for the ankle, knee, shoulder and spine are given in the relevant clinic chapters for these body parts.

References

Aagaard, P., Simonsen, E., Andersen, J. et al., 2002. Increased rate of force development and neural drive of human skeletal muscle following resistance training. *Journal of Applied Physiology* **93** (4), 1318–1326.

Alter, M.J., 1996. *Science of Flexibility*, second ed. *Human Kinetics*, Champaign, Illinois, USA.

Aman, J.E., Elangovan, N., Yeh, I.-L., Konczak, J., 2014. The effectiveness of proprioceptive training for improving motor function: a systematic review. *Frontiers in Human Neuroscience* **8**, 1075.

American College of Sports Medicine (ACSM), 1978. The recommended quantity and quality of exercise for developing and maintaining fitness in healthy adults. *Medicine and Science in Sports and Exercise* **10**, VII–X.

American College of Sports Medicine (ACSM), 1990. The recommended quantity and quality of exercise for developing and maintaining cardiorespiratory and muscular fitness in healthy adults. *Medicine and Science in Sports and Exercise* **22**, 265–274.

American College of Sports Medicine, 2002. Progression models in resistance training for healthy adults. *Medicine and Science in Sports and Exercise* **34**, 364–380.

Andersson, S.H., Bahr, R., Clarsen, B. et al., 2016, Preventing overuse shoulder injuries among throwing athletes: a cluster-randomised controlled trial in 660 elite handball players. *British Journal of Sports Medicine* **51** (14), 1073–1080.

Appell, H.J., 1990. Muscular atrophy following immobilisation: a review. *Sports Medicine* **10**, 42.

Baechle, T., Earle, R., 2015. *Essentials of strength training and conditioning*. 3rd ed. Human Kinetics. Champaign, Illinois.

Bandy, W.D., Irion, J.M., 1994. The effect of time on static stretch of the flexibility of the hamstring muscles. *Physical Therapy* **74** (9), 845–852.

Bandy, W.D., Lovelace-Chandler, V., McKitrick-Bandy, B., 1990. Adaptation of skeletal muscle to resistance training. *Journal of Orthopaedic and Sports Physical Therapy* **12** (6), 248–255.

Barnard, R.J., Gardner, G.W., Diaco, N.V., MacAlpin, R.N., Kattus, A.A., 1973. Cardiovascular responses to sudden strenuous exercise: heart rate, blood pressure, and ECG. *Journal of Applied Physiology* **34**, 883.

Barrack, R.L., Skinner, B.L., 1984. Joint kinaesthesia in the highly trained knee. *Journal of Sports Medicine and Physical Fitness* **24**, 18–20.

Barrett, D.S., Cobb, A.G., Bentley, G., 1991. Joint proprioception in normal, osteoarthritic, and replaced knees. *Journal of Bone and Joint Surgery* **73B**, 53–56.

Bartlett, M.J., Warren, P.J., 2002. Effect of warming up on knee proprioception before sporting activity. *British Journal of Sports Medicine* **36**, 132–134.

Bastide, G., Zadeh, J., Lefebvre, D., 1989. Are the 'little muscles' what we think they are? *Surgical and Radiological Anatomy* **11**, 255–256.

Beard, D.J., Kyberd, P.J., O'Connor, J.J., Fergusson, C.M., Dodd, C.A.F., 1994. Reflex hamstring contraction latency in anterior cruciate ligament deficiency. *Journal of Orthopaedic Research* **12** (2), 219–228.

Behm, D.G., Button, D.C., Butt, J.C., 2001. Factors affecting force loss with prolonged stretching. *Canadian Journal of Applied Physiology* **26**, 261–272.

Behm, D.G., Blazevich, A.J., Kay, A.D., Malachy M., 2016, Acute effects of muscle stretching on physical performance, range of motion, and injury incidence in healthy active individuals: a systematic review. *Applied Physiology, Nutrition, and Metabolism* **41**, 1–11.

Bigland-Ritchie, B., 1981. EMG and fatigue of human voluntary and stimulated contractions. In: Porter, R., Whelan, J. (eds), *Human Muscle Fatigue: Physiological Mechanisms*. Ciba Foundation Symposium 82, Pitman Medical, London.

Bouchard, C., Daw, E.W., Rice, T., 1998. Familial resemblance for VO2max in the sedentary state: the HERITAGE family study. *Medicine and Science in Sports and Exercise* **30** (2), 252–258.

Bouchard, C., Rankinen, T., 2001. Individual differences in response to regular physical activity. *Medicine and Science in Sports and Exercise* **33** (6 Suppl), S446–51.

Byrnes, W.C., Clarkson, M.C., 1985. Delayed onset muscle soreness following repeated bouts of downhill running. *Journal of Applied Physiology* **59**, 283.

Carroll, T.J., Herbert, R.D., Munn, J. et al., 2006. Contralateral effects of unilateral strength training: evidence and possible mechanisms. *Journal of Applied Physiology* **101** (5), 1514–1522.

Clark, B.C., Manini, T.M., 2012. What is dynapenia? *Nutrition* **28**, 495–503.

Clarkson, P.M., Byrnes, K.M., 1986. Muscle soreness and serum creatine kinase activity following isometric, eccentric, and concentric exercise. *International Journal of Sports Medicine* **7**, 152–155.

Comerford, M. and Mottram, S., 2013. *Kinetic control. The management of uncontrolled movement.* Churchill Livingstone. London.

Cook, J.L., Docking, S.I., 2015. "Rehabilitation will increase the 'capacity' of your …insert musculoskeletal tissue here…." Defining 'tissue capacity': a core concept for clinicians. *British Journal of Sports Medicine* **49**,1484–1485.

Costill, D.L., Fink, W.J., Getchell, L.H., Ivy, J.L., Witzmann, F.A., 1979. Lipid metabolism in muscle of endurance trained males and females. *Journal of Applied Physiology: Respiratory, Environmental and Exercise Physiology* **47**, 787.

De Jaeger, D., Joumaa, V., and Herzog, W., 2015. Intermittent stretch training of rabbit plantarflexor muscles increases soleus mass and serial sarcomere number. *Journal of Applied Physiology* **118** (12), 1467–1473.

DeLorme, T., Watkins, A., 1948. Techniques of progressive resistance exercise. *Archives of Physical Medicine and Rehabilitation* **29**, 263–273.

DeVries, H.A., 1961. Prevention of muscular distress after exercise. *Research Quarterly* **32**, 177.

Dye, S., 2005. The pathophysiology of patellofemoral pain – a tissue homeostasis perspective. *Clinical Orthopaedics and Related Research* **436**, 100–110.

Ekstrand, J., Gillquist, J., Moller, M., et al., 1983. Incidence of soccer injuries and their relation to training and team success. *American Journal of Sports Medicine* **11** (March–April), 63–67.

Emery, C.A., Roy, T., Whittaker, J.L. et al., 2015. Neuromuscular training injury prevention strategies in youth sport: a systematic review and meta-analysis. *British Journal of Sports Medicine* **49**, 865–870.

Enoka, R.M., 1994. *Neuromechanical Basis of Kinesiology*, 2nd ed., Human Kinetics. Champaign, Illinois.

Etnyre, B.R., Abraham, L.D., 1986. H-reflex changes during static stretching and two variations of proprioceptive neuromuscular facilitation techniques. *Electroencephalography and Clinical Neurophysiology* **63**, 174–179.

Etnyre, B.R., Lee, E.J., 1987. Comments on proprioceptive neuromuscular facilitation stretching. *Research Quarterly for Exercise and Sport* **58** (2), 184–188.

Farrell, P.A., Gates, W.K., Morgan, W.P., Pert, C.B., 1983. Plasma leucine enkephalin-like radioreceptor activity and tension-anxiety before and after competitive running. In: Knuttgen, H.G., Vogel, J.A., Poortmans, J. (eds), *Biochemistry of Exercise*. Human Kinetics, Champaign, Illinois.

Ferreira, R., Neuparth, M.J., Vitorino, R. et al., 2008. Evidences of Apoptosis during the early phases of soleus muscle atrophy in hindlimb suspended mice. *Physiol. Res* **57**, 601–611.

Fiatarone, M.A., 1994. Exercise training and nutritional supplementation for physical frailty in very elderly people. *New England Journal of Medicine* **330**, 1769.

Fitts, P.M., Posner, M.I., 1967. *Human Performance*. Greenwood Press, Westport, Connecticut.

Fowles, J.R., Sale, D.G., Macdougall, J.D., 2000. Reduced strength after passive stretch of the human plantarflexors. *Journal of Applied Physiology* **89**, 1179–1188.

Fradkin, A.J., Gabbe, B.J., Cameron, P.A., 2006. Does warming up prevent injury in sport? The evidence from randomized controlled trials. *Journal of Science and Medicine in Sport* **9**, 214–220.

French, D., 2016. Adaptations to anaerobic training programs. In: Haff, G.G. and Triplett,

N.T. (eds) *Essentials of Strength Training and Conditioning*. 5th ed. Human Kinetics. Champaign, Illinois.

Gabriel, D.A., Kamen, G. & Frost, G. (2006) Neural adaptations to resistive exercise. M: mechanisms and recommendations for training practices. *Sports Med.* **36**, 133.

Garber, C.E., Blissmer, B., Deschenes, M.R., Franklin, B.A., Lamonte, M.J., Lee, I.M., Nieman, D.C., Swain, D.P., 2011. American College of Sports Medicine. American College of Sports Medicine position stand. Quantity and quality of exercise for developing and maintaining cardiorespiratory, musculoskeletal, and neuromotor fitness in apparently healthy adults: guidance for prescribing exercise. *Medicine & Science in Sports & Exercise*. Jul; **43** (7):1334–1359.

Goldberg, B., Saranitia, A., Witman, P., 1980. Preparticipation sports assessment: an objective evaluation. *Pediatrics* **66**, 736–745.

Goldspink, G., 1992. Cellular and molecular aspects of adaptation in skeletal muscle. In: Komi, P.V. (ed.), *Strength and Power in Sport*. Blackwell, Oxford.

Gossman, M.R., Sahrmann, S.A., Rose, S.J., 1982. Review of length associated changes in muscle. *Physical Therapy* **62** (12), 1799–1808.

Griffiths, M.D., Szabo, A., and Terry, A., 2005. The exercise addiction inventory: a quick and easy screening tool for health practitioners. *British Journal of Sports Medicine* **39**, e30.

Grooms, D.R., Palmer, T., Onate, J.A. et al., 2013. Soccer-specific warm-up and lower extremity injury rates in collegiate male soccer players. *Journal of Athletic Training* **48** (6), 782–789.

Hartig, D.E., Henderson, J.M., 1999. Increasing hamstring flexibility decreases lower extremity overuse injuries in military basic trainees. *American Journal of Sports Medicine* **27**, 173–176.

Henneman, E., Somjen, G., Carpenter, D.O., 1965. Functional significance of cell size in spinal motoneurons. *Journal of Neurophysiology* **28**, 560–580.

Herbert, R.D., Gabriel, M., 2002. Effects of stretching before and after exercising on muscle soreness and risk of injury: systematic review. *British Medical Journal* **325**, 468–470.

Hodges, P., Gandevia, S., 2000. Activation of the human diaphragm during a repetitive postural task. *Journal of Physiology* **522**, 165–175.

Hodges, P.W., Pengel, H.M., Sapsford, R., 2007. Postural and respiratory function of the pelvic floor muscles. *Neurourology and Urodynamics* **26** (3), 362–371.

Hodges, P.W., Richardson, C.A., 1995. Neuromotor dysfunction of the trunk musculature in low back pain patients. In: *Proceedings of the World Confederation of Physical Therapists Congress*, Washington.

Janda, V., 1993. Muscle strength in relation to muscle length, pain and muscle imbalance. In: Harms-Ringdahl, K. (ed.), *Muscle Strength: International Perspectives in Physical Therapy*, 8th ed. Churchill Livingstone, Edinburgh.

Janda, V., Schmid, H.J.A., 1980. *Muscles as a pathogenic factor in backpain*. Proceeding of the International Federation of Orthopedic Manipulative therapists 4th conference. New Zealand. pp. 17–18.

Jaspers, S.R., Fagan, J.M., Tischler, M.E., 1985. Biomechanical response to chronic shortening in unloaded soleus muscles. *Journal of Applied Physiology* **59**, 1159–1163.

Jeffreys, I., 2007. Warm-up revisited: The ramp method of optimizing warm-ups. *Professional Strength Cond* **6**, 12–18.

Jeffreys, I., Moody, J., 2016. *Strength and conditioning for sports performance*. Routledge, Abingdon.

Jones, D.A., Newham, D.J., Torgan, C., 1989. Mechanical influences on long standing human muscle fatigue and delayed onset muscle pain. *Journal of Physiology* **224**, 173–186.

Jones, R.J., Wright, V., 1982. Relative importance of various tissues in joint stiffness. *Journal of Applied Physiology* **17** (5), 824–828.

Jull, G.A., 1994. Headaches of cervical origin. In: Grant, R. (ed.), *Physical Therapy of the Cervical and Thoracic Spine*. Churchill Livingstone, New York.

Jull, G.A., Janda, V., 1987. Muscles and motor control in low back pain: assessment and management. In: Twomey, L.T. (ed.), *Physical Therapy of the Low Back*. Churchill Livingstone, New York.

Kendall, F.P., McCreary, E.K., Provance, P.G., 1993. *Muscles. Testing and Function*, 4th ed. Williams and Wilkins, Baltimore.

Kennedy, J.C., Alexander, I.J., Hayes, K.C., 1982. Nerve supply of the human knee and its functional importance. *American Journal of Sports Medicine* **10**, 329.

Kenney, W.L., Wilmore, J.H., Costill, D.L., 2015. *Physiology of sport and exercise*. 6th ed. Human Kinetics, Champaign, Illinois

Koh, T.J., 1995. Do adaptations in serial sarcomere number occur with strength training? *Human Movement Science* **14**, 61–77.

Koh, T.J., Herzog, W., 1998. Eccentric training does not increase sarcomere number in rabbit dorsiflexor muscles. *Journal of Biomechanics* **31**, 499–501.

Kokkonen, J., Nelson, A.G., Cornwall, A., 1998. Acute muscle stretching inhibits maximal strength performance. *Research Quarterly for Exercise and Sport* **69**, 411–415.

Lees, A., Graham-Smith, P., 1996. Plyometric training: a review of principles and practice. *Sport Exercise and Injury* **2**, 24–30.

Lemmer, J.T., Hurlbut, D.E., Martel, G.F., Tracy, B.L., Ivey, F.M., Metter, E.J., Fozard, J.L., Fleg, J.L., Hurley, B.F., 2000. Age and gender responses to strength training and detraining. *Medicine & Science in Sports & Exercise*. Aug; **32** (8): 1505–1512.

Lephart, S.M., Fu, F.H., 1995. The role of proprioception in the treatment of sports injuries. *Sports Exercise and Injury* **1** (2), 96–102.

Lephart, S.M., Warner, J.P., Borsa, P.A., Fu, F.H., 1994. Proprioception of the shoulder in normal, unstable, and surgical individuals. *Journal of Shoulder and Elbow Surgery* **3** (4), 371–381.

Lieber, R.L., 1992. *Skeletal Muscle Structure and Function*. Williams and Wilkins, Baltimore.

Magnusson, S.P., Simonsen, E.B., Kjaer, M., 1996. Biomechanical responses to repeated stretches in human hamstring muscle in vitro. *American Journal of Sports Medicine* **24** (5), 622–628.

McArdle, W.D., Katch, F.I., Katch, V.L., 2001. *Exercise Physiology, Energy, Nutrition, and Human Performance*, 5th ed., Lea and Febiger, Philadelphia.

McBride, J.M., 1998. Effects of resistance exercise on free radical production. *Medicine and Science in Sports and Exercise* **30**, 67.

McNair, P.J., Stanley, S.N., 1996. Effect of passive stretching and jogging on the series elastic muscle stiffness and range of motion of the ankle joint. *British Journal of Sports Medicine* **30**, 313–318.

Moore, M.A., Kukulka, C.G., 1991. Depression of Hoffman reflexes following voluntary contraction and implications for proprioceptive neuromuscular facilitation therapy. *Physical Therapy* **71**, 321–333.

Morgan, D.L., Lynn, R., 1994. Decline running produces more sarcomeres in rat vastus intermedius muscle fibers than does incline running. *Journal of Applied Physiology* **77**, 1439–1444.

Nardone, A., Romanò, C., and Schieppati, M. (1989). Selective recruitment of high-threshold human motor units during voluntary isotonic lengthening of active muscles. *The Journal of Physiology*, **409**, 451–471.

Newham, D.J., 1991. Skeletal muscle pain and exercise. *Physiotherapy* **77** (1), 66–70.

Ng, G., Richardson, C.A., 1990. The effects of training triceps surae using progressive speed loading. *Physiotherapy Practice* **6**, 77–84.

Nieman, D., Pedersen, B., 1999. Exercise and immune function. *Sports Medicine* **27** (2), 73–80.

Norris C.M (2015a) *The Complete Guide to Back Rehabilitation*. Bloomsbury.

Norris, C.M (2015b) *The Complete Guide to stretching* (4th ed) Bloomsbury. London.

Norris, C.M., 1995. Spinal stabilisation. *Physiotherapy* **81** (2), 1–4.

Norris, C.M., 2001. *Acupuncture: Treatment of Musculoskeletal Conditions*. Butterworth-Heinemann, Oxford.

Olsen, O.E., Myklebust, G., Engebretsen, L., 2005. Exercises to prevent lower limb injuries in your sports: cluster randomized controlled trial. *British Medical Journal* **330**, 449–452.

Palmitier, R.A., An, K., Scott, S.G., Chao, E.Y.S., 1991. Kinetic chain exercise in knee rehabilitation. *Sports Medicine* **11** (6), 402–413.

Potteiger, J.A., 1999. Muscle power and fiber characteristics following 8 weeks of plyometric training. *Journal of Strength and Conditioning Research* **13** (3), 275–279.

Prud'homme, D., Bouchard, C., Leblanc, C., Landry, F., Fontaine, E., 1984. Sensitivity of maximal aerobic power to training is genotype-dependent. *Medicine and Science in Sports and Exercise* **16** (5), 489–493.

Richardson, C.A., 1992. *Muscle imbalance: principles of treatment and assessment.* Proceedings of the New Zealand Society of Physiotherapists Conference. Christchurch, NZ.

Richardson, C.A., Bullock, M.I., 1986. Changes in muscle activity during fast, alternating flexion–extension movements of the knee. *Scandinavian Journal of Rehabilitation Medicine* **18**, 51–58.

Richmond, S., Berg, C.V.D., Owoeye, O. et al., 2017. The efficacy of a neuromuscular training program in junior high school students. *British Journal of Sports Medicine* **51**, 379.

Röijezon, U., Clark, N., and Treleaven, J., 2015. Proprioception in musculoskeletal rehabilitation.

Part 1: Basic science and principles of assessment and clinical interventions. *Manual Therapy* Jun; **20** (3), 368–377.

Rosenbaum, D., Henning, E.M., 1995. The influence of stretching and warm up exercises on Achilles tendon reflex activity. *Journal of Sports Science* **15**, 481–484.

Safran, M.R., Garrett, W.E., Seaber, A.V., Glisson, R.R., Ribbecsk, B.M., 1988. The role of warmup in muscular injury prevention. *American Journal of Sports Medicine* **16** (2), 123–129.

Sahrmann, S.A., 1987. Posture and muscle imbalance: faulty lumbar-pelvic alignment and associated musculoskeletal pain syndromes. *Postgraduate Advances in Physical Therapy*, Forum Medicum, Berryville, Virginia.

Sahrmann, S.A., 1990. Diagnosis and treatment of movement-related pain syndromes associated with muscle and movement imbalances, course notes, Washington University.

Sahrmann, S.A., 2002. *Diagnosis and Treatment of Movement Impairment Syndromes*. Mosby, St Louis.

Sale, D.G., 1988. Neural adaptation to resistance training. *Medicine and Science in Sports and Exercise* **20** (5), 135–145.

Sale, D.G., 1992. Neural adaptation to strength training. In: Komi, P.V. (ed.), *Strength and Power in Sport*. IOC Medical Publication, Blackwell Scientific, Oxford.

Sapega, A.A., Quedenfel, T.C., Moyer, R.A., Butler, R.A., 1981. Biophysical factors in range of motion exercise. *Physician and Sports Medicine* **9** (12), 57–65.

Saunders, S.W., Rath, D., Hodges, P.W., 2004. Postural and respiratory activation of the trunk muscles changes with mode and speed of locomotion. *Gait Posture* **20**, 280–290.

Schiftan, G., Ross, L., and Hahne, A., 2015. The effectiveness of proprioceptive training in preventing ankle sprains in sporting populations: a systematic review and meta-analysis. *J Sci Med Sport* **18** (3), 238–244.

Schmidt, R.A. and Lee, T.D. (2011) *Motor control and learning* (5th ed). Human Kinetics. Champaign. Illinois.

Seward, H.G., Patrick, J., 1992. A three-year survey of Victorian football league injuries. *Australian Journal of Medicine and Science in Sport* **24** (2), 51–54.

Sipala, S., Suominen, H., 1995. Effects of strength and endurance training on thigh and leg muscle mass and composition in elderly women. *Journal of Applied Physiology* **78**, 334.

Smith, L.L., Brunetz, M.H., Chenier, T.C., 1993. The effects of static and ballistic stretching on delayed muscle soreness and creatine kinase. *Research Quarterly for Exercise and Sport* **64**, 1438–1446.

Soligard T, et al. (2016) How much is too much? (Part 1) International Olympic Committee consensus statement on load in sport and risk of injury. *British Journal of Sports Medicine* **50**, 1030–1041.

Stokes, M., Young, A., 1984. The contribution of reflex inhibition to arthrogenous muscle weakness. *Clinical Science* **67**, 7–14.

Tabary, J.C., 1972. Physiological and structural changes in the cat's soleus muscle due to immobilisation at different lengths by plaster casts. *Journal of Physiology* **224**, 231–244.

Taylor, D.C., Dalton, J., Seaber, A.V., Garrett, W.E., 1990. The viscoelastic properties of muscle-tendon units. *American Journal of Sports Medicine* **18**, 300–309.

Templeton, G.H., Padalino, M., Manton, J., et al., 1984. Influence of suspension hypokinesia on rat soleus muscle. *Journal of Applied Physiology* **56**, 278–286.

Thomason, D.B., Herrick, R.E., Surdyka, D., Baldwin, K., 1987. Time course of soleus muscle myosin expression during hind limb suspension and recovery. *Journal of Applied Physiology* **63**, 130–137.

Verhoshanski, Y., Chornonson, G., 1967. Jump exercises in sprint training. *Track and Field Quarterly* **9**, 1909.

Vujnovich, A.L., Dawson, N.J., 1994. The effect of therapeutic muscle stretch on neural processing. *Journal of Orthopedic and Sports Physical Therapy* **20** (3), 145–153.

Warren, C.G., Lehmann, J.F., Koblanski, J.N., 1971. Elongation of rat tail tendon: effect of load and temperature. *Archives of Physical Medicine and Rehabilitation* **51**, 465–474.

Wedderkopp, N., Kaltoft, M., Lundgaard, B., 1999. Prevention of injuries in young female players in European team handball. A: a prospective intervention study. *Scandinavian Journal of Medicine and Science in Sports* **9**, 41–47.

Weldon, S.M., Hill, R.H., 2003. The efficacy of stretching for prevention of exercise-related injury: a systematic review of the literature. *Manual Therapy* **8** (3), 141–150.

White, S.G., Sahrmann, S.A., 1994. A movement system balance approach to management of musculoskeletal pain. In: Grant, R. (ed.), *Physical Therapy of the Cervical and Thoracic Spine*. Churchill Livingstone, New York.

Williams, P., Watt, P., Bicik, V., Goldspink, G., 1986. Effect of stretch combined with electrical stimulation on the type of sarcomeres produced at the ends of muscle fibers. *Experimental Neurology* **93**, 500–509.

Williams, P.E., 1990. Use of intermittent stretch in the prevention of serial sarcomere loss in immobilised muscle. *Annals of the Rheumatic Diseases* **49**, 316–317.

Williams, P.E., Goldspink, G., 1978. Changes in sarcomere length and physiological properties in immobilized muscle. *Journal of Anatomy* **127**, 459–468.

Wilmore, J.H., Costill, D.L., Kenny, W.L., 2008. *Physiology of sports and exercise*, 5th ed., Human Kinetics, Champaign, Illinois.

Wolpaw, J.R., Lee, C.L., Carp, J.S., 1991. Operantly conditioned plasticity in spinal cord. *Annals of the New York Academy of Sciences* **627**, 338–348.

Zinovieff, A.N., 1951. Heavy resistance exercise, the Oxford technique. *British Journal of Physical Medicine* **14**, 129.

CHAPTER 3

The hip joint

Whereas the glenohumeral joint functions mainly in an open kinetic chain position, the hip (coxofemoral) joint functions mainly in a closed-chain position. For this reason, its structure is one of stability for weightbearing. In the standing position, however, the joint is not fully congruent, the anterosuperior portion of the cartilage of the head being exposed. It is only when the joint is taken into a position equivalent to that of the quadruped (90-degree flexion, 5-degree abduction, and 10-degree lateral rotation) that maximum articular contact of the head with the acetabulum occurs.

The femoral neck makes an angle (the angle of inclination) with the shaft of 120–130 degrees in the adult, representing the adaptation of the femur to the parallel position of the legs in gait (Fig. 3.1A). This changes from 150 degrees in the newborn to 142 degrees by age five, 133 degrees by age fifteen, and 125 degrees in the adult (Reid 1992; Palastanga, Field and Soames 2006). Greater angles than these are termed coxa valga, lesser angles as coxa vara.

Similarly, the axis of the femoral head and neck make an angle with the axis of the femoral condyles (Fig. 3.1B). This angle (angle of torsion, or angle of anteversion) is normally 10 degrees in the adult, having reduced from 25 degrees in the infant. Increased anteversion is linked to squinting or kissing patellae and this condition is twice as common in girls as in boys.

Craig's test (Fig. 3.2) may be used to assess the angle of anteversion; it compares the angle of the femoral neck to that of the femoral condyles at the knee. The patient lies prone on a couch with the knee flexed to 90 degrees. The therapist palpates the greater trochanter (posterior aspect), and the femur is medially and laterally rotated until the trochanter is parallel with the horizontal plane. The angle of anteversion is estimated from the angle of the lower leg to the vertical, and angles greater than 15 degrees are considered abnormal (Sahrmann 2002). Interestingly, this test has been found to be more reliable than radiological assessment (Ruwe et al. 1992).

Definition

In coxa vara the angle between the neck and shaft of the femur is reduced, and a knee-knee position results. In coxa valga the angle is increased and a bowleg position results.

Key point

Craig's test estimates the angle of anteversion by palpation of the greater trochanter as the femur is rotated.

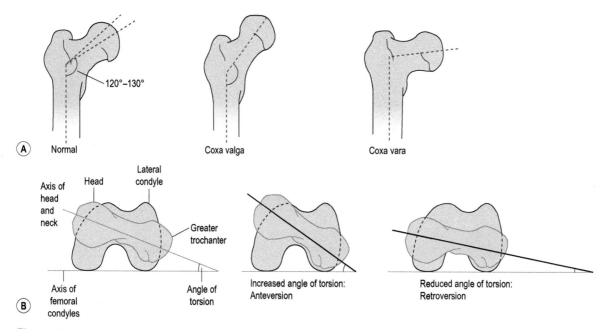

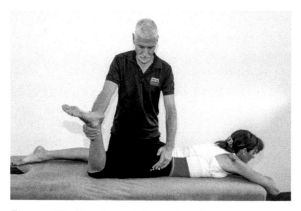

Figure 3.1 Angulation of the femoral neck. (A) Angle of inclination. (B) Angle of torsion.

Figure 3.2 The therapist palpates the greater trochanter and rotates the femur. The angle of the tibia to the vertical is compared for each side of the body.

Weightbearing

In standing, each hip takes roughly 0.3 times bodyweight, increased to 2.4 times bodyweight when standing on one leg. Weightbearing forces of up to 4.5 times bodyweight may be taken on the hip in running. In order to take weight most effectively, bony trabeculae line up in the direction of imposed stress. Two major systems exist within the femur (Fig. 3.3). The medial trabecular system travels from the medial cortex of the upper femoral shaft to the superior aspect of the head. This system takes vertically aligned forces created by weightbearing, and is aligned with the superior aspect of the acetabulum, the main weightbearing region. The lateral trabecular system begins from the lateral cortex of the upper femoral shaft, crosses the medial system, and terminates in the cortical bone on the inferior aspect of the head. The lateral system is aligned to take oblique forces created by contraction of the hip abductors during gait.

In addition to the medial and lateral trabecular systems, the upper femur is reinforced by medial and lateral accessory systems which take forces created about the trochanters. A zone of weakness is left within the femoral neck which is susceptible to bending forces and is the site of femoral neck fracture.

Hip ligaments

The hip joint is strengthened by three capsular ligaments: the iliofemoral ligament and the

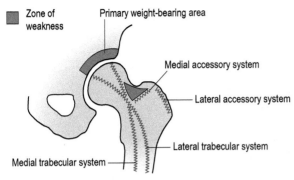

Figure 3.3 Bony trabeculae of the upper femur. After Norkin, C.C. and Levangie, P.K. (1992) *Joint Structure and Function*, 2nd edn. FA Davis, Philadelphia. With permission of the publisher, FA Davis

> **Key point**
>
> The inferior (lower) band of the iliofemoral ligament runs almost vertically. With hip extension it is under greatest tension and it limits posterior tilting of the pelvis.

During adduction, it is the turn of the superior band of the iliofemoral ligament to become tighter while the pubofemoral ligament and ischiofemoral ligament relax. In abduction the opposite occurs. In lateral rotation both the iliofemoral ligament and pubofemoral ligament are taut, while in medial rotation the ischiofemoral ligament tightens.

Screening examination

Hip conditions may refer pain anywhere within the L3 dermatome, over the front of the thigh and down to the knee. Initial observation includes resting position, muscle wasting, leg length and gait. Functional activities may also be revealing. Lying in bed with the affected side uppermost (hip adduction and medial rotation) places a stretch over the iliotibial band (ITB) and lengthens the posterior portion of the gluteus medius. This may be a consideration in ITB syndrome (IRBS) and for muscle imbalance over the

pubofemoral ligament are on the anterior aspect of the joint, while the ischiofemoral ligament is on the posterior aspect (Fig. 3.4). As the hip is flexed, all three ligaments relax. However, in extension all three ligaments are tight, with the inferior band of the iliofemoral ligament being placed under greatest tension as it runs almost vertically. It is this ligamentous band which limits posterior tilt of the pelvis.

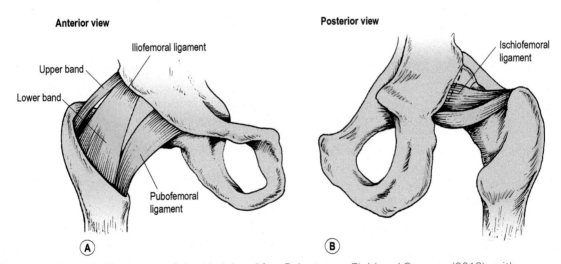

Figure 3.4 Capsular ligaments of the hip joint. After Palastanga, Field and Soames (2013), with permission

127

hip. Pain on squatting (hip flexion), as when sitting on the toilet or sitting down into a low chair, warrants closer examination of flexion movements.

Examination for range of motion (ROM) may be carried out in a supine position for flexion, abduction and adduction and both rotations. Medial and lateral rotation are best compared between the affected and unaffected hip in a prone position with the knees flexed to 90 degrees. Resisted abduction is better tested in a side-lying position with the affected joint uppermost.

Compression of the joint through the flexed knee and circumduction with compression to 'scour' the femoral head into the acetabulum is an important assessment for arthritic changes. Both the lumbar spine and the sacroiliac joints must be examined, to eliminate them as a potential cause of pain referral. The straight-leg raise and slump test should be used to eliminate the possible involvement of neural tissue. Cyriax (1982) warned that serious pathology may be present if the sign of the buttock is positive. Here, hip flexion with the knee bent is more painful and more limited than straight-leg raising. A non-capsular limitation is present, and pain may make the end-feel empty. As hip flexion in straight-leg raising is full range, the sciatic nerve is unimpinged, and the non-capsular limitation precludes the hip joint. Possibilities include an inflammatory disease state, neoplasm and fracture.

> **Key point**
>
> With the sign of the buttock, hip flexion with the knee bent is more painful and more limited than straight-leg raising. Serious hip pathology may be present and further investigation is required.

Muscle imbalance around the hip

The concept of muscle imbalance was covered in Chapter 2. In the hip region, the Thomas test and the Ober manoeuvre are used to assess for muscle tightness of the hip flexors (rectus femoris and iliopsoas) and hip abductors (tensor fascia lata and iliotibial band – TFL/ITB). Inner range holding ability of the gluteus medius is assessed with side-lying hip abduction, and of the gluteus maximus with the prone-lying hip extension movement described below. Segmental control tests include standing hip flexion, standing hip abduction and the hip hinge (see Treatment Note 3.1 and Table 3.1).

Treatment note 3.1   Muscle imbalance around the hip

Iliopsoas

The subject flexes the hip while maintaining 90-degree knee flexion so that the foot is lifted clear of the ground. Where the IP is lengthened, the thigh may drop down from the inner-range position, or more commonly the pelvis is tilted backwards while the knee position is maintained. Backward tilting of the pelvis accompanied by flattening of the lumbar lordosis moves the origin of the muscle away from its insertion and lengthens the IP.

Gluteus maximus

The subject begins in prone lying with the knee flexed to 90 degrees. Flexing the knee shortens the hamstring muscles, placing them at a physiological disadvantage and making hamstring substitution less likely. The hip is lifted to inner-range extension and held. In this position, the gluteus maximus may be palpated to determine its level of contraction (firmness) and ability to maintain the inner-range position.

Gluteus medius

The gluteus medius is tested in side lying with the knee flexed (Clamshell position). Two starting positions may be used, both with the foot supported to work the limb in closed-chain format. In the *first* the feet are placed together; in the *second* the foot of the upper leg is placed on the

Treatment note 3.1 *continued*

couch at mid-shin level. The action is to keep the foot still and lift the knee while keeping the trunk still. Rotation of the trunk at the pelvis must be avoided. The therapist should monitor the position of the greater trochanter of the upper leg and ensure that it points to the ceiling and does not move forwards or backwards.

Thomas test

The Thomas test used here is a modification of the original. With the modified Thomas test, the patient begins in crook lying at the end of the couch. The knees are brought to the chest and the back flattened to a point where the sacrum just begins to lift away from the couch surface but no further. One leg is held close to the chest to maintain the pelvic position and the other leg is straightened over the couch end. An optimal alignment exists when the femur lies horizontally, and aligned to the sagittal plane (no abduction). The tibia should lie vertically (90-degree knee flexion) and be aligned with the sagittal plane (no hip rotation). If the femur rests above the horizontal and the knee is flexed less than 90 degrees, tightness may be present in either the iliopsoas or rectus femoris. If the rectus is tight, straightening the knee will take the stretch off the muscle and the leg will drop down. If the knee is straightened and the leg stays in place, it indicates tightness in the iliopsoas. Deviation of the knee laterally (the 'J' sign) indicates a possible tightness in the iliotibial band (ITB), indicating that the Ober test should be performed to confirm the tightness.

Ober test

The modified Ober test (Ober 1936) begins in side lying. The lower leg is bent to improve stability and the therapist stabilizes the pelvis to avoid lateral pelvic dipping. The couch should be low enough to allow pressure to be placed through the iliac crest in the direction of the lower shoulder. Maintaining the neutral pelvic position, the hip is abducted and extended to 15 degrees. It is then adducted while maintaining extension. An optimal length for an athlete would be seen when the upper leg is able to lower to couch level.

Hamstring length tests

The hamstrings are assessed using the active knee extension (AKE) test. The test is performed with the subject lying supine on a couch. The knee and hip are flexed to 90 degrees and held in this position by the subject or therapist. The subject then straightens the leg using quadriceps action and holds the maximum knee extension for three to five seconds while the knee angle is measured.

Hip hinge

The hip hinge movement is the final action. It is initially performed freestanding and then using a stick. The test measures the subject's ability to isolate pelvic motion from that of the lumbar spine. Initially, forward flexion is assessed, and the relative contribution of anterior pelvic tilt to this movement is important. The subject is asked to bend forwards (hands to knee height) and the amount of anterior pelvic tilt and lumbar flexion is noted. They are then asked to perform the same action with the knee slightly bent (unlocked) and a stick held along the length of the spine to prevent lumbar flexion. Finally, they are asked to repeat the freestanding movement and attempt to replicate the second action using pelvic tilt alone. The therapist assesses (pass – fail) the subject's ability to isolate pelvic motion from lumbar motion.

Pelvic motion in the frontal plane

Pelvic motion control in the frontal plane represents the Trendelenburg sign (see also the section on lateral hip pain below). When the bodyweight is supported on one leg, the hip abductors of the supporting leg work to prevent the pelvis dipping. The subject is asked to stand on one leg and lift the contralateral knee so the foot clears the floor. The test is positive if

Treatment note 3.1 *continued*

the ipsilateral pelvis dips (Trendelenburg sign) and/or the trunk leans to the opposite side (compensated Trendelenburg). Re-education of pelvic motion control works by using the Trendelenburg test position. Initially, preventing pelvic dip during body sway (taking bodyweight from both legs to single leg) with both feet kept on the ground with the legs locked initially. This is progressed to bending one knee with both feet on the ground, and finally moving into single-knee lift actions (supported and unsupported) to mimic the Trendelenburg test.

Table 3.1 Muscle imbalance around the hip

	Muscle length	Inner range holding	Segmental control
Figure			
Test	Thomas	Gluteus medius	Standing hip flexion
Figure			
Test	Ober	Gluteus maximus	Standing hip abduction
Figure			
Test	Active knee extension (AKE)	Iliopsoas	Hip hinge

Muscle injuries

Quadriceps

On the whole, strains occur more commonly in two-joint (biarticular) muscles, due to the more complex coordination involved in controlling movement of two body segments simultaneously. Direct trauma, however, can be imposed on any muscle. In the hip region, this means that the rectus femoris, hamstrings and gracilis muscles tend to suffer strain. The more anterior position of the quadriceps, however, exposes these muscles to risk during contact sports, and to blunt trauma through collision with sports apparatus. A quadriceps contusion is often referred to colloquially as a 'dead leg' or 'charley horse'.

Initially, there is local swelling over the front of the thigh, with some superficial bruising appearing later, often tracking down to the knee. The main danger with this injury is the development of myositis ossificans traumatica (MOT). Thigh contusions may be rated as Grade I (mild), in which knee flexion beyond 90 degrees is possible, Grade II (moderate), in which motion is restricted to 45–90 degrees, or Grade III (severe), in which swelling and pain limit movement to less than 45 degrees. This grading system can be an accurate predictor of the likelihood of MOT development. Back in the early 1970s Jackson and Feagin (1973) assessed quadriceps contusions in 65 subjects, and found that none of the subjects with Grade I injuries had developed MOT. However, 13 out of 18 subjects who had been graded 2 or 3 later went on to develop the condition, so the amount of movement present in the initial stages is an important indicator of the severity of the lesion, and the prognosis.

> **Key point**
>
> Following a quadriceps haematoma or 'dead leg', myositis (muscle calcification) is more likely to occur if an injured athlete is unable to flex the knee to 90 degrees.

It is important to limit movement in Grade I and II injuries and to discourage the use of massage, vigorous stretching or exercise and ultrasound, as these are contraindicated in the early post-injury stage. The POLICE protocol is used to limit tissue damage. Cold is applied with compression with the knee and the hip flexed as far as is comfortable. Internal compression is therefore applied by fascial tightening, while external compression comes from the elastic bandage.

The athlete resuming contact sports should wear padding over the damaged area, to reduce the risk of secondary injury. It is important that full broadening of the muscle belly be obtained during rehabilitation. This will involve resisted quadriceps exercises, beginning with low intensity and building eventually to maximum voluntary contractions (MVC). This is equally important to endurance athletes as to power athletes. Often, distance runners, for example, do not use weight training, focusing instead on stretching. For this injury, however, longitudinal movement of the muscle is less important than lateral movement (broadening). This is because the rectus femoris, being a two-joint muscle, may limit movement, but the vasti, being single-joint muscles, do not. As the vasti form the bulk of the injured tissue, stretching, although important with this injury, is secondary to strength training.

In cases of MOT, calcification is slow, with fibroblasts beginning to differentiate into osteoblasts about one week after injury. Radiographic evidence of bone formation is usually visible after three weeks (Fig. 3.5). By six to seven weeks after injury, the calcified mass generally stops growing. Total reabsorption may occur with minor lesions, but more major conditions may continue to show remnants of the mass. The mass rarely interferes with muscle contraction, so excision is not normally required (Estwanik and McAlister 1990).

Rectus femoris

The rectus femoris is frequently injured by a mistimed kicking action. On examination, pain is

131

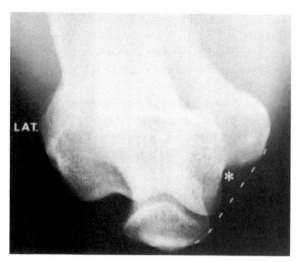

Figure 3.5 X-ray showing myositis ossificans traumatica (MOT). From Magee (2002), with permission.

Tenderness to the reflected head attaching to the anterior inferior iliac spine in a youth should raise the question of avulsion injury and may require X-ray confirmation.

Mid-belly tears are less common and are usually sited within the middle third of the thigh. Here, the muscle is subcutaneous and any swelling is immediately apparent. The athlete should flex the hip and knee to 45 degrees against resistance, and as the muscle stands out any abnormality will become apparent.

The rectus femoris can be worked concentrically by flexing the hip against a resistance supplied by a weight bag attached to the knee. Two-joint action of the muscle can be worked with the athlete in supine with the injured leg over the couch side, flexed at both the knee and hip. Manual resistance is applied to the foot of the athlete as he or she extends the knee and flexes the hip simultaneously (Fig. 3.6A).

Stretching must involve both knee flexion and hip extension and can be carried out in a side-lying position by the athlete, or by the therapist.

usually apparent to resisted knee extension and hip flexion. Passive stretch into knee flexion coupled with hip extension and adduction is also painful. Injury is usually to either the upper insertion or the mid-belly. Upper insertion injuries are palpated with the patient half-lying to relax the muscle. The area of injury is usually the musculotendinous junction approximately four finger widths below the anterior superior iliac spine.

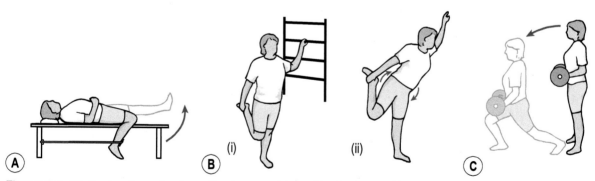

Figure 3.6 (A) Rectus femoris strengthening, combining hip flexion and knee extension against elastic band resistance. (B) Rectus stretch. (i) Correct with pelvis fixed. (ii) Incorrect, anterior pelvic tilt throws stress on lumbar spine. (C) Alternate leg lunge. Front leg stresses quadriceps and gluteals, rear leg stresses hip flexors and knee extensors.

When performing a rectus femoris stretch in standing (Fig. 3.6B), the abdominal muscles must be tightened to stabilize the pelvis before the hip stretch is applied. Failure to do so will increase the apparent range of motion by anterior tilt of the pelvis with stress thrown on the lumbar spine. Lunging actions are also useful, for both general flexibility and eccentric control (Fig. 3.6C).

> **Key point**
>
> The rectus femoris muscle must be stretched and strengthened at both the knee and hip simultaneously.

Results are generally very good, even with complete tears (Fig. 3.7), where full function may be regained even though a marked muscle deformity is present.

Sartorius

Injury to the sartorius is usually an avulsion from the anterior superior iliac spine (see also apophysitis below). There is usually immediate pain, often radiating into the anterior thigh. Swelling and bruising is seen over the iliac crest, often tracking down the thigh. Flexion/adduction of the hip with flexion of the knee causes pain. Displacement of the bone fragment may be from a few millimetres to three centimetres, but although surgical reattachment of the bone fragment has been described (Veselko and Smrkolj 1994), conservative treatment normally suffices. The athlete should be non-weightbearing initially, followed by partial weightbearing ambulation for three to six weeks, depending on the intensity of pain. Full strength and flexibility must be regained before competitive sport is resumed.

The Hamstrings

Injury incidence

Hamstring injury is common, and especially in sports, these injuries frequently recur. Up to 12 per cent of sports injuries may be to the hamstrings (Ekstrand et al. 2012), and it is the most common muscle injury in male footballers (Schuermans et al. 2014). Recurrence rates vary between 12 and 63 per cent depending on the site of injury and severity, and the first month after return to sport sees the greatest risk of re-injury (Brukner et al. 2014). High-class rehabilitation is key for hamstring injury recovery, both in sports and daily living.

The hamstrings consist of three muscles, the biceps femoris (BF) laterally, and the semimembranosus (SM) and semitendinosus (ST) medially. The BF is more commonly injured than the ST and SM, with rates of 80 per cent compared to 10 per cent respectively (Ekstrand et al. 2012). The ischial portion (vertical fibres) of adductor magnus is sometimes considered within the hamstring group, and involvement of this muscle is sometimes seen alongside hamstring injury. The anatomy of this region is an important factor in the varying injury incidence between the various hamstring components.

Anatomy

The three hamstring muscles attach to the ischial tuberosity – the SM from the superior-lateral

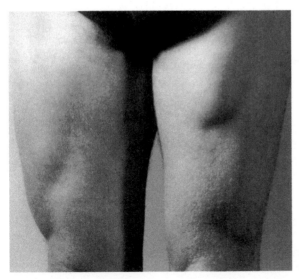

Figure 3.7 Rectus femoris tear. From Reid (1992), with permission.

aspect, the ST and BF from the infero-medial portion below the sacrotuberous ligament.

The ST and long head of BF have a combined attachment on the lower medial facet of the ischial tuberosity, the two muscles travelling together for a short distance until they form fusiform muscle bellies.

Definition

A fusiform muscle is spindle shaped, with a wide centre tapering down to narrow ends.

The ST almost instantly forms into a long slender tendon, and travels around the medial condyle of the tibia to attach to the medial surface of the tibia below gracilis. The BF has two proximal attachments; the long head, as described above, and the short head from the lower linea aspera of the femur. The muscle swings downwards and laterally across the posterior aspect of the thigh and around the lateral ligament to insert into the head of the fibula. From this point it has a strong fascial attachment to the peroneus (fibularis) longus and the iliotibial band as part of the lateral and spiral fascial lines (Myers 2014).

Key point

The semimembranosus attaches from the lateral aspect of the ischial tuberosity, the semitendinosus and biceps from the medial. At the knee the biceps are lateral, the semitendinosus (medial) is cord-like and the semitendinosus (medial) is flat.

The hamstrings as a group are innovated by the sciatic nerve (tibial branch), but the BF has a dual innervation (tibial and peroneal branch), and asynchronous stimulation of the two heads

has been described as a factor in injury (Burkett 1975). The SM comes from the lateral facet of the ischial tuberosity and travels down and medially, becoming flattened and broader as it does so. The SM is deep to both the ST and BF, and divides into five components when it reaches the knee (see Chapter 4). The principal insertion is to the posterior aspect of the medial tibial tubercle, with attachment into the oblique popliteal ligament and medial meniscus.

The proximal tendon of the BF extends into the muscle by 60 per cent of its length, and the distal tendon by 66 per cent, while for the SM the tendon extension is 78 per cent and 52 per cent (Garrett et al. 1989). The continuity between the two tendons into the centre of the muscle constitutes the central tendon (intramuscular myotendon), which is often a region of disruption in persistent injuries (Brukner and Connell 2016).

Key point

Injury to the central tendon of the biceps or semimembranosus can take longer to heal than belly tears, and may sometimes require surgical repair.

Function

The hamstrings have functions over the pelvis, hip and knee. They are two-joint (biarticular) muscles (see Treatment Note 3.2), and as with all muscles contribute force through active (contraction) and passive (recoil) means. In open-chain motion the muscles will flex the knee and extend the hip, but the short head of BF has an action (flexion) over the knee alone. When the knee is flexed, SM and ST medially rotate the tibia and the BF laterally rotates. In closed-chain action the hamstrings will assist in knee extension by drawing the femur into extension over the fixed foot.

Treatment note 3.2 Two joint muscles

The hamstrings are biarticular muscles and as such are unable to permit full movement simultaneously at both of the joints they span. Full movement may be limited during stretch (passive insufficiency), for example knee extension combined with hip extension, or contraction (active insufficiency) such as knee flexion and hip extension.

Definition

A *biarticular* muscle is one which spans two joints, a *monoarticular* muscle spans a single joint.

Biarticular muscles (Fig. 3.8) are arranged as agonist and antagonist – in the case of the thigh, the hamstrings being grouped opposite the rectus femoris. Because both biarticular muscle sets are not long enough to permit movement at both joints simultaneously, the tension in one muscle is transferred to the other. Using the hip as an example, as the hamstrings contract to extend the hip, passive tension is transmitted to the rectus femoris, creating a knee extension force. This type of action, involving either extension or flexion at both joints at the same time, is called *concurrent movement*. The muscle shortens at one end but lengthens at the other, and so maintains its length with a range of 100–130 per cent resting length to conserve tension (Burkholder and Lieber 2001). When the hip is flexed but the knee extended, the rectus femoris is shortened and rapidly loses tension, while the hamstrings are lengthened and rapidly gain tension, an example of *countercurrent movement* (Rasch 1989).

Biarticular muscles provide a number of mechanical advantages over monoarticular equivalents. First, they couple movement at both joints. For example, in the upper limb, shoulder and elbow flexion occur together in a feeding

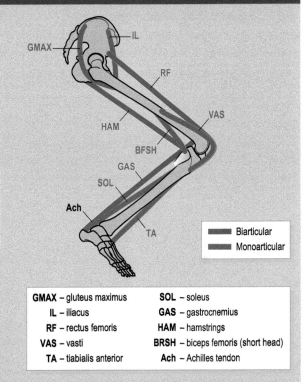

GMAX – gluteus maximus	**SOL** – soleus
IL – iliacus	**GAS** – gastrocnemius
RF – rectus femoris	**HAM** – hamstrings
VAS – vasti	**BRSH** – biceps femoris (short head)
TA – tiabialis anterior	**Ach** – Achilles tendon

Figure 3.8 Biarticular muscles of the leg.

pattern, and both actions have a contribution from biceps brachii (Enoka 1994). Biarticular muscles also allow the transfer of power from proximal to distal segments, allowing bulky musculature to be kept closer to the trunk, reducing the mass of the extremity and facilitating acceleration.

Second, the shortening velocity of a two-joint muscle is less than that of a single-joint muscle (van Ingen Schenau et al. 1990), contributing to more rapid limb movement. By shortening less than two equivalent monoarticular muscles, a biarticular muscle demonstrates lower contraction velocities and higher force development. For instance, the contraction velocity of the hamstrings during vertical jumping is said to be a quarter of that required by a monoarticular muscle. As force and velocity are linked during

Treatment note 3.2 *continued*

muscle performance (for the force–velocity relationship, see Chapter 2), biarticular muscles can generate approximately three times the force of their monoarticular counterparts (Cleather et al. 2015).

Third, two-joint muscles are said to redistribute muscle force throughout the limb (Toussaint et al. 1992). For example, if hip flexion is performed by rectus femoris, recoil of the lengthening hamstrings will tend to flex the knee. Equally, recoil of the lengthening rectus femoris in hip extension will tend to extend the knee. A biarticular muscle will also enhance joint stability by allowing co-contraction of the agonist and antagonist muscles without reducing tension, as would occur with monoarticular muscles at both joints.

The hamstrings, as biarticular muscles, have an important function during both lifting (bending) and running actions.

Bending

Forward bending is a coupled movement combining lumbar flexion and pelvic rotation (lumbar-pelvic rhythm), which results from a coordinated action between the back extensor muscles (erector spinae) and the hip extensors (gluteals and hamstrings). Towards end-range forward bending, both the back extensor muscles and the hip extensors show reduced electrical activity, a phenomenon called the flexion relaxation response (FRR). As the body bends forwards, its descent is initially controlled by eccentric action of both the spinal extensors and hamstrings, but towards the end of mid-range activity of the spinal extensors ceases and elastic resistance of the spinal extensors and posteriorly placed spinal soft tissues limits movement range. Near-end-range activity of the hamstrings also ceases and the final angle of pelvic tilt is limited by elastic resistance of these muscles and tension of other posteriorly placed soft tissues. At the initiation of body lifting, little muscle contraction is seen, the trunk being raised by elastic recoil of the posterior tissues. The point at which this occurs (critical point) varies, and the FRR of both the erector spinae and hamstrings may be altered or obliterated in subjects with chronic lower back pain (CLBP), perhaps representing an inability to relax the muscles as part of painful behaviour. EMG biofeedback training has been used to decrease lumbar paraspinal muscle activity and increase motion range in patients with chronic lower back pain. In this study, a decreased fear of movement was noted, leading the authors to suggest that initial movement limitation may have been modulated by fear avoidance (Pagé et al. 2015). Surface EMG has also successfully been used to assist a home-based stretching programme aimed at lengthening the paraspinal muscles in CLBP subjects (Moore et al. 2015), again suggesting that increased tone in these muscles may be part of the pain phenomenon of CLBP.

There are a number of important considerations with respect to injury recovery and rehabilitation with the bending action. First, the lumbar spine and pelvis have to work in a coordinated fashion, and following injury, this coordination often breaks down and must be retrained. Second, whilst both the back muscles and hamstrings must be strong enough to lift a subject's own bodyweight and the weight of any object being held (these muscles often weaken after injury) they must also be able to relax at the right point when bending. If they stay active throughout the bending action, without switching off, they will tire and become painful.

Running

During the running cycle, the hamstrings contract eccentrically to decelerate the leg in late forward swing, an action which also helps to stabilize the knee. During the support phase, they work concentrically to extend the hip, and continue to stabilize the knee by preventing knee extension. During push-off, the hamstrings and gastrocnemius, both biarticular muscles, paradoxically extend the knee.

Definition

A *paradoxical* muscle action occurs when a muscle creates the opposite movement to that which it should due to its position.

EMG studies have demonstrated differences between the medial and lateral hamstrings during knee flexion (isokinetic dynamometry), with BF showing maximal activation early on (15–30 degrees) and SM and ST later (90–105 degrees) in knee flexion (Onishi et al. 2002). BF is subjected to the greatest muscle-tendon stretch in the terminal swing phase of high-speed running, perhaps explaining the increased incidence of injury to this muscle. BF and ST are maximally active eccentrically throughout the swing phase of running, but their neuromuscular coordination patterns show BF more active in the middle to late swing and ST in the terminal swing phase only (Higashihara et al. 2010). It has been suggested that a reduced endurance capacity of the ST is compensated by increased activity of the BF, as muscle functional MRI (mfMRI) has shown increased metabolic activity in the ST compared to BF following injury (Schuermans et al. 2014).

Injury

Hamstring injuries tend to occur in two main categories, high-speed running, which typically involves the BF long head, and slower extended lengthening (high kick or splits action), which often implicates the proximal tendon of SM (Askling et al. 2012). In addition, posterior thigh pain showing no local structural injury (MRI-negative injury) may be due to referred pain from the lumbar spine or pelvis.

Key point

Hamstring injuries are typically the result of either high-speed running or over stretch (extended lengthening).

The injuries may be classified according to the Munich consensus statement (Ueblacker et al. 2013). Muscle injury may be direct or indirect, and graded from 1 to 4. Grades 1 and 2 are *functional* muscle disorders due to overexertion and/or fatigue, with grade 2 representing delayed-onset muscle soreness (DOMS) or MRI negative injury resulting from referred posterior thigh pain. Grade 3 injury is a minor or partial tear, while grade 4 is a total or complete tear or avulsion. Grades 3 and 4 represent *structural* injuries (see Chapter 1, Table 1.14).

Recovery from injury and return to the activities of daily living (ADL) or return to play (RTP) may partially be determined by the site of injury and the amount of tissue damage. However, while studies suggest that closer proximity to the ischial tuberosity is likely to imply greater recovery time (Askling et al. 2013, Silder et al. 2013), MRI and U/S studies show no association between scan findings and RTP (Reurink et al. 2015, Petersen et al. 2014). RTP before full rehabilitation has taken effect can be an important factor in re-injury. Reduction of eccentric strength and delayed rate of torque development may suggest neural function change following injury, especially at longer muscle lengths (Fyfe et al. 2013). Pain inhibition following injury may produce a structural and functional maladaptation within the muscle, meaning that early pain management may be important to reduce inhibition and encourage early muscle activation.

Key point

Pain inhibition following injury may produce functional maladaptation to the hamstrings, altering coordination.

Table 3.2 Multifactorial components of hamstring rehabilitation

Comopnent	Clinical reasoning
Biomechanics	Foot, lower limb, & limbo-pelvic alignment
Neurodynamics	SLR & slump testing
Neuromuscular control of lumbar spine	Lumbo-pelvic control and strengthening
Eccentric biased strengthening	Varying movement range & muscle length
Running overload	Varying direction and speed. Task/sport specific
Stretching	Restoration of symmetry of motion range in static and dynamic task/sport specific actions.

(After Brukner et al. 2014)

Rehabilitation

Hamstring rehabilitation is multifactorial, with a number of components identified through both research evidence and clinical experience (Brukner et al. 2014). The components are listed in Table 3.2.

Lumbo-pelvic manual therapy and neurodynamics

Addressing the lumbar spine and pelvic joints may be important as the presence of pain referred into the leg can change hamstring strength, muscle contraction timing, and willingness to bend. Manual pain provocation tests may be used to clear the lumbo-pelvic region in the hamstring injured patient, and the slump test (also see Chapter 8) may be used to differentiate hamstrings and sciatic nerve symptoms as the source of posterior thigh pain. Additionally, the slump may be used as a treatment technique to facilitate nerve length and mobility. Neural tension may both increase stretch resistance and limit total movement range.

The slump test is positive where the patient's posterior thigh pain is reproduced in the final slump position, and reduced with cervical extension. The test has been shown to be positive in sportsmen and women (rugby players) who have suffered a number of hamstring tears in the past two years (Turl and George 1998). In addition, quality of return to play is enhanced (fewer missed matches) when the test is used as a stretch within a rehabilitation programme (Kornberg and Lew 1989). Including

the slump test modified as a neuromobilization technique (slider exercise) has been recommend for athletes who have suffered a hamstring injury and feel a lack of free movement when running, even in the presence of a negative straight-leg raise (SLR) and slump test (Brukner et al. 2014).

Nerve sliding (gliding) of this type involves movement of at least two joints, with one lengthening the nerve and the other shortening it. The combination of lengthening and shortening maintains the overall nerve length but improves nerve motility. In the case of the posterior thigh, we move the distal tissues (limb) while maintaining the position of the proximal tissues (spine) and then reverse the sequence. While sustained nerve tension increases intraneural pressure and reduces local blood flow, sliding, by maintaining overall nerve length avoids these changes.

For the classic slump test or stretch the subject sits on a stool and links their arms behind their back. The action is to gently flex the spine, beginning with the neck. At the same time one leg is straightened and the foot and ankle pulled up (dorsiflexed) (Fig. 3.9). Components of this action may be used individually at first, then built up into a full sequence. If one leg is very tight, the knee on that side can be bent and gradually worked towards straightening, easing into the tightness but not forcing the movement. Supporting the foot of the tight leg on the floor by placing it on a shiny piece of paper is also helpful. With the weight of the leg taken through the floor, the subject slides the foot forwards and backwards, again gradually working

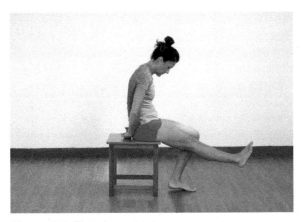

Figure 3.9 The slump test.

towards the fully extended position. Maintain this position for 20 to 30 seconds and then release.

To perform the nerve slide (seated straight-leg slider), the subject begins in the classic slump position described above, ensuring that the subject's feet are clear of the floor (Fig. 3.10A). Keeping the spine flexed throughout the exercise, the neck is bent (flexed) to bring the chin down towards the breastbone (sternum). At the same time the knee is kept bent and the toes and foot are pointed (plantarflexion). To reverse the action, straighten the knee and draw the foot and toes up (ankle dorsiflexion and toe flexion) and at the same time look up at the ceiling (cervical extension) (Fig. 3.10B). The sliding action is repeated rhythmically for ten repetitions. Where there is a high degree of tightness, or where pain occurs,

the exercise can be performed in two parts. First, keeping the head still and moving the leg, and second keeping the leg still and moving the head. When both actions are pain free the two actions may be combined.

This straight-leg sliding technique has been shown to increase range of motion of the hamstring muscles (measured by straight-leg raise) without the need for separate hamstring stretching. Looking at a group of soccer players, Castellote-Caballero et al. (2013) used straight-leg sliding for three periods over one week. Each exercise was practised for sixty seconds for five repetitions. Average scores for straight-leg raise testing for the control group (no sliding) went from 58.9 degrees to 59.1 degrees, while the intervention group (neural sliding) went from 58.1 degrees to 67.4 degrees.

Mobilization of the lumbar spine has been shown to increase motion range in the SLR test and change sympathetic nervous system activity in the limb (Szlezak et al. 2011), and it is recommended that this technique be used to modify patient symptoms with a view to pain modulation. Although lumbo-pelvic examination and treatment may be appropriate for any patient with hamstring injury, it is likely that the MRI negative patient may especially benefit due to the presence of posterior thigh pain in the absence of local tissue change.

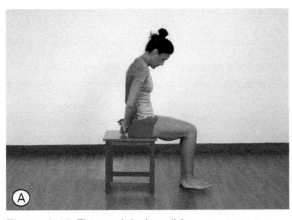
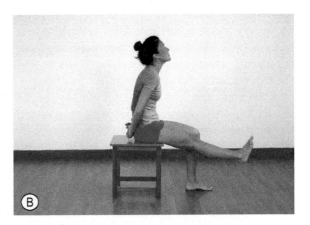

Figure 3.10 The straight-leg slider.

139

Lumbo-pelvic neuromuscular control

Improvement on lumbo-pelvic control has been suggested to reduce hamstring demand and therefore potential for injury (Brukner et al. 2014). In addition, a trunk stabilization programme has been shown to reduce hamstring injury recurrence rate (Sherry and Best 2004) and a balance training programme to reduce hamstring injury rate in women's professional football (Kraemer and Knobloch 2009). Although many athletes successfully compete at very high levels with suboptimal static and dynamic postures, in elite sport, where fractions of a second matter, optimizing control of the lumbo-pelvic region onto which the hamstrings take attachment would seem logical. Control of lumbo-pelvic alignment in the frontal plane can focus on actions based around the Trendelenburg test (pelvic alignment in single-leg standing). In the sagittal plane, forward bending and lifting actions (above) can be used to optimize pelvic tilt. These actions should be progressed in terms of overload and complexity, but must be paralleled with good exercise instruction and neurobiology re-education to reduce the chance of hypervigilance following injury (see Chapter 1).

Eccentric biased strengthening

Consistently, research studies have supported the notion that various forms of eccentric hamstring exercise are essential for prevention and rehabilitation of hamstring muscle injury. Injury commonly occurs at the end of the swing phase of sprinting, when the hamstring muscles are contracting eccentrically to decelerate the limb and are at full stretch. Rehabilitation must match this muscle contraction type and joint angle position, so eccentric work (high loads at longer muscle-tendon lengths) would seem logical.

Nordic hamstring exercise

The Nordic hamstring exercise (NHE) has been shown to reduce injuries by 60 per cent and re-injury by 85 per cent, when used in a progressive ten-week programme (Petersen et al. 2011). Progressive eccentric strengthening of this type is thought to address eccentric strength deficits, muscle tendon atrophy and scar tissue within the hamstrings (Thorborg 2012). The NHE may shift the optimum angle for torque generation towards a longer hamstring length, mimicking the limb position at terminal swing just prior to heel contact, a point at which injury has been shown to occur (Schache et al. 2010).

The NHE is an intense muscle contraction, giving rise to muscle adaptation but with the likelihood of delayed onset muscle soreness (DOMS). Progressive programmes should begin cautiously with one session each week initially (weeks 1–3) building to two sessions per week (weeks 2–5) and finally three per week (weeks 3–10), with one session per week for maintenance thereafter. Variation in the prescription is dependent on subject reaction to the exercise intervention.

Although the NHE is a vital component of rehabilitation, it should not be used in isolation as it has a number of disadvantages. In general it is practised bilaterally, not reflecting the unilateral nature of hamstring injury. Also it is a single joint (uniarticular) action whereas the hamstring muscles as a group are biarticular, and normally the NHE is performed at slow speeds. Progression of exercise must include training volume (frequency, intensity, time and type) and velocity at multiple joint angles. Slow controlled eccentrics should progress in parallel with general lower limb and lumbo-pelvic resistance training and motor control complexity. Ultimately, power- and speed-based actions (plyometrics) should be used, together with skill-based actions reflecting the sport or employment of the subject.

The NHE begins in high kneeling with the ankles fixed (Fig. 3.11A). The traditional action is to keep the hip fixed and angle the body forwards from the knee. The aim is to lower the body under control into a prone position, taking the final bodyweight of the final degrees of movement onto the hands. The action may be unloaded using a fixed strap (partner) (Fig. 3.11B), elastic powerloop (fixed point), or with

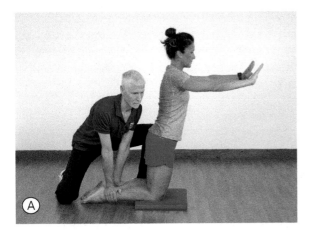

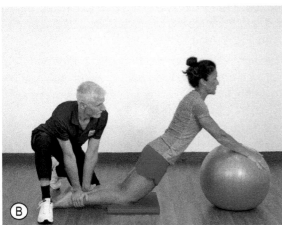

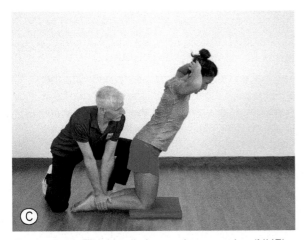

Figure 3.11 The Nordic hamstring exercise (NHE). (A) Start position in high kneeling with the ankles fixed. (B) NHE using Swiss ball. (C) Bent-knee back extension in NHE position.

the subject placing their hands on a swiss ball and rolling it away from themselves (Fig. 3.11C).

From the same starting position, a bent-knee back extension action may be performed, pulling from the hip and keeping the spine straight to begin. This action targets the hamstring higher up into the buttock, using an active pelvic tilt. It may be combined with or used separately from the traditional eccentric only version.

Deadlift variations

The straight-leg (Romanian) *deadlift* uses a fixed-leg position, either with the legs straight (knees locked) or slightly bent (knees soft). The action is to keep the spine straight and lift the body from the hip. Initially, bodyweight alone is used (arms behind the tail or behind the head), but resistance may be added from a barbell, kettlebell or dumbbells (Fig. 3.12). As an alternative, the *arabesque* may be viewed as a single-leg version of the straight-leg deadlift. The leg to be trained stays with the foot on the floor (leg vertical) and the other leg lifts (leg horizontal) (Fig. 3.13A). There are a number of versions of this action. In yoga this is one of the warrior poses, and the final position is with the lifted leg, trunk and arms horizontal to emphasize balance. This action may be performed standing on one leg with the arms lifted above the head. The movement is to keep the lifting leg, trunk and arms rigid and tip forwards into a 'T' position (Fig. 3.13B). The hands may be placed on

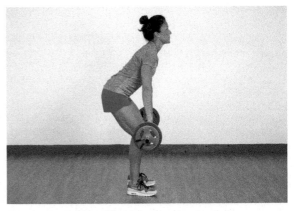

Figure 3.12 Deadlift actions using barbell.

141

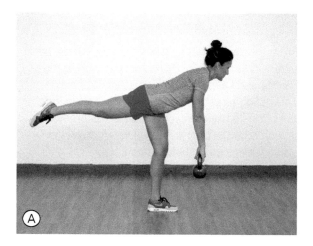

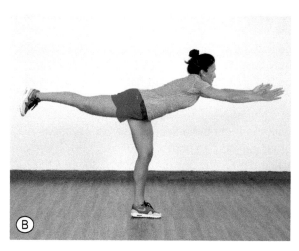

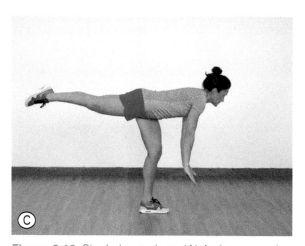

Figure 3.13 Single-leg actions. (A) Arabesque using kettlebell. (B) Warrior 3. (C) Diver.

a wall for balance. The diver is the same action, but the arms reach downwards to touch a stool or gym bench and then the body is moved back to the starting position focusing on repetitions and strength (Fig. 3.13C).

Bridge type movements

Bridging actions use the hip extensors and spine extensors from a supine lying position. For the slide board leg curl the subject lies on their back with their foot on a slide board – a piece of shiny paper on a carpet, cloth on a wooden floor, or the seat of a rowing machine. The action is to slide the foot out from a bent-knee position to straight leg and return. Single-leg or bilateral-leg action may be used (Fig. 3.14A).

The high bridge (gym ball bridge) is performed from a crook (hook) lying position, with one heel on a bench or chair, or for an unstable surface a gym ball. The action is to press the heel down to dig into the bench and lift the hips upwards. Again, unilateral or bilateral actions may both be used. Where the unilateral action is used, the pelvis must be kept level, not allowing the hip on the non-active side to trail. This action may be modified into the eccentric leg curl on a gym ball. The action now is to press the heels into the gym ball to lift the pelvis and to straighten the legs and then lower the trunk (eccentric only) or to straighten the legs and then bend them again (eccentric-concentric) (Fig. 3.14B).

The loaded bridge may be performed with the shoulders on a gym bench and the knees bent. A weight disc is placed on the lap, or a barbell is placed over the pelvis with the bar (padded) level with the top of the pelvis. The action is to lift the pelvis into a bridge position, finishing with the thigh horizontal. The foot must press directly downwards (hip extension) rather than outwards (knee extension).

Deceleration drops

Deceleration drills involve dropping into a bent hip and knee (squat) position, either unilaterally

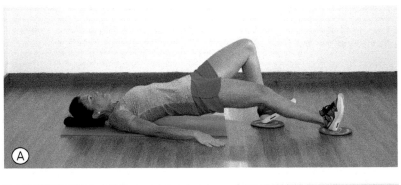

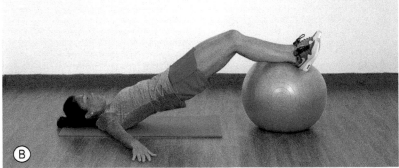

Figure 3.14 Bridging actions. (A) Using a slide board machine. (B) Bridge on Swiss ball.

or bilaterally. Initially, this may be achieved by standing tall and simply dropping into a half-squat position. First, this is performed on both legs together (squat position) and then progressed to one leg leading (lunge position). These actions may be progressed to lunge, hop and jogging actions to eventually mimic the straight-leg heel contact position of terminal swing phase of running.

The flat floor position may be changed to a box drop position, when the action is to jump down and hold the position (Fig. 3.15). This action is progressed to drop, land and move in forward, sideways or rotary actions. These actions represent in-place (staying on one spot), short response (two or three hops or steps) or long response (multiple steps or hops) plyometrics. These actions can emphasize force generation (acceleration) or force acceptance (deceleration) depending on training requirements.

HQ ratio

The ratio of the strength of the hamstrings to that of the quadriceps muscles (HQ ratio) can be an important one in determining return to sport. Normally, the quadriceps is the stronger of the two muscle groups (Table 3.3), as demonstrated by its greater volume. However, any disturbance to this natural balance may leave the weaker muscle group open to injury. The optimum value of the HQ ratio varies from 50 per cent to 80 per cent (Kannus 1989), with average values in the region of 60 per cent. After knee injury, quadriceps wasting may result in the two muscle groups producing the same power, giving an increased HQ ratio. Looking at strength imbalances in professional soccer players, Croisier et al. (2008) tested 687 players using isokinetic dynamometry. The rate of hamstring muscle injury was greater in those with strength imbalances (relative risk 4.66), and normalizing the imbalance reduced the risk for injury to that found in those players without imbalance (relative risk 1.43).

143

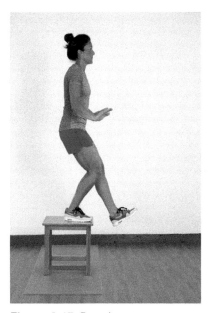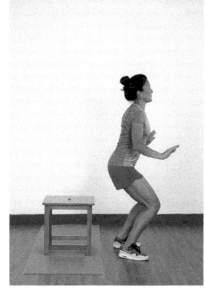

Figure 3.15 Box drop.

Table 3.3 Percentage of strength relative to quadriceps at 100%

Hamstrings	50–60%
Adductors	90%
Abductors	60%
Hip flexors	55%

From Reid (1992).

Definition

Relative risk (RR) is a statistical term comparing two groups. A relative risk of 1 means there is no difference in risk between the groups, so the risk is equal. An RR of < 1 shows the event is less likely to occur in the experimental group than in the control group, while an RR of > 1 means the event is more likely to occur, so there is greater risk.

Overload running

Initially following injury, active muscle lengthening may be imposed by walking (treadmill or set distance/time when land based). At this stage, pain tolerance can be used to limit training intensity and volume, with short timescales of five to ten minutes and pain intensity of three or four out of a maximum of ten (numerical rating scale). Early activity of this sort (from day one with more minor Grade I or II functional injuries) prevents the neuromuscular inhibition which is often seen following muscle injury. Progression can be time and/or distance, speed, stride length and incline. Table 3.4 outlines a progressive phase programme, from simply treadmill walking through to full running.

Treadmill walking gives way to gentle pain-free jogging, and scout pace (walk-jog-walk). Manual resistance is used as isometrics progress to concentrics using both bent leg (prone lying knee flexion) and straight leg (straight leg raise position) actions. The running speed increases gradually, ensuring that the subject can tolerate the increased load on the injured leg. Graded exposure is used, increasing and reducing distance and speed depending on symptoms initially. Manual concentric strength work is progressed to assisted bodyweight work using concentrics and eccentrics. Deadlift actions (straight leg and

Table 3.4 Progressive walk/run programme for hamstring rehabilitation

Phase	Activity
1	Isometrics to prevent neuromuscular inhibition
	Reduce pain maintain ROM
	Walk on treatment 4–6 mph until able to jog
2	Run at speed without symptoms – patient-led rehab
	Introduce concentrics using manual resistance bent/straight leg
	Swing through within comfortable range
	Increase running speed progressively
3	Increasing speed on treadmill to higher speed
	Concentric eccentric RDL low weight pull through with band
	NHE using swiss ball rollout
	1 k run outside
	4 mins high speed (4.5 m/s)
4	Treadmill higher speed, 30s on, 30s off, 6 reps – build to 5m/s and 6m/s
	Band assisted NHE
	Increase rate of force development using weights
5	Runway work 20m acceleration, 20m hold, 20m deceleration
	Increase speed and reduce distance to 15m then 10m
	Use acceleration/deceleration to progress rate of torque development
	Sagittal training progressing to cutting and multidirectional work
	Return to protected training and limited RTP
	Focus on load management

ROM – range of motion, NHE – Nordic hamstring exercise, RDL – Romanian deadlift, RTP – return to play.

bent leg) are performed to reduced range (bench or stool level) and using band assistance initially. Nordic hamstring curls can be begun with belt or resistance band assistance, progressing to swiss ball rollout as pain allows. Running gradually increases for pace, distance and incline. As function improves, the symptom-contingent nature of training can progress to time-contingent work (see Chapter 1).

Treadmill work gives way to normal running on a runway in the gym or sports field. Longer (50m) runs at slower pace gradually progress to shorter (30m, 20m) at increased pace. The next progression is to focus on acceleration and deceleration drills and to introduce sagittal (side step) and multidirectional (zig-zag and cutting) loading. The final progression prior to return to play (RTP) will depend on the sport and player's position, or subject's work-time and daily living actions. Functional progressions are used to replicate the actions to be encountered in sport / daily living with the aim of building final load tolerance and confidence in the limb.

Hamstring stretching

Current practice in both prevention and rehabilitation of hamstring injury places less emphasis on stretching than in previous years as the evidence for its importance is limited. Interestingly, active straight-leg raise (SLR) has been used as an assessment of both flexibility and feelings of general insecurity in the limb following injury. The test (H-test) is performed by the subject lying supine with the upper body and contralateral leg stabilized and the ipsilateral knee locked and held immobile in a brace. The subject performs a maximum number of rapid SLR actions and rates their experience on a VAS scale. The H-test was shown to be sensitive to detecting remaining signs of injury in MRI-confirmed acute hamstring strain when standard clinical examination (palpation pain, manual strength tests, passive SLR) had failed to do so (Askling et al. 2010).

Key point

The H-test consists of repeated active straight-leg raising (SLR) to rate range of motion (ROM) and feelings of limb insecurity following hamstring injury.

Table 3.5 Hamstring lengthening exercise protocol (L-protocol)

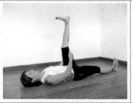

Extender: Active knee extension (AKE) exercise holding the thigh still (90° hip flexion) and extending the leg for 3 sets of 12 repetitions

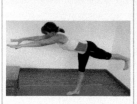

Diver: Modified arabesque exercise. Single-leg standing on injured side, with knee soft (10–20° flexion). Reach forwards, flexing at the hip, and stretch the arms out and free leg backwards, allowing back leg to bend. 3 sets of 6 reps.

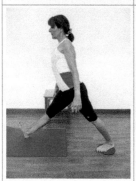

Glider: Modified front splits. Stand with the injured leg forwards holding onto a bar. Slide the unaffected leg backwards using a cloth/slide pad beneath the foot keeping the bodyweight on the front (injured) leg. Move back to the starting position using the arms, not pulling through the injured leg.

(Adapted from Askling et al. 2014)

Range of motion should be restored to that required by the subject's activities to ensure pain-free unrestricted movement. The use of range of motion combined with controlled contraction (eccentrics) more accurately reflects the functional requirements of the hamstrings than static stretching alone. A series of three lengthening actions (L-protocol) were compared to traditional contraction and static stretching (C-protocol) in elite sprinters and jumpers (Askling et al. 2014). The L-protocol gave a mean time for return to competition of 49 days, compared to 86 days for the C-protocol. The three exercises used are shown in Table 3.5 Activity-specific actions of this type can be designed using basic movement analysis of sports and daily actions, with an emphasis on 'strengthen and lengthen' exercise. These can progress to functional activities pre-competition, which involves all types of muscle work.

Where traditional stretching exercises are used, they must take account of pelvic action and the action of the two-joint muscle. In addition, relative flexibility (Chapter 2) may dictate that the majority of the stretching force is imposed on the lumbar spine in toe-touching type movements (Fig. 3.16).

Flexibility may begin with active knee extension (AKE), as described above. The advantage of this movement is the reciprocal innervation gained from quadriceps action, and the control that the athlete has over the movement. In addition, the back is supported throughout the action. The tripod stretch is also a useful exercise which requires a combination of pelvic stability with hamstring flexibility in a sitting position. The arms support the spine and encourage an upright body position.

Closed-chain actions

Closed-chain exercises for the hip extensors may be performed by modifying many common exercises. Leg rowing (Fig. 3.17A) is a useful exercise. The athlete sits on a towel (on a wooden floor) or plastic tray (on a carpeted floor) with the feet fixed. The action is to pull the body forwards

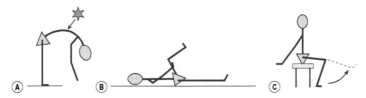

Figure 3.16 Modifying traditional hamstring stretches. (A) Relative flexibility in toe touch movement. (B) AKE action. (C) Tripod stretch.

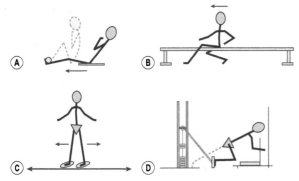

Figure 3.17 Hamstring exercises in closed kinetic chain. (A) Athlete sits on a towel on a wooden floor with feet fixed. Pull body forwards by flexing the knees and hips. (B) Sitting astride a gym bench, grip the feet against the floor and pull the body forwards. (C) Using a commercial slide trainer, straight-leg hip flexion and extension is performed. (D) Kneeling on a seated leg press machine, hip and knee extension is performed.

by hamstring action, mimicking a rowing position. Sitting astride a gym bench or 'form' (Fig. 3.17B), the athlete digs the heels into the ground and again pulls the body forwards using leg strength alone. Both of these actions may be performed unilaterally or bilaterally. The slide trainer may also be used for sagittal leg pumping actions with the knees straight or bent (Fig. 3.17C). The sitting leg press weight training apparatus may be used for the sprint kick exercise (Fig. 3.17D). Instead of sitting on the bench, the athlete turns around and places the shoulder against the chair back, and the ball of the foot on the machine pedal. The action is to press the machine pedal with a combined hip and knee extension action. Bridging actions may be performed with the foot on a moving surface (skateboard), bench or swiss ball as above for variety and resistance, increased by adding weight to the hips (barbell) and placing the shoulders on a bench.

Proximal hamstring tendinopathy

Proximal hamstring tendinopathy (PHT) may mimic a high hamstring tear. It presents as pain in the lower buttock localized to the ischial region, spreading into the upper posterior thigh. As with other types of tendinopathy, symptoms are often exacerbated by compressive forces. The subject of tendinopathy has been covered generally in Chapter 1, and specifically for the Achilles tendon in Chapter 5 and patella tendon in Chapter 4. Commonly compressive forces occur within the enthesis region of the tendon as it is compressed against underlying bone, in some cases causing inflammation of the bursa. The condition is more commonly seen in middle-distance runners, typically triggered by an increase in training volume. Symptoms are normally reproduced by compressing the common hamstring tendon onto the bone beneath, either using palpation or with static stretching (bent leg raise). Management of the condition follows that highlighted by the tendon healing phases of reactive tendinopathy, tendon disrepair and degenerative tendinopathy (Table 5.6). In the reactive phase, training modification to reduce loading is key. Subjects should avoid stretching (compression) and positions such as prolonged sitting wherever possible.

> **Key point**
>
> In the reactive (acute) phase of proximal hamstring tendinopathy, avoid stretching and limit compressive positions such as sitting.

Isometric hamstring contractions may be analgesic as with patella tendinopathy and exercises such as a prone hamstring curl with a partner or gym machine are useful. Once symptoms settle, progressive loading is used, initially with eccentric actions such as the assisted NHE described above. Exercise should avoid flexed hip positions (squat, lunge, deadlift) to minimize compressive forces and focus instead on bridging type action with the hip in neutral. As symptoms clear, hip flexion is gradually re-introduced to build load tolerance to this position. Final stage rehabilitation involves force acceptance and force development through the tendon with dynamic plyometric type actions such as jumps (standing and broad) and hops (multidimensional) as well as a progressive return to running, varying time, surface, speed and incline.

Groin injuries

Groin injury has a general incidence of between 0.5 and 6.2 per cent, with the incidence increasing to between 5 and 13 per cent in soccer (Choi, McCartney and Best 2008). Groin conditions have been categorized by the Doha agreement (Weir et al. 2015) into (i) defined clinical entities (adductor related, iliopsoas related, inguinal related and pubic related), (ii) hip-related groin pain, and (iii) other causes.

Adductor strain

Variously called groin strain and rider's strain, a tear of the adductor muscles gives pain to resisted adduction, and abduction stretch. Damage is usually to the musculotendinous junction about five centimetres from the pubis, or more rarely the teno-osseous junction, giving pain directly over the pubic tubercle (adductor longus) or body of the pubis.

The condition is more common in sports requiring a rapid change of direction, and where the adductors are used for propulsion. Pain is often experienced with sprinting, lunging and twisting on the straight leg.

In the reactive (acute) phase of the injury, rest and/ or load modification is required. Isometric exercise may be analgesic where adductor tendinopathy is present. Isometrics progress to loading exercise using both eccentrics and concentric contraction in open and closed chain.

Strength and flexibility

The adductor muscles are often neglected with respect to strengthening and flexibility, particularly in the male athlete. Sagittal plane leg movements are common in weight training, and although frontal plane actions and whole-body actions are available, they are sometimes less frequently used.

Treatment for the condition may therefore involve some stretching and a focus on strengthening the adductors. Soft tissue therapy to the region can be a useful form of pain modulation, and may change muscle tone and regional blood/fluid flow prior to exercise.

Initially, strength exercises such as side-lying (injured limb down), hip adduction with a weight bag over the knee (early) or ankle (more advanced) are useful as open-chain actions. Later, adduction may be performed using a weight and pulley apparatus (Fig. 3.18). Supported side bridge actions (Fig. 3.19) using a training partner or chair increase muscle overload. The subject begins in a splits position with the injured leg on top and supported. The action is to lift the lower leg from the ground in an attempt to bring the legs together (Copenhagen adductor exercise).

Dynamic training may be carried out by flicking a medicine ball with the foot with an adduction action. Swimming exercises, such as breaststroke, and hip adduction with a paddle secured to the lower leg are also of benefit. Closed kinetic chain actions using running, side stepping, jumping and hopping are included during late-stage rehabilitation, and whole-body actions such as squat and deadlift use the adductors as synergists.

Adductor stretching may be used for both the short adductors with the knee bent, and gracilis with the knee straight, where the demands of sport or daily activity require an increased range of motion. Stretching is not practised in the reactive phases of adductor tendinopathy to limit compressive loading on the enthesis. One common exercise is the 'tailor position' stretch (Fig. 3.20A), where the soles of the feet are together and the knees are pressed down with the hands or elbows. Although a useful movement in some cases, athletes often allow the pelvis to posteriorly tilt, flexing the lumbar spine (Fig. 3.20B). The posterior tilt of the pelvis pushes the pubic bone forwards, allowing a greater apparent range of motion and the knee to drop down further. A neutral pelvic position may be maintained by sitting on a wedge (Fig. 3.20C), or alternatively

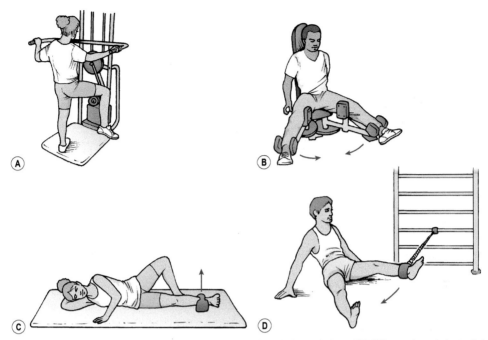

Figure 3.18 Hip adductor strengthening. (A) Unilateral weight-training. (B) Bilateral weight-training approach. (C) Weight bag. (D) Resistance tubing.

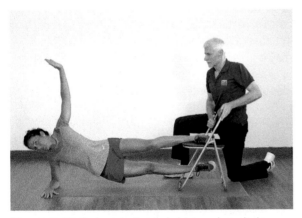

Figure 3.19 Supported side bridge using chair.

placing a rolled towel beneath the ischial tuberosities. As the knees are pressed down, the spine should be lengthened ('reach the top of your head to the ceiling'). The gracilis may be stretched in the stride sitting position with the leg straight, the same cautions concerning pelvic tilt applying. A more advanced gracilis stretch can be performed against a

wall (Fig. 3.20D). The hips are flexed to 90 degrees and the legs straight. Contract–relax (CR) stretching is performed by closing the legs (adduction resisted by limb weight) and then relaxing them into abduction. In addition, this starting position may be used to combine strength and dynamic stretch (strengthen and lengthen protocol) using the weight of the leg alone or overload imposed using a weight bag attached to the ankle.

> **Key point**
>
> When stretching the adductor muscles, take account of the degree of pelvic tilt. Posterior pelvic tilt will draw the pubic bone forwards and release tension from the adductor muscles in many stretches. Ensure that the athlete maintains lumbo-pelvic alignment throughout the stretch.

One complication of the disorder is the formation of myositis ossificans traumatica within the adductor

149

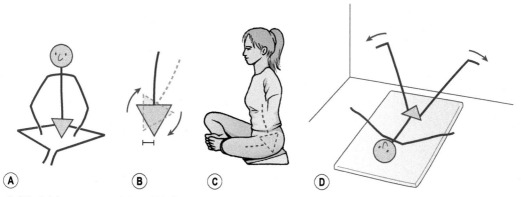

Figure 3.20 Adductor stretching. (A) Common adductor stretch. (B) Allowing the pelvis to posteriorly tilt pushes the pubis forwards. (C) Sitting on a wedge maintains the neutral lordosis. (D) Long adductor stretch.

origin. This is usually a consequence of inadequate rest during the acute stage of the condition. This condition is often described, somewhat inaccurately, under the general term 'osteitis pubis' (see below).

Iliopsoas

Pain to the anterior aspect of the groin more lateral that the adductor insertions can suggest Iliopsoas (IP) pain. While adductor pain has been shown to account for 66 per cent of athletic injuries related to kicking and change of direction, injury to the IP and proximal rectus femoris accounted for 15–25 per cent (Serner et al. 2015). IP pain may also be caused by an internal snapping hip syndrome (see below).

Symptoms are typically reproduced by resisted hip flexion and differentiated from rectus femoris by the absence of symptoms with knee extension. Palpation confirms the site of pain. Conservative treatment includes lengthening into hip extension while stabilizing the lumbo-pelvic region to avoid anterior pelvic tilt. Strengthening is by through-range hip flexor resistance against bands, building range and speed. Muscle imbalance tests to the region (see Table 3.1) may also highlight changes which may be significant if they modify symptoms.

Osteitis pubis

Several conditions may present as pubic overload in sport. True osteitis pubis is an aseptic condition affecting the pubic symphysis rather than the pubis itself, although the two conditions often coalesce. Diagnostically it is necessary to differentiate osteitis pubis from osteomyelitis pubis. The nature of osteitis pubis is inflammatory, while that of osteomyelitis pubis is infection. The most common infective agent is *Staphylococcus aureus*. This may come from infection during gynaecological or urological operations, or may be without an identifiable origin (Pauli et al. 2002).

> **Key point**
> *Osteitis pubis* is inflammatory in nature, while *osteomyelitis pubis* is an infection, most commonly of *Staphylococcus aureus* bacteria.

The clinical features of the two conditions are similar, except that osteomyelitis pubis is confirmed by biopsy and culture to identify the pathogen. Intravenous antibiotic treatment is usually effective.

With osteitis pubis, shearing stress is placed on the pubic symphysis during mid-stance as the non-weightbearing hip drops, tilting the pelvis. With distance runners, and particularly after pregnancy when the pubic symphysis is still mobile, this repetitive stress may inflame the pubic symphysis, a condition known as *pubis stress symphysitis*. Several etiological factors have been suggested, including restriction of hip mobility, hip and abdominal muscle imbalance, and sports involving repetitive twisting and cutting actions (Leblanc and LeBland 2003).

With osteitis pubis no instability of the pubic symphysis occurs, but there is tenderness over the area, with rarefaction of the pubic bones and sometimes widening of the symphysis pubis apparent on X-ray. Erosion of the superior and inferior aspects of the symphysis may also occur (Fig. 3.21). The athlete often has a waddling gait, and may describe occasional crepitus. Severe (long-term) cases may progress to sclerosis and eventual narrowing of the symphysial joint space. Bone marrow oedema may be visible on MRI scan.

Definition

Bone marrow oedema is a non-specific term describing changed signal uptake on a fluid-sensitive MRI scan. The fluid-filled region visualized may include water, blood, fibrosis or necrosis.

Palpation may be used to differentiate true osteitis pubis from tendinitis of the gracilis or avulsion injury to the gracilis attachment. The gracilis muscle attaches to the inferior aspect of the symphysis and local palpation may reveal spot tenderness (Fig. 3.22). Both of these conditions give pain to resisted adduction as well as to local palpation. Importantly, osteitis pubis often gives pain to pelvic springing tests to the iliac crest whilst gracilis conditions do not. The condition may be graded as illustrated in Table 3.6.

Key point

Palpation of the groin reveals the attachment of rectus abdominis at the top of the symphysis and adductor longus as a tight

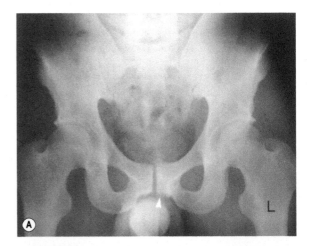

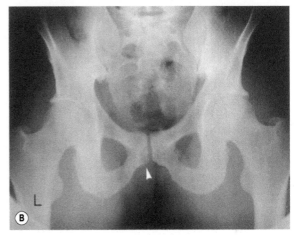

Figure 3.21 Osteitis pubis. (A) Anterior and (B) posterior view showing bone fragment. From Magee (2002), with permission.

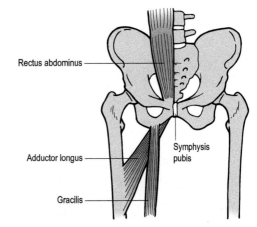

Figure 3.22 Palpation of the groin.

Table 3.6 Grading of osteitis pubis

Grade	Symptoms
I	Unilateral symptoms involving dominant leg, pain in inguinal region and adductor muscles
II	Bilateral symptoms with inguinal and adductor muscle pain
III	Bilateral inguinal pain with adductor and abdominal symptoms
IV	Adductor and abdominal pain referred to pelvis and lumbar spine. Exacerbation when walking on uneven surfaces or cough/sneeze. Limitation of ADL

ADL– activities of daily living.
After Wollin and Lovell (2006)

> cord at the bottom. Gracilis attaches to the inferior portion of the symphysis away from the mid-line.

Patients diagnosed earlier experience fewer symptoms and return to play faster. Rehabilitation focuses on core stability and strength/endurance of the muscles attaching to the pelvis. Initially, functional rest may be used, avoiding resisted exercise and ballistic stretching to the adductors and rectus abdominis. Isometric actions of the deep abdominals and pelvic floor are combined with isometric hip adduction. Fitness may be maintained with static cycling and aquajogging, providing these actions are pain free. As pain subsides, exercises progress, avoiding mid- to end-range abduction. Hip musculature may be retrained using resistance bands or pulleys. Hip stability training using single-leg standing actions to retrain the gluteus medius and core stability work are essential. Stretching, if required, must include both bent-knee and straight-leg actions. Rehabilitation progresses to skating actions on a slide board (Fig. 3.23A, B) and full-range adduction actions against resistance are used within pain tolerance (Fig 3.24A, B). Progression of both range of motion and speed of motion on a slide board are used. A rehabilitation protocol has been described by Wollin and Lovell (2006) which gives exercise suggestions and criteria for progression. This programme (Table 3.6) has been used to successfully rehabilitate young soccer players, all of whom returned to competitive sport symptom free with no recurrence reported at 12 months follow-up.

Where conservative management fails and symptoms are both severe and long lasting,

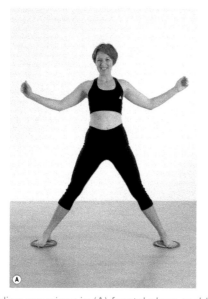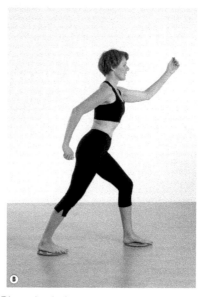

Figure 3.23 Sliding exercises in (A) frontal plane and (B) sagittal plane.

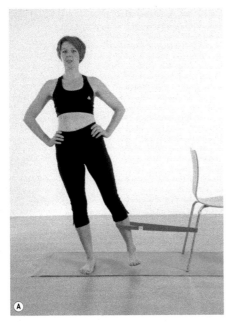

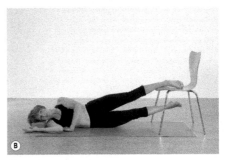

Figure 3.24 Hip adductor strength, (A) using band and (B) gravity resisted.

invasive management may be required. Injection with corticosteroid has shown a moderate success rate for return to sport (58.6 per cent with return eight weeks following injection) but a high number of athletes (20.7 per cent) may not respond (O'Connell, Powell and McCaffrey 2002). Prolotherapy using dextrose and lidocaine has shown a better success rate (91.7 per cent return to sport within nine weeks of injection), suggesting that it may be superior to corticosteroid (Topol, Reeves and Hassanein 2005). Surgery using curettage of the pubic symphysis or pubic symphysis stabilization with polypropylene mesh has also been used successfully where symptoms were long-term (17 months). Complications included haemospermia and intermittent scrotal swelling (Choi et al. 2008).

Avulsion injuries around the hip

Avulsion injuries occur when a rapid muscle contraction pulls on the bony origin of the muscle. This may occur if the contracting muscle suddenly meets an unexpected resistance, such as kicking and catching the ground. Alternatively, avulsion may occur through uncontrolled stretching, particularly unsupervised full-range ballistic stretching (Fig. 3.25). This may occur to the sartorius at the anterior superior iliac spine, the rectus femoris at the anterior inferior iliac spine, the hamstrings at the ischial tuberosity or, less commonly, to the iliopsoas at the lesser trochanter (Fig. 3.26).

Avulsion usually occurs at the apophysis in a young (14–17 years) athlete (see below). However, as the ischial apophysis unites later (20–25 years), avulsion of the hamstrings at the ischial tuberosity may be seen up until this age and has been described in judo exponents (Kurosawa et al. 1996). At this time the tenoperiosteal junction is generally stronger than the unfused growth centre. There is usually little displacement due to the thickness of the periosteum. Athletes usually complain of a sudden onset of pain with limitation of movement over the affected joint, and extensive bruising to the lower buttock. Treatment involves the POLICE protocol initially, and, importantly, protection from tension forces over the muscle. MRI is used to confirm the injury and bone healing may occur

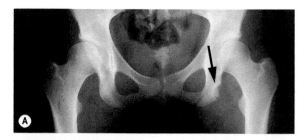

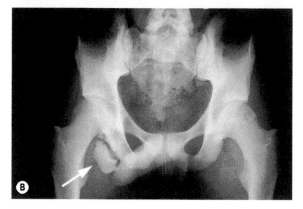

Figure 3.25 Avulsion injury around the hip. From Read (2000), with permission.

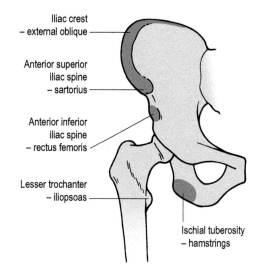

Figure 3.26 Common sites for avulsion injuries around the hip.

within three to six weeks where displacement has not occurred. With displacement of the hamstring origin, surgical management may be required (Oravo and Kujala 1995). Surgical intervention generally produces better results when the repair is performed within six weeks of initial injury (Subbu et al. 2015). The retracted portion of muscle-bone is retrieved and fastened back using synthetic sutures attached to a metal peg. Where sciatic nerve involvement is found and greater retraction has occurred, rehabilitation and RTP is longer.

Sciatic nerve involvement has also been described atraumatically. Puranen and Orava (1988) described athletes with gluteal pain radiating into the posterior thigh with no history of trauma, which they described as a *hamstring syndrome*. Pain occurred most often in the sitting position, and when stretching the hamstrings. Local tenderness was evident to the ischial tuberosity, neurological examination was normal, and extensive physiotherapy failed to remove the symptoms. At operation, tight fibrotic bands were found from

the semitendinosus and biceps femoris, close to the sciatic nerve and in some cases adhered to it. Release of the tight bands gave symptomatic relief to 52 of the 59 patients treated. The authors proposed that excessive stretching may have led to hypercompensation within the muscles, particularly in sprinters and hurdlers.

Piriformis syndrome

The piriformis muscle (Fig. 3.27) attaches from the front of the second to fourth sacral segments, the gluteal surface of the ileum and the sacrotuberous ligament. It then travels through the greater sciatic notch to attach to the upper medial side of the greater trochanter. Its position is such that the sciatic nerve rests directly on the muscle, and in 15 per cent of the population the muscle is divided into two, with the sciatic nerve passing between the two bellies.

Piriformis syndrome occurs in women more frequently than men (ratio 6:1). If the muscle is inflamed, shortened or in spasm it will impinge on the sciatic nerve, giving pain and tingling in the posterior thigh and buttock. Pain is deep and localized and examination of the lumbar spine and sacroiliac joints is unrevealing. Palpation of the

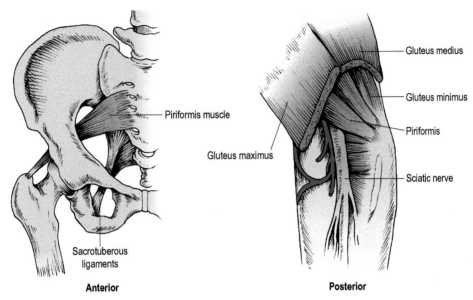

Figure 3.27 Position of the piriformis muscle.

muscle may be carried out with the patient prone in the frog position (hip flexed and abducted, bringing knee to chest), or rectally. Resisted lateral rotation of the affected hip gives pain, and passive stretch into internal rotation is painful and may be limited.

Management involves pain-relieving modalities such as acupuncture or dry needling, manual therapy and stretching to the region. A simple self-stretch can be taught to the patient. If the right hip is affected, the left hip is flexed to 90 degrees and the right foot is placed on the left knee. The right hip is pushed gently into abduction and external rotation (Fig. 3.28). Pain modulation may be produced using trigger-point self-massage using a firm ball or roller.

Lateral hip pain

Pain over the lateral aspect of the hip around the greater trochanter is a common clinical occurrence, with incidence in industrialized societies being put as high as 25 per cent of the population (Williams and Cohen 2009). Typical titles in the literature include iliotibial band syndrome (ITBS) at the hip, external snapping hip, gluteus medius

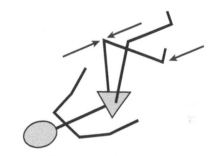

Figure 3.28 Gluteal stretch.

tendinopathy, greater trochanteric pain syndrome (GTPS) and trochanteric bursitis. These diagnoses broadly represent pathology to the same structures and may occur separately or in association with femoral acetabular impingement (FAI), degenerative changes to the joint, and labral pathology, all of which may change the quality of movement at the hip and alter muscle function, giving primary pain anteriorly and secondary pain laterally.

> **Key point**
> Lateral hip pain may occur as a single entity, or in association with other hip pathologies.

155

Lower back conditions may also refer into the lateral thigh so screening tests should rule out the lower back as a cause of pain. Compression of the lateral cutaneous nerve of the thigh (meralgia paraesthetica) close to the attachment of the inguinal ligament into the anterior superior iliac spine (ASIS) can refer pain into the lateral thigh. Impact to this area in sport (hip pointer) presenting as altered sensation warrants further investigation.

Applied anatomy

Hip joint

Alignment of the pelvis on the femur (femoropelvic alignment) in the frontal place during single-leg stance is maintained by an equilibrium of the compression forces created by weightbearing, and those of the lateral hip structures. The bodyweight acts on a resistance arm from the gravity line, passing through the centre of the sacrum to the hip joint axis. This is countered by muscle force acting on a lever from the lateral hip musculature to the hip joint axis.

This set-up subjects the hip joint to considerable forces during weightbearing. In single-leg standing, hip joint forces between 1.8 and 3.0 times bodyweight occur, while in walking these increase to 3.3–5.5 times bodyweight (Palastanga et al. 2006). The femoral head is smaller in females, while the pelvis is wider. The resistance arm from the body's line of gravity to the pelvis is therefore larger in the female (Fig. 3.29) while the lever arm from the lateral musculature to the centre of the hip joint is smaller. The combination of these two features significantly reduces the mechanical advantage of the abductor muscles. With a lower mechanical advantage, the muscles must work harder to maintain femoropelvic alignment, and this increased muscle work acting over a smaller head size results in greater femoral head pressures in females (Brinckman et al. 1981). In addition, the incidence of GTPS is four times greater in females than males (Williams and Cohen 2009).

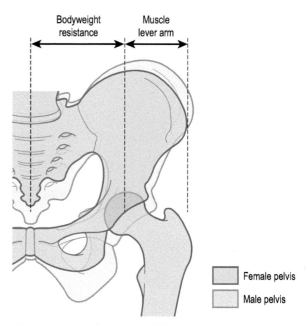

Figure 3.29 Mechanical differences between male and female pelvis.

Lateral musculature

The lateral muscles are arranged in three layers (Table 3.7) and function to control the femoral head within the acetabulum and/or to control the pelvis on the femur. Joint stability is better produced by those muscles lying close to the axis of rotation of

Table 3.7 Muscle layers of the lateral hip

Layer	Muscles	Function
1 – deep	Gluteus minimus	▶ Primary stabilizer functioning to control femoral head within acetabulum ▶ Proprioceptive role
2 – intermediate	Gluteus medius, Piriformis	▶ Significant torque producers ▶ Secondary stabilizer ▶ Low load control of pelvis on femur
3 – superficial	Tenor fascia lata (TFL), Gluteus maximus, Vastus lateralis	▶ Primary torque producers ▶ High load control of pelvis on femur

the joint (Chapter 2). Shearing (translation) force on the femoral head is therefore reduced by the deep lateral rotators (obturator externis, gamelli, quadratus femuris), gluteus minimus, iliacus and iliocapsularis. The iliacus muscle consists of two sets of fibres, with the lateral portion more active in torque production and the medial (deep) fibres being linked to stability, the medial fibres, being predominantly slow twitch in nature. The ilocapsularis (also called iliacus minor) lies beneath the rectus femoris and attaches directly to the joint capsule. It functions to tighten the joint capsule and has been shown to hypertrophy and have less fatty infiltration in cases of hip dysplasia (Ward et al. 2000, Babst et al. 2011).

Key point

The *ilocapsularis* (iliacus minor) lies beneath the rectus femoris. It attaches directly to the joint capsule, and functions to tighten it.

Failure to control translation of the head of the femur, especially in an anterior direction (anterior laxity and posterior tightness), may increase the risk of femoral acetabular impingement (FAI), particularly where an underlying bony anomaly (joint dysplasia) exists.

The gluteus medius has three distinct fascial layers (Jaegers et al. 1992), each with a separate nerve supply. The anterior and posterior portions lie deep to the middle portion. Although the gluteus medius is often considered the primary hip stabilizer and targeted by clamshell-type actions, physiologically it is unable to stabilize the pelvis on the femur in single-leg standing by itself. It has been calculated (Kummer 1993) that the abduction forces responsible for this are divided between the gluteus medius (70 per cent) and the muscles attaching to the ITB (30 per cent). The upper portion of gluteus maximus (see below) and the tensor fascia lata (TFL) both attach into the ITB and the vastus lateralis may also be considered through its fascial attachment (Birnbaum et al. 2004).

Table 3.8 Bursae around the greater trochanter (GT)

Name of Bursa	Position relative to GT	Approximate size (cm²)
Gluteus maximus	Lateral	10–15
Gluteofemoral	Caudal	10–15
Gluteus medius	Anterior to apex	1.0–1.7
Gluteus minimus	Anterolateral	2.7–4.4

(Data modified from Wollin, M., Lovell, G., 2006)

Of the hip lateral rotator group, the quadratus femoris (QF) has been shown to demonstrate the greatest differential atrophy with prolonged bed rest. In the second Berlin bed rest study, for example, the QF was shown to lose 9.8 per cent volume after 28 days and 18.1 per cent volume after 56 days of head-down tilt bed rest (Miokovic et al. 2011). The gluteus medius reduced its volume by only 3.7 per cent and no change was seen in the obturators or piriformis muscles.

Key point

Although often considered the prime stabilizing muscle of the hip, the *gluteus medius* muscle is unable to stabilize the pelvis on the femur (single-leg standing) by itself. In addition, with prolonged rest the gluteus medius wastes less than the quadratus femoris.

The lateral muscles are separated from each other and underlying structures by four main bursae (Table 3.8) each with deep, superficial and/or secondary portions. In total, synovial lined bursae around the GT have been found at ten different locations on dissection (Woodley et al. 2008).

Ilio tibial band

The deep fascia of the lower limb is collectively called the fascia lata. It attaches to the outer lip of the iliac crest along its full length, and throws branches to the sacrotuberous ligament, the ischial tuberosity, and the pubis, effectively surrounding the upper thigh. On the lateral aspect of the thigh, this fascia is thickened into two distinct layers forming a non-elastic collagen cord, the ilio tibial band (ITB).

The gluteus maximus and gluteus medius muscles insert into the ITB posteriorly and the tensor fascia lata (TFL) muscle inserts anteriorly. Some of the TFL fibres travel a third of the way down the ITB.

As the ITB travels down the lateral side of the thigh, its deep fibres form inwardly directed sheets which attach to the linea aspera of the femur, forming the medial and lateral intermuscular septa. The superficial fibres of the ITB continue downwards to attach to the lateral femoral condyle, lateral patellar retinaculum and anterolateral aspect of the tibial condyle (Gerdy's tubercle). A large amount of the lateral retinaculum of the patella actually arises from the ITB to form the iliopatellar band (Terry et al. 1986), having a direct effect on patellar tracking (see Chapter 4).

In standing, the ITB lies posterior to the hip axis and anterior to the knee axis and therefore helps to maintain hip and knee extension, reducing the muscle work required to sustain an upright stance. In running, during the swing phase the ITB lies anterior to the greater trochanter and hip flexion/extension axis, reducing the workload required for hip flexion.

The contraction of the gluteus medius and the TFL is transmitted by the ITB to control and decelerate adduction of the thigh (Fredericson et al. 1997). Where the gluteus medius shows poor endurance and control, gait alteration may occur, leading to lateral pain. In a study of distance runners (14 male, 10 female) with ITBS, significant weakness of the gluteus medius was found on the symptomatic side. Strengthening the muscle over a six-week period resulted in 92 per cent of the runners being pain free (Fredericson et al. 1997).

Muscle balance tests for the lower limb (see Table 3.1) often show a reduction in abduction endurance by the gluteus medius and compensation by overactivity of the tightening of the TFL-ITB. Although both the gluteus medius

and the TFL are able to abduct the femur, the TFL will also medially rotate the hip while the postural posterior portion of the gluteus medius is a lateral rotator (Sahrmann 2002). As a consequence, dependence on the TFL alone for abduction power during gait may favour medial rotation and adduction of the hip, increasing the valgus stress on the limb and therefore increasing passive tension in the ITB.

The Trendelenburg test

The Trendelenburg test (Fig. 3.30) is often used in the clinic to assess control of the pelvis on the femur in single-leg standing, so is perhaps the most relevant test to lateral hip pain. With a positive test, as bodyweight is taken through one leg, the pelvis dips downwards away from the weightbearing leg. This is known clinically as an uncompensated positive result. A compensated

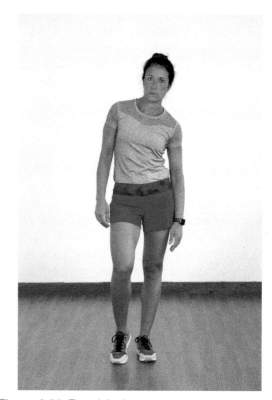

Figure 3.30 Trendelenburg test.

positive result occurs if the body is tilted (side flexed) towards the weightbearing leg. A further modification of the test is to ask the client to elevate the non-weightbearing side of the pelvis and to hold this position for 30 seconds. This modification assesses the postural endurance of the lateral hip muscles. The test is positive if the client is unable to maximally elevate the pelvis or maintain the elevation for the 30 seconds (Grimaldi 2011). The test can be refined by using goniometry to measure the pelvic to femur angle, taking a line horizontally across the anterior superior iliac spines (ASIS) and vertically down the shaft of the femur. Changes in the pelvic-femur angle can occur if the hip dips downwards (lateral pelvic tilt) or moves horizontally to the side (lateral pelvic shift). Normal values of 5-degree increase in hip adduction have been reported when moving from double- to single-leg standing (DiMattia et al. 2005).

The Trendelenburg test is not muscle specific but it does give information about the client's self-selected movement pattern, which will be influenced by factors such as pain, habit and energy expenditure, as well as muscle performance. Where subjects habitually hang on the hip (single-leg dominant swayback posture) the hip abductor muscles will lengthen. The shift into length-tension curve which occurs with posturally lengthened muscles (see Chapter 2) means that the muscle is effectively stronger in its lengthened position (peak torque at greater joint angle). As a consequence the Trendelenburg test will likely see a greater angle of hip adduction in those who demonstrate a swayback posture and favour one leg. Interestingly, in cases of hip joint degeneration, peak acetabular loading occurs at maximum gluteus medius activity rather than at peak ground reaction force, so lateral trunk movement (also called Duchenne limping) has been proposed as an offloading strategy to minimize muscle contraction (Krebs et al. 1998). Optimization of the Trendelenburg test in the clinic has been proposed (Grimaldi 2011), with actions shown in Table 3.9.

Table 3.9 Optimization of the Trendelenburg test in the clinic

Non-weightbearing leg held in 0°–30° flexion
Arms across the chest or against the body
Quantify trunk translation in the frontal plane
Measure movement of the sternal notch from the body midline (midpoint of ASIS)
Ask subject to correct bodysway to assess compensatory mechanism(s)
Is correction painful (acetabular loading/tendinopathy/bursal compression)?
Is correction not possible due to muscle condition (poor strength/inner range holding)?
Is correction simple (habitual pattern)?

(After Grimaldi 2011)

Rehabilitation

Rehabilitation aims to redress the movement dysfunction, which may be considered as a major factor in the development of lateral hip pain. Initially, the aim is to lengthen the tight lateral structures and begin building the endurance of the hip stabilizing muscles to reduce symptoms. Next, general hip and lumbo-pelvic alignment is enhanced, with an emphasis on controlling the weight shift during single-leg standing especially. Finally, more sport-specific actions are used to build control of the hip in functional sports actions. Clinically there is much overlap between each rehab stage, and the order of exercise application will be dictated by your client's symptoms.

Rehabilitation can focus on pain relief, lengthening tight tissues which restrict correct movement, retraining muscle which is underperforming (strength/endurance/power), and enhancing whole-body and segmental alignment. Where pain is a dominant feature, its reduction is important as it will have a significant effect on the quality of movement. In many cases, trigger points within a tight muscle may be a dominant feature in the production of pain and so tightness is targeted in this case. Overload of tissues and/or joints can lead to inflammation and pain, making posture the lead feature.

Treatment note 3.3   Targeting the ITB

Often with lateral hip pain the ITB becomes the focus of attention. Stretching the ITB is a subject of considerable debate. As the band attaches directly to the femur via the intermuscular septa, lengthening it would seem impossible (Mercer et al. 1998). However, clinically patients with ITBS do respond to stretching exercises, showing increased range of motion, reduced pain and an alteration in tissue tension to palpation. The superficial portion may have some independence from the deeper portions, and in addition changes in pain tolerance and alteration of muscle tone of muscle feeding into the ITB may occur.

An effective ITB stretch position must combine movement in three regions: the pelvis, hip and knee. The Ober test position is chosen in the first instance, with the affected leg uppermost. Initially, the leg is abducted (45 degrees to the horizontal) and extended (10–15 degrees behind the bodyline). The underside of the trunk is then pressed into the floor and kept in this position throughout the exercise, initially through therapist pressure (passive) and then through patient control (active). With the pelvis stable, the upper leg is lowered back towards the horizontal while maintaining the extended leg position. A useful visual cue is for the subject to look down towards their foot. If they can see their patella, the extension has been lost, if they cannot, the leg is extended and the view of the patella is blocked by the front of the pelvis. A tactile cue which may be used is to place a folded towel between the floor and the side of the body, just above the pelvis. The aim is to press down hard on the towel throughout the exercise.

The Ober stretch position targets the whole of the ITB. However, where trigger points are present within the TFL-ITB, the tissue may be placed on stretch and a self-massage technique employed. Now, the starting position is for the subject to lie on the back and to flex both the hip and knee of both legs. The unaffected leg is crossed over the affected one and the hip pulled into adduction. This places some stretch on the upper portion of the ITB and allows the subject to press into the painful area 15–25 centimetres below the greater trochanter. Where a painful trigger point is found, firm pressure should be applied and held for 30–40 seconds until the pain begins to subside.

The ITB may also be targeted using pressure from a firm ball or foam roller to modulate pain. Ball pressure may be performed by trapping the ball between the leg and a wall and moving the ball to a painful region. For foam roller pressure a side-lying position is used, with the affected leg downwards and the upper leg flexed at the knee (foot flat on the floor for support). The body is moved over the roller to target the painful region. (Fig. 3.31)

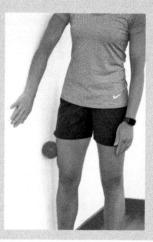

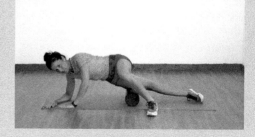

Figure 3.31 Targeting the ITB.

Open-chain exercise

Developing inner-range holding to hip abduction and external rotation can be a useful starting point for rehabilitation, and clamshell-type movements are often popular for both testing (see above) and rehabilitation. However, in cases of gluteal tendinopathy the lower position (adduction and internal rotation) may lead to compression forces which exacerbate tendinopathy pain. The full exercise is therefore modified by placing a cushion or pillow between the knees to focus on the inner-range (abduction and external rotation) position in isolation. The subject begins lying on the side with the affected leg uppermost, hip and knee flexed. Keeping the feet together, the aim is to lift the knee without allowing any trunk rotation. Many subjects with ITBS find this end position of the exercise difficult to achieve. In this case, a training partner is used to lift the leg into position and the subject tries to slowly lower the leg back to the starting position so the knee rests on the pillow between the legs (eccentric control). Once this can be performed in a controlled fashion for five repetitions, the subject should begin the movement by holding the leg in the upper position (full inner range) again for five seconds (isometric control). Finally, the subject lifts the leg (concentric control), holds it in its upper position (isometric control) and lowers it slowly (eccentric control). Once this movement can be performed for five to ten repetitions, the subject can progress to Phase II of the rehabilitation programme. This clamshell position has both advantages and disadvantages. By flexing the knee and hip, the lever arm of the leg is reduced, making the action easier to achieve for the client. Where the flexed-hip position is not tolerated, a lying scissor action (leg straight) may also be used. In both cases the non-weightbearing starting positions do not mimic the functional straight-leg weightbearing position. It is important, therefore, to progress from the clamshell or scissor muscle isolation actions to weightbearing whole-body movement as soon as the client is able.

Exercise selection

Although muscle isolation exercises have been shown to be superior to whole-body exercise at targeting the *gluteus medius* muscle, it is the side-lying hip scissor which gives the greatest work when measured as mean EMG signal amplitude expressed as a percentage of maximal voluntary isometric contraction (MVIC). Looking at 12 rehabilitation exercises for the hip, Distefano et al. (2009) found the hip scissor to give a mean of 81 per cent, compared to 40 per cent for the clam. Single-leg squat and single-leg deadlift produced values of 64 and 58 per cent respectively.

For the *gluteus maximus*, both the single-leg squat and the single-leg deadlift gave values of 59 per cent, with the lunge scoring 44 per cent and the clam 39 per cent. The forward lunge action, using a forward angulation of the trunk to bring the chest close to the thigh and hands towards the floor, has been shown to increase the workload on the hip extensors. Comparing a neutral lunge (NL) with a lunge placing the trunk forwards (LTF), Farrokhi et al. (2008) showed mean values of 18.5 and 11.9 for the gluteus maximus and biceps femoris respectively in the NL, compared to 22.3 and 17.9 for the LTF, with each score expressed as a percentage of MVIC.

Closed-chain exercise

Rehabilitation in Phase II sees the introduction of weightbearing activities maintaining lumbo-pelvic alignment as the weight is taken onto the affected leg. Exercises begin with weight-shift actions, moving the pelvis to the affected side while keeping it level and avoiding any hip 'dipping'. Once the weight can be shifted in a controlled fashion, the knee on the unaffected leg is bent to take the weight off this side and leave the affected leg taking full bodyweight. Again, control is the focus here. As the weight is shifted over the affected leg, the pelvis should remain level, and as the unaffected leg is bent, the pelvis must not dip towards this side or 'hitch' upwards. Lower-limb alignment must also be emphasized to prevent the pelvis dipping and the knee drifting inwards. The knee should remain directly over the centre of the foot, avoiding pronation (foot flattening) and hip adduction. The aim is to maintain precise alignment and to build muscle endurance. Progression is made of holding time, therefore, holding the correct alignment for 20–30 seconds and performing 5–10 repetitions.

The next stage is to perform the same alignment pattern but to allow controlled bending of the knee on the affected side using the mini-dip exercise. The subject stands with the foot of the affected leg on a small (5 cm) block. Keeping the pelvis horizontal, the weight is shifted towards the affected leg and then lowered into a single-leg squat, controlling the action and maintaining lower-limb alignment throughout the movement. This mini dip is performed for five to eight reps, emphasizing timing of the eccentric lowering aspect (five to ten seconds) rather than just the concentric lifting (two to three seconds).

Using a band around the legs at mid-thigh level, lateral walking and squat action may be performed to emphasize hip abduction and avoid an adducted and internally rotated position (Fig. 3.32A). Bridging actions performed with either one or both legs, initially with the feet on the floor, progressing to feet on a mobile platform (Fig. 3.32B), place considerable overload on the gluteal muscles and avoid hip flexion and adduction. Placing a resistance band around the knees of bilateral actions emphasizes the abduction action. A slide board or horizontal leg press machine may be used later to provide bodyweight or weight-stack resistance (Fig. 3.32C).

Classical gym-based exercises such as squats, lunges and deadlifts are useful in the final phases of rehabilitation and may be modified if required. Squat exercises may be performed freestanding (classic barbell squat) or using a frame (Smith frame) to guide the bar. Modifications include squatting with the patient's back resting on a gym ball placed on a wall, squatting onto a chair, and using dumb-bells held in each hand to the side

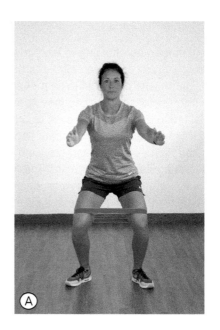

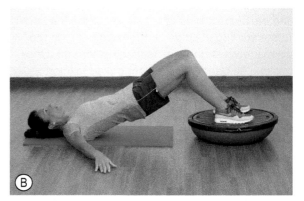

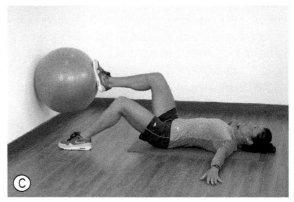

Figure 3.32 Hip strengthening. (A) Squat with band. (B) Bridge on mobile platform. (C) Horizontal leg press.

of the hip rather than a barbell held across the shoulders (dumb-bell squat).

In the classic squat the knee passes over the toes as the ankle dorsiflexes. Restricting this transverse knee movement by trying to keep the tibia vertical has been shown to reduce torque at the knee (mean value 117.3 Nm compared to 150.1Nm) but increase it at the hip (mean value 302.7NM compared to 28.2NM. In addition, restricting anterior knee motion produces a greater anterior angulation of the trunk (Fry et al. 2003). Performing a squat on a linear frame enables users to better maintain trunk alignment as the bar is unable to move forwards. In addition, the action may be changed to a semi-recumbent starting position, where the knee stays over the foot and the user sits back rather than downwards (hack squat). When performing this type of squat, the knee moment has been shown to be greater than the hip moment, with more muscle work on the knee extensors (quadriceps) than the hip extensors (gluteals and hamstrings). As the foot is moved forwards into a hack squat position, the hip moment increases and the knee moment reduces, effectively reversing the muscle emphasis, placing significantly greater work on the hip extensors compared to the knee extensors (Abelbeck 2002).

Treatment note 3.4   Trigger point treatment of buttock structures

Pain from muscle origin may be treated by direct pressure and dry needling. Dry needling or trigger point acupuncture involves inserting a sterile acupuncture needle into the muscle, which is normally overactive and may be in spasm. As the needle enters the muscle, it meets tissue resistance. The needle may gradually be pressed into the firmer tissue as the tissue gives way. Precise surface marking is required for this technique and knowledge of underlying structures is essential.

In the hip, the major hip muscles treated in this way are the piriformis, gluteus medius and quadratus femoris. The lumbar multifidus may be treated as it thickens between the sacrum and medial aspect of the ilium, an area called the multifidus triangle. In addition, the quadratus lumborum and erector spinae may be needled at their insertion onto the iliac crest (Gunn 1996, 2000).

Surface marking

To visualize important structures in the buttocks, three lines may be drawn joining the sacral dimple (posterior superior iliac spine, PSIS), greater trochanter and ischial tuberosity (Borley 1997). The sciatic nerve emerges from the pelvis midway along a line drawn from the sacral dimple and the ischial tuberosity. It then runs in a semicircle to a point halfway along a line joining the ischial tuberosity and the greater trochanter of the femur. The superior gluteal nerve and artery pass a point a third of the way along a line joining the sacral dimple to the greater trochanter. The inferior gluteal nerve and artery pass a point a third of the way along a line joining the ischial tuberosity and the sacral dimple (Fig. 3.33).

Trigger points

To facilitate palpation, the patient should be placed in side-lying, with the painful side on top and the hip flexed. The gluteus medius may be treated about five centimetres along a line from the iliac crest to the greater trochanter. It is sometimes easier to palpate the greater trochanter and allow the palpating finger to move backwards and upwards until a painful point is located. The quadratus femoris can only be located with the gluteal muscle relaxed, and it may be palpated from the posterior aspect of the greater trochanter to the lateral edge of the ischial tuberosity. As it is a lateral rotator of the hip, medially rotating the femur will place the muscle on stretch and make palpation easier. The piriformis is located along a line from the greater trochanter to the second, third and fourth sacral

---

Treatment note 3.4 *continued*

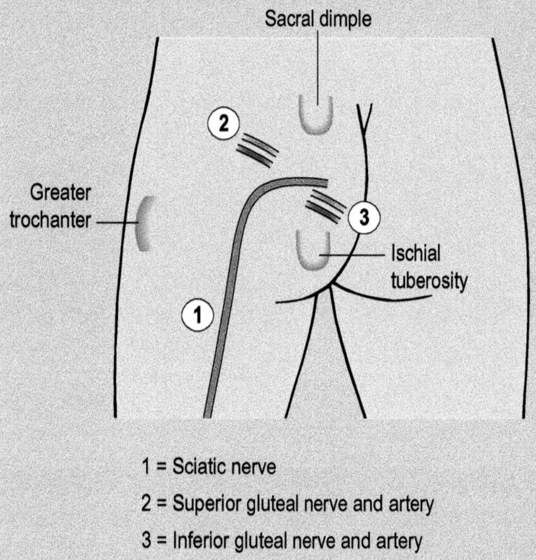

1 = Sciatic nerve
2 = Superior gluteal nerve and artery
3 = Inferior gluteal nerve and artery

Figure 3.33 Surface marking of buttock structures. From Borley (1997), with permission.

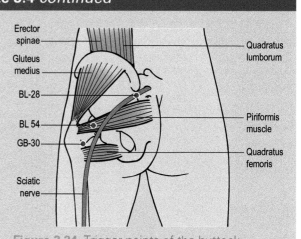

Figure 3.34 Trigger points of the buttock.

segments. If deep manual pressure is used, points within the muscles may be chosen. For dry needling, use of points close to the greater trochanter or ischial tuberosity avoids the risk of hitting the sciatic nerve.

The quadratus lumborum and erector spinae may be palpated along the iliac crest. To facilitate location, the patient should be side flexed away from the painful side to place the muscle on stretch. The multifidus is large and thick in the lumbar spine and in the area between the PSIS and sacral spines, down to a level of S4 (the multifidus triangle), and muscle may be treated for trigger points with either manual therapy or dry needling (Fig. 3.34).

Hip joint pain

The hip (coxa-femoral) joint itself may be implicated in a number of sports and work-related injuries. Arthritic changes to the joint, labral involvement and joint displacement (anterior femoral glide) causing tissue impingement are the most important hip joint conditions in this respect.

Hip arthritis

Osteoarthrosis of the hip affects between 1 and 2 per cent of the adult population, with women making up 60–75 per cent of this group. The condition often occurs secondary to other pathology, most typically osteonecrosis, Perthes' disease, developmental dysplasia, slipper femoral epiphysis, hip fracture and congenital coxa vara or valga (Fagerson 2009). X-ray shows narrowing of the joint on the weightbearing portion with osteophyte formation. Manual therapy has been shown to be of value in the non-operative treatment of hip OA, with pain, stiffness, hip function and range of motion all changing significantly (Hoeksma et al. 2004). Acupuncture may be of value to target pain (Haslam 2001), with six sessions of twenty-five minutes duration giving significant improvement of pain and function (WOMAC score), which is maintained for eight weeks after stopping treatment. Change of lifestyle is also effective, and includes weight reduction, activity modification, reduction in load carrying and use of walking aids. Clinically, a combination of initial pain relief and a progressive exercise programme to re-strengthen the supporting musculature of the hip is often effective.

Several hip arthroplasty (replacement) techniques are used, broadly falling into total and partial replacement, with and without cement. Three main incisions are used, as shown in Table 8.6, and exercise prescription should take into account the muscles affected.

Hip impingement

Impingement occurs when a structure is compressed or trapped between two surfaces. In this case it is the hip bone (femur) and hip socket (acetabulum) which are moving towards each other and impinging. Hip impingement was first discussed before the Second World War (Smith-Petersen 1936), but Femoroacetabular (FAI) syndrome itself is a comparatively new term, with surgical management reported after the millennium (Ganz et al. 2001). The condition has become more common, with 1908 patients reported in 2011 in the UK NHS (Griffin et al. 2016b).

FAI syndrome is a premature contact between the acetabulum and the proximal femur which has been defined as *a motion-related clinical disorder of the hip with a triad of symptoms, clinical signs, and imaging findings* (Griffin et al. 2016a). The condition cannot be diagnosed by imaging alone, but imaging can help guide treatment options. The term 'syndrome' is used to distinguish the condition from FAI, which may not be symptomatic, and to reflect the multifactorial nature of the condition.

Bone changes and imaging

Normally in a patient with FAI syndrome, the structure and shape (morphology) of the bones involved has altered, with the head of the femur changing from its normal ball shape to an egg shape, termed a cam. The socket (acetabulum) will typically increase the size of its lip, giving the appearance of a pincer (Fig. 3.35). Generally, pincer impingement is more commonly seen in middle-aged females (average age 40), and cam impingement is more

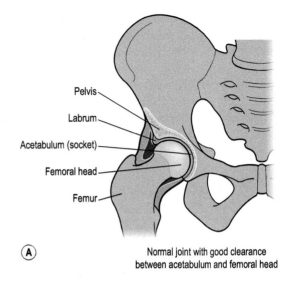

(A) Normal joint with good clearance between acetabulum and femoral head

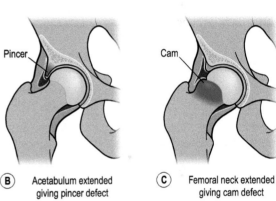

(B) Acetabulum extended giving pincer defect
(C) Femoral neck extended giving cam defect

Figure 3.35 Cam and pincer impingements.

common in young men (average age 32) (Tannast et al. 2007). These changes may be present in 30 per cent of the adult population, and not all patients with this morphology develop FAI (Dickenson et al. 2016).

> **Definition**
>
> A *cam* impingement is an alteration to the normal shape of the femoral neck. A *pincer* impingement is an alteration to the size of the lip of the acetabulum.

One or both (combination impingement) of these changes may occur and this will be visible on

X-ray. The bone change, however, may not be clinically important if asymptomatic, and represents individual bone variation. Typically, X-ray is taken in an antero-posterior (AP) and then lateral direction, and is of the hip and pelvis combined. Where associated cartilage and/or labral changes are suspected, cross-sectional imaging such as MRI or CT scan can be used to define these changes and guide treatment.

Measurement of bone alignment on X-ray may be through the α (alpha) angle, crossover sign or centre-edge angle (Radiopaedia 2016). The α angle is measured between a line from the centre of the femoral head through the middle of the neck, and a line through the femoral head–neck junction. Generally a value greater than 55 degrees is considered to show a cam impingement. The crossover sign is seen when the anterior acetabular rim projects further laterally than the posterior rim. The centre-edge angle is taken between a vertical line through the femoral head and a line to the lateral edge of the acetabulum. Values greater than 39 degrees suggest a pincer deformity.

Associated pathologies seen on imaging include labral tears (below), osteoarthritis and os acetabuli (unfused secondary ossification centres of the acetabulum).

Acetabular labrum

The labrum is a layer of fibrocartilage, triangular in cross-section, which attaches to the rim of the acetabulum (hip socket) to deepen it. It is slightly wider inferiorly (>6 mm) and slightly thicker (>5 mm) in its superior region. It is continuous with the hyaline cartilage of the acetabulum superficially and has a transition zone from its deeper aspect to the underlying bone. This direct attachment to bone allows nerves and blood vessels to cross into it (Seldes et al. 2001). The labrum surrounds the head of the femur, contributing to hip stability, and makes a seal which helps form a pressurized layer of synovial fluid to redistribute compressive loads. The labrum itself supports only 1 to 2 per

cent of forces transmitted across the hip joint when morphology is normal. In cases of hip dysplasia (growth changes), however, this can increase to 11 per cent (Bsat et al. 2016). The labrum also creates a vacuum seal between the acetabulum and femoral head, tending to resist distraction forces. The resistance it offers is shared with the joint capsule, the labrum tending to resist smaller femoral displacements in the region of 1–2 mm, while the capsule is resistant to larger forces between 3 and 5 mm (Nepple et al. 2014).

Key point

The labrum forms a seal between the femur and acetabulum, increasing fluid pressure in the joint and working with the joint capsule to resist displacement forces.

The labrum may be detached or split away from the bone rim in FAI. The loose fragment can trap within the joint on movement, and cause symptoms. Compression and shear forces generated during cam impingement may also cause the anteriorly placed articular cartilage to split away from the underlying subchondral bone, resulting in a delamination injury, described as a wave sign at arthroscopy. Additionally, linear splitting (fissure) of the cartilage may occur, causing the now exposed cartilage layer edge to catch and tear away from the underlying bone, giving a chondral flap or carpet lesion. Cartilage injury is less common with a pincer lesion, and if it occurs it is typically to the posterior articular cartilage.

Clinical examination

Clinical examination must include subjective (history) and objective (physical tests) evaluation. History of FAI is often one of catching or a clicking sensation in certain movements, suggesting a mechanical lesion rather than a disease state. Pain may occur at inner-range flexion, adduction and internal

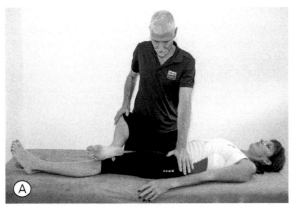 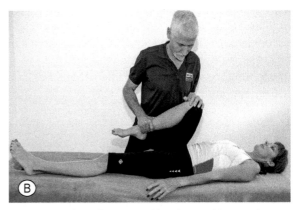

Figure 3.36 FADDIR and FABER tests. The FADDIR test (B) combines flexion, adduction and internal rotation. The FABER test (A) combines flexion, abduction and external rotation.

rotation during daily actions such as sitting in a low chair, driving and using the toilet. Active individuals may notice pain when performing squat or leg-press actions to full-range hip flexion, and when taking a high step. Hip pain is often described as 'C' shaped, meaning that anterior, lateral and posterior pain may occur on occasions. Groin pain and pain referred into the buttock are typical, with further referral into the thigh often occurring. The lower back, pelvis and sacroiliac joints should be examined and cleared, although compensatory pain is common in these regions from changes to gait pattern and daily living activities.

> **Definition**
> The 'C' sign is an indication of pain by the subject which is sited anterior, lateral and posterior.

Passive end-range hip flexion/adduction/internal rotation (FADDIR or FAIR test) or flexion/internal rotation (Flex-IR) may be used to provoke patient symptoms and to monitor treatment progress. The test may be modified into a Scour test when the movement is performed with approximation of the femur towards the acetabulum to assess osteoarthritic (OA) changes in the hip. The FABER test (flexion, abduction, external rotation) may also be used to assess inter-articular pathology at the hip and as a sacroiliac joint (SIJ) assessment. The diagnostic accuracy of several clinical tests used to diagnose FAI and labral tear has been given by Reiman et al. (2015), showing that only the FADDIR and Flex-IR tests are supported by the data as valuable screening tests for this condition (Fig. 3.36).

Treatment strategies

The Warwick Agreement of FAI syndrome (Griffin et al. 2016a) recommended a multidisciplinary approach to treatment involving conservative care, rehabilitation or surgery.

Conservative care

Conservative care involves advising the patient on what to do and what not to do. Education to explain what the condition is can be essential, and instructions on daily management and activities should be included. Activity and lifestyle changes can be used to avoid placing stress on pain-generating structures, and grading activities to increase tissue tolerance. Changing body position when sitting, standing, walking or running can avoid exacerbating the condition, and rest may be required if an action has irritated local structures. Avoiding equating 'hurt with harm' is important – patients must accept that pain may occur in the normal course of events, and a small amount (two or three out of ten on a VAS scale) does not imply tissue damage. The condition does not necessarily progress, so a process of 'watchful waiting' (monitoring the condition over a period of time) is usually appropriate.

Rehabilitation

The personalized hip therapy (PHT) programme used in the UK FASHIoN study (Wall et al. 2015) is a useful starting point for exercise selection (Table 3.10). As patients with FAI often present with alterations in muscle strength, range of motion and gait, these may form the main areas of rehabilitation focus. Close supervision is required, and a model of six therapy-led rehabilitation sessions over twelve weeks has been recommended (Wall et al. 2016). Strength and flexibility exercise may be used to target weak or inflexible regions. Muscle isolation (simple) actions progress to whole-body (complex) movements. Later, activity and/or sport-related functional movements are used and training volume is increased. Table 3.11 illustrates example exercises to target FAI.

Surgery

As with many orthopaedic procedures, surgery in FAI has been shown to improve patient symptoms, but does not always meet their expectations (Mannion et al. 2013). Both open (surgical dislocation) and keyhole (arthroscopic) techniques are described, with the recovery period from arthroscopic surgery typically being faster. Soft tissue damage to the labrum may be repaired if it is torn or detached by anchoring the labrum to the acetabulum with stiches. Unstable areas of articular cartilage may be removed (debridement)

Table 3.10 Personalized hip therapy exercise programme for FAI

▶ Exercise is individualized, progressed and supervised
▶ Phased programme begins with music control work, & progresses to stretching/strengthening with increasing ROM and resistance.
▶ Muscle control/stability exercise targets muscle of hip/pelvis/spine.
▶ Strengthening/resistance exercise begins in pain-free ROM, and targets: gluteus maximus, short external rotators, gluteus medium and abdominal muscles.
▶ Stretching exercise to improve hip external rotation and abduction in extension and flexion (avoid vigorous stretching and/or painful hard end stretching).
▶ Progress exercise intensity and difficulty, and build to activity or sport-specific exercise where relevant.
▶ Exercise programme is written and patient exercise diary encouraged.

(Data from Wall et al. 2016)

Table 3.11 Example exercises used in the rehabilitation of FAI

Non-weightbearing	Partial weightbearing	Full weightbearing
▶ Bent knee fallout	▶ Sink exercises – hip flexion/abduction/extension	▶ Lunge
▶ Shoulder bridge	▶ Step up using bannister rail	▶ Squat
▶ Clamshell	▶ Quarter squat using chair back	▶ Deadlift
▶ Kneeling leg lift	▶ Lunge using chair	▶ Step up
▶ Standing hip scissor	▶ Crook lying knee abduction using band.	▶ Side band walk
▶ Hip hitch		▶ Beam walk
▶ Gym ball leg press		▶ Star balance (in position of SEBT)
		▶ Arabesque

SEBT - star excursion balance test

to improve mechanical symptoms, and underlying bone may be microfractured to encourage new tissue formation.

Changes to bone contour such as excess bone on the rim of the acetabulum and femoral head may be removed using a burr (type of drill). The procedure on the femur is called femoral

osteochondroplasty and on the acetabulum a rim trim. Sufficient bone is removed to ensure that impingement no longer occurs within a normal motion range.

A progressive programme of rehabilitation is required following surgery.

Treatment note 3.5 Altered movement quality and hip impingement

Symptoms of both impingement and anterior labral tear may respond to correction of movement impairment/dysfunction, and should be tried prior to surgical consideration. Anterior femoral glide (Sahrmann 2002) is the most common impairment and is said to occur because the posteriorly placed hip muscles fail to posteriorly glide the femoral head during flexion. Patient groin symptoms are reproduced during flexion movements and prolonged sitting. The condition is more commonly seen in those who use hip hyperextension during their sport (dancers, yoga) or those who have an inflexible flatback posture and compensate by extending the hip instead. The position of the greater trochanter may be monitored during active hip flexion. As the hip is flexed or extended, the greater trochanter should remain in a relatively neutral position. Where anterior glide occurs, the trochanter moves forwards (glide) and inwards (medial rotation). The condition is often associated with a persistent swayback postural stance (hip extended when standing), hyperpronation of the feet and medial rotation of the femur. To palpation, the TFL muscle appears dominant over the gluteus medius in single-leg standing and hip abduction, and the hamstrings dominant over the gluteus maximus during hip extension. Underactivity of the iliopsoas during flexion and the gluteal muscles during hip extension has been shown to increase anterior hip joint force (Lewis, Sahrmann and Moran 2007). Comparison of the iliopsoas to rectus

femoris/tensor fascia lata/sartorius during hip flexion and the gluteal muscles to the hamstrings during hip extension has shown the iliopsoas and gluteal muscles to be the most important in reducing anterior hip force during flexion–extension, respectively (Lewis, Sahrmann and Moran 2009).

Key point
Preferential recruitment of the iliopsoas during hip flexion and the gluteal muscles during hip extension reduces excessive forces acting on the anterior hip.

Rehabilitation of anterior glide includes exercises to encourage posterior and inferior glide of the femoral head. Passive motion may be imposed in four-point kneeling (quadruped) with the subject rocking back towards the heels. Active use of the hip abductors using the clamshell action and hip abduction with lateral femoral rotation (see above) may also modify symptoms. Resting positions should avoid exacerbation of the condition and so swayback posture is corrected, and crossing the legs (medial rotation) avoided. Where night pain occurs, the athlete should place a pillow between their knees in lying on the side to avoid medial rotation of the hip. Key exercises during rehabilitation of anterior impingement are shown in Table 3.12.

Treatment note 3.5 *continued*

Table 3.12 Key exercises used in the management of anterior hip impingement

1. Quadruped	• Press with arms to rock the body back towards the heels • Maintain the lumbar neutral position until the last minute • Ensure that the hip flexor muscles remain relaxed. The force must come from pushing with the arms and not pulling with the hips
2. Glut med (sd ly)	• Keep the upper hip slightly forwards of the lower • Keeping the feet together, lift the upper knee
3. Hip abduction and LR (sd ly)	• Keep the upper hip directly above the lower • Use the upper hand to monitor the pelvic position throughout the exercise • Lift the upper leg upwards and slightly backwards • Rotate the leg outwards so that the toes point towards the ceiling
4. Glut max/gluteal brace (prone ly)	• Tighten the buttock muscles while slightly turning the feet outwards
5. IP –sitting with LR	• Grasp around the thigh and lift the leg (passive) to the highest comfortable position • Graduallly release the hands and hold the leg in the upper position for 5–10 seconds
6. LR with hip abducted (prone ly FROG)	• Abduct the hips so that the knees are apart just broader than hip width • Outwardly rotate the hips so that the feet touch • Contract the gluteals and press the feet together. Hold the contraction for 10–20 seconds

After Sahmann 2002

The young athlete

Pain and limitation of movement in the hip in children should always be treated with caution. The extreme forces placed on the hip by weightbearing, combined with osseous and vascular changes occurring about the joint during adolescence, can lead to a variety of serious orthopaedic conditions.

The blood supply to the femoral head may be compromised in the very young. From birth until the age of four years, blood reaches the femoral head via the metaphysis. From the age of eight years, vessels through the ligamentum teres supply the head. Between these two periods, the lateral epiphyseal vessels are the only source of blood to the femoral head. In addition, the upper femoral epiphysis does not fuse with the shaft until about twenty years of age.

Perthes' disease

Persistent hip or groin pain and/or a limp in young males (four to twelve years) may be the result of Perthes' disease, an avascular necrosis (osteochondrosis) of the femoral head. The bony nucleus of the epiphysis becomes necrosed. The upper surface of the femoral head flattens and the epiphyseal line widens, altering the biomechanical alignment of the joint. When the bone is revascularized it hardens again, leaving a permanent deformity. Objective examination often reveals slight limitation of all hip movements with protective spasm. The condition may be precipitated by joint effusion at the hip following trauma, or a non-specific synovitis.

Rest and the avoidance of high impact activity (running, jumping) is the mainstay of treatment, but surgical intervention may be required for un-resolving cases.

Slipped capital femoral epiphyses

Trauma, or more usually simply weightbearing, in the young athlete (ten to twenty years) may result in slipping of the capital (upper) femoral epiphysis (SCFE). The condition is more common in tall adolescents who have shown a rapid increase in height, and in the obese individual. In these two cases, hormone imbalance has been suggested, in the first case an excess of growth hormone and in the second an excess of sex hormone (Reid 1992).

Pain is usually felt in the hip or knee, and may begin simply as a diffuse ache to the knee alone. The epiphyseal junction may soften and, with weightbearing or trauma, may cause the head of the femur to slip on the neck, usually downwards and backwards. Slippage may compromise the blood flow to the femoral head through the neck, causing osteonecrosis with sclerosis and femoral head collapse. If left, the slipped epiphyses will fuse to the femoral neck in the abnormal position.

Objective examination often reveals limitation of flexion, abduction and medial rotation (the athlete is unable to touch the abdomen with the thigh). The leg is often rested in lateral rotation, and the gait pattern is antalgic. The condition is classified as *stable* when the patient is able to walk and *unstable* when the patient is unable to walk even with crutches.

Leg shortening up to two centimetres is common, and radiographs reveal widening and a 'woolly' appearance of the epiphyseal plate. On the X-ray, a line traced along the superior aspect of the femoral neck will reveal a step deformity (Fig. 3.37). The line remains superior to the head rather than passing directly through it (Trethowan's sign).

Treatment is through surgical pinning rather than reduction. In a study of 240 patients, 21 were found to have osteonecrosis following unstable slipped capital femoral epiphysis, while none were found from the stable group (Tokmakova, Stanton and Mason 2003). Osteonecrosis was found to be more likely in those treated with multiple pins rather than a single pin, and the risk of osteonecrosis increased where reduction of an unstable slippage was performed.

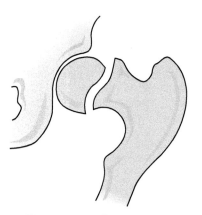

Figure 3.37 Slipped upper femoral epiphysis. The step deformity is apparent on X-ray.

> **Key point**
>
> Hip pain in the sporting adolescent must always be taken seriously, and full examination is mandatory. X-rays should be taken if hip movement range is limited with a hard end-feel and the athlete is unable to touch the abdomen with the thigh.

Apophysitis

Traction apophysitis may occur at one of several sites around the hip. The ischial tuberosity attachment of the hamstrings, anterior superior iliac spine attachment of the sartorius, anterior inferior iliac spine attachment of the rectus femoris or iliopsoas attachment to the lesser trochanter are all potential sites. Rest and activity modification normally allows symptoms to settle, and supervised re-strengthening is then given.

> **Definition**
>
> *Apophysitis* is irritation and inflammation of a secondary ossification centre (apophysis) of a bone at the insertion of a tendon.

Hip pointer

The relatively unprotected iliac crest is vulnerable to direct blows from any hard object, be it a hockey ball, boot or another player's head. Contusion is often persistent, especially if the periosteum is affected, and the condition is described as a 'hip pointer'. The pain from the injury is so severe that the trunk is flexed to the affected side. The athlete is often unable to take a breath and may panic.

Following reassurance, the iliac crest is examined and usually reveals dramatic pain but little bruising or swelling. The abdominal muscles are often rigid and the hips pulled into flexion. After 24 to 48 hours, more extensive bruising appears and local tenderness may last for weeks. A raised area may persist for many months. The POLICE protocol is used, initially to relieve pain and to protect the area with padding when the athlete resumes sport.

> **Key point**
>
> Hip pointer is a contusion of the soft tissue overlying the iliac crest.

Snapping hip syndrome

Snapping or clicking hip (Coxa Saltans) can occur to repeated flexion and extension movements. The condition is common in dancers and young athletes, and is usually painless. However, it is of obvious concern to the athlete as in some cases the sound is loud enough for others to hear.

There are two main types of clicking hip, internal and external. Although there have been many proposed causes of this condition, a common intra-articular cause of internal clicking hip is the suction phenomenon. This can occur during exercises such as sit-ups and requires reassurance rather than treatment.

Treatment note 3.6   Manual therapy techniques to the hip

The hip is a joint which responds well to manual therapy, but as the largest joint in the body, treatment can be difficult. In sports especially, it is common to have a very large sportsman such as a rugby player and a very small therapist. The answer is to use leverage and body position and a variety of seatbelt techniques to reduce the stress on the therapist.

Quadrant test

The flexion/adduction or quadrant test (Maitland 1986) is a useful test to assess the surface of the hip joint. However, the test requires that the therapist take the weight of the whole leg which, in the case of a large athlete, may be considerable. To make this test more manageable, the therapist should link the fingers over the patient's knee (Fig. 3.38) and rest the far forearm along the patient's calf. The couch should be just below hip level to allow the therapist to lean over the hip as the flexion/adduction force is

applied. In this position, a longitudinal force (axial compression) may be applied as the therapist flexes the knee slightly, and the body and forearms may be twisted to medially rotate the joint to increase the contact area of the joint.

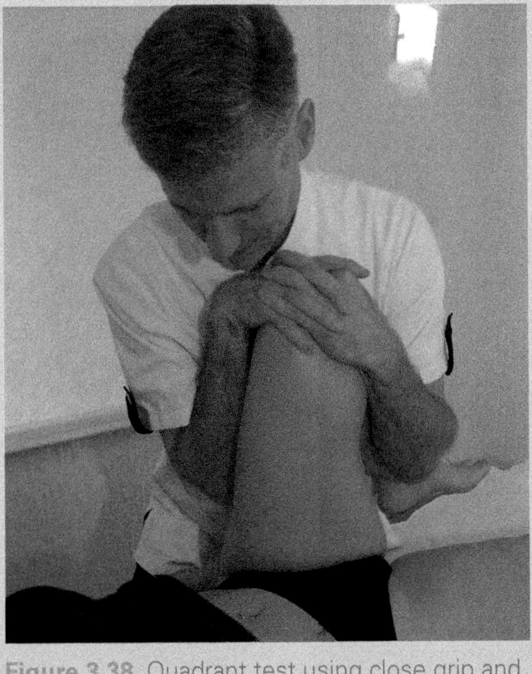

Lateral gliding

A lateral gliding (transverse) accessory movement is imposed on the joint by modifying the grip used in the quadrant test (Fig. 3.39, Fig. 3.40). The interlinked hands now grip around the patient's thigh (use a towel to protect the skin) and the side of the patient's femur rests on the therapist's chest. The action is to distract the joint using the therapist's body sway rather than arm strength. The movement should come from a slight softening of the therapist's knees together with trunk movement, rather than trunk movement alone.

Lateral glide using seatbelt

The lateral gliding motion may be increased by using a seatbelt or webbing strap. The patient

Figure 3.38 Quadrant test using close grip and bodyweight.

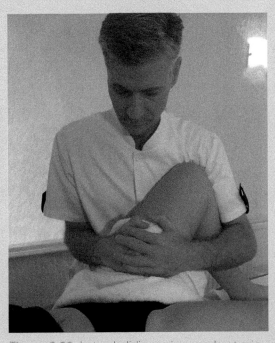

Figure 3.39 Lateral gliding using quadrant grip.

Treatment note 3.6 *continued*

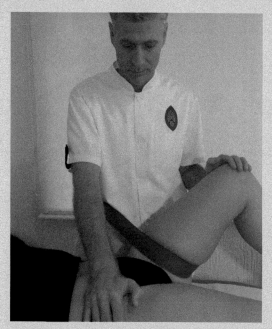

Figure 3.40 Lateral gliding in crook lying using seatbelt.

is in crook (hook) lying and a belt is fastened around the thigh and around the therapist's hip at the level of the ischial tuberosities (Fig. 3.41). The femur is stabilized by resting it against the therapist's chest and gripping around the knee with the hand. The degree of lateral glide may be assessed by palpating with the right hand. The lateral glide force is produced by the therapist leaning back slightly and softening the knee.

Hip MWM with lateral glide

A sustained lateral glide may be combined with passive flexion or rotation to produce a mobilization with movement (MWM). A towel is placed over the subject's hip to pad the area and a seatbelt surrounds the upper thigh, passing close in to the hip crease. The belt passes behind the therapist below the ischial tuberosities, so that the belt is horizontal, as above. The subject's pelvis is fixed using the leading hand against the ilium. The action is to maintain the lateral gliding pressure by the therapist sitting back into the

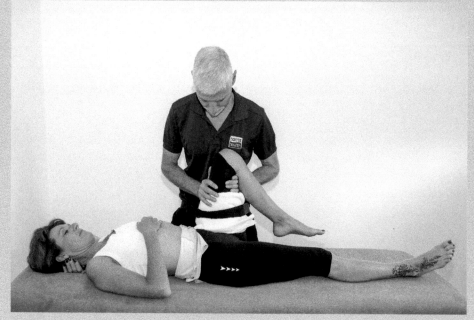

Figure 3.41 MWM for hip.

Treatment note 3.6 *continued*

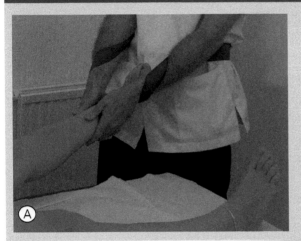

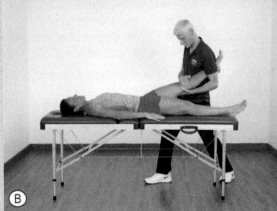

Figure 3.42 (A) Longitudinal distraction in loose pack position using seatbelt. (B) Longitudinal hip distraction using three-point contact.

belt and to use a passive motion to guide the hip into flexion by transferring bodyweight from the

trailing foot to the leading foot and side-shifting the body (Fig 3.42A). For rotation, the same body position is used to begin, but the subject's thigh is held against the therapist's chest as the therapist turns their body to impart a rotation action to the hip (Fig 3.42B)

Longitudinal distraction (hip traction)

Hip traction is one of the most relieving mobilizations for the hip joint, where capsular limitation is present. The patient is in supine and the couch positioned below the therapist (Fig. 3.42A), and the therapist takes up a stride standing position. Two techniques are useful. First, a seatbelt may be used, wound around the patient's ankle in a figure-of-eight – the patient's sock may be left on to protect the skin from abrasion. The belt passes around the therapist's lower waist and the tension is taken up. The hip is positioned in its loose pack position (flexion, abduction, lateral rotation) and the distraction force is imposed by the therapist leaning back. Either an oscillation or continuous traction may be used. To avoid imposing distraction on the knee, a three-point grip may be used on the shin and thigh. The subject's tibia is grasped under the therapist's near arm and the therapist winds their forearm beneath the subject's thigh to grasp their own far arm. Their far arm is passed beneath the subject's thigh to press the cupped hands down on top of the subject's thigh (above the knee). The action is to sit back to impose a distraction force while maintaining grip at all three points of lower limb contact (Fig. 3.42B).

Definition

The suction phenomenon is a result of pressure changes within the synovial fluid of a joint. As a joint moves, positive and negative pressures are created within the fluid. As negative pressure (suction) collapses rapidly, air bubbles are sucked into the fluid, giving a soft click.

The second cause (extra-articular) is the iliopsoas (IP) clicking across the *iliopectineal eminence*, the junction between the ilium and the superior ramus of the pubis.

Treatment aims at activity modification in the reactive phase of the condition, and later, as the subject begins the recovery phase, IP stretching may help. A half-kneeling position is taken up, with the affected leg trailing. The subject stabilizes the pelvis (avoiding anterior tilt) and moves the body forwards, pressing the trailing hip into extension. Variation in the lunge direction (straight or oblique) will change the direction of the overload from extension to extension with ab or adduction.

External clicking hip is usually a result of the gluteus maximus tendon clicking over the greater trochanter, or the iliotibial band clicking over the greater trochanter. Sometimes the click can be reproduced during examination by flexing and extending the hip in adduction, in which case tight abductors are a contributory factor. The Ober manoeuvre is often positive in these cases.

If the condition is painful, treatment designed to reduce local inflammation may be required. In painless instances, stretching of the ITB and hip abductors can help. The athlete begins in a side-lying position with the affected leg uppermost. The upper leg is abducted, and hip hitching is performed to shorten the leg (lateral tilt of the pelvis). The pelvic fixation is maintained as the upper leg is lowered into adduction.

References

Abelbeck, K.G., 2002. Biomechanical model and evaluation of a linear motion squat type exercise. *Journal of Strength and Conditioning Research* **16** (4), 516–524.

Askling, C.M., Malliaropoulos, N., Karlsson, J., 2012. High-speed running type or stretching-type of hamstring injuries makes a difference to treatment and prognosis. *British Journal of Sports Medicine* **46** (2), 86–87.

Askling, C.M., Nilsson, J., Thorstensson, A. 2010. A new hamstring test to complement the common clinical examination before return to sport after injury. *Knee Surgery, Sports Traumatology, Arthroscopy* **18** (12), 1798–803.

Askling, C.M., Tengvar, M., Tarassova, O. et al., 2014. Acute hamstring injuries in Swedish elite sprinters and jumpers: a prospective randomised controlled clinical trial comparing two rehabilitation protocols. *British Journal of Sports Medicine* **48** (7), 532–539.

Askling, C.M., Tengvar, M., Thorstensson, A., 2013. Acute hamstring injuries in Swedish elite football: a prospective randomised controlled clinical trial comparing two rehabilitation protocols. *British Journal of Sports Medicine* **47**, 953–959.

Babst, D., Steppacher, S.D., Ganz, R., Siebenrock, K.A., Tannast, M., 2011. The iliocapsularis muscle: an important stabilizer in the dysplastic hip. *Clinical Orthopaedics and Related Research* **469** (6), 1728–1734.

Birnbaum, K., Siebert, C.H., Pandorf, T., Schopphoff, E., Prescher, A. and Niethard, F.U., 2004. Anatomical and biomechanical investigations of the iliotibial tract. *Surgical and Radiological Anatomy* **26**, 433–446.

Borley, N.R., 1997. *Clinical Surface Anatomy.* Manson Publishing, London.

Brinckman, P., Hoefert, H. and Jongen, H.T., 1981. Sex differences in the skeletal geometry of the human pelvis and hip joint. *Journal of Biomechanics* **14**, 427–430.

Brukner, P., and Connell, D., 2016. Serious thigh muscle strains: beware the intramuscular tendon which plays an important role in difficult hamstring and quadriceps muscle strains. *British Journal of Sports Medicine* **50**, 205–208.

Brukner, P., Nealon A., Morgan, C., et al, 2014. Recurrent hamstring muscle injury: applying the limited evidence in the professional football setting with a seven-point programme. *British Journal of Sports Medicine* **48**: 929–938.

Bsat, S., Frei, H., Beaulé, P.E. 2016. The acetabular labrum: a review of its function. *Bone Joint Journal.* **98-B** (6), 730–735.

Burkett, L.N., 1975. Investigation into hamstring strains: the case of the hybrid muscle. *American Journal of Sports Medicine* **3**, 228–231.

Burkholder, T.J. and Lieber, R.L., 2001. Sarcomere length operating range of vertebrate muscles during movement. *J Experimental Biology* **204**, 1529–36.

Castellote-Caballero, Y., Valenza, M., Martin-Martin, L. et al., 2013. Effects of a neurodynamic sliding technique on hamstring flexibility in health make soccer players. A pilot study. *Physical Therapy in Sports* **14**, 156–162.

Choi, H., McCartney, M., Best, T., 2008. Treatment of osteitis pubis and osteomyelitis of the pubic symphysis in athletes: A systematic review. *British Journal of Sports Medicine*.

Cleather, D.J., Southgate, D. and Bull, A.M., 2015. The role of the biarticular hamstrings and gastrocnemius muscles in closed chain lower limb extension. *J Theoretical Biology* **365**, 217–225.

Croisier, J.L., Ganteaume, S., Binet, J., et al., 2008. Strength imbalances and prevention of hamstring injury in professional soccer players: a prospective study. *American Journal of Sports Medicine.* **36** (8),1469–1475.

Cyriax, J., 1982. *Textbook of Orthopaedic Medicine*, **Vol. 1**, 8th ed. Baillière Tindall, London.

Dickenson, E., Wall, P.D., Robinson, B. et al., 2016 Prevalence of cam hip shape morphology: a systematic review. *Osteoarthr Cartil* **24**, 949–961.

DiMattia, M., Livengood, A., Uhl, T., Mattaclola, C., Malone, T., 2005. What are the validity of the single-leg-squat test and its relationship to hip-abduction strength?. *Journal of Sport Rehabilitation.* **14**, 108–123.

Distefano, L.J., Blackburn, J.T., Marshall, S.W. and Padua, D.A., 2009. Gluteal muscle activation during common therapeutic exercises. *Journal of orthopaedic and Sports Physical Therapy* **39** (7), 532–540.

Ekstrand, J., Healey, J. et al, 2012. Hamstring muscle injuries in professional football: the correlation of MRI findings with return to play. *British Journal of Sports Medicine* **46**, 112–117.

Enoka, R.M., 1994. Neuromechanical Basis of Kinesiology, 2nd edn. Human Kinetics, Illinois.

Estwanik, J.J., McAlister, J.A., 1990. Contusions and the formation of myositis ossificans. *Physician and Sports Medicine* **18** (4), 52–64.

Fagerson, T., 2009. Hip pathologies: diagnosis and intervention. In: Magee, D.J., Zachazewski, J.E., Quillen, W.S. (eds), *Pathology and Intervention in Musculoskeletal Rehabilitation*. Saunders-Elsevier, St Louis, MO.

Farrokhi, S., Pollard, C.D., Souza, R.B., Chen, Y., Reischl, S, and Powers, C.M., 2008. Trunk position influences the kinematics, kinetics and muscle activity of the lead lower extremity during the forward lunge exercise. *Journal of Orthopaedic and Sports Physical Therapy* **38** (7), 403–409.

Fredericson, M., Dowdell, B.C., and Oestreicher, N., 1997. Correlation between decreased strength in hip abductors and iliotibial band syndrome in runners. *Archives of Physical Medicine and Rehabilitation* **78** (9), 1031.

Fry, A.C., Smith, J.C., and Schilling, B.K., 2003. Effect of knee position on hip and knee torques during the barbell squat. *Journal of Strength and Conditioning Research* **17** (4), 629–633.

Fyfe, J.J., Opar, D.A., Williams, M.D. et al, 2013. The role of neuromuscular inhibition in hamstring strain injury recurrence. *J Electromyogr Kinesiol* **23**, 523–530.

Ganz, R., Gill, T., Gautier, E. et al., Surgical dislocation of the adult hip. *Bone Joint Journal* **83**, 1119–1124.

Garrett, W.E., Rich, F.R., Nikolaou, P.K. et al., 1989. Computed tomography of hamstring muscle strains. *Medicine & Science in Sports & Exercise* **21**, 506–514.

Griffin, D.R., Dickenson, E.J., O'Donnell, J. et al., 2016a. The Warwick Agreement on femoroacetabular impingement syndrome (FAI syndrome): an international consensus statement. *British Journal of Sports Medicine* **50**, 1169–1176.

Griffin, D.R., Wall, P.D., Realpe, A. et al., 2016b. UK FASHIoN: Feasibility study of a randomised controlled trial of arthroscopic surgery for hip impingement compared with best conservative care. *Health Technol Assess* **20**, 1–172.

Grimaldi, A., 2011. Assessing lateral stability of the hip and pelvis. *Manual Therapy* **16**, 26–32.

Gunn, C.C., 1996. *Treatment of Chronic Pain*. Churchill Livingstone, Edinburgh.

Gunn, C.C., 2000. *The Gunn Approach to the Treatment of Chronic Pain*. Course notes, Westminster Hospital, London.

Haslam, R., 2001. A comparison of acupuncture with advice and exercises on the symptomatic treatment of osteoarthritis of the hip: a randomised controlled trial. *Acupuncture in Medicine* **19**, 19–26.

Higashihara, A., Ono, T., Kubota, J. et al., 2010. Functional differences between individual hamstring muscles at different running speeds. *Medicine & Science in Sports & Exercise* **42**, 404–410.

Hoeksma, H.L., Dekker, J., Ronday K. et al., 2004. Comparison of manual therapy and exercise therapy in osteoarthritis of the hip: a randomized clinical trial. *Arthritis and Rheumatism* **51**, 722–729.

Jackson, D.W., Feagin, J.A., 1973. Quadriceps contusions in young athletes: relation of severity of injury to treatment and prognosis. *Journal of Bone and Joint Surgery* **55A** (1), 95–105.

Jaegers, S., Dantuma, R. and deJongh, H., 1992. Three dimensional reconstruction of the hip on the basis of magnetic resonance images. *Surgical Radiologic Anatomy* 14: 241–249.

Kannus, P., 1989. Hamstring/quadriceps strength ratios in knees with medial collateral ligament insufficiency. *Journal of Sports Medicine and Physical Fitness* **29** (2), 194–198.

Kornberg, C., Lew, P., 1989. The effect of stretching neural structures on grade one hamstring injuries. *Journal of Orthopaedic and Sports Physical Therapy* **7** (2), 481–487.

Kraemer, R., and Knobloch, K., 2009. A soccer-specific balance training program for hamstring muscle and patellar and achilles tendon injuries: an intervention study in premier league female soccer. *American Journal of Sports Medicine* **37**, 1384–1393.

Krebs, D.E., Obbins, C.E., Lavine, I., Mann, R.W., 1998. Hip biomechanics during gait. *Journal of Orthopaedic and Sports Physical Therapy* **28**, (1), 51–59.

Kummer, B., 1993. Is the Pauwels theory of hip biomechanics still valid? A critical analysis based on modern methods. *Annals of Anatomy* **175** (3), 203–210.

Kurosawa, H., Nakasita, K., Saski, S., Takeda, S., 1996. Complete avulsion of the hamstring tendons from the ischeal tuberosity: a report of two cases sustained in judo. *British Journal of Sports Medicine* **30**, 72–74.

LeBlanc, K., LeBland, K.A., 2003. Groin pain in athletes. *Hernia* **7**, 68–71.

Lentell, G., Katzman, L.L., Walters, M.R. 1990. The Relationship between Muscle Function and Ankle Stability. *Journal of Orthopaedic & Sports Physical Therapy* **11** (12): 605–611.

Lewis, C., Sahrmann, S.A., Moran, D.W., 2007. Anterior hip joint force increases with hip extension, decreased gluteal force, or decreased iliopsoas force. *Journal of Biomechanics* **40** (16), 3725–3731.

Lewis, C., Sahrmann, S.A., Moran, D.W., 2009. Effect of position and alteration in synergist muscle force contribution on hip forces when performing hip strengthening exercises. *Clinical Biomechanics* **24** (1), 35–42.

Maitland, G.D., 1986. *Vertebral Manipulation*, third ed. Butterworth-Heinemann, Oxford.

Mannion, A.F., Impellizzeri, F.M., Naal, F.D. et al., 2013. Fulfilment of patient-rated expectations predicts the outcome of surgery for femoroacetabular impingement. *Osteoarthr Cartil* **21**, 44–50.

Mercer, S.R., Rivett, D.A., and Nelson, R.A., 1998. Stretching the iliotibial band: an anatomical perspective. *New Zealand Journal of Physiotherapy* **26** (2), 5–7.

Miokovic, T., Armbrecht, G., Felsenberg, D. and Belavy, D., 2011. Differential atrophy of the postero-lateral hip musculature during prolonged bend rest and the influence of exercise countermeasures. *Journal of Applied Physiology* **110** (4), 926–934.

Moore, A., Mannion, J. and Moran, R.W., 2015. The efficacy of surface electromyographic biofeedback assisted stretching for the treatment of chronic low back pain: a case series. *J Bodywork and Movement Therapies* **19** (1), 8–16.

Myers, T.W., 2014. *Anatomy Trains* (3rd ed.) Churchill Livingstone.

Nepple, J.J., Philippon, M.J., Campbell, K.J. et al., 2014. The hip fluid seal – Part II: The effect of an acetabular labral tear, repair, resection, and reconstruction on hip stability to distraction. *Knee Surgery, Sports Traumatology, Arthroscopy* **22**, 730–736.

O'Connell, M., Powell, T., McCaffrey, N., 2002. Symphyseal cleft injection in the diagnosis and treatment of osteitis pubis in athletes. *American Roentgen Ray Society* **179**, 955–959.

Ober, F.R., 1936. The role of the iliotibial band and fascia lata as a factor in the causation of low back disabilities and sciatica. *Journal of Bone and Joint Surgery.* **18**, 105–110.

Onishi H, Yagi R, Oyama M, et al., 2002. EMG-angle relationship of the hamstring muscles during maximum knee flexion. J Electromyogr Kinesiol. **12** (5), 399–406.

Oravo, S., Kujala, U.M., 1995. Rupture of the ischeal origin of the hamstring muscles. *American Journal of Sports Medicine* **23**, 702–705.

Pagé, I., Marchand, A., Nougarou, F. et al., 2015. Neuromechanical responses after biofeedback training in participants with chronic low back pain: An experimental cohort study. *Journal of Manipulative & Physiological Therapeutics* **38**, 449–457.

Palastanga, N., Field, D., and Soames, R., 2006. *Anatomy of human movement.* Elsevier.

Pauli, S., Willemsen, P., Declerck, K. et al., 2002. Osteomyelitis pubis versus osteitis pubis: a case presentation and review of the literature. *British Journal of Sports Medicine* **36**, 71–73.

Petersen, J., Thorborg, K., Nielsen, M.B. et al., 2011. Preventive effect of eccentric training on acute hamstring injuries in men's soccer: a cluster randomized controlled trial. *American Journal of Sports Medicine* **239**, 2296–2303.

Petersen, J., Thorborg, K., Nielsen, M.B. et al., 2014. The diagnostic and prognostic value of ultrasonography in soccer players with acute hamstring injuries. *American Journal of Sports Medicine* **42**, 399–404.

Puranen, J., Orava, S., 1988. The hamstring syndrome: a new diagnosis of gluteal sciatic pain, *American Journal of Sports Medicine* **16** (5), 517–521.

Radiopaedia (2016) https://radiopaedia.org/articles/femoro-acetabular-impingement accessed 03/10/2016.

Rasch, P.J., 1989. *Kinesiology and Applied Anatomy.* Lea and Febiger, Philadelphia

Reid, D.C., 1992. *Sports Injury Assessment and Rehabilitation.* Churchill Livingstone, London.

Reiman, M.P., Goode, A.P., Cook, C.E., Hölmich, P., Thorborg, K., 2015. Diagnostic accuracy of clinical tests for the diagnosis of hip femoro-acetabular impingement/labral tear: a systematic review with meta-analysis. *British Journal of Sports Medicine.* Jun; **49** (12): 811.

Reurink, G., Brilman, E.G., de Vos, R.J. et al., 2015. Magnetic resonance imaging in acute hamstring injury: can we provide a return to play prognosis? *Sports Med* **45**, 133–146.

Ruwe, P.A., Gage, J.R., Ozonoff, M.B., Deluca, P.A., 1992. Clinical determination of femoral anteversion: a comparison of established techniques. *Journal of Bone and Joint Surgery (Am)* **74**, 820.

Sahrmann, S.A. (2002) Diagnosis and treatment of movement impairment syndromes. Mosby, St Louis, USA.

Schache, A.G., Kim, H.J., Morgan, D.L. et al., 2010. Hamstring muscle forces prior to and immediately following an acute sprinting-related muscle strain injury. *Gait Posture* **32**, 136–140.

Schuermans, J., Van Tiggelen, D., Danneels, L. et al., 2014. Biceps femoris and Semitendenosus – teammates or competitors? New insights into hamstring injury mechanisms in male football players: a muscle functional MRI study. *British Journal of Sports Medicine* **48** (22), 1599–1606.

Seldes, R.M., Tan, V., Hunt, J. et al., 2001. Anatomy, histologic features, and vascularity of the adult acetabular labrum. *Clin Orthop Relat Res* **382**, 232–240.

Serner, A., Tol, J.L., Jomaah, N. et al., 2015. Diagnosis of acute groin injuries: a prospective study of 110 athletes. *American Journal of Sports Medicine* **43** (8), 1857–1864.

Sherry, M.A., Best, T.M., 2004. A comparison of 2 rehabilitation programs in the treatment of acute hamstring strains. *J Orthop Sports Phys Ther* **34**, 116–25.

Silder, A., Sherry, M.A., Sanfilippo, J. et al., 2013. Clinical and morphological changes following 2 rehabilitation programs for acute hamstring strain injuries: a randomized clinical trial. *J Orthop Sports Phys Ther* **43**, 284–299.

Smith-Petersen, M., Treatment of malum coxae senilis, old slipped upper femoral epiphysis, intrapelvic protrusion of the acetabulum, and coxa plana by means of acetabuloplasty. *J Bone Joint Surg Am* **18**, 869–880.

Subbu, R., Benjamin-Laing, H., Haddad, F., 2015. Timing of surgery for complete proximal hamstring avulsion injuries successful clinical outcomes at 6 weeks, 6 months and after 6 months of injury. *American Journal of Sports Medicine* **43** (2), 385–389.

Szlezak, A.M., Georgilopoulos, P., Bullock-Saxton, J.E. et al., 2011. The immediate effect of unilateral lumbar Z-joint mobilisation on posterior chain neurodynamics: a randomised controlled study. *Manual Therapy* **16**, 609–613.

Tannast, M., Siebenrock, K.A., Anderson, S.E., 2007. Femoroacetabular impingement: radiographic diagnosis – what the radiologist should know. *AJR Am J Roentgenol.* **188** (6): 1540–1552.

Terry, G.C., Hughston, J.C. and Norwood, L.A., 1986. The anatomy of the iliopatellar band and the iliotibial tract. *American Journal of Sports Medicine.* **14** (1), 39–45.

Thorborg, K., 2012. Why hamstring eccentrics are hamstring essentials. *British Journal of Sports Medicine* **46**, 463–465.

Tokmakova, K., Stanton, R.P., Mason, D., 2003. Factors influencing the development of osteonecrosis in patients treated for slipped capital femoral epiphysis. *Journal of Bone and Joint Surgery (America)* **85**, 798–801.

Topol, G., Reeves, K., Hassanein, K., 2005. Efficacy of dextrose prolotherapy in elite male kicking sport athletes with chronic groin pain. *Archives of Physical Medicine and Rehabilitation* **86**, 697–702.

Toussaint, H.M., van Baar, C.E., van Langen, P.P., de Looze, M.P. and van Dieen, J.H., 1992. Coordination of the leg muscles in backlift and leglift. *Journal of Biomechanics*, **25**, 1279–1289.

Turl, S.E., George, K.P., 1998. Adverse neural tension: a factor in repetitive hamstring strain? *J Orthop Sports Phys Ther* **27**, 16–21.

Ueblacker, P. et al., 2013. 'Terminology and classification of muscle injuries in sport: The Munich consensus statement', *British Journal of Sports Medicine* **47**, 342–350.

van Ingen Schenau, G.J., Bobbert, M.F. and van Soest, A.J., 1990. The unique action of bi-articular muscles in leg extensions. In: *Multiple Muscle Systems: Biomechanics and Movement Organisation* (eds J.M. Winters and S.L. Woo). Springer-Verlag, New York.

Veselko, M., Smrkolj, V., 1994. Avulsion of the anterior superior iliac spine in athletes: case reports. *Journal of Trauma* **36**, 444–446.

Wall, P.D., Dickenson, E.J., Robinson, D. et al., 2016. Personalised hip therapy: development of a non-operative protocol to treat femoroacetabular impingement syndrome in the FASHIoN randomised controlled trial. *British Journal of Sports Medicine* **50**, 1217–1223.

Ward, W.T., Fleisch, I. and Ganz, R., 2000. Anatomy of the iliocapsularis muscle. *Clinical Orthopaedics and Related Research* **374**, 278–285.

Weir, A., Brukner, P., Delahunt, E. et al., 2015. Doha agreement meeting on terminology and definitions in groin pain in athletes. *British Journal of Sports Medicine* **49**, 768–774.

Williams, B.S. and Cohen, S.P., 2009. Greater trochanteric pain syndrome: a review of anatomy, diagnosis and treatment. *Anesthesia and Analgesia* **108** (5): 1662–1670.

Wollin, M., Lovell, G., 2006. Osteitis pubis in four young football players: A case series demonstrating successful rehabilitation. *Physical Therapy in Sport* **7** (4) 153–160.

Woodley, S.J., Mercer, S.R. and Micholson, H.D., 2008. Morphology of the bursae associated with the greater trochanter of the femur. *Journal of Bone and Joint Surgery (America)* **90**, 284–294.

CHAPTER 4

The knee

The knee is the largest synovial joint in the body, consisting of the articulation between the femur and tibia (tibiofemoral joint), and that between the femur and patella (patellofemoral joint). The tibiofemoral joint is weightbearing, and consists of two articulations. The patellofemoral joint helps give a mechanical advantage to the pull of the quadriceps as it acts over the knee. In addition to these two main joints, a third – the superior tibiofibular joint – is formed between the lateral tibial condyle and the head of the fibula.

Biomechanics of the extensor mechanism

The patella is the largest sesamoid bone in the body. It is attached above to the quadriceps tendon, below to the patellar tendon, and medially and laterally to the patellar retinacula. The breadth of the pelvis and close proximity of the knee creates a valgus angulation to the femur. Coupled with this, the direction of pull of the quadriceps is along the shaft of the femur, and that of the patellar tendon is almost vertical (Fig. 4.1). The difference between the two lines of pull is known as the Q angle and is an important determinant of knee health. Normal values for the Q angle are in the region of 15–20 degrees, and knees with an angle greater or less than this can be considered misaligned.

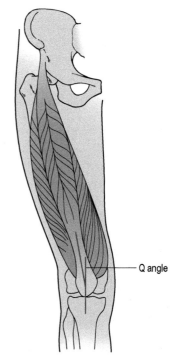

Q angle

Figure 4.1 The Q angle.

Definition

The Q angle is the difference between the direction of pull of the quadriceps along the shaft of the femur and the direction of pull of the patellar tendon, which is almost vertical.

183

As the knee flexes and extends, the patella should travel in line with the long axis of the femur. However, the horizontal force vector created as a result of the Q angle tends to pull the patella laterally, a movement which is resisted by the horizontal pull of the lower fibres of vastus medialis. This coupled pull causes the patella to follow a curved path as the knee moves from extension to flexion.

The lower fibres of the vastus medialis are sometimes considered as a functionally separate muscle, the vastus medialis oblique (VMO). The quadriceps as a whole have been shown to undergo reflex inhibition as the knee swells. However, the VMO can be inhibited by as little as 10 ml effusion, while the vastus lateralis and rectus femoris require as much as 60 ml (Arno 1990). Minimal effusion occurs frequently with minor trauma and may go unnoticed by the athlete, but this will be enough to weaken the VMO and may alter the biomechanics of the patella.

Patellar contact area

In full extension, the patella does not contact the femur but lies in a lateral position. As flexion progresses, the patella should move medially. If it moves laterally it will butt against the prominent lateral femoral condyle and the lateral edge of the patellar groove of the femur. As flexion progresses, different areas of the patella's undersurface are compressed onto the femur. At 20 degrees flexion the inferior pole of the patella is compressed, and by 45 degrees the middle section is affected. At 90 degrees flexion, compression has moved to the superior aspect of the knee. In a full squatting position, with the knee reaching 135 degrees flexion, only the medial and lateral areas of the patella are compressed (Fig. 4.2). Compression tests of the patella to examine its posterior surface must therefore be performed with the knee flexed to different angles.

Patellofemoral loads may be as high as three or four times body weight as the knee flexes in walking, and nine times body weight when descending stairs. While the posterior surface

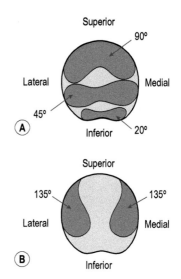

Figure 4.2 Contact areas of the patella at different angles of flexion.

of the patella is compressed, the anterior aspect receives a tensile force when seen in the sagittal plane (Fig. 4.3B). The effect of the Q angle is to create both horizontal and vertical force vectors, which tend to compress the lateral aspect of the patella but submit the medial aspect to tensile stress (Fig. 4.3A). Clearly, alterations in the Q angle will change the pattern of stress experienced by the patellar cartilage.

Knee angles in the stance phase of walking or running will be altered by foot and hip mechanics through the closed kinetic chain. Excessive foot pronation and hip internal rotation and adduction (causing a 'knock-knee' posture) have been linked to patellofemoral pain syndrome (PFPS – see below).

Patellofemoral pain syndrome

Pathology

Pain to the undersurface of the patella is variously called anterior knee pain, chondromalacia patellae, patella malalignment syndrome and patellofemoral pain syndrome (PFPS). The last term is used in this text. It is a condition affecting the posterior surface of the patella, and is sometimes attributed

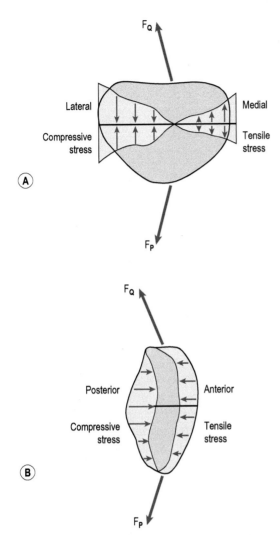

Figure 4.3 Patellar stress. (A) The Q angle causes the lateral edge of the patellar cartilage to be compressed, while the medial aspect is subjected to tensile stress. (B) The posterior surface of the patella is compressed. F_Q, quadriceps pull; F_P, patellar tendon. From Cox (1990), with permission.

to cartilage damage and, on occasion, incorrectly seen as a direct precursor to osteoarthritis. Since hyaline cartilage is aneural, changes in the patellar cartilage surface itself would not result in PFPS. Furthermore, at arthroscopy cartilage changes are often seen in patients who have no PFPS. If cartilage degeneration does occur

with this condition, it is to the ground substance and collagen at deep levels on the lateral edge of the patella. This results in a blistering of the cartilage as it separates from the underlying bone, but the cartilage surface itself is still smooth. In osteoarthritis (OA) the initial changes occur to the cartilage surface of the odd facet (medial) and are followed by fibrillation.

Patellofemoral pain (PFPS) accounts for up to 17 per cent of knee pain seen generally, and up to 40 per cent of knee problems seen in the sporting population (Crossley, Stefanik et al. 2016), with up to 7 per cent of adolescents between the ages of 15 and 19 years suffering with the condition (Rathleff 2016). The condition is more common in young adolescents, especially those active in sport, and is also seen in military recruits. In addition to active individuals, inactive adolescents who are subjected to a sudden increase in walking and/or stair climbing may also suffer. In both groups the condition represents an inability of tissue to adapt to increased loading.

> **Key point**
> PFPS represents an inability of tissue to adapt to increased loading.

The condition typically presents as a dull ache over the anterior aspect of the knee, worse following prolonged sitting and when descending stairs. Although more common in youth, the condition can occur at any age and in seniors it is typically associated with patellofemoral OA (osteoarthrosis).

The retinacula supporting the patella may be a major source of pain (Fulkerson 1982), or the subchondral bone of the odd facet. As we have seen, the odd facet is only occasionally compressed in a full squatting position and so its subchondral bone is less dense and weaker. Lateral movement of the loaded patella could pull the odd facet into rapid contact with the patellar surface of the femur, causing pain. Sources of pain are summarized in Table 4.1.

Table 4.1 Source of pain in PFPS

Articular cartilage damage (no pain) leading to synovial irritation
Mechanical and/or chemical irritation of synovium
Subchondral bone oedema and/or erosion
Lateral retinaculum tension/inflammation
Infrapatellar pad impingement/inflammation

Table 4.2 Factors associated with patella femoral pain syndrome (PFPS)

Factor	Clinical sign
Remote	
▸ Internal rotation of femur	▸ Squinting patella due to femoral internal rotation
▸ Knee valgus increased	▸ Knock-knee position, more noticeable during squatting. Often associated with poor gluteus medius tone
▸ Tibial rotation	▸ Often associated with foot biomechanics
▸ Foot (subtalar) pronation	▸ Drop foot or high arch position linked to tibial rotation
▸ Muscle flexibility	▸ Hamstrings, rectus femoris, ITB/TFL, gastrocnemius
Local	
▸ Patella position	▸ Patellar resting position and passive motion
▸ Soft tissue characteristics	▸ Compliance of medial and laterally placed tissues
▸ Muscular control of quadriceps	▸ Muscle wasting/weakness. Timing of VMO contraction. Tracking of patella

From Crossley et al. (2007).
ITB/TFL—iliotibial band/tensor fascia lata; VMO—vastus medialis obliqus.

PFPS has a multifactorial aetiology. Associated factors may be categorized as local and remote (Crossley et al. 2007). Local factors are those directly associated with the patella structure; remote factors have an effect on the patella through other structures. Table 4.2 shows some of the most common factors associated with PFPS.

Muscular factors

Flexibility and strength of the knee tissues and muscles will often reveal asymmetry, and this would need to be critically evaluated for clinical relevance. The relationship between the

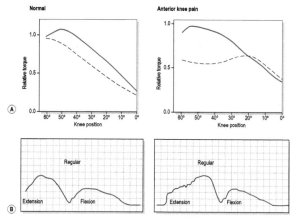

Figure 4.4 Characteristic changes in isokinetic evaluation with anterior knee pain. (A) Relative torque. (B) Shape of torque curve.

hamstrings and quadriceps (HQ ratio) can be important and may require isokinetic assessment of peak torque values if available. Isokinetic testing also demonstrates characteristic changes in the PFPS patient (Fig. 4.4). Eccentric torque production during knee extension is often poor, and the torque curve may be irregular. Both changes have been suggested to represent a deficiency in motor control, which would explain the often rapid response to quadriceps training that is achieved in these patients. One possibility is that malalignment and patellofemoral (PF) pressure alterations may result partly from subtle shifts in the timing or amount of VMO activity, in particular parts of the movement range (Reid 1992). Rehabilitation is therefore more a case of motor skill acquisition than pure strength training.

> **Key point**
>
> In PFPS, aspects of patella dysfunction may result from a shift in the timing of VMO (vastus medialis obliquus) activity during movement. Retraining depends on re-educating the motor skill involved in knee movement rather than pure strength in isolation.

Weakness or malfunction in the VMO will allow the patella to drift laterally as the quadriceps contract. Using ultrasound imaging, Herrington and Pearson (2008) were able to show medial displacement of the patella (6.8 mm) with VMO contraction and lateral displacement (5.6 mm) with vastus lateralis (VL) contraction in vivo. Normally the ratio of VMO to VL is approximately 1:1, and VMO activity is that of a stabilizing muscle in that it is tonic (Reynolds et al. 1983). In the PFPS patient, the VMO to VL ratio is less than one as the VMO weakens. In addition, its contractile nature becomes phasic as its endurance capacity is reduced.

Strengthening has traditionally been achieved by the use of short-range quadriceps exercises and straight-leg raising exercises. However, these are both open-chain movements and as the knee is in closed-chain motion during the stance phase of gait, closed-chain actions are more likely to carry over into functional activities.

Closed-chain VMO re-education may be carried out by performing limited-range squats (quarter squat exercises) or lunges moving the knee from 20–30 degrees flexion to full extension. Step-downs from a single stair are useful, as they can retrain correct knee motion. The patient should be instructed to keep the knee over the centre of the foot (avoiding adduction and medial rotation) throughout the movement. The use of surface electromyography (sEMG) can help with re-education. The sEMG electrode is placed over the VMO and the patient is taught to activate the muscle in standing and then to maintain this activation throughout the quarter squat exercise. The full motor pattern is of foot supination, slight hip abduction and external rotation while maintaining VMO contraction. This may be achieved by standing side-on to a wall, with the injured leg on the outside (Fig. 4.5). The inner knee and hip are flexed to 45 degrees and this knee presses against the wall, enabling the athlete to hold the trunk vertical while standing on one leg. This body position places significant loading on the gluteus medius of the outer leg to maintain the horizontal pelvic alignment. The foot is supinated, leg turned out and knee slightly flexed

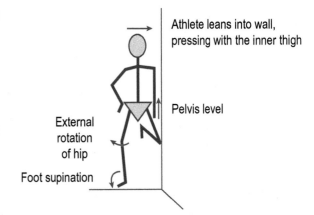

Figure 4.5 Closed-chain patellar stability re-education.

to 20 degrees. EMG biofeedback is used over the VMO, and palpation is used to facilitate gluteus medius activity (McConnell 1994).

In cases where genu recurvatum is present, strengthening of the hamstrings may be required in an attempt to correct the knee hyperextension. In addition to knee musculature, hip strength is particularly important. The hip abductors and lateral rotators warrant special attention, as weakness here has been associated with this condition (Beckman, Craig and Lehman 1989). It is common for young athletes to allow the knee to adduct and medially rotate when descending stairs. This may be due to weakness in the hip abductors, particularly gluteus medius, causing the iliotibial band (ITB) to overwork and tighten. This structure in turn pulls on the patella laterally, displacing or tilting it. Manual muscle testing of the gluteus medius in a side-lying position will often reveal weakness in the affected leg, and tightness in the ITB should be evaluated.

Evaluation of muscle tightness can be helpful, but again should only be targeted where it is related to patient symptoms. The hamstrings, ITB, quadriceps, hip flexors (iliopsoas and rectus femoris), hip rotators and gastrocnemius should all be addressed, as tightness in these structures can alter both knee alignment and gait. Tests, which may also be used as stretching exercises, are shown with average values in Table 4.3. ITB tightness may pull the patella laterally during flexion, while tight hamstrings could result in increased knee flexion and a resultant increase in patellofemoral compression forces. A tight gastrocnemius, in addition to increasing or prolonging knee flexion during gait, will also cause compensatory subtalar pronation.

> **Key point**
>
> Soft-tissue assessment and muscle-balance tests can be useful in the management of patellar pain, if related to symptoms. Clinical relevance is key.

Foot biomechanics

During normal running gait (see Chapter 7), the subtaloid joint (STJ) is slightly supinated at heel strike. As the foot moves into ground contact, the joint pronates, pulling the lower limb into internal rotation and unlocking the knee. As the gait cycle progresses, the STJ moves into supination, externally rotating the leg as the knee extends (locks) to push the body forward. This biomechanical action is combining mobility and shock absorption (STJ pronation and knee flexion) with rigidity and power transmission (STJ supination and knee extension), and shows the intricate link between foot and knee function.

If STJ pronation is excessive or prolonged, external rotation of the lower limb will be delayed. At the beginning of the stance phase, STJ pronation should have finished – but if it continues, the tibia will remain externally rotated, stopping the knee from locking. The leg must compensate to prevent excessive strain on its structures, and so the femur rotates instead of the tibia and the knee is able to lock once more. As the femur rotates internally in this manner, the patella is forced to track laterally.

In certain circumstances the patella can cope with this extra stress, but if additional malalignment factors exist, they are compounded (Fig. 4.6). Anteversion of the femur (internal rotation), VMO weakness and tightness of the lateral retinaculum

Table 4.3 Evaluation of muscle tightness

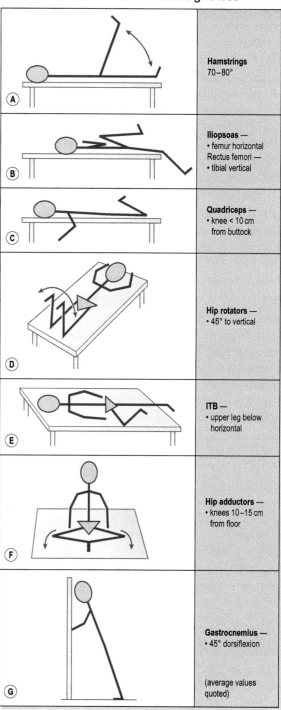

A	Hamstrings 70–80°
B	Iliopsoas — • femur horizontal Rectus femori — • tibial vertical
C	Quadriceps — • knee < 10 cm from buttock
D	Hip rotators — • 45° to vertical
E	ITB — • upper leg below horizontal
F	Hip adductors — • knees 10–15 cm from floor
G	Gastrocnemius — • 45° dorsiflexion (average values quoted)

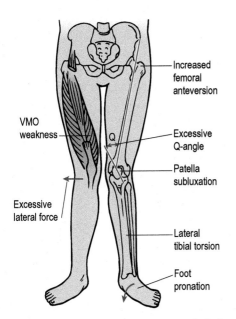

Figure 4.6 Malalignment factors in patellofemoral pain. From Magee (2002), with permission.

may all increase the lateral patellar tracking, causing symptoms. For PFPS to be treated effectively therefore, a biomechanical assessment of the lower limb is mandatory. If hyperpronation is present, it must be corrected. This will involve assessment of sports footwear, patient education and orthotic prescription.

> **Key point**
>
> Hyperpronation of the foot can be altered with an orthotic device in cases of patellofemoral pain syndrome.

Although clinically patients with PFPS often improve with the prescription of orthoses, the evidence for their use is poor. In a study comparing physiotherapy management (PF mobilization, taping, quadriceps muscle re-education) with physiotherapy and orthoses, Collins et al. (2009) studied 179 participants and found contoured foot orthosis to be superior to flat-shoe inserts in the short term, but to be no better than physiotherapy with a follow-up of 52 weeks.

In addition, not all patients with PFP benefit from foot orthosis. Benefit can be predicted by greater midfoot mobility, reduced dorsiflexion motion range and immediate PF pain improvement when performing a single-leg squat while wearing an orthotic (Crossley, Stefanik et al. 2016).

> **Key point**
>
> Orthotics are more likely to be useful in the treatment of PFPS if immediate symptom change occurs when they are worn to perform a previously painful quarter-squat action.

Patella position

A number of forces are imposed on the patella as a result of active and passive structures (Fig. 4.7). The vastus lateralis pulls at 12–15 degrees to the long axis of the femur, while the vastus medialis longus pulls at 15–18 degrees and the VMO at 50–55 degrees. The medial and lateral retinacula, if tight, may tilt the patella. The ITB attaches to the patella via a small slip from its lower end called the iliopatellar band, and in addition has a connection to the biceps femoris through the lateral intermuscular septum. Loading the ITB has been shown to both displace the patella laterally and move the contact area of the patellofemoral joint laterally. In addition, the pull of the ITB imparts a lateral rotation stress onto the tibia. Subjects with PFPS have been

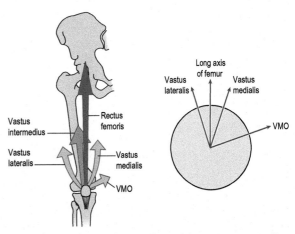

Figure 4.7 Angle of pull of quadriceps onto patella.

189

shown to have a significantly tighter ITB on their symptomatic side (Hudson and Darthuy 2009). Lateral patella displacement has been shown to correlate with ITB length when measured using a modified Ober test, where the upper leg is straight and pelvic position is monitored using pressure biofeedback (Herrington, Rivett and Munro 2006).

Quantifying the position of the patella can be important because, as we have seen above, excessive pressure on the odd facet may result if the patella position is changed and produces symptoms. McConnell (1986) described four different patellar position faults which could be assessed with the patient in the supine position with the quadriceps relaxed. By using the patellar poles as landmarks and comparing their position to the planes of the femur, any malalignment becomes evident. In addition, accessory patellar movements can be assessed with particular emphasis on medial and lateral gliding.

Patellar glide occurs when the patella moves from a neutral position. The distance from the centre of the patella to the medial and lateral femoral condyles is assessed. A difference in the medial

distance compared to the lateral of greater than 0.5 cm is significant (Fig. 4.8A). Tightness in the lateral retinaculum, a frequent occurrence in PFPS sufferers, will cause lateralization of the patella. Patellar tilt evaluates the position of the medial and lateral facets of the patella, with PF pain patients frequently showing a more prominent medial facet with difficulty actually palpating the lateral and posterior edge of the patella (Fig. 4.8B). Patellar rotation occurs when the inferior pole of the patella deviates from a neutral position. Medial (internal) rotation occurs when the inferior pole of the patella lies medial to the long axis of the femur. Lateral (external) rotation is present when the inferior pole of the patella lies lateral to the long axis of the femur (Fig. 4.8C). Anteroposterior (AP) tilt exists when both the superior and inferior poles are not clear to palpate, indicating that one is lower in the surrounding soft tissue (Fig. 4.8D).

Clinical measurement of patella position has been shown to be reliable and valid. Using 20 experienced manual therapists, Herrington (2000) was able to show good agreement between testers when assessing medial and lateral orientation of the patella (r = 0.91 medial measurement, r = 0.94 lateral measurement). In addition, validity has been assessed using MRI as the criterion measure, and a good correlation found between clinical examination and MRI measurement (McEwan, Herrington and Thom 2007).

Measurement of patellar glide is made easier and more accurate by placing a piece of zinc oxide tape over the patella (Fig. 4.9). The knee is flexed to 20 degrees to fix the patella in the trochlea groove of the femur. The medial and lateral epicondyles are marked on the tape together with the mid position of the patella. The tape is removed and the distance between the patella central position and the epicondyles measured.

Alternative measurements of patellar position

Arno (1990) attempted to quantify the patellar position clinically with a description of the A angle.

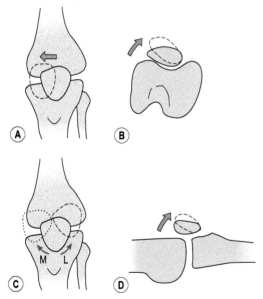

Figure 4.8 Patellar position. (A) Medial and lateral glide. (B) Medial and lateral tilt. (C) Rotation – M: medial, L: lateral. (D) Anteroposterior tilt.

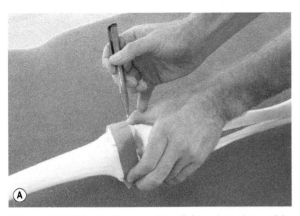

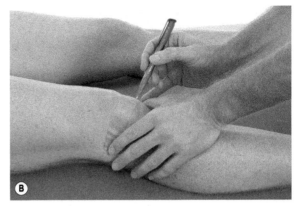

Figure 4.9 Assessing patellar glide using zinc oxide taping.

This relates patellar orientation to that of the tibial tubercle. The poles of the patella are palpated and a line is drawn bisecting the patella. Another line is drawn from the tibial tubercle to the apex of the inferior pole of the patella, and the angle of intersection forms the A angle (Fig. 4.10). The same author argued that an A angle greater than 35 degrees constituted malalignment when the Q angle remained constant.

Radiographic assessment of patellar position is more reliable than clinical measurements. Three common measurements are used (Fig. 4.11). Patellofemoral congruence angle (PFCA) is the angle formed between a line bisecting the sulcus angle and a line connecting the apex of the sulcus to the lowest aspect of the patellar ridge. Lateral patellofemoral angle (LPFA) is the angle between lines drawn joining the summits of the femoral condyles and the patellar poles. Lateral patellar displacement (LPD) is the distance between the highest point of the medial femoral condyle and the most medial border of the patella.

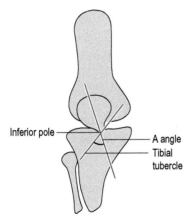

Figure 4.10 The A angle. From Arno, S. (1990) The A angle: a quantitative measurement of patella alignment and realignment. *Journal of Orthopaedic and Sports Physical Therapy*, **12**(6), 237–242. With permission.

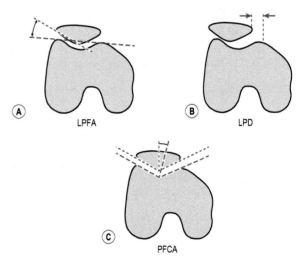

Figure 4.11 Radiographic measurements of patellar position. Modified from Crossley et al. (2000) with permission.

Using these measurements, patellar malalignment is considered to exist when the LPD is greater than 1 mm, the PFCA is < +5 degrees or the LPFA equals 1 degree (Crossley et al. 2000).

Patient examination

Subjective examination typically presents as a diffuse ache over the anterior aspect of the knee. The pain may be worse with loading in a bent-knee position with pain onset on rising from prolonged sitting or with stair climbing. Typically, descending stairs is worse than ascending. There is rarely a history of specific injury, rather a history of symptom exacerbation when loading is increased – for example through training increase, competition or an increase in knee-loading activity during daily living.

PFPS must be differentiated from Patellar tendinopathy, Osgood-Schlatter's syndrome and Sinding-Larsen-Johannsen (SLJ) disease. Patellar tendinopathy is more common with jumping actions and commonly presents with pain localized to the inferior pole of the patella (insertion) or patella tendon proper (body). In Osgood-Schlatter's syndrome, pain is normally restricted to the tibial tubercle. In SLJ disease there is normally point tenderness to the inferior pole of the patella, as with insertional tendinopathy, but X-ray reveals subtle changes with calcification over longer term. The condition must be distinguished from traumatic avulsion fracture, which shows a definite history of injury.

Key point
PFPS must be differentiated from Patellar tendinopathy, Osgood-Schlatter's syndrome and Sinding-Larsen-Johannson disease.

PFPS is reproduced in 80 per cent of patients when performing a squatting action, and tenderness to the patellar edges is seen in 71–75 per cent (Nunes et al. 2013), making these two clinical tests important in objective examination. Traditional grinding tests (patellar compression during quadriceps contraction) have low sensitivity and diagnostic accuracy in PFPS (Crossley, Stefanik et al. 2016).

Patellar taping

Pain relief may often be provided by temporarily correcting any underlying fault in patella position through taping. Exercising with this taping in place may re-educate correct muscle sequencing to improve patellar alignment (McConnell 1994), or simply modulate pain by changing patella loading temporarily to allow recovery. Initially, open-web adhesive taping is applied to protect the skin against excessive tape drag. The pull of the final taping is applied using 5 cm zinc oxide tape. Decreased medial glide (most common) is corrected by pulling a piece of tape from the lateral border of the patella (Fig. 4.12A). The soft tissue over the medial femoral condyle is lifted towards the patella to give a skin-bunching appearance. Lateral tilt is corrected again by a medially orientated tape. This time, however, the tape covers only the medial half of the patellar face, and again the medial soft tissue is lifted towards the patella (Fig. 4.12B). Rotation is corrected by pulling the patella around its central axis. Internal rotation is corrected by attaching the tape to the upper inner quadrant of the patella. The tape is pulled down medially to rotate the patella clockwise (Fig. 4.12C). External rotation is corrected by placing the tape over the lower inner quadrant of the patella and pulling anticlockwise. A posterior tilt of the inferior pole should be corrected first to elevate the pole away from the fat pad. The tape is placed over the upper pole of the patella and the patella is taped medially (Fig. 4.12D).

Evidence exists to support the clinical use of patellar taping. Roberts (1989) found a change in LPFA (1.2 degrees) and a reduction in LPD of 1.1 mm in taped knees. Somes et al. (1997) showed a significant improvement in LPFA in weightbearing, but none in non-weightbearing with taped knees. Larsen et al. (1995) showed improved PFCA in healthy subjects with taped knees, but

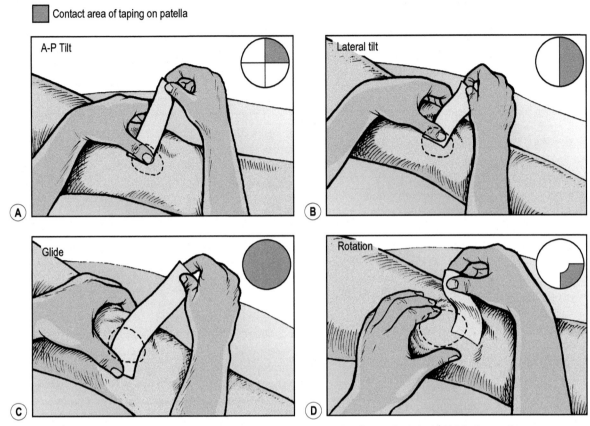

Contact area of taping on patella

Figure 4.12 Correction of patellar position using tape. After McConnell, J. (1992) McConnell Patellofemoral Course, London. With permission.

this change lessened after 15 minutes of vigorous exercise.

One of the functions of patellar taping is to facilitate selective recruitment of the VMO in the belief that patellar pain patients contract their VMO after the VL (McConnell 1986). Some studies have supported this hypothesis (Millar et al. 1999), but others have not (Herrington and Payton 1997). Interestingly, patellar taping seems to enhance proprioception, but only in those subjects where proprioception is poor to begin with (Callaghan et al. 2000).

Fat-pad impingement (Hoffa's syndrome – see below) may coexist with PFP. In standing the patella rests on the fat pads, and if the pad is enlarged, patella alignment may change. Relief of fat-pad related pain may often be given using a 'V' taping attached from the tibial tubercle to run either side of the patella. The action is to draw the taping upwards so the patella is cradled in the base of the 'V' (Fig. 4.58).

Rehabilitation

Exercise therapy which combines hip and knee actions (rather than knee movement in isolation) is a mainstay of treatment with this condition, both to reduce pain and increase function in the short, medium and long term (Crossley, Stefanik et al. 2016).

Where individuals get pain on assessment of a single-leg squat, lower-limb alignment may be addressed as part of motor-control training in the short term to modify symptoms. If patients show a Trendelenburg sign (hip adduction, tibial medial rotation and foot pronation), this movement should be modified using a temporary orthotic and patient re-education to determine if symptoms reduce.

Enhancing hip strength can be achieved by both open- and closed-chain actions. Closed kinetic chain (CKC) is more functional, mimicking the weightbearing action which loads the leg. However, leg loading in the early stages of the condition may exacerbate symptoms, and so open chain may be used until pain settles. Additionally, CKC actions will work the hip and knee together, which may not be required in the present of irritable knee structures. Open-chain gluteal actions such as the traditional clamshell in crook side-lying, and the fire hydrant, and donkey kick in kneeling together with hip scissor actions are useful starting points (Fig. 4.13). Motion range and resistance are progressed, with the aim of reducing pain intensity and frequency during daily living actions and enhancing tissue load tolerance. CKC actions can be begun, with partial weightbearing progressing to full weightbearing. Single-leg squat, step-down (eccentric) and full step (concentric-eccentric) exercises may all be performed initially holding a wall bar in the gym, or a chair back or pole at home. Focusing on lower-limb alignment to avoid excessive hip adduction may reduce symptoms, and the symptom-free movement range and type should initially be chosen. As tissue tolerance is enhanced, both range and alignment should be varied to increase movement variability. Varying training in this way may avoid building fear of certain movement types and encouraging behaviours which avoid actions out of fear of symptom reproduction (hypervigilance).

Resistance should be increased to build lower-limb strength, and specific motor-control actions may give way to more traditional, gym-based lower-limb exercises such as leg presses, squat variations, deadlifts (bent-leg and straight-leg) and lunge actions, with increasing weight and varying motion ranges and speed. Sport-or task-specific movement should also be incorporated to regain confidence in the limb.

Surgery

Before surgery is considered, conservative management must be attempted. Even in the late 1970s clinicians were recommending that surgery was only indicated when continuous pain limited normal activities for at least six months and the condition had not responded to conservative management (Insall 1979).

> ### Key point
> Surgery for patellar pain should only be considered after conservative management has been tried and has failed.

The complex aetiology of the condition has led to a number of different surgical procedures (Fig. 4.14). Release of tight lateral retinaculum is performed through a small incision or arthroscopy to divide the retinaculum from the lower fibres of the vastus lateralis. Although this technique may be used to decrease a patellar tilt greater than 12 degrees (Zachazewski, Magee and Quillen 1996), the procedure has been shown to be ineffective at treating subluxation (Post and Fulkerson 1992) or articular degeneration (Shea and Fulkerson 1992).

Patellar debridement/shaving has been carried out to remove degenerate articular cartilage on the patella undersurface. Small areas of cartilage may be removed en bloc, or larger areas shaved (chondroplasty).

Realignment procedures involve structural transfer to reduce or alter compression forces on the patella. The Maquet operation elevates the tibial tubercle to reduce patella reaction forces, and the Hauser manoeuvre uses distal and medial transfer to reduce the valgus vector acting on the patellofemoral joint. The Goldthwait procedure involves release and transfer of part of the patellar tendon. Proximal realignment, by moving the attachment of the vastus medialis, aims at increasing the mechanical advantage of the

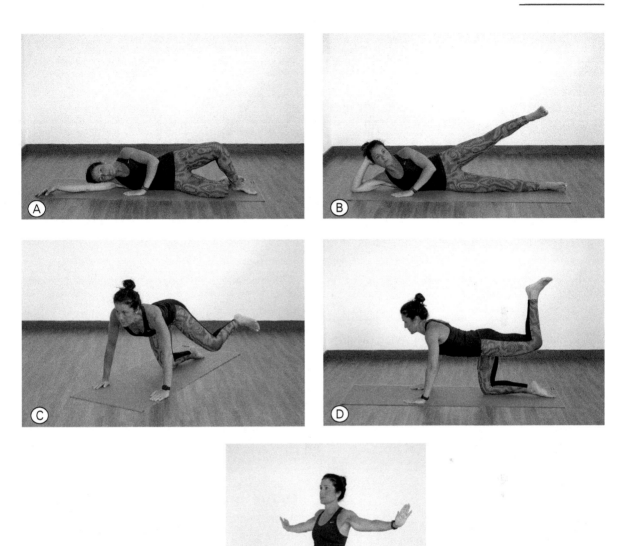

Figure 4.13 Gluteal actions in PFPS rehabilitation (A) clamshell, (B) hip scissor, (C) fire hydrant, (D) donkey kick, (E) step down.

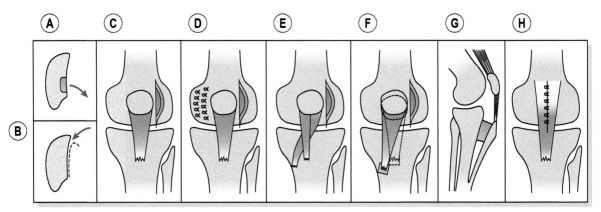

Figure 4.14 Surgical procedures used in anterior knee pain treatment. (A) Excision of diseased area (chondroplasty). (B) Shaving (debridement). (C) Lateral release. (D) Lateral release and medial reefing. (E) Release and transfer of part of tendon (Goldthwait). (F) Release and transfer of entire extensor insertion (Hauser). (G) Tibial tubercle elevation (Maquet). (H) Patellectomy. From Apley and Solomon (1993), with permission.

VMO. This technique is used in the young, where alteration of the tibial tuberosity will detrimentally affect the apophysis. Facetectomy involves excision of all or part of a single patellar facet, and patellectomy entails excision of the whole patella. It should be noted that the results for surgical treatment of PFPS are generally poor (Crossley et al. 2007).

Patellar fracture

Patellar fractures in sport occur most frequently in adolescent athletes, usually as a result of jumping. Fracture may occur at the pole of the patella, or as transverse, vertical or comminuted injuries. In the young, the bony fragment may pull off a substantial amount of articular cartilage from the patella undersurface, giving a 'sleeve' fracture. Stress fracture at the distal third of the patella has been reported after sprinting (Jerosch, Castro and Jantea 1989). Conservative treatment, consisting of immobilizing the limb in a cast for two to three weeks, is sufficient in 50–60 per cent of cases (Exler 1991). Surgical treatment involves internal fixation of the patellar fragments, and hemipatellectomy or total patellectomy in the case of comminuted injuries, combined with immobilization in a cast.

Following immobilization, mobility exercises and quadriceps strengthening are started. Strengthening begins with quadriceps setting (QS) exercises and straight-leg raising. An extension lag is common in these patients. The leg is locked from a long sitting position, and as it is raised, the tibia falls 2–3 cm as the patient is unable to maintain locking.

Definition

An extension lag occurs when the straight (locked) leg is lifted from a sitting position and the tibia drops slightly. The leg continues to lift but the unlocked position is maintained, because the quadriceps are unable to pull the leg into its final degrees of extension and initiate the screw-home effect.

Re-education of the knee-locking mechanism may be achieved in a side-lying (gravity eliminated) position. This is followed by knee bracing with a rolled towel under the knee, the patient being instructed to push down on the towel with the back of the knee and, at the same time, to lift the heel from the couch surface. Short-range movements over a knee block using a weight bag is the next progression. When 60–90 degree knee flexion is achieved, light-weight training on a universal machine with a relaxation stop, or isokinetic training, is used before closed-chain activities.

Patellar dislocation

Patellar dislocation may occur traumatically with any athlete, but is more frequently seen in children between the ages of eight and fifteen years and in middle-aged women who are overweight and have poor muscular development of the quadriceps. Biomechanically, individuals are more susceptible to this condition if they demonstrate genu valgum, femoral anteversion or external rotation of the tibia, and if the VMO is weak. Patellar mobility may be assessed by lateral gliding. If the patella is divided into quadrants (Fig. 4.15), reduced mobility occurs when the patella can only glide laterally by one quadrant. Increased mobility and therefore susceptibility to dislocation is present when the patella glides by two quadrants or more. In this case, more than half of the patellar surface moves over the femoral condyle (Magee 2002).

The injury usually occurs when the knee is externally rotated and straightened at the same time, such as when the athlete turns to the left while pushing off from the right foot. In this position the tibial attachment of the quadriceps moves laterally in relation to the femur, increasing the lateral force component as the muscle group contracts. The patella almost always dislocates laterally and is accompanied by a ripping sensation and excruciating pain, causing the knee to give way. As the knee straightens, the patella may reduce spontaneously with an audible click.

> **Key point**
> Patellar dislocation usually occurs when an athlete turns and pushes off at the same time, combining external rotation and extension of the knee.

Swelling is rapid due to the haemarthrosis, causing the skin to become taut and shiny. Bruising forms over the medial retinaculum, and the athlete is normally completely disabled by pain and quadriceps spasm. On occasion, the VMO may avulse from the patella revealing a hollow, and little tissue resistance to palpation, along the medial edge of the patellofemoral joint.

Initial treatment is to immobilize the knee completely and apply the POLICE protocol. Aspiration may be required if pain is intense, but usually swelling abates with non-invasive management. Quadriceps re-education plays an important part in the rehabilitation process, with VMO strengthening being particularly important. The medial retinaculum must be allowed to heal fully, and it is a mistake to allow these athletes to mobilize unprotected too soon. Only when 90 per cent knee flexion is achieved and the patient is able to perform a straight-leg lift with 30–50 per cent of the power of the uninjured leg are they ready to walk without support.

Early quadriceps exercises

The question of which quadriceps exercise to use at the beginning of rehabilitation is one of considerable debate within physiotherapy. The decision depends on a number of factors including PF reaction forces, the efficiency of an exercise

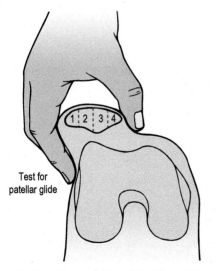

Figure 4.15 Test for patellar glide. From Magee (2002), with permission.

Test for patellar glide

1 2 3 4

to emphasize the VMO and the relevance of an exercise movement to functional requirements (see Specificity of strength training, Chapter 2).

The choice is often between open- and closed-chain movements, and bracing or lifting leg actions. In the gait cycle, the quadriceps are active during leg loading as the opposite leg moves into the swing phase, and to a lesser extent at the beginning of toe-off. In jumping, these muscles create very large concentric and eccentric forces in closed-chain format. In a fast kicking action they work in an open-chain action, but most of the work is from the two-joint rectus femoris (Richardson and Bullock 1986). Both open-chain and closed-chain actions are important, but for early-stage rehabilitation, closed-chain action emphasizing stability is more appropriate.

Comparing the leg extension with the leg press, Steinkamp et al. (1993) found PF joint stress, PF reaction force and quadriceps force to be significantly greater in a leg-extension exercise from 0 to 30 degrees, but significantly greater in a leg-press action from 60 to 90 degrees. These authors concluded that the leg press was more appropriate, because it placed minimal stress on the PF joint in the functional range of motion and simulated normal movement patterns.

Key point

Closed-chain movements reduce patellofemoral (PF) joint forces during inner range of the quadriceps. In addition, they are more functional than open-chain actions because they simulate the normal weightbearing activities of daily living.

It is often argued that QS with isometric hip adduction will increase the recruitment of the VMO because some of the VMO fibres originate from adductor magnus. However, Karst and Jewett (1993) compared quadriceps setting (QS), straight-leg raising (SLR), SLR with the hip laterally rotated, and SLR with isometric hip adduction with resistance equivalent to 5 per cent bodyweight.

These authors found that QS elicited a greater degree of activity than SLR. In addition, SLR with either hip adduction or lateral rotation failed to increase emphasis on the VMO over that of the rest of the quadriceps.

Ilio tibial band syndrome (ITBS)

The iliotibial band (ITB) is a non-elastic collagen cord stretching from the pelvis to below the knee. At the top it is attached to the iliac crest, where it blends with the gluteus maximus and tensor fascia lata. As the tract descends down the lateral side of the thigh, its deep fibres attach to the linea aspera of the femur. The superficial fibres continue downwards to attach to the lateral femoral condyle through fibrous bands, lateral patellar retinaculum and anterolateral aspect of the tibial condyle (Gerdy's tubercle) and to the head of the fibula. A large amount of the lateral retinaculum actually arises from the ITB to form the iliopatellar band, having a direct effect on patellar tracking.

In standing, the ITB lies posterior to the hip axis and anterior to the knee axis, and therefore helps to maintain hip and knee extension, reducing the muscle work required to sustain an upright stance. As the knee flexes to 30 degrees, the ITB passes posterior to the knee-joint axis, and in so doing it appears to glide over the lateral femoral condyle. Anatomical dissection (Fairclough et al. 2006) has shown the ITB to be firmly attached to the distal femur by fascial bands, which act as tendon entheses. Deep into these bands lies fat which is richly innervated and vascularized. The presence of nerve sensors (Pacinian corpuscles) within this fat may suggest a proprioceptive role for the ITB.

Key point

A highly innervated and vascularized fat pad lies beneath the ITB insertion to the distal femur.

There is no separate bursa beneath the distal ITB (Nemeth and Sanders 1996), but the lateral recess (an invagination of the knee joint capsule) of the knee will often be visible on an MRI scan. Two portions of the ITB are visible in a well-defined subject (low percentage body fat). A tendinous part lies proximal to the lateral femoral epicondyle and a ligamentous part passes between the femoral epicondyle and Gerdy's tubercle on the tibia. During knee movement, different parts of the distal ITB are placed under tension. In knee flexion the posterior bundles of the ITB tighten, while during extension the anterior portion is tense. This alternating anterior-posterior tissue tension gives the appearance of the ITB sliding forwards and backwards. However, true AP movement cannot occur due to the tight fibrous bands binding the ITB to the femur (Fairclough et al. 2006).

> **Key point**
>
> During knee movement different bundles of the distal ITB are placed under tension, but true antero-posterior (AP) movement of the ITB across the distal femur does not occur.

Aetiology

ITBS can occur in a number of subject groups. The tall, lanky teenager who has recently undergone the adolescent growth spurt may experience pain if soft-tissue elongation lags behind long-bone development, and tightness in adolescent females is a consistent factor in patella femoral pain syndrome (PFPS). In runners, particularly those who cover longer distances, a number of factors can contribute to the condition. Running on cambered roads and using shoes worn on their lateral edge will increase varus knee angulation and may change loading through the ITB. Rapid increases in tissue loading with speed or hill work may challenge the tissue's ability to adapt quickly enough.

Pain can occur over the lateral hip (trochanteric region) or lateral knee (femoral condyle) (Fig. 4.16). Pain is experienced to palpation, but also to limited-range squats or lunges on the affected leg. As the knee flexes and the ITB passes over the lateral femoral condyle, fat compression rather than friction may occur (Fairclough et al. 2007). Flexibility tests, particularly the Ober manoeuvre and Thomas test, often reveal pain and a lack of flexibility. In addition, compressing the ITB over the proximal part of the lateral femoral condyle with the knee flexing and extending to 30 degrees may elicit pain. Where passive adduction (Ober test) is limited, active abduction is often also affected, and so rehabilitation must address pelvic control over the fixed foot as part of a multimodal treatment programme.

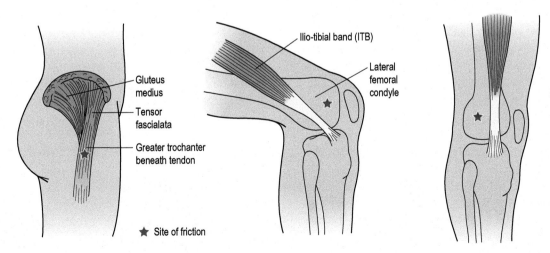

Figure 4.16 Iliotibial band friction syndrome.

Management

As with many types of tendinopathy, there is little inflammation in this condition. Enlargement of the distal structures normally reflects increased blood flow and fluid retention within the underlying fat layer, rather than an active process involving swelling. The small amount of inflammation which is present produces chemical irritants to activate the local neural sensors (nociception). To reduce tissue irritation, loading must be reduced initially. Modifications include alterations of running surface and footwear, gait modification and changes to training intensity, frequency, duration and content.

Stretching

Where limited-range motion is identified, stretching procedures may be pain modulating, although any improvement in motion range will be from alteration in muscle tone rather than overall lengthening of the ITB itself. Static stretching into hip extension and/or adduction may be used for subject self-management and will often ease pain and stiffness. These actions should be practised first thing in the morning where an athlete finds the condition stiff on rising, and after prolonged sitting. As compression is one of the factors in the condition, repeated stretches may increase irritation, so the condition should be monitored throughout rehabilitation.

Three stretch positions may be useful: the Ober test position, half kneeling, and a modified straight-leg raise using a belt.

In the Ober test position (side-lying on non-painful side), the pelvis is stabilized by the subject flexing and holding the lower knee. The affected upper leg is initially abducted and extended at the hip and flexed at the knee. From this position, hip extension is maintained and the leg is pushed downwards into adduction, and held for 30–60 seconds, with the stretch being repeated four or five times. As adduction commences, the subject's pelvis will tend to tilt and an assistant should press down on the rim of the ilium to stabilize the pelvis and increase the stretch. Rather than a passive stretch this involves eccentric action of the hip

abductors followed by isometric contraction of the adductors (Fig. 4.17a).

In a half kneeling position with the unaffected leg forwards, the body is lunged forwards and outwards to carry the trailing leg into hip extension and adduction. Side flexing the trunk away from the painful leg encourages pelvic lift to avoid dipping towards the affected leg and releasing the stretching force (Fig. 4.17b).

Lying on the back, the affected leg is lifted straight and a webbing belt (yoga belt) is looped over the forefoot and held in both hands. Initially the belt is used to draw the leg towards the head (hamstring stretch) and then the belt is transferred into the contralateral hand and the straight leg is drawn across the body moving the hip into adduction (Fig. 4.17C).

Between treatment sessions the subject should attempt these procedures at home. The weight of the leg may be used to press it into adduction, and a weight bag on the knee will assist this. In addition, a training partner or family member can be taught to help maintain lumbo-pelvic stability.

Passive techniques

Passive techniques including self-massage, trigger point release and foam roller techniques do little to the structure of the tissues themselves, but may offer pain relief reducing the requirement for medication. In some instances the technique may allow subjects to train without pain; however, caution must be used if passive techniques are disguising underlying pain due to tissue weakness. Foam rolling and trigger point release are used to target the muscles (tensor fascial lata and gluteals) attaching into the ITB and the tender areas mid-way down the outer thigh. As ITBS is caused by compression of the fat at the insertion of the ITB, compressing this area further with a foam roller is likely to increase pain.

To perform foam rolling, lie on your side (painful side down) with a foam roller beneath your hip or upper leg. Bend your top leg, placing your foot on the floor and use it and your hands to control your

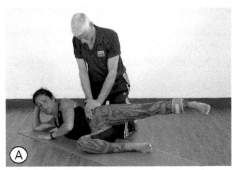

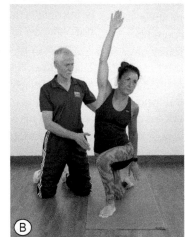

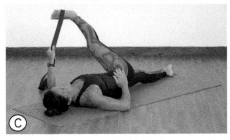

Figure 4.17 ITB stretch positions. (A) Ober test position, (B) half kneeling, (C) belt assistance.

movement. Move your body up and down to roll the tissues and reduce pain. Where trigger points are targeted use you hand or a trigger point tool / firm ball to press into the painful spots. Build up the pressure gradually aiming to relieve pain.

Deep tissue massage or acupuncture techniques may also be used to further target pain (Norris 2003). Again, the effect won't be on the fascia itself, simply to the pain. It is the rehab that you do to strengthen the muscles around the hip and alter loading on the ITB which ultimately will help with the condition longer term.

Strengthening

Weakness in the hip abductors may allow the pelvis to tilt or 'dip' during the stance phase of walking or running. This often gives the impression of a mild Trendelenburg gait, and may be habitual following lower limb injury. Gait re-education and abductor strengthening may be helpful, and these may be performed in combination with muscle lengthening (eccentric contraction). The abductors may be strengthened from an open-chain or more functional closed-chain starting position.

Open-chain strengthening is performed using a weight bag in a side-lying hip abduction (scissor) exercise with the knee extended, or classic clamshell where the knee is bent.

Side-lying hip abduction is performed lying on the non-affected side. A weight bag is placed on the affected leg at the knee (less leverage) or ankle (greater leverage). The action should be pure hip abduction with the greater trochanter (GT) facing towards the ceiling, rather than flexion-abduction with the GT facing slightly backwards. This movement can also be modified to incorporate ITB stretching for pain modulation. In this case, the subject lies on their side at the front edge of a bench or bed. The leg is held in a flexed position at the hip with a weight

bag on the ankle. The action is to lift into abduction and then lower into adduction below couch level to impart the stretch. This movement uses an eccentric action to strengthen and lengthen the hip abductor muscles; a standard hip scissor action may be used for strengthening alone (Fig. 4.18A).

The clamshell exercise is an isolation action for the side-hip musculature, and often the exercise of choice for the gluteus medius muscle in popular exercise such as Pilates. Interestingly, however, it is the side-lying hip abduction (above) which has been shown to produce the greatest contraction of this muscle in EMG (Distefano et al. 2009).

The subject lies on their side with feet and knees together (placing a folded towel between the feet aids grip). The action is to keep the feet together and lift the top knee. When the abductor muscles weaken, the leg cannot be lifted as high, so it is useful to have a training partner lift the knee as high as it

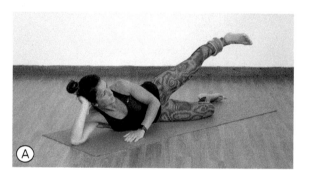
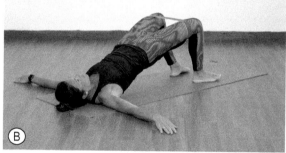
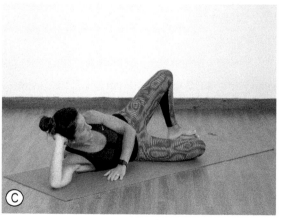
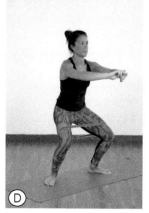
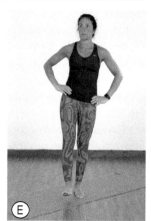

Figure 4.18 Hip abductor strengthening in ITBS. (A) Weighted hip scissor, (B) bridge using resistance band, (C) clamshell, (D) squat with resistance band, (E) single-leg quarter squat.

will go. The subject attempts to hold this high position (isometric hold) and lower the leg under control (eccentric action). The aim is to eventually be able to lift the knee to its full inner range position (Fig. 4.18B).

Closed-chain strengthening is carried out with the athlete standing on the affected leg, or using a bridging action. The shoulder bridge is used to target the gluteus maximus. It is performed lying on the back with the feet hip width apart and hands on the floor. The action is to lift the hips up until the knee, hip and shoulder form a straight line. The exercise intensity is increased by placing a weight on the pelvis, or by performing the single-leg version. For the single-leg bridge the feet are together, the bridging action is performed and then the unaffected leg is straightened to take full bodyweight on the affected leg alone. The exercise intensity of both versions may also be increased by placing the feet on a lift (step or bench). Gluteus medius activity may be increased in the bridge by placing a resistance band around the knee and pressing the knees apart (against band resistance) throughout the movement (Fig. 4.18C).

The pelvic drop action targets the gluteus medius in a functional standing position which mimics the action seen in the Trendelenburg test. In this test, as the bodyweight is taken onto the affected leg and the other leg lifted, the pelvis drops towards the better leg. The drop occurs because the hip abductor muscles are not strong enough (or lack endurance) to hold the pelvis aligned. In this exercise, the subject stands on a step on the weaker leg and allows the pelvis to drop. The action is to keep both legs straight and to hitch the hip up to lift the pelvis and make the leg appear shorter. The action is made harder by standing on an uneven surface (a balance cushion), as balance is additionally challenged, increasing demand on the hip musculature to maintain hip-pelvic stability (Fig. 4.18D).

The side-lying plank exercise begins in a similar side-lying position to the hip scissor action above. This time the subject's affected (weaker) leg is underneath, however. The action is to form a side plank (elbow or hand) and then to lift the top leg in a scissor action, to place a significantly greater demand on the hip abductor muscles of the lower leg. This action has been shown to work the gluteus medius muscle to 103 per cent of maximal voluntary isometric contraction (MVIC) using EMG (Boren et al. 2011).

The resistance band side walk (lateral band walk) is performed with a resistance band around the knees and the knees slightly bent. The action is to sidestep in one direction, stop and then sidestep back facing the same way. In each case the leading leg works the muscles hard concentrically initially, while the trailing leg works eccentrically at first. As the direction is changed the muscle work is reversed. The resistance band position may also be used in a squat action to encourage hip abductor action and correct a knock-knee position often seen when a novice begins squatting (Fig. 4.18E).

Squatting actions are useful to target all of the lumbo-pelvic musculature, and are functional actions used in daily living to sit and rise from a chair, for example, or when lifting (also see deadlift below). Subjects can begin in a quarter or three-quarter squat to limit range and use a high or low bench to touch down onto. Range of motion can increase, and full squats have uses for lower limb rehab, although tension in the patellar tendon may be a consideration where weighted squats are used. Full-range squats may be performed holding a single dumb-bell upright in both hands (the Goblet squat). Hip stability is targeted further in single-leg squats again to a greater or lesser range, and with more or less support to challenge balance. Single-leg squats have been shown to work the gluteus medius at 82 per cent of MVIC (Boren et al. 2011). The squatting action may also be progressed to deadlifts, where the muscle work of the legs is similar to that of the squat but upper body and trunk work is increased.

Gait retraining

Changing the running pattern permanently is difficult to do and could be unwise if it impacts on a subject's performance. The reason is simply that most people run in a way that suits their body, and many Olympic athletes have gait patterns that would seem to be less than optimal – yet they work! However, a suboptimal gait pattern may place excessive stress on a tissue and be a co-factor for tissue irritation. If changing a gait pattern temporarily eases pain and allows recovery while tissue resilience is being enhanced, it can be a useful element of a progressive training programme. Two gait modifications have been shown to be successful in the management of ITBS, step width and cadence.

Some subjects with ITBS exhibit a crossover gait pattern when they run. Here, as the foot is lifted from the ground at toe-off (leg and foot moving behind you), the foot is flicked into adduction and crosses the midline of the body. This often occurs in parallel, with the pelvis dipping down on the trailing leg, lengthening through the side of the body and leg. Step width may be targeted using the resistance band side walk shown above and using cueing techniques, such as running with the feet slightly further apart. Greater strain in the ITB has been shown in narrower step widths (Meardon et al. 2012), so altering step width would seem a logical method of modifying symptoms in those with this condition. Even when this modification is not maintained, it may be one factor that allows subjects to self-manage the condition.

Hip adduction and pelvic drop has been shown to reduce with gait retraining (Noehren et al. 2011). External cues in the laboratory can include electrogoniometry and video feedback, while for the average user, mirror feedback on the gym treadmill may prove useful. Cadence may be changed using a simple metronome app on a smartphone. High cadence (a greater number of steps) means that each step is shorter, reducing ground contact time and total load on the weightbearing leg. Subjects have been shown to increase step rate (7.5 per cent), and to reduce vertical load rate (17.9 per cent) and peak hip adduction (2.9 degrees), following an eight-session training programme using a simple wireless accelerometer of the type found in a smartphone or sports watch (Willy et al. 2016). Thus the results of laboratory investigations have made their way directly into the field to help subjects performing recreational sport.

Collateral ligament injuries

The medial collateral ligament (MCL) is a broad, flat band about 8 or 9 cm in length. It travels downwards and forwards from the medial epicondyle of the femur to the medial condyle and upper medial shaft of the tibia. At its femoral attachment some fibres continue into the adductor magnus muscle. The ligament has both deep and superficial fibres, with the deep fibres attaching to the medial meniscus and the superficial fibres extending below the level of the tibial tuberosity. The posterior border of the deep ligament is associated with an expansion from the semimembranosus muscle, adding strength to this portion of the joint capsule. The superficial fibres have anterior, middle and posterior portions.

Key point

The medial collateral ligament has both deep and superficial fibres. The deep fibres attach to the medial meniscus. The superficial fibres have anterior, middle and posterior portions which must all be considered in treatment.

When the knee is in full extension, it is in close-pack formation. The medial femoral condyle is pushed backwards and the medial epicondyle lifts away from the tibial plateaux, tightening the posterior part of the MCL. As the knee is flexed, the posterior part of the ligament relaxes, but the anterior and middle parts remain tight. By 80–90 degrees flexion the middle of the ligament is still tight, but the anterior and posterior portions are lax. In this way, the strong middle section of the ligament remains tight for most of the range of movement. The changing distribution of tension strain in the ligament means that the section which is affected through injury will depend on the knee-joint angle when the injury occurred, so an accurate history is extremely helpful.

The lateral collateral ligament (LCL) is a round cord about 5 cm long, which stands clear of the joint capsule. It travels from the lateral epicondyle of the femur to the lateral surface of the head of the fibula. In some subjects the ligament is continuous with the peroneus longus muscle. The ligament splits the tendon of the biceps femoris, and is separated from the joint capsule by the popliteus muscle and the lateral genicular vessels and nerve. The lower end of the lateral ligament is pulled back in extension, and forwards in flexion of the knee.

Damage to the MCL can result from excessive valgus angulation of the knee coupled with external rotation, while LCL damage is normally through varus strains coupled with internal rotation. MCL damage usually gives pain over the medial epicondyle of the femur, the middle third of the joint line or the tibial insertion of the ligament. With LCL damage, pain is normally over the head of the fibula or lateral femoral epicondyle.

Palpating the collateral knee structures

The joint line of the knee can be found by sliding one finger up the patellar tendon and palpating the apex (lower part) of the patella. Rest one finger horizontally across this point, and the joint line lies at the lower edge of the fingertip.

> ### Key point
>
> To find the knee joint line, slide one finger up the patellar tendon until it touches the lower part of the patella. Rest the finger horizontally across this point, and the joint line is felt as a shallow groove at the lower edge of the fingertip.

Palpation of the medial aspect of the knee is made easier by dividing the area into thirds (Fig. 4.19). The anterior third comprises the edge of the patellar tendon and extensor retinaculum, and the superficial border of the MCL. Inferior and medial to the tibial tubercle are the insertions of semi-tendinosus, sartorius and gracilis (pes anserine structures). The middle third comprises the MCL and the coronary ligaments. The posterior third comprises the deep part of the MCL and the diverse expansion from the semimembranosus.

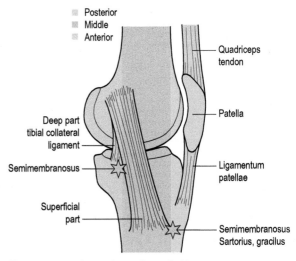

Figure 4.19 Palpation of medial knee structures.

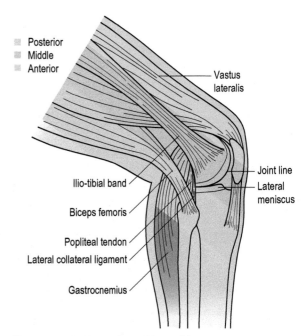

Figure 4.20 Palpation of lateral knee structures. Adapted from Reid (1992), with permission.

Palpation of the lateral aspect of the knee may be similarly divided into thirds (Fig. 4.20). The anterior third consists of the lateral edge of the patellar tendon and the lateral retinaculum. The middle

205

third is dominated by the ITB, and the posterior third consists of the fibular collateral ligament, the tendon of biceps femoris, the lateral head of gastrocnemius and popliteus.

Ligament tests

The integrity of the ligaments is tested by applying a varus and valgus stress to the knee flexed to 30 degrees. Performing the same test with the knee locked is ineffective as this is the close-pack position, and nearly 50 per cent of medial and lateral stability is provided by the cruciate ligaments and joint capsule.

Pain and/or laxity to valgus and varus stress implicates structures other than the collateral ligaments. Valgus (abduction) stresses place tension on the MCL, posterior oblique ligament and posteromedial capsule. Varus (adduction) stress places tension on the lateral collateral ligament, posterolateral capsule, arcuate ligament and ITB. Diagnosis must therefore be made using several tests and the patient's history.

The easiest way to perform the varus/valgus test is with the patient's hip abducted, the thigh supported on the couch or a rolled towel, and the lower leg over the couch side. Where a lower couch is used, the practitioner may need to use his/her own thigh to rest the patient's leg (Fig. 4.21). The practitioner's hands are positioned for maximum leverage, with pressure coming through the forearms rather than from the hands alone. The limb is tightly controlled by holding close to the joint line and supporting the leg against the practitioner's body.

First-degree and second-degree injuries are generally treated conservatively. Third-degree injuries (complete rupture) have been treated surgically, but some authors argue that stability of the knee is not improved to a greater extent than with non-operative intervention (Keene 1990). First-degree injuries are generally treated partially or fully weightbearing, with the ligament supported by strapping. Second-degree and third-degree injuries are managed non-weightbearing.

Initially, the aim is pain relief, swelling reduction and the start of mobile scar formation. Isometric quadriceps drill is begun and modalities used to reduce pain and swelling (Table 4.4). At night, a knee brace may be used to protect the ligament. By the third or fourth day after injury (sometimes earlier with a first-degree and later with a third-degree injury) gentle mobility exercises are begun, either in a side-lying starting position or in the pool. Gentle transverse frictions may be used with the aim of encouraging mobile scar formation. The sweep should be quite broad and a large section of the ligament treated. Free or light-resisted exercises are begun to the knee, hip and calf musculature within the pain-free range. Isokinetics may be used with the aim of restoring the HQ ratio to that of the uninjured limb.

When 90 degrees of pain-free movement is obtained (usually 10–14 days after injury with a grade 3 sprain), the rehabilitation programme can be progressed further to include more vigorous activities, and increased mobility and strength training. An exercise cycle or light jogging may be used, and swimming (not breaststroke) started.

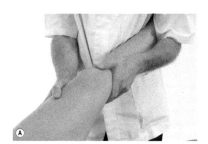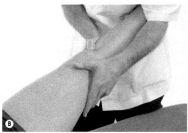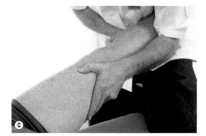

Figure 4.21 Collateral ligament tests: (A) valgus, (B) varus and (C) using practitioner support.

Table 4.4 Guidelines for medial collateral ligament rehabilitation

Phase I (0–7 days) POLICE Protocol
Knee immobilizer (Grade II/III injuries) or knee sleeve (Grade I injury) Modalities to reduce pain and inflammation 2–7 days Active knee mobility exercises within pain-free range Progress to static cycle (high saddle) Deep transverse frictions at multiple joint angles Avoid valgus stress Begin hip adductor strengthening with resistance above knee Begin quadriceps and hamstring strengthening, open and closed chain
Phase II (7–14 days)
Increase resistance on open-chain isotonic exercise Progress closed-chain exercise to quarter squat (partial weight-bearing if still painful) Increase range motion using active assisted and automobilization exercises Begin proprioceptive work
Phase III (14 days onwards*)
Progress all strength exercise Obtain final degrees of motion range Progress proprioceptive work Introduce acceleration/deceleration work Multi-direction agility skills (sports specific), e.g. zig-zag run, shuttle run, plyometric exercises (Use aerobic/upper limb activities throughout programme)

*Criterion for progression to Phase III: no joint effusion; minimal pain to direct ligament palpation; full or near full painless range of motion; knee stable to hop/hop and turn tests. After Reid (1992), with permission.

Weight training is progressed to use leg machines, and some power training is added. Towards the end of this period, depending on pain levels, shallow jumping, bench stepping, circle running and zig-zagging in the gym are used to gradually introduce rotation, shear and valgus stress to the knee. In addition to improving strength and power, these exercises build confidence and provide an assessment of knee stability.

Occasionally, anteroposterior X-ray will show a bony plaque under the femoral attachment of the MCL (Pellegrini-Stieda disease). The attachment of the adductor magnus onto the adductor tubercle may also be partially avulsed. The condition is normally due to ossification of the haematoma formed at the time of injury, and MCL injuries which do not improve or get worse with treatment should be examined radiographically to check for this condition. Infrequently it may occur in the absence of apparent trauma. The condition will normally resolve with rest, but where pain is continuous, surgical removal is required.

Definition

Pellegrini-Stieda disease is an ossification of the haematoma formed when the medial collateral ligament (MCL) is injured. The attachment of the adductor magnus onto the adductor tubercle may also be partially avulsed.

Cruciate ligaments

Structure and function

The cruciate ligaments are strong, rounded cords within the knee-joint capsule, but outside its synovial cavity. The ligament fibres are 90 per cent collagen and 10 per cent elastic, arranged in two types of fasciculi. The first group travels directly between the femur and tibia, as would be expected, but the second set spiral around the length of the ligament. This structure enables the ligament to increase its resistance to tension when loaded. Under light loads only a few of the fasciculi are under tension, but as the load increases the spiral fibres unwind, bringing more fasciculi into play and effectively increasing the ligament strength.

The anterior cruciate ligament (ACL) is attached from the tibia, anterior to the tibial spine. Here, it blends with the anterior horn of the lateral meniscus and passes beneath the transverse ligament. Its direction is posterior, lateral and proximal to attach to the posterior part of the medial surface of the lateral femoral condyle. As it travels from the tibia to the femur, the ligament twists in a medial spiral. The ligament consists of two bundles, the posterolateral bundle of the ACL, which is taut in extension, and the anteromedial bundle, which is lax. In flexion, all of the fibres except the anteromedial portion are lax.

The posterior cruciate ligament (PCL) arises from the posterior intercondylar area of the tibia and travels anteriorly, medially and proximally, passing medial to the ACL to insert into the anterior portion of the lateral surface of the medial femoral condyle. The majority of the PCL fibres are taut in flexion, with only the posterior portion being lax, and in extension the posterior fibres are tight but the rest of the ligament is lax.

The ACL provides 86 per cent of the resistance to anterior displacement and 30 per cent to medial displacement, while the PCL provides 94 per cent of the restraint to posterior displacement and 36 per cent to lateral stresses (Palastanga, Field and Soames 1989).

Injury

Of the two ligaments, the ACL is far more commonly injured in sport, with over 70 per cent of knee injuries with acute haemarthrosis involving ACL damage. The athlete has often participated in either a running/jumping activity or skiing. The history is usually of a non-contact movement such as rapid deceleration, a 'cutting' action in football or a twisting fall. The combination is frequently one of rotation and abduction, a similar action to that which causes MCL or medial meniscus damage, and the three injuries often coalesce to form an 'unhappy triad'. The mechanism of ACL injury falls into two distinct categories, therefore: firstly a cutting-type action (sidestep), and secondly a single-leg landing. The action usually combines a valgus force with internal hip rotation while the body is decelerating in preparation for the subject making a sudden direction change. This position,

known as functional valgus, sees the knee being pushed medial to the hip and foot.

Following injury, swelling is usually immediate as a result of haemarthrosis, leaving a hot, tense, inflamed knee within one or two hours after injury. This contrasts with simple effusion which may take many hours to form (normally overnight). In addition, the athlete often describes 'something going', 'popping' or 'ripping' inside the knee as it gave way. Rapid swelling, a feeling of internal tearing and giving way are essential elements of the history of injury with this condition. The classic anterior drawer test is often negative at this stage due to hamstring muscle spasm and effusion. The high strain rates encountered in sports situations cause the majority of injuries to occur to the ligament substance rather than the osseous junction, and so X-ray is usually unrevealing.

Manual testing

Diagnosis relies heavily on clinical history and tests for instability, the latter being the subject of some debate. The two most common tests are the anterior drawer test and modifications of this, and the pivot shift.

The classic anterior drawer test (Fig. 4.22) involves flexing the patient's knee to 90 degrees and stabilizing the foot with the examiner's bodyweight. The proximal tibia is pulled anteriorly and the amount of movement compared to the 'normal' value of the uninjured leg. Various grades of movement may be assessed, grade one being

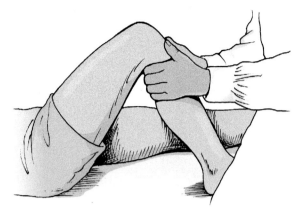

Figure 4.22 Anterior drawer test.

up to 5 mm of anterior glide, grade two 5–10 mm and grade three over 30 mm. The test can, however, give false negatives if haemarthrosis prevents the knee being flexed to 90 degrees. Movement can also be limited by protective hamstring spasm or if the posterior horn of the medial meniscus wedges against the medial femoral condyle.

> **Key point**
>
> The classic anterior drawer test can give a false negative result if haemarthrosis prevents the knee being flexed to 90 degrees. Movement can also be limited by protective hamstring muscle spasm.

Lachman test

The Lachman test, a modification of the anterior draw, has been shown to be highly reliable (Donaldson, Warren and Wickiewicz 1985). The test is performed with the patient lying supine. The examiner holds the patient's knee in 20-degree flexion, minimizing the effect of hamstring spasm and reducing the likelihood of meniscal wedging. The reduced angle of flexion compared with the anterior drawer test is less painful for the patient, and comfort can be further enhanced by placing the knee over a pillow. One hand stabilizes the femur and the other applies an anterior shearing

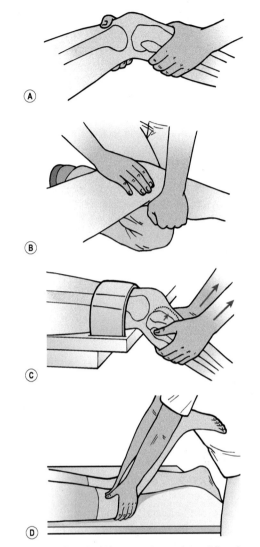

Figure 4.23 The Lachman test and modifications. (A) Standard test. (B) Patient's leg supported over the therapist's knee. (C) Patient's leg over couch end and supported by a strap. (D) Reverse Lachman's.

force to the proximal tibia, avoiding medial rotation (Fig. 4.23A).

Clinically, the test may be modified in a number of ways to avoid holding the weight of the whole leg. The therapist may place his or her flexed knee on the couch and rest the patient's leg over it (Fig. 4.23B). Alternatively, the patient's femur may

209

be supported on the couch with the tibia over the couch end. The femur is stabilized with a strap, leaving both of the therapist's hands free to shift the tibia (Fig. 4.23C). If anterior translation of the tibia is felt, the test is positive. The movement is compared to the uninjured knee, both for range and end-feel, an ACL tear giving a characteristically soft end-feel. The same grading system is used as with the anterior drawer test.

With the anxious patient who is unable to relax, the reverse-Lachman test may be used. Here, the patient is lying prone with the knee flexed to 20 degrees. The examiner grasps the patient's tibia, with the forefingers over the tibial tubercle and the thumbs over the politeal fossa (Fig. 4.23D). Anterior displacement, rather than being felt (as in the classic Lachman test), is actually seen with this modified test.

Pivot shift tests

Another frequently used test is the pivot shift, and its adaptations. These work on the basis that the ACL-deficient knee will allow the lateral tibial plateau to sublux anteriorly (Fig. 4.24). By applying forces to enforce this and then moving the knee, the tibia can be made to reduce rapidly, causing a 'thud'. The pivot-shift test starts with the affected leg in *full extension*. The examiner grasps the ankle of this leg with his or her distal hand, and the outside of the ipsilateral knee with his or her proximal hand. The ankle and tibia are forced into *maximum internal rotation*, subluxing the lateral tibial plateau anteriorly. The knee is slowly flexed as the proximal hand applies a valgus stress. If the test is positive, tension in the ITB will reduce the tibia at 30–40 degrees, causing a sudden backward 'shift'. The major disadvantage with this test is that the patient must be relaxed throughout the manoeuvre, a situation often not possible because of pain. Donaldson, Warren and Wickiewicz (1985) tested over 100 ACL-deficient knees preoperatively and found the pivot shift test to be positive in only 35 per cent of cases. The same examination carried out under anaesthesia (muscles completely relaxed) gave 98 per cent positive results.

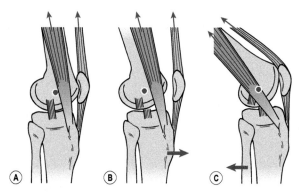

Figure 4.24 The pivot shift test. (A) In the normal knee at rest, anterior pull of the quadriceps and iliotibial band (ITB) is resisted by the intact anterior cruciate ligament (ACL). The ITB lies in front of the knee pivot point. (B) In the ACL-deficient knee the tibia is drawn forwards, pushing the ITB anterior to the pivot point of the knee. (C) In the ACL-deficient knee the pivot point of the knee moves backwards (closer to the ITB) allowing the tibia to reduce with a thud. From Reid (1992) with permission.

> **Key point**
>
> The pivot-shift test is only accurate if the patient remains relaxed throughout the movement. Accuracy is increased from 35 per cent for the conscious patient to 98 per cent when the test is performed under anaesthetic.

This test is reversed in the jerk test (Table 4.5), while the flexion rotation draw (FRD) test eliminates the need for a valgus force by using gravity to sublux the tibia. A reliability of 62 per cent has been reported for the FRD, rising to 89 per cent with the anaesthetized patient (Jensen 1990). The Slocum test uses a side-lying position to perform a pivot shift and is particularly suitable for heavier patients.

Since the ACL has two functionally separate portions (see above), depending on the knee angle at the time of injury, only one portion may be damaged, resulting in a partial ligament tear. If the anteromedial band is damaged but the posterolateral portion is intact, the Lachman test

Table 4.5 Manual laxity tests of the knee

Anterior draw	Knee flexed to 90°, foot stabilized, tibia drawn forwards
Lachman	Knee flexed to 20°, femur stabilized, tibia drawn forwards
Pivot shift (MacIntosh)	Knee extended, foot/tibia internally rotated, valgus strain on knee as it is flexed
Jerk (reverse pivot shift)	Knee flexed to 90°, valgus stress on knee, internally rotate tibia and extend knee
Flexion/rotation drawer	Leg held by tibia only, knee in 20° flexion posterior force on tibia, then flex knee
Slocum	(i) Knee and hip flexed, anterior drawer test in 30° external rotation. AMRI if medial condyle still moves forwards
	(ii) Patient on uninjured side, pelvis rotated posteriorly. Ankle on couch. Knee flexed to 10°, apply valgus stress and push further into flexion. Tests for ALRI. Knee flexed to 45°, tibia externally rotated.
Losee	Knee extended, and valgus force applied, allowing tibia to internally rotate

Adapted from Jensen (1990). Manual laxity tests for anterior cruciate ligament injuries. *Journal of Orthopaedic and Sports Physical Therapy,* **11**(10), 474–481.

AMRI—anteromedial rotary instability, ALRI—anterolateral rotary instability.

may be negative but the anterior draw positive. This is because the anteromedial portion is tightened as the knee flexes, and so will be tighter (and therefore instability will be more apparent) with the 90-degree knee angle of the anterior draw. Similarly, if the posterolateral band is disrupted (the more usual situation), the anterior draw may be negative but the Lachman positive, as this portion of the ligament becomes tighter as the knee approaches extension.

Partial tears usually remain intact and show good long-term results. However, Noyes et al. (1989) argue that progression to complete deficiency, although unlikely in knees which have sustained injury to one quarter of the ligament, may be expected in 50 per cent of knees with half ligament tears and 86 per cent of those with three-quarter tears.

Combined instabilities

Most ligament tests assess instability in only one plane, but various combinations of instability exist in two or more planes (Fig. 4.25). The two most common instabilities are anteromedial, in which the medial tibial plateau moves anteriorly on the femur, and anterolateral, where the lateral tibial plateau moves anteriorly. Movement of the lateral tibial plateau posteriorly (posterolateral instability) or

the medial tibial plateau posteriorly (posteromedial instability) may also occur. Anteromedial instabilities may be assessed using a modified anterior draw and anterolateral instabilities by the pivot shift (above).

For the modified anterior drawer test or Slocum, the patient sits with the hip and knee flexed. The test is to perform the anterior draw initially with the tibia in neutral, and then with tibial rotation. The degree of anterior movement of the medial tibial condyle is assessed using the standard draw test, and then the tibia is externally rotated to 15–30 degrees. The external rotation tenses ('winds up') the anteromedial structures, and if the tibial rotation *fails to reduce the anterior movement of the medial condyle* the test is positive.

Arthrometer testing

An arthrometer measures joint motion. The most commonly reported arthrometer in the literature for assessing knee-joint motion is the KT-1000 (Med Metrics Corp. Inc., San Diego, California, USA). To perform anteroposterior testing, patients are placed in the Lachman-test position (see above) with the knee flexed to 30 degrees. In this position the patella is engaged in the trochlea, so that it does not move during assessment of tibial movement relative to the femur. The arthrometer unit is placed

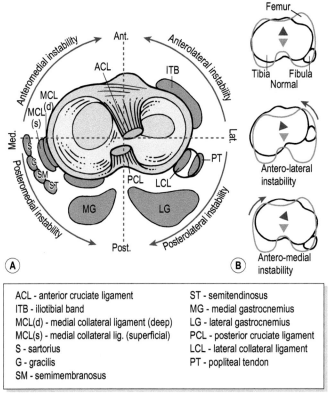

ACL - anterior cruciate ligament
ITB - iliotibial band
MCL(d) - medial collateral ligament (deep)
MCL(s) - medial collateral lig. (superficial)
S - sartorius
G - gracilis
SM - semimembranosus

ST - semitendinosus
MG - medial gastrocnemius
LG - lateral gastrocnemius
PCL - posterior cruciate ligament
LCL - lateral collateral ligament
PT - popliteal tendon

Figure 4.25 (A) Structures contributing to combined instabilities of the knee. (B) Movement directions. From Magee (2002), with permission.

on the anterior tibia and held in place with Velcro straps around the calf. Leg rotation is avoided by supporting the heel in a shallow rubber cup on the couch.

The arthrometer handle applies a force to the tibia, usually of 67 N (15 lb) and 89 N (20 lb). The difference in anterior displacement between the two forces is called the 'compliance index' and is a frequently quoted measure of knee-joint stability. Alternatively, maximal manual force may be used and the injured and non-injured legs compared (side-to-side measurement). Tibial translation (to the nearest 0.5 mm) is measured by the change in relative alignment of pads placed on the tibial tuberosity and patella. However, the translation values seen with arthrometry do not represent actual bony motion specifically. When arthrometer readings are compared with

stress radiographs, different values are obtained, suggesting that an amount of tissue compression is occurring.

Arthrometer measurement has been found to be consistently accurate. Using maximal manual testing and side-to-side measurement, 90 per cent of conscious and 100 per cent of anaesthetized patients with acute ACL tears had measurements greater than 3 mm. Using 141 uninjured subjects, Bach, Warren and Wickiewicz (1990) showed 99 per cent to have side-to-side measurements less than 3 mm using a force of 89 N.

A number of factors can influence measurement consistency and accuracy. First, muscle relaxation must be obtained. Comparing conscious and anaesthetized patients at force values of 67 N and 136 N, Highgenboten, Jackson and Meske (1989) found side-to-side differences greater than 2 mm in

64 per cent and 81 per cent in conscious patients, but 72 per cent and 83 per cent in anaesthetized patients, respectively. Greater muscle relaxation can be obtained as patients become familiar with the testing procedure, and repeated measurements have certainly been shown to be more effective than isolated tests (Wroble et al. 1990). In addition, arthrometer measurement has been found to be operator dependent. Consistently accurate results will only be obtained with trained testers who have gained significant expertise. Larger testing forces tend to produce better reproducibility, with maximal manual testing giving the most accurate results with all instruments (Torzilli 1991, Anderson et al. 1992).

Management

First-degree and second-degree injuries may be immobilized initially and then subjected to intense rehabilitation to re-strengthen the supporting knee musculature. A de-rotation brace may be used to protect the knee until muscle strength is sufficient. Third-degree injuries, with marked instability, may be treated surgically, although some authors argue that rehabilitation alone is the better solution (Garrick and Webb 1990).

General guidelines of indications for surgery include combined injuries (ACL, MCL and/or meniscus), and high degrees of anterior shear. Isolated injuries treated conservatively seem to remain functional. Jackson, Peters and Marczyk (1980) reported a retrospective study with a mean follow-up of ten years. Of those patients treated non-operatively, 80 per cent of isolated ACL injuries had no functional deficit, compared to only 10 per cent of those with combined injuries. In a later study (Evans et al. 2001), 90 per cent of those with isolated injuries who were treated non-operatively reported that they were satisfied with the result, compared to 60 per cent for those with combined injuries.

Patients treated non-operatively are often presumed to be at risk of developing meniscal injury and joint degeneration. However, X-ray examination and bone scan of patients treated both operatively and non-operatively has shown an increased incidence of degenerative joint disease in the surgically treated group. However, the explanation for this finding is the subject of debate (Woo et al. 1994).

Surgery

Surgery involves repair and reconstruction, most authors agreeing that the latter is more appropriate. Reconstruction techniques may be either extracapsular, intracapsular or a combination of the two. In the UK, 58 per cent of orthopaedic surgeons use bone-patellar tendon autografts and 33 per cent semitendinosis/gracilis autografts (Kapoor et al. 2004). Less commonly, extracapsular reconstruction is performed using a 10 x 1 cm strip of the ITB is passed beneath the fibular collateral ligament, under the lateral attachment of the gastrocnemius, and then looped back on itself. The knee is flexed to 60 degrees and the leg externally rotated, before the ITB is pulled tight and secured with sutures.

For bone-patellar tendon graft, a section is taken from the middle third of the patellar tendon, to include both non-articular patellar and tibial tubercle bone. This has the advantage that it leaves other structures around the knee intact. Tunnels are then drilled in the tibia and femur, travelling through the attachments of the ACL. The graft is passed through the bone tunnel and attached to the lateral aspect of the lateral femoral condyle and the tibial tubercle. The graft is secured with cancellous screws and sutures. This procedure gives a very strong graft, but may have the complication of patellar pain following surgery. Flexion contraction (5 degrees or more) and PF irritability may be present post-operatively. Where contracture is a likelihood, rehabilitation should place a greater emphasis on maintaining full knee extension.

For a hamstring graft, a bundle is taken from the semitendinosis and gracilis and passed through a tunnel as above. This avoids the patellar complications described above, but obtaining sufficient tendon material may be difficult in smaller subjects, and hamstring strength recovery may be problematic during rehabilitation.

Synthetic tissues such as polytetrafluoroethylene (PTFE) may also be used, and mobility may be attained more rapidly following surgery using these materials. However, synthetics are generally only used where intra-articular reconstructions have failed. Bovine substances have been used, but problems have been caused by reactive synovitis following these operations. Allogenic tendon grafts from cadavers and amputation specimens have been used to good effect with patients suffering chronic ACL insufficiency.

Guidelines for rehabilitation following ACL reconstruction

Rehabilitation will depend very much on the particular surgical procedure that has been performed. As synthetic grafts do not need to redevelop a blood supply, they can be rehabilitated more quickly than autogenous grafts. Intra-articular repairs weaken with revascularization, so the repairing ligament will reach only 25–50 per cent of its ultimate strength by 6–12 weeks following surgery. In contrast, extra-articular grafts regain approximately 75 per cent of their original strength in the same time (Reid 1992). Tendon grafts often suffer fewer complications, and the patellofemoral joint remains mobile, while extracapsular grafts require more restraint on movement. Patellar tendon reconstructions tend to be the strongest grafts, but cause greater morbidity due to the anterior surgical approach (Briggs, Sandor and Kenihan 1995). Arthroscopic repairs will recover more quickly than open repairs, as the knee joint is less affected. There is less swelling and a reduced likelihood of complications.

The dichotomy is that immobilization is thought desirable for healing of the graft, but early mobility is required to avoid cartilage degeneration, soft-tissue contracture and muscle atrophy. To overcome the combined problem of healing and mobility, the subject is mobilized early, providing the movement used does not overly stress the graft.

> **Key point**
> Early mobilization is required to avoid cartilage degeneration, soft-tissue contracture and muscle atrophy. However, any movement used must not overly stress the graft.

Early rehabilitation (0–3 days) focuses on avoiding the standard complications following general surgery, and reducing pain and swelling, and an example rehabilitation protocol is shown in Table 4.6. Simultaneous contraction of the hamstrings and quadriceps (closed chain) are used to aid the leg-muscle pump, but isolated quadriceps exercises and straight-leg raising (open chain) are avoided. From 0–2 weeks, as the scar settles, manual therapy to the patella may be required and prone-lying leg hanging (Fig. 4.26A) is a useful exercise for regaining terminal extension while placing minimal stress on the healing tissues. The patient lies prone, with the thigh supported on a folded towel, leaving the anterior knee free. The weight of the tibia presses the knee into extension. Resistance may be supplied by a small weight bag attached to the heel, as tolerated. The patient then performs eccentric hamstring actions, allowing the tibia to lower as far as pain will allow. A wedge may be used below the tibia as a relaxation stop. Before progressing to the next stage of rehabilitation the aim is to achieve full knee extension and 90–120-degree knee flexion. Full quads contraction with no extensor lag is also required.

From two to six weeks, co-contraction activities of the quadriceps and hamstrings are performed by using simple closed-chain actions. Co-contraction of the hamstrings and quadriceps has been shown to place 15 per cent of the quadriceps tension on the ACL at 5-degree knee flexion. By the time flexion has increased to a mean angle of 7.4 degrees, this force is reduced to zero. As the angle of flexion increases still further, a posterior draw force is imposed (Yasuda and Sasaki 1987).

Closed-chain terminal leg extension is a useful exercise for co-contraction of the quadriceps

Table 4.6 Example rehabilitation protocol following ACL reconstruction

Timing	Activity
0–3 days	▶ Monitor skin condition and swelling. Pain management and use of POLICE protocol as required. ▶ Isometric quads/gluts/hamstring exercise ▶ Knee range of movement exercises to achieve full range of extension and approximately 90° flexion ▶ Ankle ROM, contralateral limb and upper body exercise to maintain CV condition ▶ CKC quads work ▶ Gait re-education using crutches/walking aid brace
0–2 weeks	▶ Skin and swelling management as above ▶ Gait re-education & posture work as required ▶ Knee ROM exercise into flexion ▶ Static cycle with minimal resistance ▶ Strengthen knee-stabilizing muscles in closed chain ▶ Soft tissue techniques and patella mobilization
2–6 weeks	▶ Stationary cycling with increasing resistance ▶ Swimming/hydrotherapy exercise, providing wound well healed, and avoid breaststroke kick ▶ Treadmill with increasing walking speed ▶ Resistance training in CKC ▶ Balance and proprioceptive work work – stable/unstable BOS and COG shift ▶ Core stability and gluteal work ▶ Stretches of tight structures as appropriate. ▶ Manual therapy of soft tissue and joint structures as required ▶ Single-leg squat and step up with focus on knee valgus ▶ Increase ROM to flexion ▶ Supervised exercise without brace progressing to self-monitored work without brace.
6–12 weeks	▶ Static cycle and rowing machine with increasing resistance ▶ Speed-walk progressing to slow jog on treadmill ▶ Balance/proprioception to progress to single leg with unstable BOS and COG shift ▶ Progress strengthening with movement variety ▶ Brace not used once proprioceptive control and knee stability in single-leg standing regained
12 weeks – 1 year	▶ Increase jogging pace on treatment ▶ Jogging progressing to change of direction and rotation component as appropriate ▶ Swimming breaststroke kick from 16 weeks ▶ Introduce bilateral jump progressing to single leg ▶ Progress hopping and plyometrics (straight line/sidestep/zigzag/twist) ▶ Progress strengthening through range to include OKC actions for kicking sports

CKC – closed kinetic chain. OKC – open kinetic chain. ROM – range of motion. POLICE – protect, optimal loading, ice, compression, elevation. BOS – base of support. COG – centre of gravity.

☐ Early ☐ Intermediate ☐ Late

and hamstrings (Fig. 4.26B). The athlete stands predominantly on the unaffected leg (partial weight bearing), placing sufficient weight on the injured leg to prevent the foot from moving. An elastic resistance band attached to a wall bar is placed around the mid-thigh, and the action is to extend the hip and knee simultaneously. Adding trunk flexion (Fig. 4.26C) has been shown to increase hamstring activity on surface EMG (Ohkoshi et al. 1991).

The heel slide against a wall or on the floor is also useful at this stage (Fig. 4.27A). This exercise may be progressed by performing it against isometric resistance using a large diameter Swiss ball or isotonic resistance against rubber tubing. Leg-press and shuttle exercises may be used on a sliding platform or low-friction surface. A declined bench is useful, and a linoleum surface or the 'slide trainer' used in popular exercise classes, both providing suitable low-friction

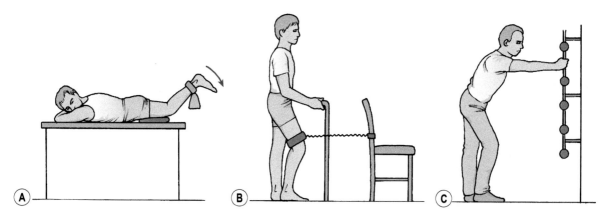

Figure 4.26 Staged anterior cruciate ligament (ACL) exercises. (A) Prone leg hang – to regain terminal extension while working the hamstring muscles. (B) Closed-chain co-contraction of quadriceps and hamstrings. (C) Adding trunk flexion increases hamstring muscle work.

surfaces. Static cycles and step machines provide useful closed kinetic chain actions in a partial weightbearing starting position, and will also improve cardiopulmonary fitness. From six to twelve weeks, treadmill walking can progress to slow jogging, and the subject is gradually weaned off the knee brace as proprioception and knee stability improve. Traditional exercises such as squat, deadlift and lunge can be used modified, and double-leg squat progressed to single-leg. Variations in base of support and body centre of gravity are used to overload proprioception.

> **Key point**
>
> Closed-chain activities using quadriceps/hamstring co-contractions are more functional and place less stress on the graft than isolated muscle contractions.

From 12 weeks to 1 year the subject is introduced back into normal sports or daily-living actions, monitoring valgus control of the knee and hip alignment (avoiding Trendelenburg sign). Leg strength is increased to 100–125 per cent of the uninjured side, and a variety of progressive plyometric actions are used including double-leg/single-leg hopping and jumping in multiple directions.

Rehabilitation of the ACL repaired knee has been described in six stages by a consensus group (Herrington et al. 2013), shown in Table 4.7.

Progress through rehabilitation may be monitored in terms of both quantity and quality. Reaction to loading stress imposed on the knee may be judged by both swelling and pain. Assessment of knee circumference at the mid patella has been shown to be a reliable and sensitive measure, with increases greater than 1 cm being clinically significant (Jakobsen et al. 2010). Subjects should measure knee circumference first thing in the morning and at the end of the day, and load should be reduced if a greater than 1 cm knee circumference change has occurred (Herrington et al. 2013). Measurement of pain on a commonly used ten-point numerical rating scale (NRS) is useful, with a one-point change regarded as clinically important. Any pain generated by rehabilitation activities should reduce to within one point of the previous day's score. A greater than one point day-to-day change requires rest until recovered.

Lack of neuromuscular control when landing from a single-leg jump is considered a significant risk factor for re-injury following ACL repair (Paterno et al. 2010), with increases in knee

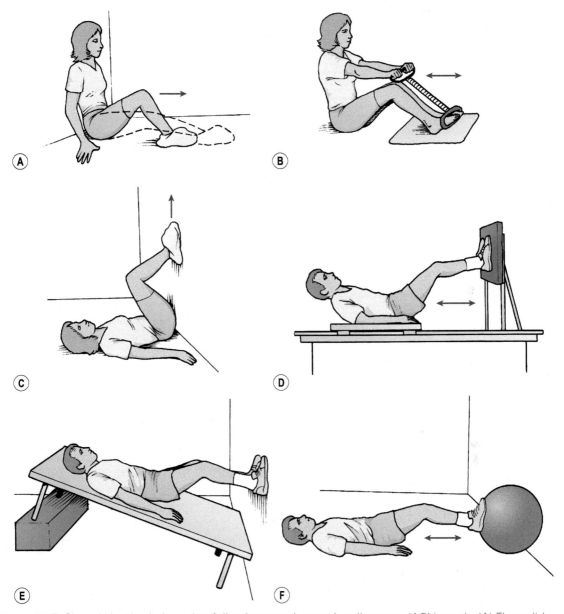

Figure 4.27 Closed kinetic chain action following anterior cruciate ligament (ACL) repair. (A) Floor slide. (B) Slide against resistance tubing. (C) Wall slide. (D) Shuttle. (E) Declined bench. (F) Gym ball pass.

abduction and/or body sway being key factors to note during rehabilitation. Optimal and sub-optimal performance in single-leg loading may be monitored at different body parts using the qualitative analysis of single-leg loading score (QASLS) described by Herrington et al. (2013).

The scoring system (Table 4.8) assesses ten components on a pass (0 – appropriate movement) or fail (1 – inappropriate movement) basis, with the best overall score being 0 and the worst 10. The scale may be used as part of progress monitoring during ACL rehabilitation.

217

Table 4.7 Stages of ACL rehabilitation

Stage	Key criteria
Pre-operative	Prepare for surgery by minimizing swelling, activating the quadriceps musculature and normalizing gait.
Post-operative	Overcome the effects of surgery by regaining movement range and muscle activation, controlling swelling and normalizing walking gait.
Progressive limb loading	Progress from bilateral to unilateral weightbearing activity. Begin load acceptance actions and progress strength training and work capacity.
Unilateral load acceptance	Progress from bilateral to unilateral load acceptance actions in multiple motion planes. Continue progression of strength/force development and work capacity.
Sport-specific task loading	Improve capacity for unilateral load acceptance in multiple planes with a reactive element. Multidirectional running and landing tasks appropriate to individual sporting needs.
Unrestricted sport-specific loading	Progressive return to sport matching rehabilitation and sport-specific skills.

(Data from Herrington et al. 2013)

Table 4.8 Qualitative analysis of single-leg loading score (QASLS)

Date: Patient:

Condition: Left   Right   Bilateral

QASLS	Task: Single leg squat Single leg step down Single leg hop for dist	Left	Right
Arm strategy	Excessive arm movement to balance		
Trunk alignment	Leaning in any direction		
Pelvic plane	Loss of horizontal plane		
	Excessive tilt or rotation		
Thigh motion	WB thigh moves into hip adduction		
	NWB thigh not held in neutral		
Knee position	Patella pointing towards 2nd toe (noticeable valgus)		
	Patella pointing past inside of foot (significant valgus)		
Steady stance	Touches down with NWB foot		
	Stance leg wobbles noticeably		
	Total		

(From Herrington et al. 2013)

Muscle imbalance and proprioception in the ACL deficient knee

Excessive hypertrophy of the quadriceps relative to the hamstrings can lead to a muscle imbalance which may alter ACL loading (Fig. 4.28). The normal, even distribution of pressure on the femoral articular surface seen with balanced musculature has been shown to change to a focused, high-pressure point in the absence of opposing hamstring coactivation (Baratta et al. 1988).

However, functional return is not related directly to hamstring strength, but rather to reflex contraction (Seto, Orofino and Morrissey 1988). Co-contraction of the agonist and antagonist muscles of a joint will enhance stability. As the knee extends, the muscle spindles in the hamstrings will be stretched, leading to mild hamstring contraction. In addition,

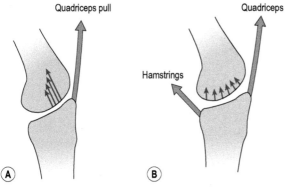

Figure 4.28 Articular surface pressure distribution with muscle co-activation. (A) Focused high pressure point at the anterior articular surface in the absence of opposing hamstring co-activation. (B) Low, evenly distributed articular surface pressure with hamstring co-activation. After Baratta, R. et al. (1988) Muscular coactivation: the role of the antagonist musculature in maintaining knee stability. *American Journal of Sports Medicine*, **16**, 113–122. With permission.

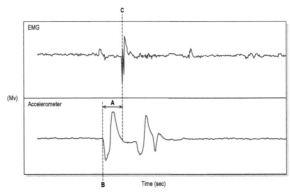

Figure 4.29 Reflex hamstring contraction latency is the time interval between the initial tibial displacement and the first measurable reaction of the hamstrings. A. Reflex hamstring contraction latency. B. First recorded displacement of the tibia (accelerometer). C. First reflex reaction of the hamstrings (EMG). Adapted from Beard et al. (1994) with permission.

mechanical stress on the ACL has an inhibitory effect on the quadriceps, but will simultaneously excite the hamstrings (Baratta et al. 1988). A reflex arc from the ACL mechanoreceptors may allow dynamic torque regulation during ligament loading, and mechanoreceptor stimulation from muscles and the joint capsule causes hamstring stimulation to stabilize the knee (Reid 1992).

Both tension and mechanoreceptors are present in the ACL. Failure of the feedback system from these structures can result in a loss of reflex muscular splinting and the increased likelihood of re-injury. Normally there is a minimal, 2 per cent, variation in the threshold to detection of passive movement (TTDPM) between the two knees. With ACL-deficient knees, variation values as high as 25 per cent have been found (Kennedy, Alexander and Hayes 1982). The proprioceptive deficit seems to be increased at near terminal range of motion. Lephart and Fu (1995) reported longer TTDPM in the involved knee tested at 15-degree knee flexion, but no significant difference when tested at 45 degrees.

Hamstring contraction of ACL-deficient patients occurs earlier in the gait cycle and is of longer duration (Sinkjaer and Arendt-Nielsen 1991). Clinically, ACL-deficient patients have an increased hamstring contraction latency – the time interval between displacement of the tibia and reflex reaction of the hamstrings (Fig. 4.29). ACL-deficient patients have been found to have a mean contraction latency of 90.4 ms, compared to the normal, uninjured knee with a mean latency of 49.1 ms (Beard et al. 1994).

Definition

Hamstring contraction latency is the time interval between displacement of the tibia and reflex reaction of the hamstrings attempting to stabilize the knee.

Quadriceps exercises using short range (from 45 degrees to full extension) should be preceded by isometric hip extension to facilitate hamstring contraction (Seto, Brewster and Lombardo 1989). The use of a standard leg-extension regime in open-chain position places considerable anterior shear on the knee, and may stretch an ACL graft. When performing leg extension on an isokinetic dynamometer, an anti-shear device will greatly reduce shear forces generated with the exercise. When using weight training, however, closed-chain motions such as the squat or leg-press movement are more appropriate during rehabilitation, especially as they produce co-contraction of the quadriceps and hamstrings to reduce shear.

Proprioceptive exercises for the knee include three components. First, sudden alterations in joint position are employed to retrain reflex stabilization. Secondly, general posture and balance activities are used. Finally, joint-positioning skills form the basis of retraining for automatic motor control.

Definition

Proprioceptive exercises for the knee use:
(i) sudden alterations in joint position,
(ii) general posture and balance activities, and
(iii) joint-positioning skills.

Single-leg standing activities begin the training, progressing from positions with the eyes open to those with eyes closed. These activities may be performed on an uneven surface (thick mat and then mini trampette), and later in combination with trunk and upper-limb movements. Reflex hamstring contraction may be performed in crook-sitting (Fig. 4.30A). A towel is placed under the patient's heel. The patient must hold the towel in place with a sudden downward pressure (hip extension and knee flexion) as the therapist pulls on the towel suddenly. Similar actions may be performed on a low stool (Fig. 4.30B). The patient stands on the affected leg only, eyes closed. The therapist produces a very small but sudden displacement of the stool. Partner activities include single-leg standing (eyes closed) with a partner suddenly pushing on the patient's shoulders from any direction. Again, the movement, while rapid, is of small amplitude.

Posture and coordination activities include backward walking, zig-zags, crossover drills of

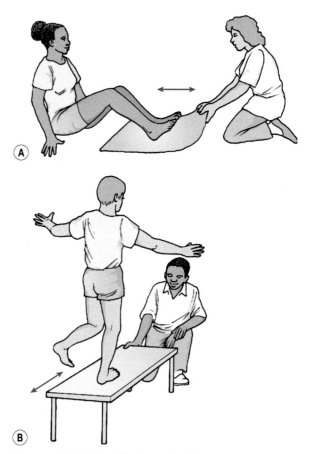

Figure 4.30 Rehabilitation of reflex hamstring contraction. (A) Therapist pulls towel suddenly, athlete must rapidly flex knee to stop movement. (B) Therapist minimally displaces stool suddenly, athlete must maintain balance.

varying complexity and figure-of-eight running. Running on uneven surfaces and lateral step-ups are useful, as is speed walking and uphill walking. Multidirectional running skills based on the functional tests used for the knee also form part of the rehabilitation at this stage.

Accurate static joint repositioning uses cognitive skills and is helpful at various stages of rehabilitation. This may be performed by passive movement on a one-to-one basis with the therapist, or on a dynamometer which shows a display for range of motion. In each case, the patient is encouraged to reposition the joint exactly in the range that the limb rested in before movement began.

A variety of apparatus is useful for proprioceptive rehabilitation. Rocker boards, wobble boards, balance cushions, etc. – used so frequently for ankle re-education – are also of use for the knee. Proprioceptive training using balance boards has also been shown to reduce the incidence of ACL injuries in soccer players. In a study of 600 soccer players, those who included 20 minutes per day of a progressive regime of five different proprioceptive exercises (Table 4.9) had an incidence of 0.15 ACL injuries per team year, compared to 1.15 in the control group (Caraffa et al. 1996).

Table 4.9 Proprioceptive training to prevent ACL injuries in soccer players

Phase	Exercise
1	Single-leg standing for 2.5 min four times each day
2	Single-leg training (half step exercise) on a rocker board for 2.5 min
3	Single-leg training on balance board
4	Single-leg training, combined rocker and balance board
5	Single-leg training on BAPS board

From Caraffa, A. et al. (1996) Prevention of anterior cruciate ligament injuries in soccer. *Knee Surgery, Sports Traumatology and Arthroscopy*, **4**, 19–21. With permission.

> **Key point**
>
> Proprioceptive exercises used for ACL rehabilitation have also been shown to reduce the incidence of ACL injuries. They should therefore form a part of a general training programme for 'at risk' sports, and are used to help protect the knee from ACL injury.

The early stages of rehabilitation emphasized hamstring activity to reduce shear forces imposed on the knee. Now, any imbalance between the quadriceps and hamstring muscle groups must be corrected with both concentric and eccentric quadriceps training. Again, the emphasis is on closed-chain activity, but limited open-chain activity may be introduced. With all activities, the shearing stress placed on the knee must be considered (Fig. 4.31), noting that downhill running and

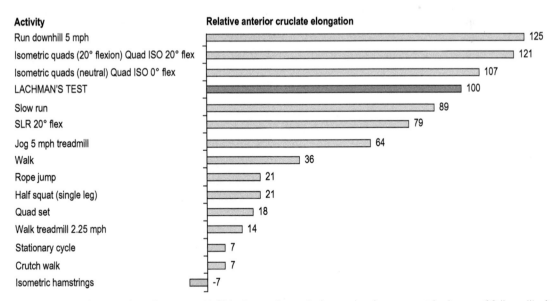

Figure 4.31 Anterior cruciate ligament (ACL) elongation relative to Lachman test (using an 80 lb pull). After Henning, C.E. (1988) Semilunar cartilage of the knee: function and pathology. *Exercise and Sport Sciences Review*, **16**, 67–75. With permission.

resisted isometric quadriceps activity at 20 degrees flexion, for example, produce the greatest ACL elongation (Henning, Lynch and Glick 1985).

It must be remembered that following knee injury, there is a selective atrophy of type I muscle fibres, so endurance ability must be regained to ensure joint stabilization. Patients have been shown to be able to restore quadriceps strength six weeks after surgery (on a leg extension bench) but to still have a 20 per cent deficit in endurance capacity (Costill, Fink and Habansky 1977).

Neuromuscular training for knee-injury prevention

Neuromuscular training (NT) has been used successfully in the prevention of knee injury. In a study of 457 floorball (indoor hockey) players followed up for six months, the NT group suffered 20 injuries against a control group of 52 injuries. The injury rate per 1,000 hours was 0.65 and 2.08 for intervention (NT) and control group (normal sport training) respectively. The risk of non-contact leg injury was 66 per cent lower in the NT group (Pasanen et al. 2008). Four exercise types may be used for NT in the prevention of knee injury: balance and movement control, running skills/footwork, specific strengthening and plyometrics (Table 4.10). The emphasis is on correct movement and alignment. For example, during knee-flexion actions such as lunges, squats and jumps, the knee should pass over the centre of the foot rather than in inner aspect. Jumps should encourage shock absorption through the foot, knee and hip, and should not be performed stiff-legged. The hip hinge action is emphasized when angling the body forwards rather than lumbar flexion alone. Where movements are limited by flexibility issues (hamstring tightness in forward bending for example) stretching is used in parallel with movement re-education. Training is periodized. The total training period for NT is 20–30 minutes 2 or 3 times per week during the non-competitive season, and a single weekly maintenance period is used during the competitive season.

Table 4.10 Neuromuscular training for knee injury prevention

Balance and movement control	Running skills/footwork	Specific strengthening	Plyometrics
Double-leg squat Single-leg squat Balance board double/single-leg Single-leg throw/catch with partner	Backwards running Sidestep Carioca Zigzag Walking lunge (knee over centre of foot) Combination hops	Squat Lunge and multidirectional lunge Nordic hamstring Single-leg shoulder bridge	In-place jump Forward jump Side jump Box jump

Modified from Pasanen et al. (2008)

Treatment note 4.1   The squat exercise in knee rehabilitation

The squat is a controversial exercise in both rehabilitation and general training. Generally, the parallel squat (to a point where the femur is horizontal) rather than the full squat (buttock to heel) is often recommended (Baechle 1994), as it is claimed that less stress is placed on the knee using the reduced range of motion. When performing this exercise, less skilled individuals have been shown to produce a large initial drop velocity, to bounce in the low position, and to lean the trunk forwards while pushing the hips back. The more skilled individual, by limiting trunk extension, places more stress on the quadriceps and reduces the leverage effect on the lower spine.

The squat has the advantage of being a closed-chain activity, but is often said to 'overstretch the knee ligaments' and so is frequently

Treatment note 4.1 *continued*

Table 4.11 Common errors when performing a squat

Error	Technique modification
Knees move inwards (knock-knee)	Foot may be flattening too much (pronation). Wear more supporting shoes and practise the movement in front of a mirror. Aim to keep the knee over the foot.
Knees stay behind feet throughout movement	Ankle forward bending (dorsiflexion) may be limited. Place a 1–2 cm wooden block beneath the heels. Squat onto a bench without a weight and practise pressing the knee forwards.
Back angles too far forward	Keep the spine more vertical and monitor your posture by standing side-on to a mirror.
Spine flexes between the shoulders (thoracic region)	Press the breastbone (sternum) forwards and draw the shoulder blades (scapulae) down and in using a bracing action.
Lower back hollows excessively (increased lumbar lordosis)	Tighten the abdominal muscles and hold them tight throughout the movement. Practise hip flexor muscle stretching.
Heel lift	Position the squat in front of a mirror and use a horizontal line drawn on the mirror to line up the bar.
Bar dips to one side	Practise the squat in front of a mirror and use a horizontal line drawn on the mirror to line up the bar.
Bouncing in the low position	Practise squatting onto a bench and gradually lower the weight into the final position.

From Norris, C.M. (2003) *Bodytoning*, A&C Black, Oxford.

derided. The squat has been shown to work the quadriceps, but significant co-contraction of the hamstrings has been questioned (Gryzlo et al. 1994). Heavy-resistance squatting (130–200 per cent bodyweight) used over a 21-week training period has not been shown to increase knee laxity (Panariello, Backus and Parker 1994). Ligament stability was assessed in 32 professional football players using an arthrometer at 30 degrees and 90 degrees flexion after 12 and 21 weeks. Table 4.11 details common errors when performing a squat. They broadly fall into two categories: (i) lower-limb alignment, and (ii) lumbo-pelvic alignment. The foot should be turned out slightly (Fick angle) by about 15 degrees.

Key point

The Fick angle is formed by the long axis of the foot (second toe to mid heel), relative to the sagittal axis of the body. Normal range is 5–18 degrees.

As the knee bends, the patella should face forwards and outwards slightly but not pull inwards (knock-knee) or outwards (bow-legged) excessively. To check this position, ensure that the knee moves over the centre of the foot and not over the outer or inner edge. The spine should stay relatively upright and straight. There is often a tendency to angle forwards as the weight is lowered and extend the spine as the weight is lifted (Fig. 4.32). Where this happens, the weight is generally too heavy and the spinal extensor muscles are being used excessively.

The knee should pass over the foot, showing that the ankle has dorsiflexed. Where the ankle is stiff, the shin may remain vertical. To maintain the line of gravity through the base of support, the individual will be forced to angle the trunk forwards. This situation is corrected by placing a block beneath the heels.

In some individuals the trunk may lose alignment, either flexing at the lumbar (Fig. 4.33) or thoracic (Fig. 4.34) spine or hyperextending at the lumbar spine, a position accompanied by anterior pelvic tilt (Fig. 4.35).

Treatment note 4.1 *continued*

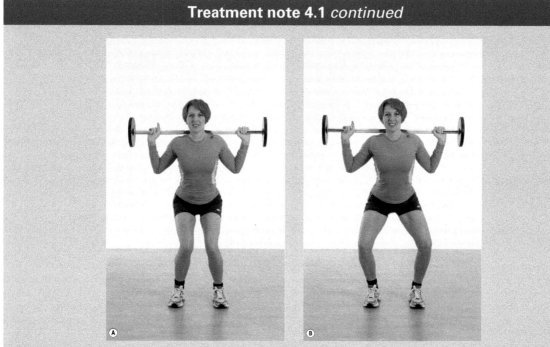

Figure 4.32 Knee position: (A) knock-knee; (B) bow-legged.

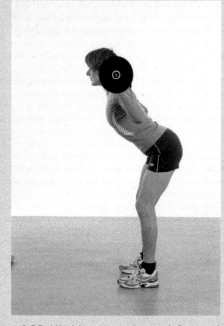

Figure 4.33 Hip hinge – angle trunk forwards excessively.

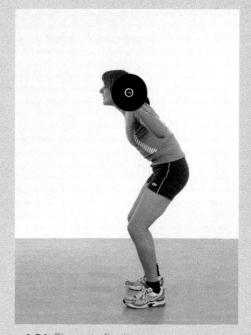

Figure 4.34 Thoracic flexion.

Treatment note 4.1 *continued*

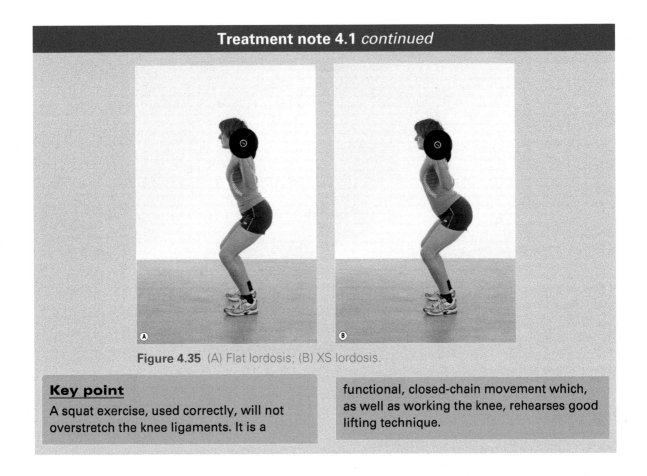

Figure 4.35 (A) Flat lordosis; (B) XS lordosis.

Key point

A squat exercise, used correctly, will not overstretch the knee ligaments. It is a functional, closed-chain movement which, as well as working the knee, rehearses good lifting technique.

Knee stiffness

Knee stiffness is a common problem following ACL surgery. There are a variety of possible causes, including adhesions within the suprapatellar pouch and/or patellofemoral joint, quadriceps contracture and retraction of the alar folds. Furthermore, patients have been described with an involvement of the infrapatellar fat pads, producing infrapatellar contracture syndrome (Paulos, Rosenberg and Drawbert 1987).

Initially, stiffness begins with inflammation, immobility and quadriceps weakness. Patients are unable to gain full extension and may complain of excessive pain. Patellar glide is restricted and pain may be located around the patellofemoral joint. Later, fat-pad involvement may be noted and the patellar tendon may become rigid. Patellar mobility is virtually eliminated and both active and passive knee motion is severely restricted. Flexion contracture is often present by this time, and the patient walks with an apparent 'short leg'.

If progress in regaining knee mobility begins to slow, this must be recognized immediately and acted upon. Intense rehabilitation is the key to preventing development of this condition. Patellofemoral joint mobilization and the restoration of full knee extension is vital.

Posterior cruciate damage

The PCL (as with the ACL) has two bundles, but in this case it is said to be the strongest ligament in the knee and is much less frequently damaged in sport than the ACL. When an injury does occur,

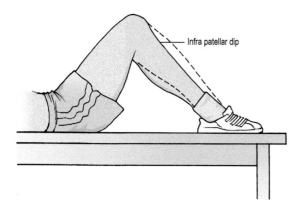

Figure 4.36 Posterior sag with posterior cruciate ligament (PCL) deficient knee.

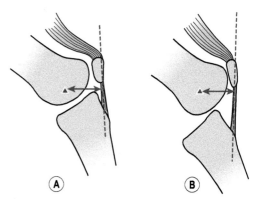

Figure 4.37 Alteration in mechanical advantage of the knee following posterior cruciate ligament (PCL) rupture. (A) Normal knee: axis of rotation to patellar tendon distance gives mechanical advantage. (B) PCL deficient knee: tibial shift gives reduced mechanical advantage.

it may be the result of a posteriorly directed force onto a flexed knee (typically a road-traffic accident), forced hyperextension, or forced flexion where the athlete falls into a kneeling position, pressing the ankle into plantarflexion. Unlike ACL injury, the athlete with a damaged PCL can usually continue playing and may only notice minimal swelling, but there is marked pain on the posterior aspect of the knee.

Posterior subluxation of the tibia often occurs during walking and standing. It may be seen clinically from the side if the knee is flexed to 90 degrees (Fig. 4.36). This may be accentuated if the patient contracts the quadriceps against a resistance provided by the examiner. The patient is asked to 'slide the foot down the couch' (Daniel et al. 1988) as the examiner stabilizes the ankle. If not viewed from the side, the subluxation may be missed and the injury wrongly diagnosed as an ACL tear, the tibia moving forwards to reduce and mimicking an anterior drawer sign.

The posterior shift of the tibia moves the patellar tendon closer to the axis of rotation of the knee, reducing the mechanical advantage of the quadriceps (Fig. 4.37). The change in quadriceps muscle efficiency is reflected in the gait cycle. With the PCL-deficient knee, athletes demonstrate quadriceps activity before heel strike, in contrast to normal individuals who show this contraction after heel strike (Reid 1992).

Rehabilitation

As with ACL damage, conservative treatment involving intensive muscle strengthening is tried first. Isolated hamstring contractions will cause posterior shear of the tibia on the femur, and so should be avoided. In addition, excessive external rotation of the tibia as the knee approaches full extension will stress the repaired tissue. As with ACL rehabilitation, co-contraction exercises should be favoured, with a greater emphasis on quadriceps rather than hamstring contractions where isolation movements are used.

The PCL is contained within a synovial sheath, which enhances its ability to heal in continuity. Reconstruction may be attempted using a similar patellar tendon graft to that described above. This time, the graft is positioned lateral to the tibial attachment of the PCL and travels through the femur at the junction of the medial condyle and the intercondylar notch.

The knee with isolated PCL insufficiency producing unidirectional instability generally does well when treated conservatively, but when PCL damage is associated with additional tissue damage which results in multidirectional instability, surgery should be considered. In a study investigating the long-term effects of non-operative management of PCL damage, Parolie and Bergfeld (1986) assessed 25 athletes on average 6.2 years after injury. Of these, 84 per cent had returned to their previous sport. Importantly, those who were not satisfied with their knee had less than 100 per cent strength compared to the undamaged knee (measured as mean torque on an isokinetic dynamometer at varying angular velocities), and those who were satisfied had strength values greater than 100 per cent. The importance of maintaining superior muscle strength following PCL injuries is therefore clear. Shelbourne et al. (1999) found that half of all patients treated non-operatively returned to the same sport at the same or even higher levels of activity. Those with greater PCL laxity do not generally have lower functional rating scores (Shelbourne and Muthukaruppan 2005). The same authors found that even after long-term follow-up (7.8 years) 16 per cent of patients were still improving, 40 per cent scored excellent, 10 per cent good and 6 per cent fair, measured on the Noyes knee survey.

Of those patients who are symptomatic enough to seek treatment, damage to the medial compartment is more common with chronic injuries, and to the lateral compartment with acute injuries. Damage includes meniscal tears and articular cartilage defects.

Functional testing of the cruciate ligament deficient knee

Functional testing may be used to assess stability, pain and confidence in the knee. Tests normally aim to reproduce some key aspect of a sport to enhance specificity. In each case, the injured and uninjured sides of the body are compared.

For the crossover test the athlete stands on the affected leg and uses the unaffected leg to step in front and behind the injured one, imparting multiplane stress on the knee (Fig. 4.38). The test may also be performed with the injured leg on a small stool to increase flexion stress on the knee.

The single-leg hop test measures the distance obtained on the injured side and divides this figure by that obtained for the uninjured side to obtain a 'hop ratio', which may be recorded throughout treatment (Reid 1992). Combining straight hopping with hop-and-turn activities increases and varies the stress imposed on the knee, as does hopping down or up from a low stool.

Figure-of-eight, slalom and slope/stair running circuits are also useful. The figure of eight may be performed with a gradual curve or a sharp one, to impose more or less stress on the knee. The knee on the outside of the circle is exposed to a varus stress as the body leans inwards. The slalom or zig-zag run imposes sudden direction changes and shear on the knee. This test is particularly suitable for assessing function in sports which involve 'cutting' actions. Slope/stair running may be performed on an inclined or declined surface, or on a camber. In each case, repetitive shearing stress is imposed on the knee.

The menisci

The menisci are fibrocartilage structures which rest on the tibial condyles. They are crescent-shaped when viewed from above, but triangular in cross-section. Their peripheral border is formed from fibrous tissue and attached to the deep surface of the joint capsule. These same fibres attach the menisci to the tibial surface, forming the coronary ligaments. Anteriorly, the two menisci are joined by the transverse ligament, a posterior transverse ligament being present in 20 per cent of the population.

The medial meniscus is the larger of the two, semicircular in shape, and broader posteriorly. Its anterior horn is attached to the front of the intercondylar area of the tibia in front of the ACL. The posterior horn attaches to the posterior intercondylar area between the PCL and the lateral meniscus. It has an attachment to the MCL and the oblique popliteal ligament coming from semimembranosus (Fig. 4.39A). The upper part of the meniscus is firmly attached to the MCL, the fibres here forming the medial meniscofemoral

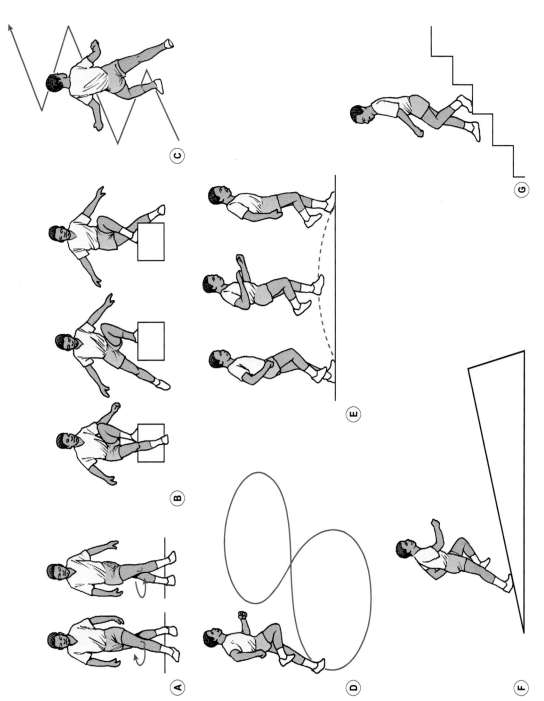

Figure 4.38 Functional testing of the knee. (A) Crossover. (B) Crossover on box. (C) Zig-zag. (D) Figure-of-eight. (E) Single-leg hop. (F) Slope running. (G) Ascending and descending stairs.

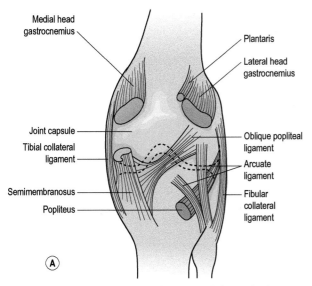

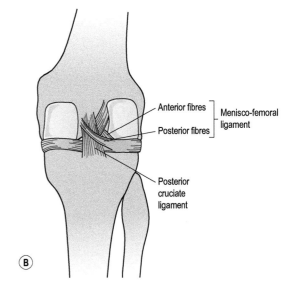

Figure 4.39 Attachments of the medial menisci.

ligament (Fig. 4.39B). The lower part, attached to the coronary ligament, is more lax. This has important functional consequences, because the medial meniscus is anchored more firmly to the femur than to the tibia. In flexion/extension the femur is thus able to glide on the tibia, while in rotation the meniscus can slide over the tibial plateau.

The lateral meniscus is more circular and has a uniform breadth. Its two horns are attached close together, the anterior horn blending with the attachment of the ACL. The posterior horn attaches just anterior to the posterior horn of the medial meniscus. The meniscus has a posterolateral groove which receives the popliteus tendon, and a few fibres from this muscle attach to the meniscus itself. In addition, the tendon of popliteus partially separates the lateral meniscus from the joint capsule, a configuration which makes the lateral meniscus more mobile than its medial counterpart. The posterior part of the lateral meniscus has two ligamentous attachments, the anterior and posterior meniscofemoral ligaments (Fig. 4.40). These divide around the PCL, and in extreme flexion, as the PCL tightens, so do the anterior and posterior meniscofemoral ligaments. The lateral meniscus is thus pulled back and medially.

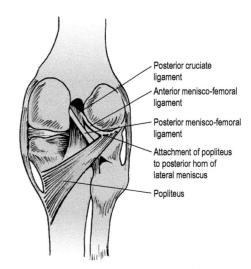

Figure 4.40 Posterior aspect of the left knee.

Key point
Because the lateral meniscus attaches through the meniscofemoral ligaments to the posterior cruciate, it is more mobile than the medial meniscus and so less likely to be trapped and torn.

The menisci receive blood flow from the inferior genicular arteries which supply the perimeniscal plexus (Fig. 4.41). Small, penetrating branches from

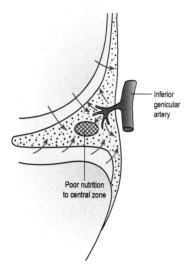

Figure 4.41 Perimeniscal plexus. After Reid (1992), with permission.

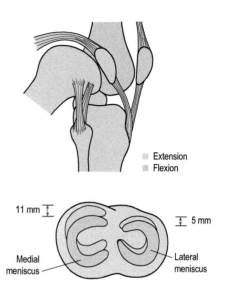

Figure 4.42 Movement of the menisci with flexion and extension of the knee.

this plexus enter the meniscus via the coronary ligaments. Up until the age of about 11 years the whole meniscus has a blood supply, but in the adult only 10–25 per cent of the periphery of the meniscus is vascular. The anterior and posterior horns are covered by vascular synovium and have a good blood supply. The peripheral vessels are within the deeper cartilage substance, the surface receiving its main nutrition via diffusion from the synovial fluid. A few myelinated and non-myelinated nerve fibres are found in the outer third of the menisci, but no nerve endings.

Because the menisci are held more firmly centrally, they are able to alter their shape and move forwards and backwards over the tibial plateau. The lateral meniscus has a greater amount of movement, and is often 'pulled away from trouble', leaving the medial meniscus to be more commonly injured in association with the MCL and ACL, to which it has attachments.

In flexion, the lateral meniscus is carried backwards onto the steep posterior slope of the lateral tibial plateau, and with extension it moves forwards again. In flexion/extension the medial meniscus is held firm until the last 20 degrees of extension, when the knee begins to rotate (screw-home

mechanism). As this happens, the medial meniscus is carried backwards. The lateral meniscus has the greater movement therefore – approximately 11 mm versus only 5 mm for the medial. In extension, the menisci are squeezed and elongated in an anteroposterior direction, and in flexion they become wider (Fig. 4.42).

The menisci enlarge the tibiofemoral contact area, thus spreading the pressure taken by the subchondral bone (Fig. 4.43). It has been estimated that the menisci disperse between 30 per cent and 55 per cent of the load across the knee (Kelley 1990). When only a portion of the meniscus is removed, the joint surface contact forces may increase by 350 per cent (Seedhom and Hargreaves 1979).

The menisci contribute substantially to knee stability. In the ACL-deficient knee, the anterior drawer test may be positive in only 35 per cent of knees with an intact medial meniscus, but in 83 per cent when the meniscus is removed (Levy, Torzilli and Warren 1982). The menisci limit sagittal gliding of the femur over the tibial plateau, a movement greatly increased in patients who have undergone meniscectomy. In addition, they allow a dual movement to occur, normally only possible in joints

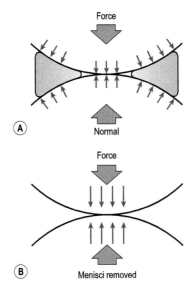

Figure 4.43 The effect of cartilage removal (meniscectomy) on the knee. (A) Forces on the normal knee. (B) Menisci removed. The bones take more jarring strain.

which are far more lax. The menisci also aid joint lubrication by spreading the synovial fluid over the surface of the articular cartilage.

> **Key point**
>
> When a portion of the meniscus is removed, the joint surface contact forces may increase by 350 per cent. Following meniscectomy, bone adaptation will take time and weightbearing should be progressed slowly.

Injury

It has been estimated that meniscal injury has a frequency of 61 per 100,000 individuals. The condition is three times more prevalent in males than females, with the medial meniscus being injured four times as often as the lateral (Kelley 1990).

With ageing, degeneration and asymptomatic splitting occurs. The incidence of slowly forming degenerative lesions to the meniscus (usually horizontal cleavage) increases from

25 per cent in those aged 50–59 to 45 per cent in the 70–79 age group. In patients with concomitant OA the incidence may be as high as 75–95 per cent, and most findings are incidental (ESSKA 2017).

In the active athlete, the history of injury is usually one which combines twisting on a semi-flexed knee with the foot fixed on the ground. The onset is sudden, and pain is felt deep within the knee, the patient often saying they 'felt something go'. Effusion may be extensive after injury, and haemarthrosis may result if the injury occurs in combination with ACL or MCL damage. Tears may be to the periphery or body of the meniscus, running horizontally or vertically (Fig. 4.44). A longitudinal tear (bucket handle) of the medial meniscus may allow its lateral portion to slip over the dome of the medial femoral condyle causing blocked extension (true locking). Shakespeare and Rigby (1983) reviewed 272 patients found to

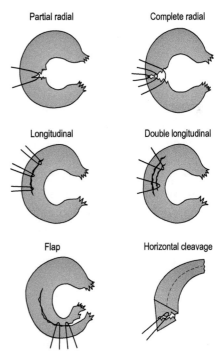

Figure 4.44 Common meniscal tears. The longitudinal tear may extend anteriorly to form a bucket-handle tear. From Zuluaga, Briggs and Carlisle (1995), with permission.

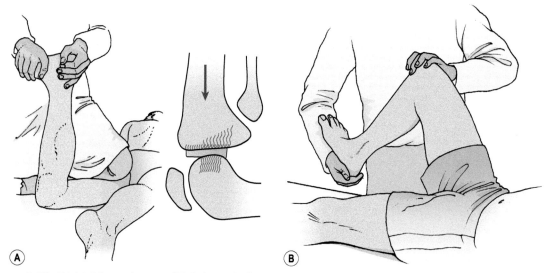

Figure 4.45 (A) McMurray's test. (B) Apley grinding test.

have bucket-handle tears at operation. Of these, 43 per cent presented with true locking. When the knee unlocks, either spontaneously or through manipulation, anterior extension of the bucket-handle tear, rather than meniscal relocation, may occur.

On examination, effusion is apparent and tenderness is often found over the joint line, most usually medially. A capsular pattern may be noticeable (see Table 1.9), and terminal extension is often blocked with a springy end-feel if muscle spasm is not present. Various tests are used to assess the problem, of which the two most common are McMurray's and Apley's.

McMurray's test (Fig. 4.45A) requires full flexion of the knee and so is not suitable for the acute joint. The medial joint line is palpated and from the fully flexed position the knee is externally rotated and extended, as a slight varus strain is applied. If positive, a painful click or thud is felt over the medial meniscus. The lateral meniscus can be similarly tested by extending the knee with internal rotation and a valgus strain, although the value of lateral testing in this way is questionable (see below). In each case only the middle and posterior portion of the meniscus is tested, and so a negative McMurray's sign does not preclude

meniscal damage, but when positive the test is clinically revealing.

The McMurray's test has been shown to be useful only with medial meniscal tears (Evans, Bell and Frank 1993). In this evaluation, the authors found that a thud elicited on the medial joint line was the only significant sign to correlate with meniscal injury. They showed the test to have a positive predictive value of 83 per cent and a specificity of 98 per cent.

Apley's grinding test (Fig. 4.45B) involves placing the patient in a prone-lying position, flexing the knee to 90 degrees, rotating the tibia and compressing it against the femur in an attempt to elicit a popping or snapping sensation. It is important not to force the movements too far, as this may further tear the already damaged meniscus. The intention with this test is to help differentiate between meniscal and MCL damage at the joint line. Symptoms will be present as the knee is compressed when the meniscus is damaged, but not if the MCL alone is injured because this structure will be relaxed by the compression force. Conversely, a distraction force stretches the ligament but disengages the meniscus, so giving pain where MCL damage has occurred in isolation.

The results of meniscal tests combined with the clinical history will indicate if damage is likely, in which case arthroscopy is called for to confirm the findings.

Management

If a meniscal tear is present, the choice is either non-operative management or surgical intervention involving removal or repair of the injured meniscus.

Non-operative management

Historically, Henning (1988) argued that meniscal tears of less than 10 mm in length, and partial thickness injuries involving 50 per cent or less of the vertical height of the meniscus, could be treated non-operatively providing the ACL was undamaged. Weiss et al. (1989) reported that stable vertical longitudinal tears in the vascular outer area of the meniscus had a good potential for healing, whereas stable radial tears did not. They performed a repeat arthroscopy on 32 patients (on average 26 months after the first procedure) and found that 17 longitudinal tears had healed completely. Five radial tears showed no evidence of healing, and one had extended. No degenerative changes were found in the adjacent articular cartilage of the stable lesions.

Looking at a group of 146 patients (35 to 65 years) with degenerative meniscal tears but without OA, Sihvonen et al. (2013) found no difference between arthroscopic partial meniscectomy and sham surgery. Kise et al. (2016) examined a group of 140 adults (mean age 49.5 years) to compare the results of exercise therapy versus arthroscopic partial meniscectomy for degenerative meniscal tears with no history of OA. They found a superior result in terms of muscle strength

with the exercise group at three months, and no difference in overall outcome at two-year follow-up. Interestingly, 19 per cent of subjects in the exercise therapy group chose to cross over to surgery during the two year follow-up, but showed no additional benefit.

Meniscal repair

The peripheral part of the meniscus has a blood supply sufficient to support healing. Initial healing in this region is by fibrosis, with vessels from the capillary plexus and synovial fringe penetrating the area. Fibrous healing may be complete within ten weeks, and the scar tissue can be remodelled into normal fibrocartilage within several months. Tears to the peripheral third of the meniscus may be sutured, and healing improved by abrading the parameniscal synovium. Weightbearing or full-range motion will deform the menisci and so pull on the scar site. For this reason, rehabilitation of the repaired meniscus is much less intense than that of a patient who has undergone meniscectomy. General recommendations for rehabilitation include the restriction of weightbearing for six weeks, with no flexion allowed for the first two weeks. After two weeks, 20–70 degrees flexion is allowed, with free motion allowed four weeks after surgery. Full weightbearing is allowed, and resistance exercises are progressed. Return to full sports is not permitted for six weeks.

For successful repair, DeHaven and Bronstein (1995) produced a number of recommendations. First, that the tear should lie within 3 mm of the meniscosynovial junction and that the overall contour of the meniscus should be normal. In addition, these authors stated that the tear should be at least 7 mm long and making the meniscus unstable. For tears further than 4 mm from the meniscosynovial junction and those with deformity, healing enhancement using fibrin clot was recommended. In general, tears greater than 3 cm and transverse tears do not heal. Repair is either from the outside or inside of the meniscus. The 'outside in' procedure uses needles passed through the joint capsule, but placement of sutures is less precise. The 'inside out' procedure uses sutures placed arthroscopically from inside the knee.

DeHaven, Black and Griffiths (1989) reported follow-up results on 80 repaired menisci on average 4.6 years after surgery. Of these, 11 per cent had torn again (only three at the repair zone), and these authors recommended meniscal repair in view of the degenerative changes following meniscectomy.

Meniscectomy

Degenerative changes following total meniscectomy, including joint narrowing, ridging and flattening, were first described following the Second World War (Fairbank 1948). Follow-up after meniscectomy (Jorgensen, Sonne-Holm and Lauridsen 1987) has shown patients to be increasingly dissatisfied with the knee. Incidence of complaint grew from 53 per cent after 4.5 years to 67 per cent after 14.5 years. A positive anterior draw sign was demonstrated in 10 per cent after 4.5 years and 36 per cent after 14.5 years, with 34 per cent of the latter group giving up sport as a result of knee symptoms (Table 4.12).

Where the meniscus is grossly damaged and the knee is unstable, however, a partial or total meniscectomy may be required, the minimum amount of tissue being removed to reduce the biomechanical impairment to the joint. Arthroscopic removal of all, or part, of the meniscus is normally performed through an anterolateral or anteromedial approach, depending on which compartment of the knee the lesion lies in. The knee is held in 10-degree flexion and the joint is gapped by applying a valgus or varus stress. The joint is distended with fluid to allow easier inspection of the tissue surfaces. An initial incision is made into the anterior part of the meniscus, and the incision is then extended into the middle and posterior segments. The posterior horn is released, followed by the anterior horn, and the meniscus is removed. In cases where only part of the meniscus is removed, the edge of the remaining tissue is trimmed.

Results of arthroscopic partial meniscectomy are generally good, but are dependent on the amount of

Table 4.12 Follow-up after complete meniscectomy

	4.5 years (n 5 131)%	14.5 years (n 5 101) %
Symptoms		
Swelling	19	29
Pain		
Weightbearing	38	30
On stairs	15	23
When first walking	–	23
At rest	12	13
Sensation of instability	20	21
Signs		
Crepitus	18	38
Quadriceps wasting	7	12
Positive anterior drawer	10	36
Joint-line tenderness	10	12
Activity		
Unchanged	53	19
Reduced because of knee	12	12
No sport because of knee	15	34

After Jorgensen, U. et al. (1987) Long term follow up of meniscectomy in athletes: a prospective longitudinal study. *Journal of Bone and Joint Surgery*, **69**, 80. With permission.

tissue damage which occurred at the time of injury. Investigating 67 patients on average 12.2 years after arthroscopic partial meniscectomy, Higuchi, Kimura and Shirakura (2000) found 79 per cent to have a satisfactory outcome (52 per cent excellent, 27 per cent good, 10.5 per cent fair). Osteoarthritic deterioration was noticed in 48 per cent of patients, the amount being dependent on the amount of cartilage degeneration noticed at the time of surgery. Of the original group, 39 had normal knee cartilage and 28 had articular degeneration.

The use of arthroscopy with local anaesthesia is steadily increasing, and obviously removes the risk inherent in any procedure involving a general anaesthetic. In addition, complication rate is lessened, cost is reduced and the patient is discharged significantly earlier than when general anaesthesia is used. The skin puncture sites are injected with lidocaine (lignocaine) or similar, and

Table 4.13 Example rehabilitation protocol following meniscus repair

Timing	Activity
0–2 weeks	▶ Limb circulation exercise for general surgical recovery ▶ Monitor skin condition ▶ 0°–90° progressive knee ROM exercises ▶ Patellar mobilization ▶ Re-strengthen knee musculature OKC to progress to CKC ▶ Ensure full-knee extension (no lag) using quadriceps setting initially ▶ Crutch walking with toe-touch as initially required
2–6 weeks	▶ ROM exercise to continue ▶ CKC exercise such as leg-press with band, wall slides ▶ Begin proprioceptive work, double-leg progressing to single-leg ▶ Gait and posture optimization ▶ Treadmill walking progresses speed walk
6–12 weeks	▶ Progress to full ROM ▶ Introduce static cycle/cross-trainer/rowing ▶ Wall squat/mini squat/leg press ▶ Proprioceptive work progresses to single-leg and changing BOS/COG
12–36 weeks	▶ Regain full ROM ▶ Increase strength aiming to equal contralateral leg ▶ Running programme ▶ Progressive jumping and hopping ▶ Plyometrics

CKC – closed kinetic chain. OKC – open kinetic chain. ROM – range of motion. BOS – base of support. COG – centre of gravity.

Early   Intermediate   Late

the joint is distended with saline and anaesthetic solution. Studying 400 patients in total, Jacobson, Forssblad and Rosenberg (2000) compared results from elective knee arthroscopy using either local, general or spinal anaesthesia and obtained a 92 per cent success rate using local anaesthesia in 200 of the patients. They concluded that the use of local anaesthesia was superior to either spinal or general anaesthetic in this group.

Following meniscectomy of any type, the initial aim is to limit effusion and pain. As this is achieved, the leg musculature is progressively built up. Initially, open-chain movements are used within the pain-free range, to protect the joint from excessive loading. Range of motion is gradually increased, and as this is achieved, closed-chain movements are introduced. Once strength equals that of the contralateral limb, functional activities and power training are used in later-stage rehabilitation, with sports-specific progressions forming the mainstay of pre-competitive work. An example post-operative rehab protocol following meniscus repair is shown in Table 4.13, and this progression is shorter for meniscectomy.

Meniscal cysts and discoid meniscus

The discoid meniscus (Fig. 4.46) is more usually seen on the lateral side than the medial. Even so, the condition is unusual. When this shape remains later in life, the discoid meniscus is said to be present.

Definition

The meniscus of the knee in an unborn child is disc shaped rather than moon shaped. When this shape remains later in life, a discoid meniscus is present.

Discoid menisci may be classified as complete, incomplete (partial) or Wrisberg type. In the latter type the posterior osseous attachment of the meniscus is absent, leaving it attached only by the meniscofemoral ligament (Wrisberg's ligament).

The abnormal shape of the meniscus subtly alters both the contact area between the tibia and femur and joint mobility. In the young, the discoid meniscus may be asymptomatic, with 65 per cent of those who present with symptoms being over

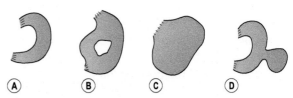

Figure 4.46 Meniscal abnormalities. (A) Normal. (B) Partial discoid. (C) Complete discoid. (D) Cyst.

18 years old. A clunk may be felt in the knee at 110 degrees as it is bent, and at 10 degrees as it is straightened again. Surgical treatment may be by meniscectomy or repair.

Meniscal cysts (ganglia) are again more common in the lateral meniscus, with the posterior and mid-portion of the meniscus being affected. The cyst is associated with a horizontal tear and may be the result of infiltration of synovial fluid through the tear, with the edge of the tear acting as a one-way valve. In a series of 18 patients with MRI-documented cysts, all were found to have horizontal cleavage tears at arthroscopy (Ryu and Ting 1993).

The cyst generally begins as a small pedicle and gradually enlarges, the size fluctuating with varying activities. It is more easily seen with the knee flexed to 45 degrees. Arthroscopic repair of the tear site is possible, allowing the cyst to decompress into the joint. Where no tear is identified, removal of the cyst is attempted. The meniscal rim is scarified and the perimeniscal tissue reattached, leaving the meniscus proper fully intact. Some cysts respond to direct aspiration.

Jumper's knee

Jumper's knee is traditionally described as a patellofemoral pain syndrome (PFPS) affecting the teno-osseous junctions of the quadriceps tendon as it attaches to the superior pole of the patella, and the patellar tendon as it attaches to the inferior pole of the patella and tibial tuberosity. It is, therefore, an insertional tendinopathy resulting in derangement of the bone-tendon unit.

Definition

Jumper's knee is patellar pain traditionally described as affecting the insertion of the patellar tendon into either the patella itself or the tibial tuberosity. Histologically it is a tendinopathy of the patellar tendon.

Jumper's knee occurs more frequently in athletes who regularly impose rapid eccentric loading on the extensor mechanism of the knee, especially on hard surfaces. On examination, quadriceps wasting is sometimes apparent in long-standing cases and pain occurs to resisted extension, with slight soreness to full passive flexion. Some swelling may be noticed around the patellar tendon in acute cases, with fluctuance present if the condition is severe. A non-capsular pattern is found, and the VISA-P (Victorian Institute of Sports Assessment for the Patellar tendon) questionnaire is useful to monitor progress through the rehabilitation programme. VISA-P is available to download at http://www.ouh.nhs.uk/oxsport/information/documents/TheVISAscore.pdf. One of the key findings on objective assessment is reproduction of symptoms on a single-leg decline squat (Fig 4.46A). The subject keeps their upper body vertical while performing the single-leg squat on a 25-degree decline board. Maximum joint angle and pain (VAS scale) is compared to the contralateral side. Hop tests (vertical and broad jump) and take-off/landing drills can also be used as part of a functional assessment. As jumping involves movement through the ankle and foot as well as the knee, these areas should also be assessed. Limited-range dorsiflexion at the ankle and hallux limitus will reduce the shock-attenuating properties of the lower limb, throwing more stress onto the knee.

Palpation is performed with the knee in full extension to relax the patellar tendon. Palpation to the lower pole of the patella is best performed by pressing with the flat of the hand onto the upper surface of the patella to tilt it. This brings the lower pole into prominence and enables the practitioner to reach the part of the T/O junction which lies on the undersurface of the angular lower pole. This area is tender in most subjects, so it is important to compare any tenderness to the contralateral side.

Imaging, including ultrasound and MRI, can show disorganization within the tendon, and radiographic changes may be apparent where symptoms have been present for more than six months. An elongation of the involved pole of the patella may be seen, with calcification of the affected tendon matrix. Bone scan can indicate increased blood pooling and concentration of radioactive tracer in the affected area. However, imaging findings are often not directly related to symptoms, and subjects can demonstrate pain in tendons that appear normal on scanning.

Aetiology

Both intrinsic and extrinsic factors have been implicated as possible causes. Intrinsic factors include biomechanical alterations in the extensor mechanism, such as hypermobility, altered Q angle and genu valgum or genu recurvatum. Changes in the HQ ratio and hamstring flexibility may also have a part to play and should be examined. Muscle imbalance, consisting of weakness of the glutei, hamstrings and abdominals, combined with hip-flexor shortening, has been noted. In addition, on landing, players who are susceptible to this condition have a greater tendency to adduct the knee and internally rotate the leg, giving a functional valgus appearance.

Extrinsic factors include frequency and intensity of training (most important), training surface, and footwear (less important). Ferretti (1986) showed a correlation between jumper's knee and both hardness of playing surface and training frequency. In his study, 37 per cent of players (matched for sport, playing position, and training type) using cement surfaces suffered from the condition, compared to only 5 per cent of those using softer surfaces (Fig. 4.47A). In addition, the percentage of players affected by the condition escalated as the number of training sessions per week increased. Only 3.2 per cent of those with the condition trained twice each week, whereas nearly 42 per cent trained four times or over (Fig. 4.47B).

Tendon overload is a key factor in the development of this condition. An activity which exceeds the capacity of the tendon will cause tissue breakdown rather than adaptation (see Chapter 1). The aim of treatment in the short term is to reduce the overload by reducing activity and off-loading the tendon. In the mid to long term, the tendon must be loaded to cause adaptation that allows it to cope with the new stresses imposed by the increased workload.

Pathological tendon changes

The subject of tendinopathy was covered in Chapter 1 and Chapter 5, and the continuum model of the patho-aetiology of tendinopathy was illustrated in Table 5.6. The continuum model presents three interrelated stages – reactive tendinopathy, tendon disrepair and degenerative

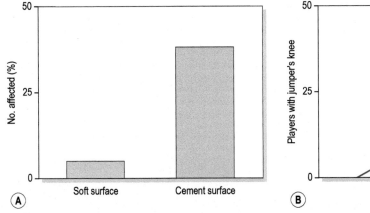
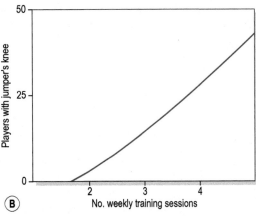

Figure 4.47 Incidence of jumper's knee. Data from Ferretti, A. (1986) Epidemiology of jumper's knee. *Sports Medicine*, **3**, 289–295. With permission.

Table 4.14 Main pathological features of patellar tendinopathy

Feature	Characteristic
▶ Deterioration of collagen bundles	▶ Transverse disruption of collagen fibres and separation of bundles, leading to reduction of cross-links and weakening
▶ Increased ground substance	▶ Gap in collagen bundles filled with ground substance. Increased volume of ground substance and change in type (larger molecules)
▶ Activation of cellular components	▶ Tendon cells activate and myofibroblasts migrate into tendon
▶ Vascular proliferation	▶ New vessels are thick-walled with a small lumen

From Cook et al. (2001)

tendinopathy – and often pathological tendons present a mixture of states, for example a degenerative tendon that is now reactive (acute or chronic). Subjects have been shown to progress and regress along the continuum (Rudavsky and Cook 2014). Four main pathological features can be present in patella tendinopathy, affecting the tendon collagen, ground substance, cells and blood vessels (Table 4.14). The affected region of the patella tendon demonstrates mucoid degeneration, being a dull, brownish tissue rather than the white, glistening appearance characteristic of normal tendon tissue. Instead of the parallel fibres of a healthy tendon, pathological tendons can demonstrate disorganized fibre arrangement with microtearing, some necrotic fibres and vascular ingrowth, which can be visualized on Doppler ultrasound.

Key point

Mucoid degeneration is a biological degrading of connective tissue into a gelatinous, mucus-like substance.

Management

The general principles of tendinopathy management were introduced in Chapter 1 and expanded in the section on Achilles tendinopathy in Chapter 6. As with any overuse syndrome, part of the early management of the condition involves avoidance or modification of training. The volume of training/daily activity that drives symptoms should be reduced. This may mean reducing running and jumping activity, stair climbing and

prolonged sitting/driving in daily living. Footwear should incorporate shock-absorbing materials, either by choosing sports footwear with greater shock absorption and/or using shock-absorbing heel pads. Where taping modifies symptoms it should be considered. Local soft-tissue techniques such as transverse frictional massage can be effective at modulating pain in some cases. Frictions to the T/O junction attaching to the patella (infrapatellar tendon) are performed with the patella tilted and pressure from the therapist's finger is directed at a 45-degree angle to the long axis of the femur, rather than straight down. There is some Level I evidence to support this. Deep-tissue mobilization of this type has been shown to be beneficial in the treatment of tendon pathology in the rat model. Increased fibroblast recruitment has been demonstrated following three minutes of soft-tissue mobilization over four treatments (Davidson et al. 1997). Use of heavy pressure during soft-tissue mobilization has been shown to significantly increase the fibroblast number compared to light pressure (Gehlsen, Ganion and Helfst 1999).

Exercise therapy is by far the most important treatment clinically. Sustained isometric contractions (70 per cent MVC held for 45–60 sec and repeated 4 times) can reduce pain in some cases for up to 8 hours (Rudavsky and Cook 2014). Isometrics may be used in isolation or as a precursor to loading during a rehabilitation programme. Sustained heavy loading follows as pain allows, initially with slow-speed eccentrics followed by concentric-eccentric and slow-speed. As symptoms settle, slow-speed actions give

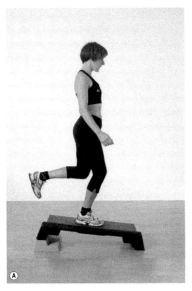
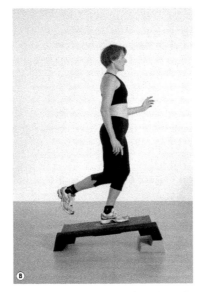
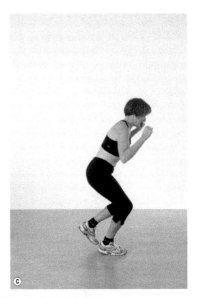

Figure 4.48 Exercise therapy for knee extensor mechanism: (A) decline board, (B) incline board and (C) hop.

way to stretch–shortening cycle (SSC) actions, advancing to full plyometrics (see below).

Exercise on a decline board (Fig. 4.48A–C) targets the extensor mechanism of the knee (Purdam et al. 2003). During a standard squat, tension in the calf musculature increases as the dorsiflexion angle of the ankle increases. This increased calf tension reduces the required workload of the quadriceps, as the elastic response of the gastrocnemius will tend to lock the knee during the final degrees of extension. The eccentric squat should be used as a progression from a *flat* surface to *decline* and finally as a *hop* action, in each case initially practised with both legs and then with a single (affected) leg. The single-leg decline squat is an intense action which has been shown to be an accurate test to detect change in pain with a better discriminative ability than the standard squat (Purdam et al. 2003).

Key point

The decline-squat action should be used as a progression in patella tendinitis from (i) flat, to (ii) decline and (iii) hop, in each case from double-leg to single-leg.

The shock-attenuating function of the leg musculature must be enhanced, and re-education of correct lower-limb alignment during take-off and landing patterns is useful. Any muscle imbalance must be identified and corrected. Eccentric loading is increased through progressive closed-chain activities, using 'drop and stop' exercises of varying intensities. These are progressed initially to slow concentric-eccentric coupling, and eventually to plyometrics. For further details, see the section on tendinopathy rehab in Chapter 5.

Arthritis

Knee pain is a common complaint, especially in the over-fifties. Studies have shown almost half of the over-fifties complain of pain in the knee, and in about 25 per cent this lasts for a prolonged period, being considered chronic. Chronic knee pain can lead to a significant reduction in quality of life (QOL) and difficulty carrying out common activities of daily living. Although the condition can progress, many risk factors of progression are modifiable. Exercise therapy can improve muscle strength and control of movement, and increase range of motion. Strength

239

exercise may increase muscle mass and muscle recruitment, providing the overload on the muscle tissue is great enough. Strength increase to the knee musculature may lessen internal knee forces, modify biomechanics, decrease rate of joint loading and reduce articular cartilage stress (Fransen et al. 2015). Overload during strength exercise may be reduced where pain is a barrier to exercise performance leading to exercise under dosage, often making pain management early on in the condition especially important. Exercise in general may improve QOL, increasing the number and variety of daily living tasks and improving physical function, these factors in turn having positive psychological benefits. One of the most common diagnoses of chronic knee pain through imaging is osteoarthritis (OA). The pathological processes involved in OA were covered in Chapter 1. Here, we will look at the relevance of OA to the knee in sport especially.

Arthritis secondary to sports injury

Joint cartilage is continually subjected to impact stress in sport and recreational exercise. For example, when running a marathon an athlete is said to take 38,000 steps and each time to subject the knee joint to between 4 and 8 times their bodyweight, which equates to almost 5,000 tons of force. After a 20 km run, cartilage volume is seen to reduce by 8 per cent in the patella, 10 per cent in the meniscus and 6 per cent on the tibial plateau, with all cartilage volumes returning to normal within 1 hour of cessation of exercise (Hohmann 2006). Joint cartilage is open to continuous micro-damage. However, providing the cartilage repair mechanisms (synthesis) outweigh the damage process (degradation), the joint will remain healthy.

If these repair mechanisms break down, however, the joint will degrade. The repair mechanism is carried out by chondrocytes, which are responsible for secreted proteoglycans and collagen. Some of the changes which occur in OA, if detected early enough, may be reversible. Altered biomechanics of a joint, if corrected, can result in regrowth of fibrocartilage. However, subtle alterations in normal joint mechanics, which may remain long after an injury has 'resolved', may be largely undetectable to a patient or physician. It is not until these changes are well developed and limit physiological joint movement or cause deformity that they become readily apparent. Accessory movements, however, when limited, are detectable to a therapist. As an example of the importance of this principle, note an early study by Sharma et al. (2001) which showed that a small change in alignment of the knee (10 per cent increase in varus angle) changed the peak contact force from 3.3 times bodyweight to 7.4 times bodyweight, more than doubling the forces acting on the knee during running. These changes may be relevant if they drive symptoms, and the use of this type of assessment may be particularly useful in the early stages of rehabilitation to modulate pain in preparation for reconditioning.

Joint loading

Animal studies have often been used to examine the effect of exercise and loading on the synovial joint. Radin et al. (1979) found no evidence of cartilage deterioration in sheep forced to walk for 4 hours daily on concrete for 12 and 30 months. Videman (1982) found that running did not affect the development of OA in rabbits. Experimentally induced OA was not increased when the animals were forced to run over 2,000 m per week for 14 consecutive weeks. Studies on runners have also failed to show any significant difference from non-runners. Puranen et al. (1975) found less hip OA in Finnish distance runners than in non-runners of a similar age. Panush et al. (1987) found no greater clinical or radiological evidence of OA in male runners of average age 55 years, and Lane et al. (1998) concluded that runners and non-runners showed similar evidence of hip and knee OA.

Although chronic mechanical loading may be detrimental to the knee, evidence suggests that recreational running is not a cause of knee OA (Leech et al. 2015) and may even be used therapeutically in OA patients (Lo et al. 2014). Chronic knee stress that may be imposed by elite-level running is less clear cut. A systematic review of 19 studies looked at MRI scans of knees of distance runners and found no irreversible effects other than temporary proteoglycan depletion, which took more than 3 months to recover to baseline. The authors were unable to conclude if this represented permanent structural damage (Hoessly and Wildi 2015).

Maintaining the normal mobility and strength of a joint throughout life, and maintaining a healthy BMI (body mass index), could help maintain the health of the joint structures and perhaps delay the onset of OA. Many forms of exercise, including running, are helpful in doing this. Certainly, obese individuals have been shown to be more likely to develop OA, the increased risk being 4.8-fold in men and 4.0-fold in women. In addition, it has been suggested that obesity increases the risk of the development of bilateral rather than unliteral OA (Felson 1997).

Arthritis and obesity

Obesity is steadily increasing in the Western world: 55–60 per cent of adults in the USA are overweight (with a BMI of 25 or more) and 20–25 per cent are clinically obese (with a BMI of 30 or more) (ACSM, 2001). As well as having an important effect on cardiovascular health, obesity has an effect on joints. A high percentage of subjects with end-stage hip OA have been shown to be overweight, with a mean BMI of 28.8 (Marks and Allegrante 2002).

The weightbearing joints of the lower limb (hip, knee and ankle) are especially at risk from obesity. Obese patients with arthritis of these joints should therefore be helped to lose weight, as this may significantly help the condition.

Definition

Body mass index (BMI), or 'Quetelet index', is a measure of body bulk. BMI is obtained by dividing a person's weight (in kilograms) by their height (in metres) squared. A BMI below 20 is considered underweight, 20–25 normal, 25–30 overweight and over 30 obese.

Stages of Osteoarthritis

Osteoarthritis is normally categorized (stages or grades) as 1–4 in terms of severity, with 0 being a normal joint. Stage 1 is often asymptomatic, but on X-ray mild cartilage changes may be detected, often as a result of an X-ray being taken for another condition such as a ligament injury. Osteophytes may be seen but do not affect joint function. Stage 2 pathology shows more changes on X-ray with greater osteophyte formation and change in subchondral bone density. Bone will often appear whiter on X-ray (sclerosis) and bone cysts may sometimes be seen, and occasional cartilage thinning may be noted. Symptoms may occur on severe joint loading, and muscle wasting may be noted where mild pain has encouraged reduced activity. Stage 3 injury will show more severe osteophyte formation and joint-space narrowing. Overall bone shape may change, and cartilage erosion is noted in patches down to subchondral bone. Muscle-wasting and joint stiffness are common, and should be addressed by rehabilitation. Joint stiffness is seen following prolonged rest (on rising from a chair or waking, for example). Stage 4 OA is severe and can often show complete loss of joint space with severe bone-end deformity. Pain is common following rest and joint loading. Movement range is severely limited and muscle-wasting marked.

Imaging for OA knee

X-rays and scans will often look for two essential signs in the presence of OA in the knee, osteophytes and joint-space narrowing. Some individuals who show marked changes on X-ray report very little pain, while others with obvious pain show few radiographic changes (Urquhart et al. 2015). The changes on an X-ray which together indicate the presence of OA sometimes explain less than 20 per cent of the pain (Wylde et al. 2016). A positive X-ray does not indicate that the condition is untreatable, and usually patients can expect significant improvement in their symptoms with treatment such as muscle strengthening, active general exercise and weight loss.

A number of features on X-ray may be used to guide treatment. Firstly, we can look at bone alignment. Pain that is driven by excessive valgus angulation may be reduced by using a shoe insert, a procedure which may be used as a temporary or longer-term measure.

Secondly, joint space (the gap between the bones) is assessed. This gap is filled with cartilage, which does not show up on X-ray, and where the joint space is reduced, either between the knee bones themselves or between the femur and patella, this is an indication that the cartilage has thinned. When looking for OA in the knee, a number of X-ray views are normally taken, including one to show the condition of the patello-femoral joint. An antero-posterior (AP) view looks straight onto the knee, while the lateral view looks from the side, and both may be taken weightbearing or with weight off the knee. A skyline view (infer superior) looks between the thighbone and the kneecap. Cartilage has a number of functions, one of which is to absorb and redistribute shock. If the cartilage has worn, shock absorbing heel pads or springy shoes may be used to compensate and de-load the joint.

The X-ray will also show if another injury coexists (co-morbidity), such as a hairline fracture if the subject has had a fall, and if there is effusion within the knee that will take time to settle. Following trauma, joint fluid may also contain a small amount of blood (haemarthrosis), which acts as an irritant, giving rise to peripheral nociception. The health of the knee-joint bones is also important, and the bone density can be assessed from an X-ray and Dexa bone scan.

Treatment of the osteoarthritic knee

Cartilage repair

Articular cartilage damage is common in the general population, with over 60 per cent of patients showing damage on arthroscopic

Table 4.15 Criteria for autologous chondrocyte implantation (ACI)

Inclusion criteria	Exclusion criteria
Focal defect larger than 1 cm Age range 15–55 Commitment to rehabilitation	Advanced osteoarthritis Rheumatoid arthritis Total meniscectomy Ligament instability

investigation. Of these, just over 10 per cent may be suitable for cartilage repair (Aroen, Loken and Heir 2004). Damage may occur through trauma, including contact sports, chronic repetitive trauma (overuse in the presence of biomechanical malalignment), or through disease states such as osteoporosis and osteoarthrosis.

Several surgical techniques may be used to aid repair of injury to articular cartilage (see Table 4.15). The joint surface may be debrided (scraped) and the joint itself washed out (lavaged) to remove fragments of cartilage or subchondral bone. Damaging enzymes produced through cartilage degeneration are also removed. New cartilage cells may be introduced into the damaged area to stimulate healing. Osteochondral grafts of this type may be taken from the patient (autografts) or from cadaveric donors (allografts). A number of tissues have been used for autografts, including rib perichondrial cells, periosteum and chondrocytes themselves. The technique involves two surgical procedures. First the cells must be removed, then they must be allowed to grow in a laboratory, and finally they must be replanted into the damaged cartilage. Allograft techniques can result in high degrees of rejection as a complication (Wroble 2000), but only involve a single surgical procedure.

Definition
Autografts involve implanting cells or tissue taken from the patient. Allografts are taken from a cadaver (dead body).

Drilling, abrasion and microfracture all work by penetrating the subchondral bone and stimulating cell regrowth. The aim is to allow a conduit for clot formation containing mesenchymal stem cells capable of forming repair tissue (Steadman, Rodkey and Singleton 1997). Unfortunately, fibrocartilage rather than renewed hyaline cartilage is produced by these procedures, and this is less durable than hyaline cartilage.

The most commonly used technique for articular cartilage repair is autologous chondrocyte implantation (ACI), and Table 4.15 shows general indications for this type of surgery. This technique was developed in the 1980s and is now the most commonly used technique. In the first stage of the procedure, a biopsy of cartilage is taken from a non-weightbearing area and the harvested tissue is sent to a laboratory where new chondrocyte cells are grown from it. As this is the patient's own tissue, rejection is avoided. On average, one million such cells are required per centimetre of chondral defect. In the second surgical stage, a collagen membrane is sutured to the defect site to create a watertight region and the cultured cells are implanted into the hollow.

Outcome ratings are best for procedures involving the medial femoral condyle, with patella and trochlea regions being less successful. Treatment failure can occur, especially if high-impact sport is begun too early, and standard surgical complications to arthroscopy apply.

Rehabilitation following cartilage repair

Maturation and remodelling of the graft can continue for up to 24 months following surgery, an important factor to consider when structuring a rehabilitation programme. Return to weightbearing activities must be progressive, and both range of motion and strengthening exercise is required. Intensity of rehabilitation is dependent on defect size, larger defects clearly having more tissue. The graft is at most risk for the first 12 weeks following surgery, and is especially vulnerable to shearing stresses.

During rehabilitation there must be a balance between *protection* of the joint and encouraging *function*. Joint motion, intermittent loading

(progressive) and tissue adaptation is encouraged, while repetitive friction, shearing stress and either overload or underload of the repaired joint are restricted (Hambly 2009). In the initial post-surgical stage, reduction in swelling and pain are key components of rehabilitation while the joint is protected. A knee brace is worn, and the patient may be non-weightbearing on crutches for two to four weeks. Gentle range-of-motion exercises are encouraged, but rotation actions on the knee such as kneeling or squatting are prohibited to prevent imparting shear forces onto the new tissue. Cartilage reattachment can take between 8 and 12 weeks, and during this time a progressive programme from non-weightbearing to partial weightbearing is used. Early full weightbearing (avoiding shearing) may be desirable. A study comparing an 11-week programme of full weightbearing to an accelerated 8 week programme (Ebert et al. 2008) showed that patients in the accelerated group achieved greater six-minute walking distances and better improvement in knee pain, measured using the Knee Injury and Osteoarthritis Outcome Score. The programmes caused no adverse effects in either group when investigated using MRI.

Sports that involve twisting and pivoting actions are generally limited for three to five months following surgery, depending on the type of surgery performed. Small, isolated defects will recover, while larger defects, and those associated with other structural faults of the knee (traumatic debridement accompanied by cruciate or meniscal injury, for example), will take longer.

Non-weightbearing activity should include general mobility, such as static cycling and pool exercise, while specific work addresses muscle imbalance around the hip and knee. Imbalance exercises such as the clamshell, hip hitch and mini squat are used, together with walking re-education. It is also important to reinforce an appreciation of the amount of weight being taken through the limb in partial-weightbearing activities. This can be achieved by having the athlete stand on two sets of scales (Hambly 2009) and gradually increasing and reducing the amount of weight taken. As with all knee injuries requiring the athlete to walk with crutches, part of the training should be education on three-point and then four-point walking with correct heel-toe action and whole-body alignment.

Hyaluronic acid injections

The use of hyaluronic acid (HA) injections of the knee is now widespread. Its use is based on the fact that in OA, the synovial fluid of the knee decreases in both elasticity and viscosity, as a result of a lowering of the molecular weight of the naturally occurring hyaluronic acid. The aim of HA injection is to counteract this effect. HA is a glycosaminoglycan (GAG), which acts as a lubricant and shock absorber. It supports the normal effect of GAG within the cartilage ground substance produced by chondrocytes. This has the effect of acting as a 'molecular sponge', as its molecules repel each other to form a lattice which attracts water into itself (Jackson, Sheer and Simon 2001). Injection of HA into a joint is claimed to have a viscosupplementing effect (Wright, Crockett, and Dowd 2001). However, the half-life of HA has been shown to be less than 24 hours in sheep, suggesting that other effects may be important.

It is thought that injected HA may stimulate the natural production of hyaluronate by synoviocytes, and that HA has a direct anti-inflammatory effect by blocking prostaglandin production and reducing levels of inflammatory mediators (Bobic 2002). In addition, pain relief occurs, possibly by inhibition of substance P (Watterson and Esdaile 2000). Side effects are typical of any joint injection and include redness, local pain and effusion lasting two to three days. The risk of infection and synovitis also exists, but is minimized by clean technique. A Cochrane review (Bellamy et al. 2006) of 76 trials of viscosupplementation concluded that the technique was an effective treatment for OA of the knee. Pain on average changed by 26 per cent from baseline, and function improved by 23 per cent from baseline, during weeks 5–13 post-injection. There was a longer-term benefit compared to interarticular injection of corticosteroids.

Interestingly, the use of oral supplementation with glucosamine shows similar results. A Cochrane review of the use of glucosamine therapy (500 mg three times daily) for treating osteoarthritis (Towheed et al. 2008) demonstrated a reduction in pain of 22 per cent from baseline, and an improvement of function of 11 per cent from baseline.

Treatment note 4.2   Manual therapy techniques for the knee

Manual therapy techniques around the knee can be used either to relieve pain or to mobilize a stiff joint. The aim is to use either a sustained stretch or a small amplitude oscillation; for manipulation, a high-velocity, low-amplitude movement is used at end-range.

Abduction/adduction in extension

The patient lies supine with the couch raised to the hip level of the therapist. The therapist grasps the patient's leg, tucking the shin beneath their arm and gripping it into the side of their body with the elbow (Fig. 4.49). The leg is then supported with the hands either side of the knee, thumbs resting loosely over the top of the patella, fingers curled over the popliteal area of the knee. The action is to impart an abduction and adduction oscillation with the knee extended or minimally unlocked. The valgus stress to the knee can be increased by drawing the inner hand distally and the outer hand proximally, and gapping the joint. Similarly, a varus stretch may be applied by moving the inner hand proximally and the outer hand distally.

Abduction/adduction in flexion

The therapist moves close into the couch and grips the patient's ankle with the inner hand,

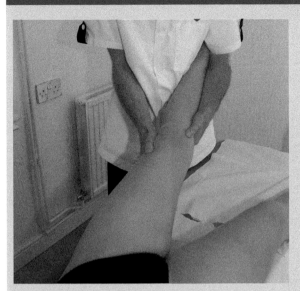

Figure 4.49 Abduction/adduction in extension.

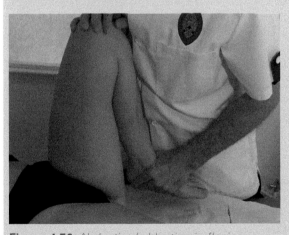

Figure 4.50 Abduction/adduction in flexion.

and rests the outer hand on the lateral aspect of the knee. The movement is one of flexion by pressing the heel towards the buttock (Fig. 4.50). An abduction force is applied by drawing the heel laterally, or an adduction force by drawing the heel medially. These movements may be combined with either a lateral rotation (abduction) or medial rotation (adduction) by surrounding the calcaneus in the cup of the hand and using the fingers for leverage.

Anteroposterior (AP) glide

The patient's thigh (femur) is placed on a block leaving the tibia free. The therapist lowers the couch below waist height and uses the heel of the hand to impart an AP glide to the tibia while the femur is blocked. For low-grade movements, both hands may be used surrounding the tibia; for high-grade movements the motion is imparted through the straight arm (Fig. 4.51).

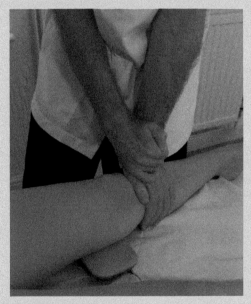

Figure 4.51 Anteroposterior (AP) glide using block.

Posteroanterior (PA) glide

The patient is supported in crook-lying with the knee flexed between 45 degrees and 90 degrees. The therapist lightly sits on the patient's foot to prevent it slipping. The patient's shin is gripped with the heel of the hands on the anterior aspect of the tibia, and the fingers curled around the back of the calf (Fig. 4.52). The PA draw is performed by drawing the tibia forwards, and may be combined with either external rotation (foot turned out) or internal rotation (foot turned in).

Treatment note 4.2 *continued*

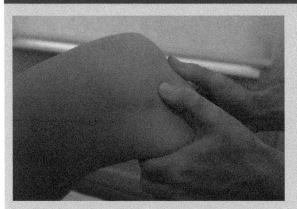

Figure 4.52 Posteroanterior (PA) glide in crook lying.

Lateral glide

In the crook-lying position, a webbing belt is placed around the patient's tibia and the therapist fixes the belt around his or her own waist, standing to the side of the patient. The tibia is supported with one hand and the femur with the other (Fig. 4.53). The lateral-glide movement is instigated by the therapist swaying backwards;

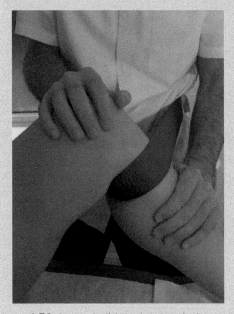

Figure 4.53 Lateral glide using seatbelt.

movement may be monitored using the thumb over the lateral joint line.

Capsular stretch

A joint distraction or capsular stretch to flexion may be imposed using the therapist's forearm as a pivot. The couch is raised above waist level and the patient sits in crook-lying. The therapist places his or her arm under the popliteal area of the patient's knee, and the distal arm contacts the tibia. The action is to apply flexion against the pivot point of the forearm in a 'nutcracker' action (Fig. 4.54). The flexion movement may be combined with internal or external rotation simultaneously.

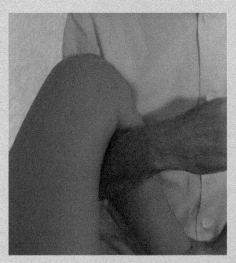

Figure 4.54 Capsular stretch.

Joint distraction

The couch is raised above waist height and the knee is placed in its open-pack position of slight flexion. The patient's shin is fixed beneath the therapist's arm, and the action is a distraction movement which is brought on by swaying the body back (Fig. 4.55).

For higher-grade distraction movements, the patient begins side-lying with the femur supported against the headboard of the couch. The therapist

Treatment note 4.2 *continued*

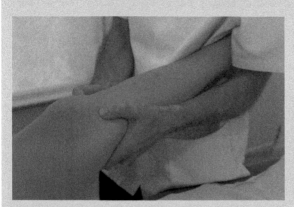

Figure 4.55 Joint distraction gripping patient's tibia beneath arm.

grasps the patient's ankle and leans back with their full body weight to impart a distraction force (Fig. 4.56). This distraction has also been used combined with rotation of the tibia to perform a loose-body manipulation of the knee (Cyriax and Cyriax 1983).

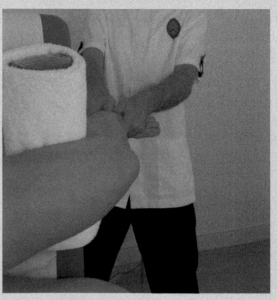

Figure 4.56 Joint distraction using couch headboard.

Manual therapy, exercise therapy and acupuncture

Manual therapy (see Treatment note 4.2), exercise therapy and acupuncture are techniques commonly used within physiotherapy for treatment of OA of the knee. Exercise (muscle strengthening and aerobic fitness) were recommended as core treatments for OA, while manual therapy was recommended as an adjunctive treatment in the NICE guidelines on osteoarthritis (NICE 2014). Two manual therapy techniques are especially useful for OA, the capsular stretch (see Fig. 4.52) and joint distraction (see Fig. 4.53). Marked pain reduction and increased movement usually result from these procedures where flexion is substantially limited and pain occurs through prolonged standing especially.

Exercise therapy for pain reduction includes pendular swinging, where the patient sits on a high bench with their feet off the ground.

The action is to rhythmically swing the legs within mid-range (knee flexion and extension). The exercise is continued for two to three minutes, until pain reduces and the patient feels movement loosening. The capsular stretch mobilization may be followed up using a self-mobilization technique and home exercise. For the knee-flexion self-mobilization, the patient places a soft, rolled towel into the popliteal region of their knee. Overpressure is then placed on the knee by flexing the knee passively, either using the hands holding the shin in lying, or pressing into flexion from a long sitting position. The kneeling sit-back exercise is used as a follow-up procedure when pain has subsided below two to three on a visual analogue scale (VAS) and there is no visible swelling. The patient kneels (four-point kneeling) on a mat or cushion, taking their weight mostly on the hands and uninjured knee. The action is to gradually press the hips backwards towards the heels (auto-assisted knee flexion), easing into the movement gradually rather than forcing the motion range.

Acupuncture is often used by physiotherapists in the treatment of the osteoarthritic knee, and the results are generally good. In a systematic review of seven trials (393 patients), Ezzo et al. (2001) concluded that acupuncture was effective for both pain relief and restoration of function, and that real acupuncture was better than sham acupuncture. In a later systematic review of 13 RCTs (1334 patients), White et al. (2007) concluded that acupuncture was superior to sham acupuncture for improving pain and function with chronic knee pain. Effective treatment of pain and function is dependent on adequate treatment, which normally includes more than 10 treatment sessions of 30 minutes' duration, use of an appropriate treatment protocol, the patient feeling a dull aching sensation (deqi) travelling from the needling site, and electrical stimulation of the needles (electroacupuncture). The current NICE guidelines do not recommend acupuncture for knee arthritis (NICE 2008, 2014) but a network meta-analysis from the NIHR stated that acupuncture could be considered as one of the more effective physical treatments for alleviating osteoarthritis knee pain in the short term (Corbett et al. 2014).

Sinding-Larsen-Johansson disease

In this condition, the secondary ossification centre on the lower border of the patella is affected in adolescents. The epiphysis is tractioned, leading to inflammation and eventual fragmentation. Avascular necrosis is not usually present, but a temporary osteoporosis has been described (Traverso, Baldari and Catalani, 1990) during the adolescent growth spurt.

Definition

Sinding-Larsen-Johansson disease affects the secondary ossification centre on the lower border of the patella in adolescents. Inflammation, bone fragmentation and occasionally temporary (transient) osteoporosis may occur.

Sinding-Larsen-Johansson (SLJ) disease can easily be confused with chondromalacia on first inspection, as it gives pain to the lower pole of the patella, especially when kneeling. However, on closer examination the differences are soon apparent, and X-ray confirms the bony change. Initially, no abnormalities are seen on X-ray, but after two to four weeks, irregular calcification is noted at the inferior pole. The calcifications are seen to coalesce later, and may finally be incorporated into the patella, so are largely clinically non-significant.

The condition may exist with Osgood-Schlatter's syndrome, and the conservative management of the two syndromes is largely the same, involving the use of pain relieving/anti-inflammatory modalities initially. The condition usually represents a patellar tendinopathy with non-significant imaging findings, and so training modification followed by a progressive reintroduction to loading is normally key to management (see above).

Osgood-Schlatter's syndrome

This condition affects adolescents, especially males. Most often the patient is an active sportsperson who has recently undergone the adolescent growth spurt. With Osgood-Schlatter's syndrome, traction is applied to the tibial tubercle, eventually causing the apophysis of the tubercle to separate from the proximal end of the tibia. Initially fragmentation appears, but with time the fragments coalesce and further ossification leads to an increase in bone. This gives the characteristic prominent tibial 'bump' often noticeable when the knee silhouette is compared to that of the unaffected side.

The infrapatellar tendon shows increased vascularization and, particularly where radiographic changes are not apparent, soft-tissue swelling and infrapatellar fat-pad involvement is noted.

Pain is highly localized to the tibial tubercle and exacerbated by activities such as running, jumping and descending stairs. The condition may coalesce with patellar malalignment faults such as patella infera and patella alta. Initial management is by limiting activity in the acute phase. Some pain relief and reduction of inflammation may be obtained by using electrotherapy modalities or medication. An infrapatellar strap to reduce the pull of the quadriceps onto the tibial tubercle has been used with some success (Levine and Kashyap 1981).

Assessment of the lower-limb musculature often reveals hypertrophy and inflexibility of the quadriceps. When passive knee flexion is tested, intense pain precludes the use of quadriceps stretching. However, when pain has subsided, flexibility of this muscle group must be regained. Where prolonged rest has given rise to muscle atrophy, strengthening exercises are indicated. Ice packs may be used to limit pain or inflammation following activity. Restoration of acceleration/deceleration mechanics in jumping and landing (closed chain) is as for jumper's knee (see above).

Synovial plica

The synovial plica is a remnant of the septum that separates the knee into three chambers until the fourth intrauterine month. Three types of plica are seen. The infrapatellar plica (ligamentum mucosum) lies within the intercondylar notch and runs parallel to the anterior cruciate ligament. The suprapatellar plica is found on the medial aspect of the suprapatellar pouch, lying proximal to the superior pole of the patella. The mediopatellar plica extends from the medial suprapatellar pouch over the medial femoral condyle and onto the synovium covering the infrapatellar fat pad (Fig. 4.57). The mediopatellar plica is by far the most important in terms of pathology.

> **Definition**
> A synovial plica is a remnant of the tissue that separates the knee into three chambers in

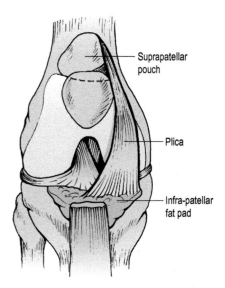

Figure 4.57 The mediopatellar plica. After Reid (1992), with permission.

> the unborn child. A mediopatellar plica is the most common type to give problems in sport.

A mediopatellar plica may be present in some 20–60 per cent of knees (Amatuzzi, Fazzi and Varella 1990), but does not necessarily cause symptoms. In a series of 3,250 knee disorders, Koshino and Okamoto (1985) found only 32 patients to have the complaint (1 per cent). The structure separates the knee joint into two reservoirs, one above the patella and the other constituting the joint-cavity proper. The normal plica is a thin, pink, flexible structure, but when inflamed it becomes thick, fibrosed and swollen, losing its elasticity and interfering with patellofemoral tracking.

These tissue changes are often initiated by trauma that results in synovitis, and are more common in athletes. Pain is usually intermittent and increases with activity. Discomfort is experienced when descending stairs and may mimic PFPS. However, pain of plical origin normally subsides immediately when the knee is extended. In addition, the 'morning sign' may be present. This is a popping sensation that occurs as the knee is extended, particularly on rising, but disappears throughout the day. The popping may be accompanied by giving way, and is caused by the thickened plica passing over the medial femoral condyle. As the day progresses, joint effusion pushes the plica away from the condyle. This sign may be reproduced with some patients by extending the knee from 90-degree flexion while internally rotating the tibia and pushing the patella medially. The pop is usually experienced between 45-degree and 60-degree flexion.

> **Key point**
>
> A popping sensation may be caused as the plica passes over the medial femoral condyle when the knee is extended. This may be reproduced by: (i) extending the knee from 90-degree flexion while (ii) internally rotating the tibia and (iii) pushing the patella medially.

Conservative treatment has been found to be effective in 60 per cent of cases (Amatuzzi, Fazzi and Varella 1990), and aims at reducing the compression over the anterior compartment of the knee by using stretching exercises. The length of the hamstrings, quadriceps and gastrocnemius muscles should be assessed, and these muscles stretched if noticeable shortening is found. Where conservative treatment fails and symptoms limit sport or daily living, arthroscopic removal may be required.

Tendinitis

Tendinitis (inflammation within the tendon substance) and tendinopathy (swelling around but not within the tendon) of the knee occurs most commonly within the patellar tendon (jumper's knee, see above), the semimembranosus and the popliteus.

Semimembranosus has a complex insertion consisting of five slips onto the proximal tibia (Williams 1995), making direct palpation of an inflamed area difficult. The five insertions are:

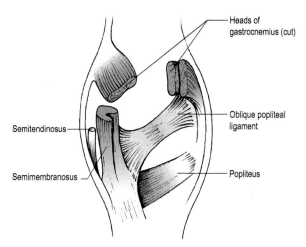

Figure 4.58 Extensive insertion of semimembranosus.

1. into a small tubercle on the posterior aspect of the medial tibial condyle (the tuberculum tendinis)
2. the medial margin of the tibia immediately behind the medial collateral ligament
3. a fibrous expansion to the fascia covering popliteus
4. a cord-like tendon to the inferior lip of the medial tibial condyle below the MCL
5. the oblique popliteal ligament passing upwards and laterally (Fig. 4.58).

Tendinopathy of this muscle gives a persistent ache over the posteromedial aspect of the knee. It occurs as the semimembranosus tendon slides over the medial corner of the medial femoral condyle, and is distinct from semimembranosus bursitis which affects the area of the medial tibial condyle. Pain may occur within the tendon substance itself, or over the teno-osseous junction, when an insertional tendinopathy is present. Increased tracer uptake has been noted on bone scan with this latter condition (Ray, Clancy and Lemon 1988).

Popliteus tendinopathy can be related to increased pronation of the STJ and excessive internal rotation of the tibia (Brody 1980). The increased internal rotation causes traction on the popliteus attachment to the lateral femoral condyle. The popliteus acts with the PCL to prevent forward displacement of the femur on the flexed tibia, and so will be overworked with downhill running. On examination, tenderness is revealed over the popliteus just anterior to the fibular collateral ligament. The patient is examined in a supine position with the injured knee in the 'figure of four' position, that is, affected hip flexed, abducted and externally rotated, knee bent to 90 degrees and foot placed on the knee of the contralateral leg. The condition is differentiated from ITB friction syndrome by testing resisted tibial internal rotation with the knee flexed, and palpating the popliteus while internal rotation is resisted in extension.

Snapping-knee syndrome

Tendinopathy of the semitendinosus and gracilis is a cause of snapping-knee syndrome. Here, a snapping sensation occurs over the posteromedial aspect of the knee, normally following intense training. The condition is rare and must be differentiated from synovial plica (see above) through imaging. Cadaveric studies have revealed that the semitendinosus fibres fan out to hold the tendon within its groove at the posteromedial

corner of the tibia. Both the semitendinosus and gracilis have aponeurotic expansions (accessory tendinous bands) attaching into the fascia cruris and gastrocnemius forming the tensor fascia cruris muscle (Mochizuki et al. 2004). The bands arise 5–9 cm proximal to the pes anserinus, insert into the gastrocnemis (Candal-Couto and Deehan 2003) and act as an additional medial stabilizer when the knee is fully extended. Repetitive, high-intensity actions in athletes where the knee hyperextends may stress the region excessively and result in pathology.

Treatment for tendinopathy involves rest, anti-inflammatory modalities and load modification. Flexibility of the knee musculature and the biomechanics of the lower limb should be assessed and corrected as necessary. Surgery may be required where tendinous subluxation does not resolve.

Bursitis

The knee joint has on average 14 bursae (Table 4.16) in areas where friction is likely to occur, between muscle, tendon, bone and skin. Any of these can become inflamed and give pain

Table 4.16 Bursae around the knee

Bursa	Lying between
Subcutaneous pre-patellar	Lower patella/skin
Deep infrapatellar	Upper tibia/patellar ligament
Subcutaneous infrapatellar	Lower tibial tuberosity/skin
Suprapatellar	Lower femur/deep surface of quadriceps (communicates with joint)
No specific name	Lateral head of gastrocnemius/capsule
	Lateral collateral ligament/tendon of biceps femoris
	Lateral collateral ligament/popliteus
	Popliteus tendon/lateral condyle of femur
	Medial head of gastrocnemius/capsule
	Medial head of gastrocnemius/semimembranosus
Pes anserine	Superficial to medial collateral ligament/sartorius, gracilus, semitendinosus
No specific name	Deep medial collateral ligament/femur, medial meniscus
Semimembranosus	Semimembranosus/medial tibial condyle, gastrocnemius
No specific name	Semimembranosus/semitendinosus

when compressed through muscle contraction or direct palpation. Those most commonly injured in sport include the pre-patellar, pes anserine and semimembranosus.

Pre-patellar bursa

The pre-patellar bursa is usually injured by falling onto the anterior aspect of the knee, or by prolonged kneeling (housemaid's knee). Haemorrhage into the bursa can cause an inflammatory reaction and increased fluid volume. Enlargement is noticeable, and the margins of the mass are well defined, differentiating the condition from general knee effusion or subcutaneous haematoma. Knee flexion may be limited, the bursa being compressed as the skin covering the patella tightens.

> **Key point**
>
> Falling directly onto the point of the knee may cause housemaid's knee (pre-patellar bursitis). Only the anterior aspect of the knee is swollen, and pain is increased by knee flexion as the bursa is compressed.

Septic bursitis may result by secondary infection if the skin over the bursa is broken by laceration or puncture wound. If the condition becomes chronic, the bursa may collapse and the folded walls of the thickened bursal sac appear as small, hardened masses on the anterior aspect of the knee. In these cases, erythema and exquisite tenderness are usually present.

Minor cases normally respond to rest and ice, but more marked swelling requires aspiration. Aspiration is carried out under sterile conditions, and a compression bandage applied.

Semimembranosus and pes anserine bursae

Semimembranosus bursitis gives rise to pain and swelling over the lower posteromedial aspect of the knee. Pain may be made worse by hamstring or gastrocnemius contraction against resistance, and in activities involving intense action of these muscles, such as sprinting and bounding.

Pes anserine bursitis gives pain and swelling over the metaphyseal area of the tibia, sometimes referred to the medial joint line. The bursa may be injured by direct trauma (hitting the knee on a hurdle) or by overuse of the pes anserine tendons.

With both of the latter causes of bursitis, rest and anti-inflammatory modalities are required. Biomechanical assessment of the lower limb and analysis of the athlete's training regime is also useful where there is no history of injury.

Baker's cyst

One condition often referred to as 'bursitis' is a Baker's cyst (popliteal cyst). This is actually a posterior herniation of the synovial membrane into the bursa lying between semimembranosus and the medial head of the gastrocnemius (Fig. 4.59).

The mass bulges into the popliteal space, and occurs particularly in rheumatoid arthritis. The posterior knee ligaments weaken and fail to support the joint capsule, allowing the herniation

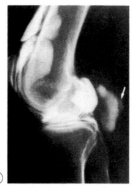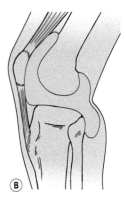

Figure 4.59 Baker's cyst. From Reilly, B.M. (1991) *Practical Strategies in Outpatient Medicine*. W.B. Saunders, Philadelphia. With permission.

to occur. The cyst can be palpated over the medial side of the popliteal space beneath the medial head of the gastrocnemius.

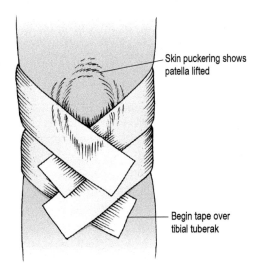

Skin puckering shows patella lifted

Begin tape over tibial tuberak

Figure 4.60 Fat pad unloading using taping.

> **Definition**
>
> A Baker's cyst is a bulging (herniation) of the synovial membrane backwards into the bursa lying between semimembranosus and the medial head of the gastrocnemius.

When painless, the condition may be managed conservatively, but it is essential to trace the pathology which has given rise to the increased volume of synovial fluid within the knee as a precursor of the condition. Removal of the cause of the swelling (for example, traumatic arthritis) will often allow the Baker's cyst to resolve spontaneously. The cyst may rupture during heavy activity or exercise, giving sudden and severe knee pain. Bruising may track down the leg and appear at the ankle (von Schroader et al. 1993) with blood coming from the cyst wall where it is haemorrhagic. Where the enlargement compromises venous return or causes severe pain, aspiration or excision of the mass is called for.

Fat pads

Fat pads consist of fat cells (adipose tissue) packed closely together and separated from other tissues by fibrous septa. They have an abundant blood supply and are well innervated. Most significant to the knee is the infrapatellar fat pad, lying beneath the patellar tendon and in front of the femoral condyles. The fat pad is intracapsular but extrasynovial, and a piece of synovial membrane (ligamentum mucosum, see above) may pass from the pad to the intracondylar notch of the femur. When the knee is fully flexed, the infrapatellar fat pad fills the anterior aspect of the intercondylar notch. As the knee extends, the fat pad covers the trochlear surface of the femur within the patellar groove.

The usual pathology of the infrapatellar fat pad is irritation and enlargement causing increased pressure with resultant pain (Hoffa's disease). Direct trauma can cause haemorrhage and local oedema, but more normally impingement occurs with hyperextension of the knee. Patients typically present with a history of pain inferomedial, and sometimes inferolateral, to the patella. On examination, impingement pain is present deep to the inferior pole of the patella at 20 degrees flexion with resisted quadriceps contraction.

Relief of mild compression pain may be achieved with V taping, which begins over the tibial tubercle and extends laterally and medially. The tape is placed under traction to lift the patella in a cephalic direction. This effectively forms a sling to prevent the patella pressing into the fat pad to allow recovery (Fig. 4.60).

References

Amatuzzi, M.M., Fazzi, A., Varella, M.H., 1990. Pathologic synovial plica of the knee. *American Journal of Sports Medicine* **18** (5), 466–469.

American College of Sports Medicine (ACSM), 2001. Intervention strategies for weight loss and prevention of weight regain for adults. *Medicine and Science for Sports and Exercise* **33**, 2145–2156.

Anderson, A.F., Snyder, R.B., Federspiel, C.F., Lipscomb, A.B., 1992. Instrumented evaluation of knee laxity: a comparison of five arthrometers. *American Journal of Sports Medicine* **20**, 135–140.

Arno, S., 1990. The A angle: a quantitative measurement of patella alignment and realignment. *Journal of Orthopaedic and Sports Physical Therapy* **12** (6), 237–242.

Aroen, A., Loken, S., Heir, S., 2004. Articular cartilage lesions in 993 consecutive knee arthroscopies. *American Journal of Sports Medicine* **32** (1), 211–215.

Bach, B.R., Warren, R.F., Wickiewicz, T.L., 1990. Arthrometric evaluation of knees that have a torn anterior cruciate ligament. *Journal of Bone and Joint Surgery* **72A**, 1299.

Baechle, T.R., 1994. *Essentials of Strength Training and Conditioning.* Human Kinetics, Champaign, Illinois.

Baratta, R., Solomonow, M., Zhou, B.H., et al., 1988. Muscular coactivation: the role of the antagonist musculature in maintaining knee stability. *American Journal of Sports Medicine* **16**, 113–122.

Beard, D.J., Kyberd, P.J., O'Connor, J.J., et al., 1994. Reflex hamstring contraction latency in anterior cruciate ligament deficiency. *Journal of Orthopaedic Research* **12** (2), 219–227.

Beckman, M., Craig, R., Lehman, R.C., 1989. Rehabilitation of patellofemoral dysfunction in the athlete. *Clinics in Sports Medicine* **8** (4), 841–860.

Bellamy, N., Campbell, J., Welch, V., et al., 2006. Viscosupplementation for the treatment of osteoarthritis of the knee. http://www.cochrane.org/reviews/en/ab005321.html (accessed April 2009).

Bobic, V., 2002. Viscosupplementation for osteoarthrosis of the knee. International Society for Arthroscopy, Knee Surgery and Orthopaedic Sports Medicine. http://www.isakos.com/innovations/bobic2.aspx (accessed April 2009).

Boren, K., Conrey, C., Le Coguic, J., Paprocki, L., Voight, M., & Robinson, T. K., 2011. Electromyography analysis of gluteus medius and gluteus maximus during rehabilitation exercises. *International Journal of Sports Physical Therapy* **6** (3), 206–223.

Briggs, C., Sandor, S.M., Kenihan, M.A.R., 1995. The knee. In: Zuluaga, M. (ed.), *Sports Physiotherapy.* Churchill Livingstone, London.

Brody, D.M., 1980. Running injuries. *Clinical Symposia* **32** (4), Ciba Pharmaceutical Company.

Callaghan, M.J., Selfe, J., Bagley, P.J., Oldham, J.A., 2000. Effects of patellar taping on knee joint proprioception. *Physiotherapy* **86** (11), 590.

Candal-Couto, J.J., and Deehan, D.J., 2003. The accessory bands of gracilis and semitendinosus: an anatomical study. *Knee* **10** (4): 325–328.

Caraffa, A., Cerulli, G., Projetti, M., Aisa, G., 1996. Prevention of anterior cruciate ligament injuries in soccer. *Knee Surgery, Sports Traumatology and Arthroscopy* **4**, 19–21.

Collins, N., Crossley, K., Beller, E., et al., 2009. Foot orthoses and physiotherapy in the treatment of patellofemoral pain syndrome: randomized clinical trial. *British Journal of Sports Medicine* **43**, 169–171.

Corbett, M.S., Rice, S.J., et al., 2014. Acupuncture and other physical treatments for the relief of pain due to osteoarthritis of the knee: network meta-analysis. National Institute for Health research accessed 11/2016.

Costill, D.L., Fink, W.J., Habansky, A.J., 1977. Muscle rehabilitation after knee surgery. *Physician and Sports Medicine* **7**, 71.

Crossley, K., Cook, J., Cowan, S., McConnell, J., 2007. Anterior knee pain. In: Brukner, P., Khan, K. (eds), *Clinical Sports Medicine*, 3rd ed. McGraw Hill, Sydney, pp. 506–537.

Crossley, K., Cowan, S.M., Bennell, K., McConnell, J., 2000. Patellar taping: is clinical success supported by scientific evidence? *Manual Therapy* **5** (3), 142–150.

Crossley, K.M., Stefanik, J. et al., 2016. Patellofemoral pain consensus statement from the 4th International Patellofemoral Pain Research Retreat, Manchester. Part 1: Terminology, definitions, clinical examination, natural history, patellofemoral osteoarthritis and patient-reported outcome measures. *British Journal of Sports Medicine* **50** (14), 839–843.

Cyriax, J.H., Cyriax, P.J., 1983. *Illustrated Manual of Orthopaedic Medicine*. Butterworths, London.

Daniel, D.M., Stone, M.L., Barnett, P., Sachs, R., 1988. Use of the quadriceps active test to diagnose posterior cruciate ligament disruption and measure posterior laxity of the knee. *Journal of Bone and Joint Surgery* **70A**, 386–391.

Davidson, C., Ganion, L., Gehlsen, G., Verhoestra, B., 1997. Rat tendon morphologic and functional changes resulting from soft tissue mobilization. *Medicine and Science in Sports and Exercise* **29** (3), 313–319.

DeHaven, K.E., Black, K.P., Griffiths, H.J., 1989. Open meniscus repair: technique and two to nine year results. *American Journal of Sports Medicine* **17**, 788–795.

DeHaven, K.E., Bronstein, R.D., 1995. Injuries to the menisci of the knee. In: Nicholas, J.A., Hershman, E.B. (eds), *The Lower Extremity and Spine in Sports Medicine*, 2nd ed. C.V. Mosby, St Louis.

Distefano L.J., Blackburn J.T., et al., 2009. Gluteal muscle activation during common therapeutic exercises. *Journal of Orthopaedic & Sports Physical Therapy* **39** (7), 532–540.

Donaldson, W.F., Warren, R.F., Wickiewicz, T., 1985. A comparison of acute anterior cruciate ligament examinations. *American Journal of Sports Medicine* **13**, 5–10.

Ebert, J.R., Robertson, W.B., Lloyd, D.G., Zheng, M.H., 2008. Traditional vs accelerated approaches to post-operative rehabilitation following matrix induced autologous chondrocyte implantation. *Osteoarthritis Cartilage* **16** (10), 1131–1140.

ESSKA (2017) http://c.ymcdn.com/sites/esska.site-ym.com/resource/resmgr/docs/2016-meniscus-consensus-proj.pdf. Accessed 17/04/2017.

Evans, N.A., Hall, F., Chew, W.D., Stanish, M.D., 2001. The natural history and tailored treatment of ACL injury. *Physician and Sports Medicine* **29** (9), 70–84.

Evans, P.J., Bell, G.D., Frank, C., 1993. Prospective evaluation of the McMurray test. *American Journal of Sports Medicine* **21**, 604–608.

Exler, Y., 1991. Patella fracture: review of the literature and five case presentations. *Journal of Orthopaedic and Sports Physical Therapy* **13** (4), 177–183.

Ezzo, J., Hadhazy, V., Birch, S., et al., 2001. Acupuncture for osteoarthritis of the knee: a systematic review. *Arthritis and Rheumatism* **44** (4), 819–825.

Fairbank, T.J., 1948. Knee joint changes after meniscectomy. *Journal of Bone and Joint Surgery* **30B** (4), 664–670.

Fairclough, J., Hayashi, K., et al., 2006. The functional anatomy of the iliotibial band during flexion and extension of the knee: implications for understanding iliotibial band syndrome. *Journal of Anatomy* **208** (3), 309–316.

Fairclough, J., Hayashi, K., et al., 2007. Is iliotibial band syndrome really a friction syndrome? *Journal of Science and Medicine in Sport* **10** (2), 74–76; discussion 7–8.

Felson, D.T., 1997. Understanding the relationship between bodyweight and osteoarthritis. *Clinical Rheumatology* **11**, 671–681.

Ferretti, A., 1986. Epidemiology of jumper's knee. *Sports Medicine* **3**, 289–295.

Fransen, M., McConnell, S., Harmer, A.R., et al., 2015. Exercise for osteoarthritis of the knee. *Cochrane Database of Systematic Reviews* Issue 1. Art. No. CD004376.

Fulkerson, J.P., 1982. Awareness of the retinaculum in evaluating patello-femoral pain. *American Journal of Sports Medicine* **10**, 147–149.

Garrick, J.G., Webb, D.R., 1990. *Sports Injuries: Diagnosis and Management*. W.B. Saunders, London.

Gehlsen, G., Ganion, L., Helfst, R., 1999. Fibroblast responses to variation in soft tissue mobilization pressure. *Medicine & Science in Sports and Exercise* **31** (4), 531–535.

Gryzlo, S.M., Patek, R.M., Pink, M., Perry, J., 1994. Electromyographic analysis of knee rehabilitation exercises. *Journal of Orthopaedic and Sports Physical Therapy* **20**, 36–43.

Hambly, K., 2009. Knee articular cartilage repair and athletes. *Sportex Medicine* **39**, 17–21.

Henning, C.E., 1988. Semilunar cartilage of the knee: function and pathology. *Exercise and Sports Science Review* **16**, 67–75.

Henning, C.E., Lynch, M.A., Glick, K.R., 1985. An in vivo strain gauge study of elongation of the ACL. *American Journal of Sports Medicine* **13**, 34–39.

Herrington, L., 2000. The inter-tester reliability of a clinical measurement used to determine the medial/lateral orientation of the patella. *Manual Therapy* **7** (3), 163–167.

Herrington, L., Myer G., Horsley I., 2013. Task based rehabilitation protocol for elite athletes following anterior cruciate ligament reconstruction: a clinical commentary. *Physical Therapy in Sport* **14**, 188–198.

Herrington, L., Payton, S., 1997. Effects of corrective taping of the patella on patients with patellofemoral pain. *Physiotherapy* **83** (11), 566–572.

Herrington, L., Pearson, S., 2008. The applicability of ultrasound imaging in the assessment of dynamic patella tracking: a preliminary investigation. *The Knee* **15**, 125–127.

Herrington, L., Rivett, N., Munro, S., 2006. The relationship between patella position and length of the iliotibal band as assessed using Ober's test. *Manual Therapy* **11**, 182–186.

Highgenboten, C.L., Jackson, A., Meske, N.B., 1989. Genucom, KT-1000, and Stryker knee laxity measuring device comparisons: device reproducibility and interdevice comparison in asymptomatic subjects. *American Journal of Sports Medicine* **17**, 743.

Higuchi, H., Kimura, M., Shirakura, K., 2000. Factors affecting long term results after arthroscopic partial meniscectomy. *Clinical Orthopedics* **377**, 161–168.

Hoessly, L.H., Wildi, L.M., 2015. Magnetic resonance imaging findings in the knee before and after long distance running – documentation of irreversible structural damage? *American Journal of Sports Medicine* **45** (5), 1206–1217.

Hohmann, E., 2006. Long distance running and arthritis. *Sportex Medicine* **30**, 10–13.

Hudson, Z., Darthuy, E., 2009. Iliotibial band tightness and patellofemoral pain syndrome: A case control study. *Manual Therapy* **14**, 147–151.

Insall, J., 1979. Chondromalacia patellae: patellar malalignment syndrome. *Orthopaedic Clinics of North America* **10**, 117–127.

Jackson, D.W., Sheer, M.J., Simon, T.M., 2001. Cartilage substitutes: overview of basic science and treatment options. *Journal of the American Academy of Orthopedic Surgeons* **9**, 37–52.

Jackson, R.W., Peters, R.I., Marczyk, R.I., 1980. Late results of untreated anterior cruciate ligament rupture. *Journal of Bone and Joint Surgery* **62B**, 127.

Jacobson, E., Forssblad, M., Rosenberg, J., 2000. Can local anesthesia be recommended for routine use in elective knee arthroscopy? *Arthroscopy* **16**, 183–190.

Jakobsen, T., Christensen, M., Christensen, S., Olsen, M., Bandholm, T., 2010. Reliability of knee joint range of motion and circumference measurements after total knee arthroplasty. *Physiotherapy Research International* **15**, 126–134.

Jensen, K., 1990. Manual laxity tests for anterior cruciate ligament injuries. *Journal of Orthopaedic and Sports Physical Therapy* **11** (10), 474–481.

Jerosch, J.G., Castro, W.H.M., Jantea, C., 1989. Stress fracture of the patella. *American Journal of Sports Medicine* **17**, 4.

Jorgensen, U., Sonne-Holm, S., Lauridsen, E., 1987. Long term follow up of meniscectomy in athletes: a prospective longitudinal study. *Journal of Bone and Joint Surgery* **69**, 80.

Kapoor, B., Clement, D., Kirkley, A., Maffuli, N., 2004. Current practice in the management of anterio cruciate ligament injuries in the United Kingdom. *British Journal of Sports Medicine* **38**, 542–544.

Karst, G.M., Jewett, P.D., 1993. Electromyographic analysis of exercises proposed for differential activation of medial and lateral quadriceps femoris muscle components. *Physical Therapy* **73**, 286–299.

Keene, J.S., 1990. Ligament and muscle tendon unit injuries. In: Gould, J.A. (ed.), *Orthopaedic and*

Sports Physical Therapy, 2nd ed. C.V. Mosby, St Louis, pp. 137–165.

Kelley, M.J., 1990. Meniscal trauma (of the knee) and surgical intervention. *Journal of Sports Medicine and Physical Fitness* **30** (3), 297–306.

Kennedy, J.C., Alexander, I.J., Hayes, K.C., 1982. Nerve supply of the human knee and its functional importance. *American Journal of Sports Medicine* **10**, 329.

Kise, N.J., Risberg, M.A., Stensrud, S., et al., 2016. Exercise therapy versus arthroscopic partial meniscectomy for degenerative meniscal tear in middle-aged patients: randomised controlled trial with two-year follow-up. *British Medical Journal* **354** : i3740.

Koshino, T., Okamoto, R., 1985. Resection of painful shelf (plica synovialis mediopatellaris) under arthroscopy. *Arthroscopy* **1**, 136–141.

Lane, N.E., Oehlert, J.W., Bloch, D.A., Freis, J.F., 1998. The relationship of running to osteoarthritis of the knee and hip and bone mineral density of the lumbar spine: a 9 year longitudinal study. *Journal of Rheumatology* **25**, 334–341.

Larsen, B., Adreasen, E., Urfer, A., Mickelson, M.R., 1995. Patellar taping: a radiographic examination of the medial glide technique. *American Journal of Sports Medicine* **23** (4), 465–471.

Leech, R.D., Edwards, K.L., Batt M.E., 2015. Does running protect against knee osteoarthritis? Or promote it? Assessing the current evidence. *British Journal of Sports Medicine* **49** (21), 1355–1356.

Lephart, S.M., Fu, F.H., 1995. The role of proprioception in the treatment of sports injuries. *Sports Exercise and Injury* **1** (2), 96–102.

Levine, J., Kashyap, S., 1981. A new conservative treatment of Osgood-Schlatter's disease. *Clinical Orthopaedics and Related Research* **158**, 126–128.

Levy, I.M., Torzilli, P.A., Warren, R.F., 1982. The effect of medial meniscectomy on anterior-posterior motion of the knee. *Journal of Bone and Joint Surgery* **64**, 883–888.

Lo, G., Driban, J., Kriska, A., et al., 2014. Habitual running any time in life is not detrimental and may be protective of symptomatic knee osteoarthritis: data from the osteoarthritis initiative, *Arthritis & Rheumatology* **66**, 1265–1266.

Magee, D.J., 2002. *Orthopedic Physical Assessment*, 4th ed. W.B. Saunders, Philadelphia.

Marks, R., Allegrante, J.P., 2002. Body mass indices in patients with disabling hip osteoarthritis. *Arthritis Research* **4** (2), 112–116.

McConnell, J., 1986. The management of chondromalacia patella: a long term solution. *Australian Journal of Physiotherapy* **31**, 214–223.

McConnell, J., 1992. McConnell Patellofemoral Course, London.

McConnell, J., 1994. McConnell Patello-femoral Course, London.

McEwan, I., Herrington, L., Thom, J., 2007. The validity of clinical measures of patella position. *Manual Therapy* **12**, 226–230.

Meardon S.A., Campbell S., Derrick T.R., 2012. Step width alters iliotibial band strain during running. *Sports Biomech* **11** (4), 464–472.

Millar, A.L., Berglund, K., Blake, B., Amstra, C., 1999. Effects of patellofemoral taping on knee pain and EMG activity of the quadriceps. *Medicine and Science in Sports and Exercise* **31** (Suppl. 5), s207.

Mochizuki, T., Akita, K., Muneta, T., Sato, T., 2004. Pes anserinus: layered supportive structure of the medial side of the knee. *Clinical Anatomy* **17** (1), 50–54.

Nemeth W.C., Sanders B.L., 1996. The lateral synovial recess of the knee: anatomy and role in chronic iliotibial band friction syndrome. *Arthroscopy* **12**, 574–580.

NICE [National Institute for health and Care Excellence], 2008. NICE guidelines on osteoarthritis. Clinical Guideline - CG59.

NICE [National Institute for health and Care Excellence], 2014. Osteoarthritis: care and management. Clinical Guideline - CG177.

Noehren, Scholz, J., Davis, I., 2011. The effect of real-time gait retraining on hip kinematics, pain and function in subjects with patellofemoral pain syndrome. *British Journal of Sports Medicine* **45**, 691–696.

Norris, C.M., 2001. *Acupuncture: Treatment of Musculoskeletal Conditions*. Butterworth-Heinemann, Oxford.

Noyes, F.R., Mooar, L.A., Moorman, C.T., McGinniss, G.H., 1989. Partial tears of the anterior cruciate ligament: progression to complete ligament deficiency. *Journal of Bone and Joint Surgery* **71B**, 825–833.

Nunes, G.S., Stapait, E.L., Kirsten, M.H., et al., 2013. Clinical test for diagnosis of patellofemoral pain syndrome: systematic review with meta-analysis. *Physical Therapy in Sport* **14**, 54–59.

Ohkoshi, Y., Yasuda, K., Kaneda, K., et al., 1991. Biomechanical analysis of rehabilitation in the standing position. *American Journal of Sports Medicine* **19**, 605–611.

Palastanga, N., Field, D., Soames, R., 1989. *Anatomy and Human Movement*. Butterworth-Heinemann, Oxford.

Panariello, R.A., Backus, S.I., Parker, J.W., 1994. The effect of the squat exercise on anterior-posterior knee translation in professional football players. *American Journal of Sports Medicine* **22**, 768–773.

Panush, R.S., Brown, D.G., 1987. Exercise and arthritis. *Sports Medicine* **4**, 54–64.

Parolie, J.M., Bergfeld, J.A., 1986. Long term results of nonoperative treatment of isolated posterior cruciate ligament injuries in the athlete. *American Journal of Sports Medicine* **14**, 53–58.

Pasanen, K., Parkkari, J., Pasanen, M., et al., 2008. Neuromuscular training and the risk of leg injuries in female football players: cluster randomised controlled study. *BMJ.* **337**, a295.

Paterno, M., Schmitt, L., Ford, K., Rauh, M., Myer, G., Huang B, Hewett, T.E., 2010. Biomechanical measures during landing and postural stability predict second anterior cruciate ligament injury after anterior cruciate reconstruction and return to sport. *American Journal of Sports Medicine* **38**, 1968–1978.

Paulos, L.E., Rosenberg, T.D., Drawbert, C.W., 1987. Infrapatellar contraction syndrome: an unrecognised cause of knee stiffness with patellar entrapment and patella infera. *American Journal of Sports Medicine* **15**, 331.

Post, W., Fulkerson, J., 1992. Distal realignment of the patellofemoral joint. *Orthopaedic Clinics of North America* **23**, 6–11.

Puranen, J., Ala-Ketola, L., Peltokalleo, P., Saarela, J., 1975. Running and primary osteoarthritis of the hip. *British Medical Journal* **1**, 424–425.

Purdam, C., Cook, J., Hopper, D., Khan, K., 2003. Discriminative ability of functional loading tests for adolescent jumper's knee. *Physical Therapy in Sport* **4** (1), 3–9.

Radin, E.L., Eyre, D., Schiller, A.L., 1979. Effect of prolonged walking on concrete on the joints of sheep. Abstract. *Arthritis and Rheumatism* **22**, 649.

Ray, J.M., Clancy, W.G., Lemon, R.A., 1988. Semimembranosus tendinitis: an overlooked cause of medial knee pain. *American Journal of Sports Medicine* **16**, 4.

Reid, D.C., 1992. *Sports Injury Assessment and Rehabilitation*. Churchill Livingstone, London.

Reynolds, L., Levin, T., Medeiros, J., Adler, N., Hallum, A., 1983. EMG activity of the vastus medialis oblique and vastus lateralis and their role in patellar alignment. *American Journal of Physical Medicine* **62** (2), 61–71.

Richardson, C., Bullock, M.I., 1986. Changes in muscle activity during fast, alternating flexion-extension movements of the knee. *Scandinavian Journal of Rehabilitation Medicine* **18**, 51–58.

Roberts, J.M., 1989. The effect of taping on patellofemoral alignment: a radiological pilot study. Manipulative Therapists Association of Australia Conference, Adelaide, pp. 146–151.

Rudavsky A., Cook, J., 2014. Physiotherapy management of patellar tendinopathy (jumper's knee). *Journal of Physiotherapy* **60** (3),122–129.

Ryu, R.K.N., Ting, A.J., 1993. Arthroscopic treatment of meniscal cysts. *Arthroscopy* **9**, 591–595.

Seedhom, B.B., Hargreaves, D.J., 1979. Transmission of the load in the knee joint with special reference to the role of the menisci. Part II: Experimental results, discussion and conclusions. *Engineering Medicine* **8**, 220–228.

Seto, J.L., Brewster, C.E., Lombardo, J., 1989. Rehabilitation of the knee after anterior cruciate ligament reconstruction. *Journal of Orthopaedic and Sports Physical Therapy* **10**, 8.

Seto, J.L., Orofino, A.S., Morrissey, M.C., 1988. Assessment of quadriceps/hamstring strength, knee ligament stability, functional and sports activity levels five years after anterior cruciate ligament reconstruction. *American Journal of Sports Medicine* **16**, 170–180.

Shakespeare, D.T., Rigby, H.S., 1983. The bucket handle tear of the meniscus: a clinical and arthrographic study. *Journal of Bone and Joint Surgery* **65**, 383.

Sharma, L., Song, J., Felson, D.T., Cahue, S., 2001. The role of knee alignment in disease progression and functional decline in knee osteoarthritis. *Journal of the American Medical Association* **286** (7), 792.

Shea, K., Fulkerson, J., 1992. Pre-operative computed tomography scanning and arthroscopy in predicting outcome after lateral release. *Arthroscopy* **8**, 327–334.

Shelbourne, K.D. Muthukaruppan, Y., 2005. Subjective results of nonoperatively treated acute isolated posterior cruciate ligament injuries. *Arthroscopy* **21** (4), 457–461.

Shelbourne, K.D., Davis, T.J., Patel, D.V., 1999. The natural history of acute, isolated nonoperatively treated posterior cruciate ligament injuries: a prospective study. *American Journal of Sports Medicine* **27** (3), 276–283.

Sihvonen, R., Paavola, M., Malmivaara, A., et al., 2013. Arthroscopic partial meniscectomy versus sham surgery for a degenerative meniscal tear. *The New England Journal of Medicine* **69** (26), 2515–2524.

Sinkjaer, T., Arendt-Nielsen, L., 1991. Knee stability and muscle coordination in patients with anterior cruciate ligament injuries: an electromyographic approach. *Journal of Electromyography and Kinesiology* **1**, 209–217.

Somes, S., Worrell, T.W., Corey, B., Ingersol, C.D., 1997. Effects of patellar taping on patellar position in the open and closed kinetic chain: a preliminary study. *Journal of Sports Rehabilitation* **6**, 299–308.

Steadman, J., Rodkey, W., Singleton, S., 1997. Microfracture technique for full-thickness chondral defects. *Operative Techniques in Orthopaedics* **7** (4), 300–304.

Steinkamp, L.A., Dillingham, M.F., Markel, M.D., Hill, J.A., Kaufman, K.R., 1993. Biomechanical considerations in patellofemoral joint rehabilitation. *American Journal of Sports Medicine* **21**, 438–444.

Torzilli, P.A., 1991. Measurement reproducibility of two commercial knee test devices. *Journal of Orthopaedic Research* **9**, 730.

Towheed, T., Maxwell, L., Anastassiades, T.P., et al., 2008. Glucosamine therapy for treating osteoarthritis. http://www.cochrane.org/reviews/en/ab002946.html (accessed April 2009).

Traverso, A., Baldari, A., Catalani, F., 1990. The coexistence of Osgood-Schlatter's disease with Sinding-Larsen-Johansson's disease. *Journal of Sports Medicine and Physical Fitness* **30** (3), 331–333.

Urquhart, D.M., Phyomaung, P.P., Dubowitz, J. et al., 2015. Are cognitive and behavioural factors associated with knee pain? A systematic review. *Seminars in Arthritis and Rheumatism* Vol. 44 (4) p. 445–455.

Videman, T., 1982. The effect of running on the osteoarthritic joint: an experimental matched pair study with rabbits. *Rheumatology and Rehabilitation* **21**, 1–8.

Von Scroeder, H., Ameli, F.M., Piazza, D., Lossing, A.G., 1993. Ruptured Baker's cyst causes ecchymosis of the foot. *Journal of Bone and Joint Surgury* [Br] **75-B**: 316–317.

Watterson, J.R., Esdaile, J.M., 2000. Viscosupplementation: Therapeutic mechanisms and clinical potential in osteoarthritis of the knee. *Journal of the American Academy of Orthopedic Surgeons* **8**, 277–284.

Weiss, C.B., Lundberg, M., Hamberg, P., et al., 1989. Non-operative treatment of meniscal tears.

Journal of Bone and Joint Surgery **71A**, 811–822.

White, A., Foster, N., Cummings, M., Barlas, P., 2007. Acupuncture treatment for chronic knee pain: a systematic review. *Rheumatology* **46** (3), 384–390.

Williams, P.L., 1995. *Gray's Anatomy*, 38th ed. Churchill Livingstone, Edinburgh.

Willy R.W., Buchenic, L., Rogacki, K., Ackerman, J., Schmidt, A., Willson, J.D., 2016. In-field gait retraining and mobile monitoring to address running biomechanics associated with tibial stress fracture. *Scandinavian Journal of Medicine and Science in Sports* **26** (2), 197–205.

Woo, S.L.-Y., Ohno, K., Weaver, C.M., et al., 1994. Non-operative treatment of knee ligament injuries. *Sports Exercise and Injury* **1** (1), 2–13.

Wright, J.M., Crockett, H.C., Dowd, M., 2001. The role of viscosupplementation for the osteoarthritis of the knee. *Orthopaedic Special Edition* **7**, 15–18.

Wroble, R.R., 2000. Articular cartilage injury and autologous chondrocyte implantation – which patients might benefit? *Physician and Sportsmedicine* **28** (11), 43–49.

Wroble, R.R., Van Ginkel, L.A., Grood, E.S., et al., 1990. Repeatability of the KT-1000 arthrometer in a normal population. *American Journal of Sports Medicine* **18**, 396.

Wylde, A., Sayers, A., Odutola, R. et al., 2016. Central sensitization as a determinant of patients' benefit from total hip and knee replacement. *European Journal of Pain* **1**, 1–8.

Yasuda, K., Sasaki, T., 1987. Muscle exercise after anterior cruciate ligament reconstruction: biomechanics of the simultaneous isometric contraction method of the quadriceps and hamstrings. *Clinical Orthopaedics and Related Research* **220**, 266–274.

Zachazewski, J.E., Magee, D.J., Quillen, W.S., 1996. *Athletic Injuries and Rehabilitation*. Saunders, Philadelphia.

CHAPTER 5

The shin

Shin splints

The term 'shin splints' is often used as a blanket description of any persistent pain occurring between the knee and ankle in an athlete. The condition has a number of names including Exercise Induced Leg Pain (EILP), Chronic Exertional Compartment Syndrome (CECS), Exertional Lower Limb Pain (ELLP), and Biomechanical Overload Syndrome (BOS). The term CECS with be used in this text.

The condition presents as a gradually increasing cramping or aching pain (fullness) along the side of the shin, and can be due to stress on several structures, including bone, nerve, muscle and fascia.

> **Definition**
> Chronic Exertional Compartment Syndrome (CECS) is a cramping or aching sensation along the side of the shin bones.

Originally called 'fresher's leg', a more accurate description of this type of exercise-induced leg pain comes with the various 'compartment syndromes' which identify the anatomical structures affected. The lower leg contains four compartments containing the structures outline in Table 5.1. The structures overlie and take attachment from

Table 5.1 Compartments of the lower leg

Compartment	Structures contained
Anterior	▶ Tibialis anterior, Extensor Hallucis Longus (EHL), Extensor Digitorum Longus (EDL) and Peroneus Tertius. ▶ Anterior tibial artery and vein ▶ Deep perineal nerve
Lateral	▶ Peroneus Longus, Peroneus brevis ▶ Superficial perineal nerve
Superficial posterior	▶ Gastocnemius, Soleus, Plantaris ▶ Branch of tibial artery and vein ▶ Sural nerve
Deep posterior	▶ Flexor Hallucis Longus (FHL), Flexor Digitorum Longus (FDL), Tibialis posterior and Politeus ▶ Posterior tibial artery and vein ▶ Peroneal artery and vein ▶ Tibial nerve

the tibia, while the deep and superficial posterior compartments are separated by the deep transverse fascia of the leg (Fig. 5.1).

Several structures may be implicated in CECS (Table 5.2). Direct bone pain may occur with a stress fracture or stress reaction, and indirect bone pain can come from traction through muscle fascia causing inflammation of the periosteum. Periosteal inflammation (periosteal contusion) may also be instigated by direct trauma such as a kick to the shin. Muscular pain may be acute immediately following exertion, or chronic building over time.

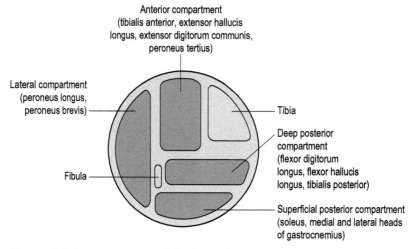

Figure 5.1 Compartments of the lower leg.

Table 5.2 Structures affected in compartment syndrome

- ▸ Bone – local stress fracture
- ▸ Osteofascia – periostitis or MTSS
- ▸ Muscle – tibialis anterior, peronei, extensor hallucis
- ▸ Nerve (local) – compression of superficial peroneal or posterior tibial nerves
- ▸ Nerve (root) – referred pain from sciatic compression
- ▸ Blood vessel – popliteal artery compression

MTSS – medial tibial stress syndrome.

Chronic pain may eventually become noticeable, even at rest. Neural compression may be local or pain referred from nerve root compression in the lumbar sacral spine. Finally, vascular signs may exist in cases of popliteal artery entrapment.

The pathophysiology of the condition is generally thought to include a sudden increase in muscle bulk in parallel with reduced compartment compliance due to stiffening and thickening of the connective tissue forming the compartments. Although muscle hypertrophy is a key feature of CECS, it is not the only cause. Bodybuilders rarely suffer from the condition, so the rate, rather than the amount, of muscle hypertrophy may be important. Vascular congestion results from reduced microcirculation and vascular congestion through a reduction in venous return. Intercompartment volume increases faster than the ability of the compartment wall to adapt. The resultant changes in oxygen balance to nerve and muscle, direct sensory nerve stimulation of fascia or periosteum and kinin release have all been proposed as sources of pain (Rajasekaran et al. 2012).

Anterior compartment syndrome

Anterior compartment syndrome involves pain in the anterior lower leg (Fig. 5.2A), which is increased in resisted dorsiflexion. There is usually a history of a sudden increase in training intensity, frequently involving jumping or running on a hard surface. The anterior compartment muscles swell, and in some cases hypertrophy occurs, giving a tense drum-like feel to palpation. The fascia covering the muscles may be too tight and inflexible to accommodate the increase in size. As a consequence, when the muscles relax, their intramuscular pressure remains high and fresh blood is unable to perfuse the tissues freely. This decrease in blood flow leads to ischaemia with associated pain and impairment of muscle function – resisted dorsiflexion often scoring lower than the unaffected limb.

Usually, when a muscle contracts, its blood flow is temporarily stopped. Arterial inflow occurs once more between the muscle contractions as

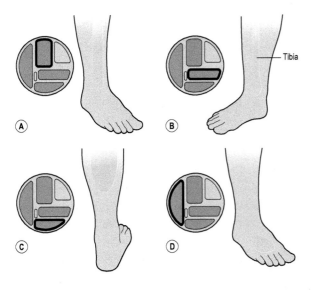

Area of pain/altered sensation

Figure 5.2 (A) Anterior compartment syndrome. Pain on the anterolateral aspect of the lower leg. (B) Deep posterior compartment syndrome (medial tibial stress syndrome). Pain over distal third of tibia. (C) Superficial posterior compartment syndrome. Pain within the calf bulk. (D) Lateral compartment syndrome. Loss of sensation over the dorsum of the foot.

the intramuscular pressure falls. Normal resting pressure within the tibialis anterior in the supine subject is about 5–10 mmHg, increasing to as much as 150–250 mmHg with muscle contraction. Muscle relaxation pressure, that which occurs between repeated contractions, is between 15 and 25 mmHg in the normal subject, but in athletes with anterior compartment syndrome pressures may rise to 30–35 mmHg and take up to 15 minutes to return to normal values (Styf 1989).

> **Key point**
>
> In anterior compartment syndrome, the resting pressure within the tibialis anterior can be 50 per cent greater than normal.

The intracompartment pressure (ICP) may be measured using several invasive techniques,

including mamometry (side-ported, split catheter, or standard needle) and solid-state transducer intracompartment catheters (Hislop and Tierney 2011). Non-invasive techniques are also available using a small (5 mm diameter) indenter to measure quantitative hardness of the shin compartment as an objective measure of tissue tension (Steinberg 2005).

Lateral compartment and superficial peroneal nerve

This is a less common cause of shin pain and occurs when the peroneal muscles are affected, often by hyperpronation. The condition may have existed for some time but is brought to the fore when running begins. Again, there is ischaemia and pain, but in addition the superficial peroneal nerve may be compressed as it emerges from the lateral compartment.

The superficial peroneal nerve lies deep to the peroneus longus and then passes forwards and downwards between the peronei and the extensor digitorum longus. It pierces the fascia in the distal third of the leg, where it divides into medial and lateral branches to enter the foot. Entrapment may occur if muscle herniation or fascial defects exist. In addition, ankle sprain, fasciotomy and an anomalous course of the nerve have been suggested as contributory factors (Styf 1989). Clinically, the patient presents with loss of sensation over the dorsum of the foot, especially the second to fourth toes (Fig. 5.2D). Certain resting positions may compress the nerve and bring on the symptoms. To test the nerve, it is compressed over the anterior intermuscular septum 8–15 cm proximal to the lateral malleolus while the patient actively dorsiflexes and everts the foot. Tinel's sign, involving local percussion over the compression site, may be positive.

> **Key point**
>
> With lateral compartment syndrome the superficial peroneal nerve may be compressed, giving loss of sensation over

the dorsum of the second, third and fourth toes. To test the nerve, compress it 8–15 cm proximal to the lateral malleolus while the patient actively dorsiflexes and everts the foot.

Posterior compartment

The superficial posterior compartment contains the soleus and gastrocnemius (together with plantaris). These muscles are usually affected by trauma rather than ischaemia. Pain occurs within the calf bulk (Fig. 5.2C) and is increased with resisted plantarflexion.

The deep posterior compartment contains tibialis posterior, flexor digitorum longus (FDL) and flexor hallucis longus (FHL), and is a common site for CECS in distance runners. Pain in this region is usually experienced over the distal third of the medial tibia (Fig. 5.2B), either within muscle or directly over bone. The latter is described as medial tibial stress syndrome (MTSS). The exact site of pain will vary depending on the specific structures affected, with bone shaft being deeper than periosteum or muscle.

Medial tibial stress syndrome

Medial tibial stress syndrome (MTSS) is shin pain over the distal third of the inner aspect of the tibia. The disorder is a traction periostitis, and pain in this region must be differentiated from CECS of the deep posterior compartment (above).

Definition

Medial tibial stress syndrome is pain over the distal third of the inner aspect of the tibia. The disorder may affect the bone, periosteum (bone membrane), fascia or muscles.

Type I MTSS involves microfractures or stress fracture of the bone itself. The patient is usually a runner who has recently increased his or her mileage. The stress imposed by the sport exceeds the ability of the bone to adapt and remodel. The condition may present as a stress fracture, showing a concentrated positive uptake in a single area on bone scan and point tenderness to palpation, or as a diffuse area along the medial edge of the tibia, giving more generalized pain. In chronic conditions which have existed for some time, the tibial edge may be uneven due to new bone formation (Fig. 5.3A).

Type II medial tibial stress syndrome involves the junction of the periosteum and fascia, and occurs particularly in sprinters and those involved in jumping activities. Pain is maximal just posterior to the bone, and has often persisted for a number of years. Initially, pain occurs only with activity, but as the condition progresses discomfort is felt with walking and even at rest. In this condition, compartment pressures may not be elevated, and the periosteum is unchanged. During the chronic stage of this condition, adipose tissue has been found, during surgery, between the periosteum and underlying bone (Detmer 1986). In the early stages of the condition, the periosteum may heal back with rest, but when the condition becomes chronic it is unable to heal, and continues to cause pain when stressed by activity.

The Type III condition involves ischaemia of the distal deep posterior compartment and presents as a dull ache over the posterior soft tissues brought on by exercise. Intramuscular pressures are elevated and remain elevated after exercise (Fig. 5.3B).

Traction from muscle attachment is the most likely cause of the condition, the attachment of tibialis posterior normally being associated with the condition. However, both the soleus and flexor digitorum longus may also be implicated. The medial fibres of soleus and the attached fascia extend over the deep posterior compartment, forming a region known as the soleus bridge, an area implicated in MTSS. Excessive pronation is thought to be a significant factor in the development of the condition. The muscles attaching to the posterior border of the tibia become overactive in an attempt to slow the rate of pronation and limit its degree. This deceleration

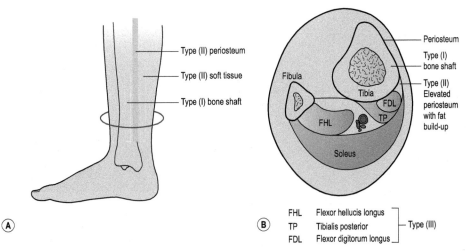

Figure 5.3 Medial tibial stress syndrome. (A) Painful areas of palpation. (B) Cross-section of structures affected. After Detmer, D.E. (1986) Chronic shin splints: classification and management of medial tibial stress syndrome. *Sports Medicine*, **3**, 436–444. With permission.

results in eccentric overload and the consequent traction stress, which may be higher in those who overpronate (Bradshaw et al. 2007).

The condition usually demonstrates a clear X-ray, but bone scan can show patchy diffuse areas (bone stress reaction) rather than the focal uptake of stress fracture, although asymptomatic individuals can also demonstrate these appearances (Batt et al. 1998), showing that diagnosis must be multifactorial.

Management

Initial management of shin pain includes a reduction of the stresses which caused the condition in the first place. This involves accurately identifying the structures affected and taking a thorough history of causal factors, particularly stresses imposed during training. Temporary pain relief may be achieved using deload taping to limit the fascial traction thought to be part of the pathology. Taping is applied in a spiral, beginning on the lateral aspect of the ankle just above the lateral malleolus. The tape is wound around the shin, going behind the calf and emerging once more onto the front of the tibia. As the tape is applied, it is pulled proximally to unload the fascia

(Fig. 5.4A). Another approach is to place anchors just below the knee and just above the ankle, and connect the anchors with two or three strips of zinc oxide taping, gathering the skin up to take tension away (Fig. 5.4B). Both tapes alter the fascial loading and give temporary relief only.

K tape (kinesiology tape) has been shown to decrease the rate of medial loading in athletes with MTSS (Griebert et al. 2016). A single Y-strip is applied, with the base of the Y at the superomedial aspect of the tibia. The Y tails travel down the medial tibia, passing anterior and posterior to the medial malleolus to the arch of the foot (Fig. 5.4C). A higher time to peak force (TTPF) was seen in healthy volunteers and those with MTSS following K tape application, demonstrating a slower rate of medial loading.

Biomechanical assessment of the lower limb is often helpful and prescription of orthotics should be made where necessary. An increased navicular drop (reduction of the medial arch height on weightbearing) has been linked with the development of MTSS (Hamstra-Wright 2015). Correction of overpronation and reduced medial arch height would therefore seem appropriate, at least in the short term, to reduce symptoms.

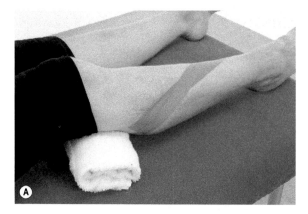

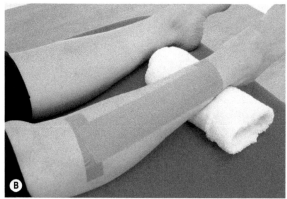

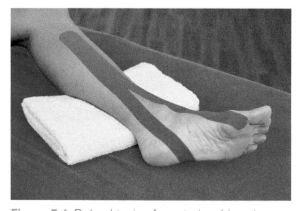

Figure 5.4 Deload taping for anterior shin pain: (A) spiral (B) strip (C) K tape.

Initially, rest and anti-inflammatory modalities may be used to allow the acute inflammation to settle, but external compression and elevation of the limb can exacerbate the problem in some athletes so symptom reaction should be monitored. Some athletes report anecdotal improvement using compression socks, however. If training stresses can be modified, and the condition has been identified early enough, this may be all that is required.

One of the key points about bone pain in shin splints is that the bone is reacting to stress (see also overtraining syndrome, Treatment Note 2.1). All tissues react to a stressor (overload), be it impact, weight training or stretching. The demand placed on the tissue challenges it and stimulates adaptation. If the tissue stress is not great enough, no adaptation will occur, but if the stress is excessive, the breakdown of tissue will be greater than its ability to adapt, and the condition will progress to overtraining, and pathology.

The initial management of shin pain is to reduce loading on the tissues. This may mean complete rest if the condition is very painful, or just reducing running mileage if there is less pain. Unloading the tissue with taping or changing footwear or running surface may also help. Once pain begins to subside, tissue loading should resume, but be graded. Simply to rest until pain has eased and then return to running at the same level will challenge the now-weakened tissue too much. The subject should begin at a level which does not cause an excessive reaction. If the next day there is no bone pain, gradually build up the tissue loading (mileage, changing surface, speed work, hill work) while monitoring the body reaction. With time, subjects will be able to do more before pain onset. Eventually the damaged tissues will have been strengthened sufficiently to return to full pain-free training.

In chronic conditions in which conservative management has failed, decompression by fasciotomy or fasciectomy may be called for. With fasciotomy the fascia of the affected compartment is surgically split along its length. The procedure is often performed on an outpatient basis, with two incisions being made, at the junction of the proximal and middle third of the leg and the middle and distal third. Subjects mobilize early and are often able to resume running after three weeks. Where fasciotomy fails, fasciectomy may be performed. Here, a longer open incision is made and a ribbon of fascia is removed. Because a longer incision is made, there is an increased risk of infection and dehiscence (incision bursting open). A longer rehabilitation period may be required, depending on incision healing time. Full return to sport may be expected in eight to twelve weeks.

> **Definition**
> *Fasciotomy* is surgical splitting (cutting) of the fascia to reduce pressure within the fascial compartment. *Fascietomy* is the surgical removal of a ribbon of fascia.

Running re-education

Running form can be used effectively as part of the management of CECS. Several common errors may occur. First, control of the pelvis over the lower limb in the frontal plane is important. A positive Trendelenburg sign (pelvis dipping down as one leg is lifted from the ground) suggests weakness or lack of control over the hip abductor muscles. Viewing the subject from behind when running often shows excessive pelvic dip and/or wide foot stance (feet apart). Overstriding (each step too

long) coupled with a slow gait cycle may also be seen. Shorter steps and increasing cadence (using a metronome beat on a smartphone) can alter tissue loading sufficiently to modify symptoms and speed recovery. Excessive hip flexion will increase loading on the anterior tibials at heel strike compared to a reduced hip flexion and more vertical orientation of the tibia (midfoot strike). This action will be coupled with a faster cadence, as above.

Postural optimisation may also be helpful. Although many top runners demonstrate what would normally be considered a 'poor posture' (round shoulders, tight hips, asymmetry of arm and/or leg action), optimising posture may modify symptoms sufficiently for the condition to resolve. A subject should try to run more upright (tall rather than slouched) and correct any glaring asymmetries such as one foot turning out further than the other or one hip hitching. Video the subject from behind and from the side and see if changing obvious postural features affects shin pain. The table below shows some factors to consider. Remember, though, that while postural features may help to change your symptoms, there is really no good and bad posture – only one which works best for you. Table 5.3 summarises key aspects of running re-education in CECS.

Table 5.3 Aspects of running re-education in CECS

Action	Justification
Bent knee at heelstrike	▶ Tibia more vertical reducing vertical reaction force ▶ Quads less active allowing lower limb shock attenuation
Reduce overstrike	▶ Shorter cadence (more steps) ▶ Foot further under hip ▶ Mid-foot contact rather than heel strike
Quicker cadence	▶ Produce of feature above ▶ Use metronome and add 1 beat per minute (BPM) each week upto 80-90 BPM
Relaxed posture	▶ Knees and hips softer ▶ Shoulders and jaw released ▶ Forearms and hands lower
Body alignment	▶ Trunk for upright 'think tall' ▶ Pelvis neutral ▶ Shoulders further back to open chest
Strength & stretch	▶ Lower limb, trunk, and arm?shoulder strength important ▶ Flexibility of hips/ankles/feet

Treatment note 5.1 Manual therapy for shin pain

Trigger point massage

Trigger point (TrP) massage for anterior compartment syndrome focuses on the tibialis anterior and the extensor digitorum longus. The TrP for the tibialis anterior is located approximately a third of the way distally from the knee and to the lateral side of the tibia. A muscle-stripping technique can be used, starting from half way down the tibia and progressing up towards the knee in a slow movement, gradually progressing in depth (Fig. 5.5). The thickness of the muscle means that both thumbs must be used simultaneously or a pressure tool where ischaemic compression is used. The elbow is the tool of choice, direct compression is given and maintained for three to ten seconds or until pain subsides.

The long toe extensors (extensor digitorum longus (EDL) and extensor hallucis longus (EHL)) may be similarly treated. The EDL TrP is located approximately eight centimetres distal and slightly anterior to the head of the fibula. The EHL is located at the junction of the middle of the distal thirds of the lower leg (Fig. 5.6). Home stretching may again be used, this time forcing the foot into plantarflexion and the distal toes into flexion.

For lateral compartment syndrome, the peroneus longus and peroneus brevis muscles are targeted.

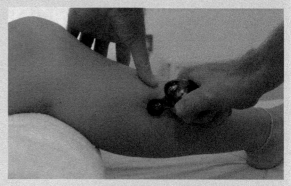

Figure 5.6 Trigger points of the long toe extensors.

The TrP for peroneus longus is approximately two to four centimetres distal to the fibular head, close to the shaft of the fibular itself, while that of the peroneus brevis is located at the junction of the middle and distal third of the lower leg.

Ischaemic compression may be used with the thumbs, and ice stretch may again be given, this time stretching the foot into plantarflexion and inversion (Fig. 5.7).

Posterior compartment syndrome and medial tibial stress syndrome require treatment of the flexor digitorum longus (FDL) and tibialis posterior along the lower third of the posterior edge of the

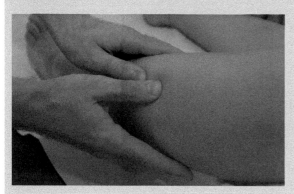

Figure 5.5 Muscle stripping technique for tibialis anterior trigger point.

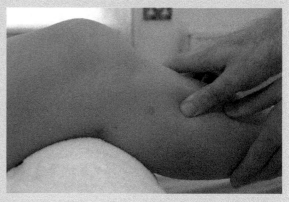

Figure 5.7 Trigger points of the lateral compartment muscles.

Treatment note 5.1 *continued*

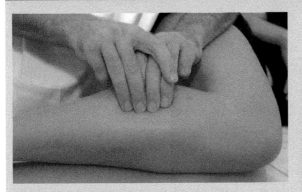

Figure 5.8 Trigger points of the posterior compartment.

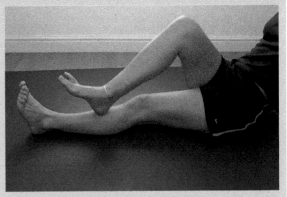

Figure 5.9 Self-treatment of the tibialis anterior using the heel.

tibia. Where the muscle itself is stressed, the TrP is targeted on the medial border of the upper tibia. The patient lies in crook, side-lying, and the palpation point is between the medial edge of the tibia and the gastrocnemius muscles (Fig. 5.8). The gastrocnemius is pushed posteriorly and the pressure is then applied downward and then laterally. For the flexor hallucis longus (FHL), the patient may be treated in prone and this time the thumb is positioned lateral to the mid-line, pressing on the edge of the soleus at the junction between the middle and lower thirds of the lower leg.

Self-help trigger point methods

The athlete may be taught to use trigger-point therapy as a self-treatment to relieve pain as it occurs. For the tibialis anterior, the easiest method is to use the heel of the opposite foot (Fig. 5.9). The movement is on the lateral edge of the tibia and begins at mid-shin level, the pressure being in a continuous sweep towards the lateral edge of the knee.

For the peroneal muscles, pressure may be given by the index finger, supported by the middle finger or by a single flexed knuckle (Fig. 5.10). For the flexor digitorum longus and tibialis posterior, one or two fingers may suffice. Alternatively, hands may wrap around the shin

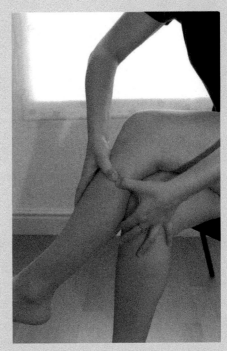

Figure 5.10 Self-treatment of the peroneus longus using both hands.

and both thumbs may be used to apply to the peroneus longus.

Use of massage tools and foam rollers may also be of use in some cases, and so athletes should be taught the correct method of application and

Treatment note 5.1 *continued*

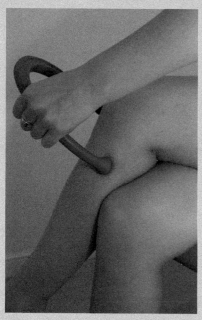

Figure 5.11 Creating more force by using the 'backnobber' apparatus. Pressure Positive Co., with permission.

incorporate this intervention as part of a broader treatment programme (Fig 5.11).

Dry needling techniques for trigger-point therapy

For anterior tibial syndrome, traditional acupuncture points on the stomach meridian may be used. Point ST. 36, located three finger breadths below the lateral aspect of the knee, and point ST. 40, located midway between the lateral maleolus and the knee joint line, may be used. Lateral compartment syndrome responds to needling along the gall-bladder meridian. GB 34, located distal and lateral to the head of the fibula, and GB 39, located three finger breadths above the apex of the lateral maleolus on the edge of the tibia, may be used.

For medial tibial stress syndrome, the point Sp. 6 may be used; located three finger breadths above the apex of the medial maleolus on the edge of the tibia, this point is directly opposite GB 39 (Fig. 5.12). See Norris (2001) for specific details.

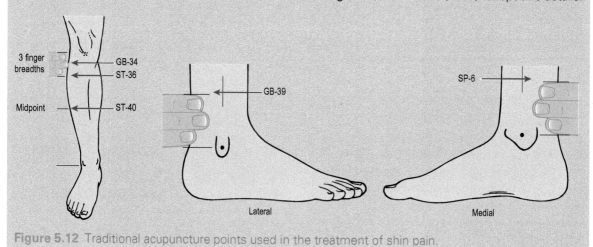

Figure 5.12 Traditional acupuncture points used in the treatment of shin pain.

Stress fractures

Over 50 per cent of all stress fractures occur to the tibia and fibula with the remaining sites being mostly to the lower limb (Fig. 5.13). Stress fractures are usually the end point in a sequence of overuse. A number of causal factors usually coexist to begin the development of the condition. Training errors may account for 60 to 75 per cent of such injuries in runners (McBryde 1985). Common

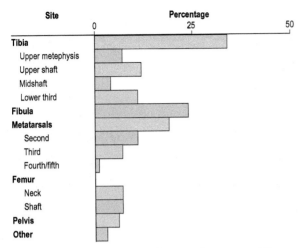

Figure 5.13 Distribution of stress fractures. After McBryde (1985), with permission.

faults include high-intensity work carried out for too long with an inadequate recovery, for example a distance runner who suddenly increases mileage. Faulty footwear which fails to attenuate shock and exercising on unforgiving surfaces will also contribute to lower limb pathology. These factors, coupled with an underlying malalignment problem of the lower limb, may exacerbate the problem. With novice runners, an additional factor is muscular weakness in the lower extremity, leading to a reduction in shock-absorbing capacity of the soft tissues. In each case, the overload on the tissues exceeds the elastic limit, causing a plastic deformation of bone.

Very often, the stress fracture is a direct result of a change of some type – in the athletes themselves, in the environment in which they train, or in the activity. In terms of the athlete, stress fractures often emerge following the onset of a growth spurt or at the menopause as a result of the major body adaptations occurring at these times. Similarly, following illness, the body must be allowed time to readapt to training demands. Environmental changes, such as new clothing (shoes) or a new playing surface, will also require time to allow tissue adaptation, and failure to allow for this may lead to tissue breakdown, of which stress fractures are one type. Finally, alterations in the quality or

quantity of a training programme itself will require a period of adaptation.

Far from being inert, bone is a dynamic tissue which is continually remodelling in response to mechanical stress. A balance usually exists between bone proliferation and reabsorption, which maintains the bone integrity. The result of athletic activity is normally that bone strengthens, but if unbalanced stresses cause bone reabsorption to exceed proliferation, the bone weakens.

> **Key point**
> Exercise (loading) normally causes microscopic damage within bone, and the body responds by producing stronger bone material. If the amount of damage caused by loading is greater than the ability of the bone to restrengthen, stress fracture occurs.

Examining excessive running and jumping in rabbits, Li et al. (1985) demonstrated that osteoblastic activity occurred from seven to nine days later than osteoclastic activity. Remodelling began on day two, with the haversian blood vessels dilating, and by day seven osteoclastic activity was noted in the bone cortex. New bone formation began in the periosteum by the fourteenth day of excessive stress. The adaptation to this excessive stress was reabsorption, which occurred for some time before the formation of new cortical bone, thus weakening the bone structure. Abnormal X-rays were not found until day 21 after the stress was imposed.

Angular stresses, in particular, may cause failure of the bone, with a resultant stress fracture. Two theories are generally accepted for the mechanisms by which stress affects bone. The first (fatigue) proposes that training which is too intense causes the muscles to fatigue so that they are no longer able to support the skeleton and absorb shock. The strain passes to the bone, causing the fracture. The second theory (overload) suggests that when certain muscles contract, they cause the bones to bend slightly. Training which is too intense will exceed the capacity of the bone to recover from this stress.

Signs and symptoms

The main symptom of a stress fracture is pain. This has been categorized into four types, depending on its characteristics (Puffer and Zachazewski 1988). With Type I pain, the athlete only feels discomfort after activity. With Type II and III pain, discomfort is felt while training, but with Type II this does not restrict activity. Type IV pain is chronic and unremitting in nature. Further symptoms include warmth and tenderness over the injured area, made worse by sporting activity and better with rest. Swelling may be evident in the later stages of the condition if the bony surface is superficial. Accuracy of palpation when assessing bone pain is vital. The tenderness of a stress fracture is usually well localized, whereas that of compartment syndrome is more diffuse. Initially, radiographs are usually negative – it takes at least two weeks for X-ray changes to be apparent. Local periosteal reaction and new bone growth may be seen after six weeks in long bone and compressive stress fractures in cancellous bone are sometimes visible after twenty-four hours (Puddu et al. 1994). Taunton and Clement (1981) found radiographs to be positive in only 47.2 per cent of their cases, while bone scan was accurate in 95.8 per cent. Bone scan is normally revealing at the onset of symptoms and is generally more reliable. Phosphate labelled with technetium-99 m is incorporated into osteoblasts and a hot spot appears over the active area, 6 to 72 hours after the onset of pain (Puddu et al. 1994).

Pain may be produced over the superficial fracture site by vibration. This may be produced from a tuning fork or ultrasound unit, and is generally of more use in low-risk areas, such as the foot and shin. Where there is a risk of complication through displacement (such as in the neck of the femur) bone scan with possible surgical intervention may be more appropriate (Fig. 5.14).

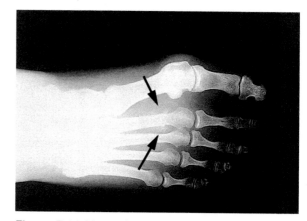

Figure 5.14 X-ray of stress fracture. From Read (2000), with permission.

Treatment

Treatment of a stress fracture is primarily rest. As a general guide, with Type I or II pain the workload should be reduced by 25 per cent and 50 per cent, respectively. Total rest is called for where Type III pain is experienced, and Type IV pain requires immediate medical investigation (Table 5.4). In the more severe conditions, rest should be total, because even allowing an athlete to train the upper body will often result in 'just trying the leg out' in the gym. Training should not resume until the athlete has been totally pain free for ten days. It should be emphasized to the athlete that this means that at the end of each day he or she should

Table 5.4 Pain classification

Classification	Characteristics	Action
Type I	Pain only after activity	↓ workload by 25%
Type II	Pain during activity but not restricting performance	↓ workload by 50%
Type III	Pain during activity restricting performance	Total rest
Type IV	Chronic unremitting pain at rest	Splint/cast Medical investigation

After Puffer and Zachazewshi (1988).

go to bed having felt no pain over the injured area during that day.

The timescale of healing will vary depending on the site of injury. With reduced activity, fibular stress fractures will normally heal in four to six weeks, tibial stress fractures in eight to ten weeks and femoral neck stress fractures in twelve to sixteen weeks.

When activity is resumed, the athlete should be closely monitored, and activities stopped if any pain occurs. Return to sport should be progressive and varied. Different speed, running surfaces and activities should all be used to spread the emphasis of training. Alternative training should be used to reduce the weightbearing on the limb. Swimming and cycling may be utilized to restore cardiopulmonary fitness, for example.

Tennis leg

Of the sural muscles, it is the gastrocnemius which is usually injured. The soleus is infrequently affected by trauma, being a single-joint muscle, but is more usually the victim of temporary ischaemia, giving rise to superficial posterior compartment syndrome. Both conditions must be differentiated from neural and vascular conditions. Pain in the calf may be referred from the lumbar spine or entrapment of the sciatic nerve further down, the S2 dermatome referring into the back of the thigh and calf. An inability to raise onto the toes of one foot in standing is a test for S1-2 nerve root entrapment (tibial nerve) in a case of lower-back history in the absence of calf symptoms. Neural involvement can be differentiated using the straight-leg raise variations and slump test (see Chapter 8). Vascular symptoms include claudication, usually from popliteal artery entrapment (see below), although in older patients calf and thigh claudication may occur in the presence of atherosclerotic disease.

True tennis leg is a strain of the gastrocnemius muscle itself, normally involving the medial head at its musculotendinous junction with the Achilles tendon. The history of injury is usually a sudden

propulsive action, such as a lunge or jump, as the athlete pushes off from the mark. Women are more commonly affected than men, and the athlete is typically over 30 years of age. The condition is often described as a rupture of the plantaris, more by tradition than anything else, because this muscle is rarely the cause of symptoms. A gastrocnemius strain usually occurs between the middle and proximal third of the muscle, with the medial belly more often affected. Palpation reveals a painful area, and with injuries affecting larger areas of the muscle, palpable scarring may be felt as tissue repair progresses.

> ### Key point
> Calf muscle strain usually affects the gastrocnemius muscle rather than the soleus. The medial head of the muscle is more commonly affected, at the junction of the middle and proximal third.

The athlete often feels something 'go' in the back of the leg, as though he or she were hit from behind. Pain and spasm occur rapidly, preventing the athlete from putting the heel to the ground. Later, swelling and bruising develop distal to the injury site, peaking at 48 hours after injury. There is local tenderness over the medial head of gastrocnemius at the junction between the middle and proximal third of the calf. Pain to passive stretch is worse with the knee straight than with it flexed.

Initial treatment is to immobilize the calf to prevent further tissue damage. Some authorities recommend a plantarflexed position with a 2–4 cm heel lift, while others claim that a 90-degree neutral ankle position gives a better result by preventing contraction and tightening the fascia to limit the spread of bruising. Pain and the amount of tissue damage is usually the deciding factor. Partial ruptures are best immobilized non-weightbearing in plantarflexion to approximate the tissue, whereas less serious injuries can be prevented from shortening by adopting a neutral resting position. Taping has been shown to reduce gastrocnemius activity (Alexander et al. 2008). Applying undertaping and taping reduced the muscle activation measured by the Hoffman reflex (H-reflex) by 19 per cent for the medial gastrocnemius and 13 per cent for the lateral gastrocnemius.

Compression from an elastic bandage limits the formation of swelling, and strength and flexibility is maintained by starting rehabilitation early. Massage involving calf kneading and transverse frictions can aid broadening of the muscle fibres. Stretching to the gastrocnemius begins in the long sitting position. A towel or band is placed over the foot and the athlete gently pulls the foot into dorsiflexion. Stretching with the toes on a block in a partial, and later full, weightbearing position is the exercise progression. Strength is regained by utilizing a comparable long sitting position but substituting an elastic band for the strap. The foot is pressed into plantarflexion against the resistance of the band. Heel raises are performed in a standing position, initially from the floor and later with the heel on a 2–3 cm block. Strength should be increased to that of the uninjured leg.

Gait re-education is used to encourage equal stride length and the adoption of a normal heel-toe rhythm avoiding external rotation of the leg. When the calf is pain free, strength activities give way to power movements, to build up the fast twitch nature of the muscle (Ng and Richardson 1990). Gentle jogging, jumping and skipping are used and progressed to plyometrics. The athlete should be instructed to jump and land correctly. The toes should be the last point to leave the floor in a jump and the first to contact the floor on landing. Toe contact is followed by progressive lowering through the foot, with the knee and hip flexing as the heel touches the floor to minimize shock. Flat-foot landing and remaining on the toes must be avoided (Fig. 5.15). Slow squats raising up onto the toes at the top point give way to toe-springing actions with and without weight resistance (dumbbells or a weighted jacket). Leg drives from a mark are useful, as are 'side hops' and 'hop and twist' actions over a bar.

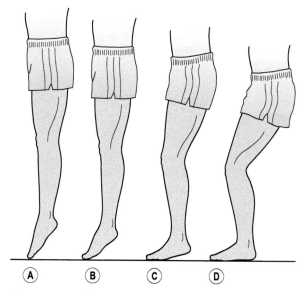

Figure 5.15 Correct landing action from a jump. (A) Toe contacts floor first. (B) Foot flexes to absorb shock. (C,D) Knee and hip flex ('give') as heel touches ground.

Popliteal artery entrapment

Popliteal artery entrapment syndrome (PAES) may be either structural or functional in nature (Stager and Clement 1999). Structural changes (Fig. 5.16) include abnormal attachment of the medial head of gastrocnemius and additional tendinous remnants derived from the medial head. In long-standing cases, arterial wall degeneration may occur. Functional entrapment occurs when the popliteal structures appear normal, but compression occurs during activity. Differentiation of PAES during exercise-induced calf pain must be made from compartment syndrome. Pain occurs during exercise in both conditions, but with PAES pain stops immediately on cessation of exercise, whereas compartment syndrome pain typically dies down slowly, taking 30–60 minutes to ease after exercise. Functional PAES is more normal with younger strength-trained athletes and it is thought that plantarflexion compresses the artery between the underlying bone and muscle in the presence of hypertrophy of the gastrocnemius

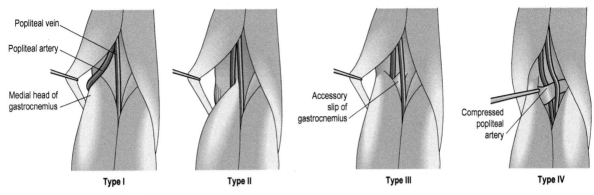

Figure 5.16 Structural variation in popliteal artery entrapment. From Pillai (2008).

muscle. Prevalence of functional PAES has been estimated to be as high as 50 per cent in the normal population (Pillai 2008).

Although pain is the prevalent symptom, signs of ischaemia such as temperature changes, paraesthesia and skin discolouration may also occur. Initially, evaluation is through the absence of distal pulses after exertion. Further information may be gained using the *ankle to brachial pressure index* (ABPI), the ratio of the blood pressure (BP) in the lower legs to that of the arms. The patient rests for 20 minutes (supine lying) and then an automatic blood pressure monitor (sphygmomanometer) is used to test systolic brachial pressure (arm) and systolic ankle pressure. The presence of the pulse is registered using Doppler ultrasound, and the BP at the point when the pulse is first detected is used. The ABPI index is calculated by dividing the ankle systolic BP by the *higher* of the two brachial systolic BPs. Normal index values are 0.90–1.0, with lower values representing moderate (0.75–0.90) or severe (0.75–0.50) disease. Values less than 0.50 are said to represent limb-threatening vascular disease (Taylor and Kerry 2002). Full examination is by angiography, but the condition may be missed if these tests are not carried out in resisted plantarflexion. Training modification is the treatment of choice initially, with surgical division of fascial bands in extreme cases.

Treatment note 5.2 Treatment of gastrocnemius tear

Taping

Anchors are placed over the heel and the back of the knee (Fig. 5.17A). Zinc oxide tape is then applied, pre-stretched, between the heel and posterior knee (Fig. 5.17B).

Massage

The patient lies prone with the foot over the couch end and the lower shin supported on a rolled towel or block to unlock the knee. Effleurage is applied using the flat palm (Fig. 5.18A) or webspace (Fig. 10.18B). Deep pressure may be applied using the supported fingers (Fig. 5.18C) and fascial stretch using the forearm placed across the muscle (Fig. 5.18D).

Exercise therapy

Stretching for the gastrocnemis is performed with the knee straight, taking the bodyweight against a wall (Fig. 5.19A). The stretch is increased by placing the toes on a slim book or block (Fig. 5.19B). Dynamic stretching is performed in a 'sprint start' position, alternately plantarflexing and dorsiflexing the ankle (Fig. 5.19C). Heel-raise

Treatment note 5.2 *continued*

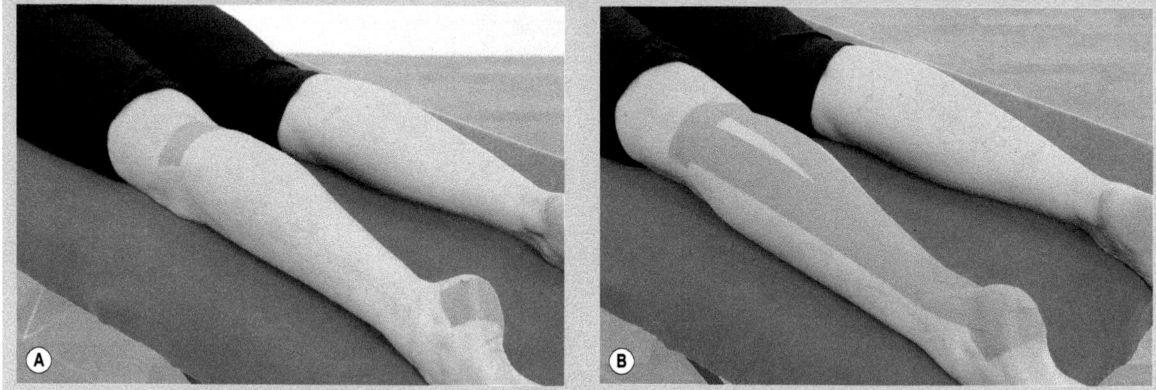

Figure 5.17 Calf taping (A) anchors (B) reins.

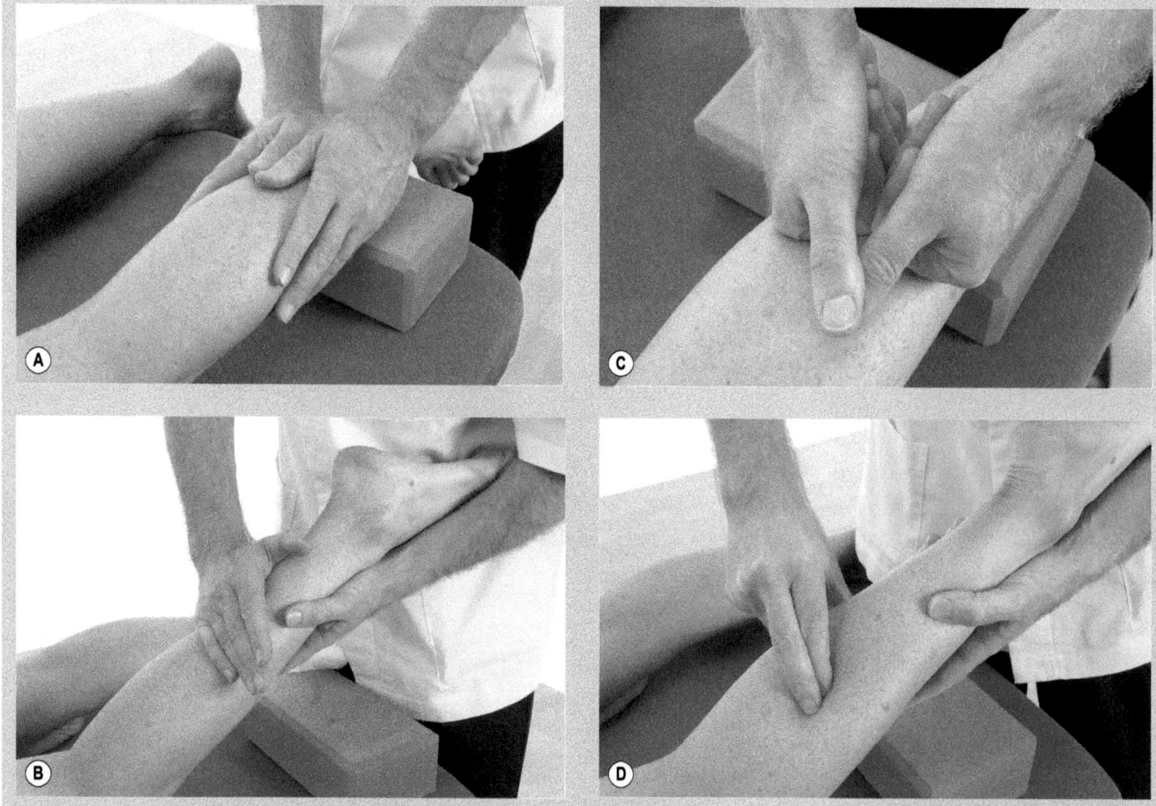

Figure 5.18 Example massage techniques for the calf.

activities using a dumbbell (Fig. 5.19D) may be used to strengthen the muscle, and light jogging progresses to running, sprinting, jumping and bounding.

Treatment note 5.2 *continued*

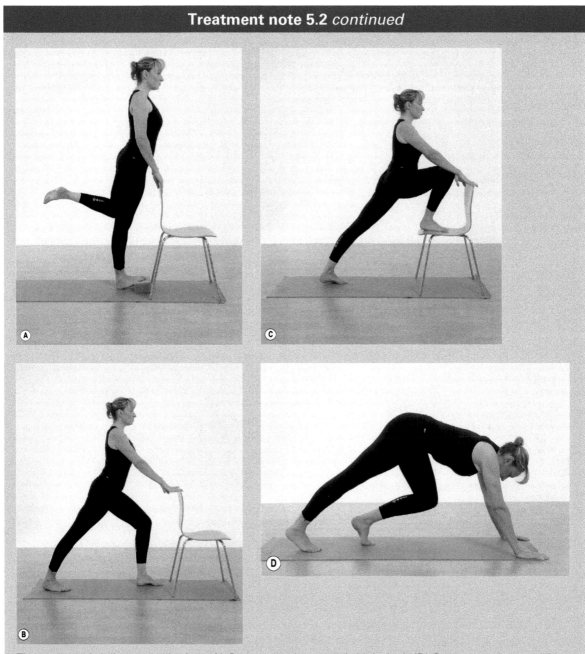

Figure 5.19 Achilles rehabilitation. (A) Gastrocnemius stretch (right leg). (B) Gastrocnemius stretch (right leg). (C) Soleus stretch (right leg). (D) Sprint start position.

Achilles tendon

Achilles tendon pain (achillodynia) is a common condition in sport, with the incidence in runners being as high as 9 per cent (Lysholm and Wiklander 1987). Interestingly, the condition was relatively uncommon until the 1950s; the increased incidence of Achilles tendon rupture may be a result of the increasingly sedentary lifestyles seen in Western industrialized countries (Kvist 1994).

The Achilles tendon is the largest tendon in the body, being some 15 cm long and about 2 cm thick. It is able to sustain loads of up to 17 times bodyweight while utilizing only 13 per cent of the oxygen supply of a muscle (Khan and Maffulli 1998). The tendon consists of connective tissue containing fibroblasts (tenoblasts) in a ground substance. The main extracellular component (80 per cent of the dry weight of the tendon) is collagen, predominently Type I, with a small amount of Type III. The ground substance consists of proteoglycans and glycosaminoglycan (GAG) chains. In a normal tendon, the amount of ground substance is minimal and not visible using light microscopy (Cook, Khan and Purdam 2002).

Definition

Type I collagen is white and glistening and consists of large-diameter fibres. It is found predominantly in skin and tendon. Type III collagen forms a delicate supporting network and is more common in young and repairing tissue. It is found commonly in skin and blood-vessel walls.

Analysis of normal and ruptured Achilles tendon has shown that ruptured tendon has a greater percentage of Type III collagen, making the tendon less resistant to tensile forces and increasing the risk of rupture (Maffulli, Ewen and Waterston 2000).

The tendon originates from the musculotendinous junction of the calf muscles, the soleus inserting lower down on the deep surface of the tendon. The Achilles tendon gradually becomes more

Table 5.5 Structures to consider in differential diagnosis of Achilles tendon pain

- ▶ Sural (short saphenous) nerve
- ▶ Lumbar referral (L4–S2)
- ▶ Foot and toe tendons (especially medial)
- ▶ Ankle impingement (especially posterior)
- ▶ Retrocalcaneal bursitis
- ▶ Haglund's deformity
- ▶ Tarsal tunnel structures
- ▶ Kager's fat pad (triangle)

rounded as it travels distally, and flares out to insert into the posterior aspect of the calcaneum. The tendon is separated from the calcaneum by the retrocalcaneal bursa and from the skin by the subcutaneous calcaneal bursa. The tendon blood supply enters via the deep surface, making injection of any vessel abnormality with sclerosant more difficult than in other regions. Several structures are within the same body part and so should be considered in the differential diagnosis of Achilles tendon pain (Table 5.5).

Key point

The retrocalcaneal bursa separates the Achilles tendon from the calcaneum (heel bone). The subcutaneous calcaneal bursa separates the tendon from the skin.

The force from the Achilles tendon is delivered not through its insertion into the calcaneum, but via the point of contact on the posterior aspect of the calcaneum over the retrocalcaneal bursa. With increasing plantarflexion, the tendon 'unrolls' in such a way that this contact point moves lower down. In this way, the lever arm is maintained throughout the range of motion (Fig. 5.20).

The whole tendon rotates through 90 degrees as it descends, so that the medial fibres become posterior by the time the tendon attaches to the calcaneum. This rotation is thought in part to account for the elastic properties of the tendon, giving it an elastic recoil when stretched. In the running action, as the lower limb moves from heel strike to mid-stance, the Achilles tendon is

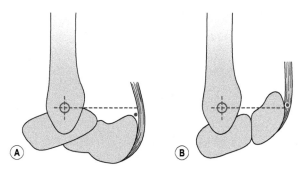

Figure 5.20 Contact point of Achilles tendon moves downwards as plantarflexion increases.

stretched, storing elastic energy. At toe-off, the tendon recoils, releasing its stored energy and reducing the work required from the calf muscles to propel the body forwards.

The Achilles tendon is surrounded by a soft membranous paratenon (peritendon), which is continuous proximally with the muscle fascia and distally with the calcaneal periosteum. The paratenon consists of the epitenon or inner layer, which lies directly over the Achilles tendon itself, and the paratenon proper, which comprises the outer layer. The paratenon does not have a synovial layer, in contrast to the tendon sheaths of the hand, for example.

On the medial and lateral aspects of the dorsal surface there are thin spaces between the tendon and skin. These spaces are filled with thin gliding membranes covered in lubricating mucopolysaccharides. The membranes move freely over each other and greatly reduce friction. On the ventral side of the tendon there is fatty areolar tissue and connective tissue containing blood vessels.

The blood supply to the tendon is from either end and from the paratenon itself, but a relatively avascular zone exists between two and six centimetres proximal to the tendon insertion. Under normal circumstances, blood vessels do not travel from the paratenon to the tendon substance, and removal of the paratenon does not seem to compromise the blood supply. Tendon tissue in general has a low metabolic rate, and this, coupled with the poor blood supply to the tendon, means that the structure has a slow rate of healing. Although anatomically the blood flow to the tendon seems poor, investigation using laser Doppler has found that the blood supply is actually of a similar volume throughout its length (Astrom and Westlin 1994). Changes in tendon blood flow are, however, important to tendon pathology (Malliaras et al. 2008).

Injuries to the Achilles tendon fall broadly into one of two categories. First, those which affect the tendon substance (partial or complete rupture), and, second, injury to the surface of the tendon and its covering (tendinopathy or peritendinopathy).

Tendinopathy

The term tendonitis implies an inflammation within the tendon substance. However, the pathology of chronic exercise-induced tendon injury is that there is no triphasic inflammatory response, and inflammatory cells are rarely found. As such, the term *tendinopathy* is now used to describe local pain and swelling around but not within the tendon. *Tendinosis* is a term used to refer to histological changes which have been confirmed using biopsy or scanning.

> **Definition**
>
> Tendinopathy refers to a combination of tendon pain and local swelling. Tendinosis is present when these changes are verified on tendon biopsy or through ultrasound scanning.

Tendinopathy presents as pain and thickening of the Achilles tendon of gradual onset, and may occur in the mid substance of the Achilles, in which case tensile overload appears to be an important factor (Cook et al. 2017), occurring as part of the energy storage function of the tendon. Where pain is at the teno-osseous (T/O) junction, pathology may be due to compression and shear rather than tensile force. The T/O junction (*enthesis*) sees the tendon compressed against the bone, giving a mechanical advantage. The compression forces are reduced by fibrocartilage within the tendon, and the presence of the bursa between the tendon and bone.

> **Definition**
>
> An *enthesis* is a connective tissue region between tendon or ligament and bone. The enthesis may be fibrous or fibrocartilaginous.

Tendinopathy is said to develop along a continuum (Cook and Purdam 2009), with three interrelated phases – reaction, repair, and degeneration (Table 5.6). Histological changes show a failed healing response, which leaves the tendon open to further injury. The condition (reactive tendinopathy) is a non-inflammatory response where tendon cells activate and produce more proteoglycan. The proteoglycan in turn increases the amount of bound water within the tendon, thickening it. This change is visible on MRI and US scanning, which also demonstrates that there is little collagen fibre disruption. Additionally, the thickened tendon is often visibly and palpably different to the contralateral side.

Tendon disrepair demonstrates greater extra-cellular matrix (ECM) breakdown and tendon cells taking on a more rounded appearance. Collagen and proteoglycans increase, causing collagen to separate and the ECM to become disorganized,

with ingrowth of small nerve fibres and blood vessels. Sonography reveals hypoechoic areas, with some increased vascularity and nerve-fibre ingrowth.

Degenerative tendinopathy represents the final stage in a progressive degenerative process. Areas of tendon cell death (apoptosis) may be present, with large areas of disordered ECM filled with cells, vessels and disorganized collagen (Warden, Cook, and Purdam 2017).

Collagen bundles may vary, with the relative amount of Type I collagen reducing and that of Type III increasing. This latter type is thought to be produced as a response to injury (Cook, Khan and Purdam 2002), but its structure is thinner and weaker than Type I, hence the tendon has reduced load tolerance and an increased risk of further disruption. Fibroblast cells migrate from the peritenon into the tendon substance and the total number of tenocytes (tendon cells) increases. As mentioned above, the cells become more rounded in appearance and are metabolically active, having an increased number of protein-synthesizing organelles.

Clinically, as well as thickening, focal nodular regions are often seen interspaced with normal tendon, and the risk of tendon rupture is increased. Overload to this type of tendon can cause a reactive change in the non-degenerative portions of the tendon (acute on chronic).

The increased vascularity is most easily seen on colour Doppler ultrasound, with the new vessels

Table 5.6 Phases of tendinopathy

Reactive tendinopathy	Tendon disrepair	Degenerative tendinopathy
▸ Tenocyte activation ▸ Proteoglycan increase ▸ Increased bound water concentration ▸ Increased tendon volume ▸ Little significant collagen fiber disruption ▸ Little significant inflammation	▸ Greater ECM breakdown ▸ Tendon cells take on a more rounded appearance ▸ Collagen & proteoglycan increase ▸ Collagen separation ▸ ECM disorganized ▸ Possible ingrowth of small nerve fibers & blood vessels. ▸ Hypoechoic areas on U/S	▸ Areas of tendon cell death ▸ Large regions of disordered ECM ▸ ECM filled with cells, vessels, & disorganized collagen ▸ Focal nodular regions interspaced with normal tendon ▸ Increased risk of tendon rupture ▸ Significant blood vessel ingrowth ▸ Large focal hypoechoic regions.

ECM – extracellular matrix, U/S – ultrasound,
(Cook and Purdam 2009, Warden, Cook and Purdam 2017)

having a small lumen and a twisted appearance. In peritendinitis, the paratenon is inflamed and often thickened, and there is local oedema and crepitus. The condition can exist in isolation to tendinopathy and is normally due to repeated actions, especially with tendon compression. Kager's triangle (the space between the inner surface of the Achilles tendon, the deep flexors and the calcaneus) is obliterated. Hard-scarred bands appear within the paratenon and adhesions develop between the Achilles tendon and surrounding tissue. Fatty tissue surrounding the tendon may remain thickened up to two years after the onset of paratenonitis (Kvist et al. 1988). Connective tissue has increased, and local blood vessels have degenerated or been obliterated, suggesting the presence of immature scar tissue.

Tendon examination

Specific examination of the Achilles tendon is carried out with the patient in prone, lying with the foot over the couch end (shin supported on a rolled towel) and in standing and/or the position which reproduces pain (sprint start, for example). Tendon rupture is discounted from the history (sudden onset/trauma for rupture, gradual onset/overuse for tendinopathy) and using the calf squeeze test (see below). The tendon sheath can be differentiated from the tendon proper using the 'painful arc' sign (Williams 1986). Using a pincer grip (Fig. 5.21),

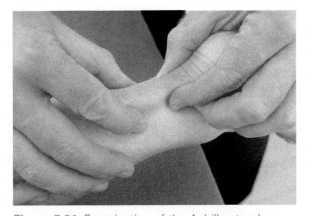

Figure 5.21 Examination of the Achilles tendon palpation for thickening.

the painful area of the tendon is palpated while the foot is actively plantarflexed and dorsiflexed. As the tendon moves through the sheath, the sheath will stay still as the foot is moved, but the tendon will move away from the palpating fingers. The painful arc test is positive (confirming tendinopathy) if the pain moves away from the fingers. For the posterior impingement test the pain in midrange plantarflexion is compared to that of full range plantarflexion. The therapist places one hand beneath the patient's forefoot to resist plantarflexion and load the tendon. Pain which occurs in a midrange position is compared to that of full plantarflexion, which compresses the posterior structures. The impingement test is positive if Achilles pain is increased with resisted plantarflexion.

Management

Initial management of tendinopathy or peritendinitis aims at reducing pain. Rest and cold application can be used in conjunction with modalities and/ or medication. Ice must be used with caution due to the risk of producing an ice burn over the tendon or malleoli. Wet ice enclosed in a moist cloth is preferable to an ice pack. Commercial ice packs should never be placed directly onto the skin.

Several forms of manual therapy may be useful to modulate pain. *Transverse friction* massage has been used for both insertional and mid-substance pain. Traditionally, tendon insertion is frictioned with the patient prone and the foot plantarflexed (Fig. 5.22A). The therapist uses the side of his or her flexed forefingers to impart the friction, pulling the hands distally against the curved insertion of the Achilles tendon into the calcaneum. The musculotendinous junction is frictioned with the foot dorsiflexed, and the tendon gripped from above between the finger and thumb. The movement is perpendicular to the tendon fibres (Fig. 5.22B). The tendon sheath may be treated by placing the length of the finger alongside the tendon and pressing inwards. The forearm is pronated/supinated to impart the friction

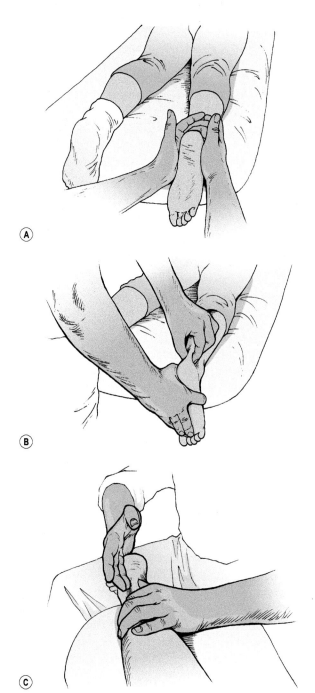

Figure 5.22 Transverse frictional massage for the Achilles tendon. (A) Teno-osseous junction. (B) Musculotendinous junction. (C) Tendon sheath/underside.

(Fig. 5.22C). In each case it is unlikely that the massage has any effect on the tendon tissue, but pain modulation may enable earlier tendon loading, which is key to this condition.

General massage may be used, focusing on effleurage to the calf muscle and circular frictions along the tendon itself. Specific wringing actions (see Figs 5.18A,B and C) are useful both to test the tendon compliance as part of tissue assessment and for treatment itself. Specific soft tissue mobilization (SSTM) has been described (see Chapter 1), and its use shown to be effective in the treatment of Achilles tendinopathy. The direction of the soft tissue mobilization was determined by reproduction of symptoms. A medial glide was used with the Achilles on stretch. This was progressed to gliding during isometric loading, and then gliding during dynamic through-range loading against resistance (Christenson 2007). Figure 5.23 shows SSTM of the Achilles.

A heel raise is used to reduce the stretch on the tendon, and the calf may be strapped in plantarflexion. If pain is intense, the subject should initially be non-weightbearing. A heel raise (built into an orthotic) may also be useful as the athlete returns to sport. Raising the heel can reduce the rate of eccentric loading during gait, as well as the range of motion, and may affect the strain response of the tendon. In addition, a medial heel post (wedge) used to control excessive subtalar pronation may reduce the shear stress on the tendon. In a study comparing lower-limb kinematics of those with chronic Achilles tendon pain to controls, Donoghue et al. (2008a) found greater eversion and ankle dorsiflexion and less leg abduction in the symptomatic group. In a separate study of rear-foot control for patients with Achilles tendon injury, Donoghue et al. (2008b) found a 92 per cent reduction in symptoms when using a rear-foot orthotic designed to reduce pronation. The fact that an orthotic changes foot motion may be enough to alter tissue loading and modify symptoms.

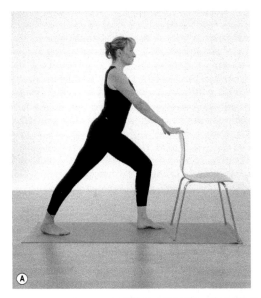

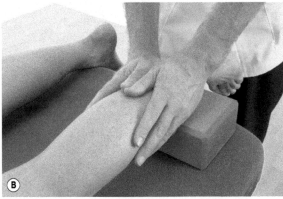

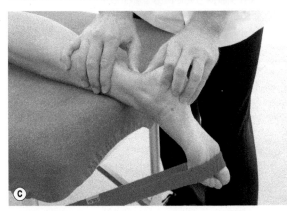

Figure 5.23 SSTM of the Achilles.
(A) Gastrocnemius and Achilles stretch (used with caution). (B) Calf muscle massage. (C) SSTM during resisted plantar flexion.

Eccentric exercise in the management of tendinopathy

The use of eccentric loading in the treatment of Achilles tendinopathy was popularized in the late 1980s. The aim was to increase the tensile strength of the tendon by subjecting it to active lengthening and high tensile forces. Eccentric exercise also prepares the tendon for rapid unloading, which has been associated with injury. However, eccentric loading in isolation will fail to prepare the tendon for functional tasks requiring concentric-eccentric coupling. MRI has been used to assess Achilles tendon following eccentric loading. Shalabi, Kristoffersen-Wilberg and Svensson (2007) tested 25 subjects (mean age 51 years) using a three-month eccentric calf-muscle stretching training programme, and showed a 14 per cent decrease in tendon volume. Collagen fibre synthesis has also been shown to change. Langberg et al. (2007) used a twelve-week programme of heavy eccentric training in elite soccer players. Markers of Type I collagen were measured using microdialysis, and increased from 3.9 μg/L prior to training to 19.7 μg/L. Sagittal thickness of the Achilles has been shown to reduce as a result of eccentric loading, and eccentric loading has been shown to induce a fourfold greater thickness reduction than concentric training (Grigg, Wearing, and Smeathers 2009). In this study, average sagittal thickness reduced by 20 per cent (4.4 mm to 3.5 mm) following eccentric training, and by 5 per cent (4.5 mm to 4.3 mm) following concentric training. Tendon thickness did not return to post-treatment values until 24 hours after treatment. Training, which involves cyclic loading of this type, has been shown to exude water from the tendon core to the peritendinous space through straightening of crimped collagen fibres and reducing the interfibrillar space (Cheng and Screen 2007).

Key point
Eccentric exercise causes the Achilles to exude water from the tendon core to the periphery, reducing cross-sectional area for up to 24 hours.

Treatment note 5.3   Early work on eccentric training

Eccentric training was a focus of rehabilitation for a number of years. In a study of 200 Achilles tendinopathy patients treated by eccentric loading, 44 per cent had complete pain relief and 43 per cent showed a marked decrease in their symptoms (Stanish, Robinovich and Curwin 1986). Comparing concentric to eccentric protocols, Niesen-Vertommen et al. (1992) showed better subjective pain scale scores for the eccentric group. Heavy eccentric loading has also been shown to be superior to surgery. The eccentric group achieved full function in 12 weeks compared to the surgery group timescale of 24 weeks, and pain response and strength deficit were better in the eccentric group (Alfredson et al. 1988).

Eccentric training may be given by performing a heel raise, rising on the uninjured leg and lowering on the injured side, both with the leg straight (gastrocnemius) and then bent (soleus). This type of programme has been shown to give relief in 90 per cent of patients with mid-tendon

pain and pathology (Roos et al. 2004). Forty-four patients (mean age 45 years) were given a twelve-week eccentric training programme and the results were measured using the Foot and Ankle Outcome Score. Significant pain reduction occurred, which lasted for one year follow-up. As pain eases, functional progression may be made using speed and power actions.

Application

Eccentric training for the Achilles is performed using a step. The athlete lifts his or her bodyweight using both legs by plantarflexing the ankle. Weight is transferred to the painful side and the non-injured knee is flexed. Bodyweight is then lowered using the painful leg alone. Ideally, athletes should perform 3 × 15 repetitions, twice daily on each day of the week (90 repetitions for each of the two exercises, giving 180 in total). Exacerbation of pain is to be expected as tissue repair is stimulated within the tendon. If pain does not occur, loading is likely to be suboptimal and more resistance should be applied.

Tendinopathy rehab

Current tendinopathy rehabilitation progresses from the use of isometrics for pain relief in a reactive tendon, through to isotonics to enhance strength and load the tendon. Final rehab progressions are targeted at the energy-storage and release-capacity function of the tendon.

Isometrics

Isometrics have been shown to be better at producing pain relief than isotonics in patellar tendinopathy (Rio et al. 2015), and about the same with Achilles tendinopathy (O'Neal et al. 2016). They are especially useful in the early stages of recovery if a subject is unable to practice isotonics, and have the advantage that they are easily incorporated into daily living. They may also be

used prior to isotonics to reduce pain in the early transition stage back into training. In the reactive phase of an injury, pain relief may be gradual, with some subjects responding in days and others taking weeks depending on pain intensity. Four to five repetitions of a 30- to 45-second hold are generally used, with contraction intensity at 60 to 80 per cent of maximal voluntary contraction (MVC). Training of this type is likely to be effective at modulating pain, and altering aberrant motor control if externally paced (e.g. metronome) rather than self-paced (e.g. set number of reps), and has been termed *tendon neuroplastic training* or TNT (Rio et al. 2016).

An isometric exercise example is to perform a calf raise on a lift, initially against bodyweight resistance and then using weight resistance with the knee flexed (bent-knee calf raise) and then extended (straight-leg calf raise), with the top position of the exercise held to isometric contraction.

Isotonics

Isotonic training is generally used as a progression once pain has eased or has reached a stable level. The action should be slow, using heavier resistances to minimize limb movement but maximize tendon overload. Eccentric action is emphasized with a timing of 2-3 seconds lift, pause, and then 4-5 seconds lowering. The isotonic protocol is continued to target both pain and strength deficit. Maximal loading will not be achieved in the presence of pain inhibition, so isometrics may be used prior to isotonics for pain relief. The affected limb may be compared to the unaffected and strength training continued until symmetry is regained, and stretch matches the requirements of activities to be undertaken by the subject in work, daily living and sport. An isotonic example of the calf-raise action may be performed with bent or straight knee, as above, to place focus on the Soleus and Gastrocnemius muscles respectively.

Energy storage and release

Energy storage and release works on the stretch shortening cycle (SSC, see Chapter 2), where the musculotendinous unit (MTU) is lengthened (wind-up) and then recoils (released). The eccentric action is to wind up the MTU and the concentric action begins slowly and progresses in speed. Actions such as the calf raise, above, may be used initially with more rapid movements than in the isotonic example. These can progress to jumps and hops, moving from limited range to full range. Final progressions include isolated plyometric actions and then sports/task-related plyometrics.

Tendon substance

Focal degeneration (tendonosis) may occur in the tendon with athletes in their early thirties. The onset is usually gradual, giving highly localized pain. Microscopically, there is proliferation of capillary cells and lacunae along the tendon fibres, giving a loss of the normal wavy alignment of collagen. As we have seen, this is a non-inflammatory condition resulting in haphazard collagen fibre orientation and relative absence of tenocytes, increased interfibrillar glycosaminoglycans (GAG) and scattered vascular in-growth. Collagen fibres fray and thin, losing their orientation, and the quantity of Type III collagen increases. There may be a reduction in fibre cross-linkage, reducing the tensile properties of the tendon.

Tendon rupture generally occurs later in an athlete's life, being more common from the late thirties to mid forties, with a male to female ratio of 10:1. With partial rupture, a few fibres or nearly all of the tendon may be affected. The characteristic history is one of sudden onset. There is swelling, pain on resisted movement and the patient is unable to support his or her weight through the toes of the affected foot.

In complete rupture there is usually a single incident where the patient feels a sudden sharp 'give' in the tendon, as though he or she had been struck from behind. Immediately afterwards there may be little pain but gross weakness. The patient is unable to take the weight through the toes, and the foot will hang straight downwards rather than being pulled into relaxed plantarflexion by calf muscle tone. Active plantarflexion is minimal, being accomplished by the peronei and posterior tibial muscles only. Often a subject can walk quite well using these muscles, but will be unable to lift up onto their toes. The calf squeeze (Thomson) and gap tests are useful to establish whether imaging may be required. For the *calf squeeze* the patient is prone with the foot over the couch end. The calf is squeezed, and where the foot fails to plantarflex the test is positive (Fig. 5.24). Closer examination reveals a depression (the Toygar angle) visible in the normal smooth contour of the Achilles tendon, and this is the basis of the *gap test*. With this test, identification of the gap and determination of its size manually or using ultrasound scanning indicates the severity of the lesion. If the athlete is not seen for a number of days, this gap will have

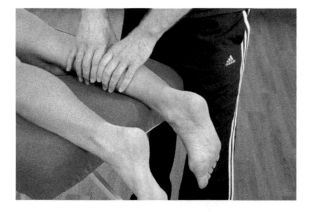

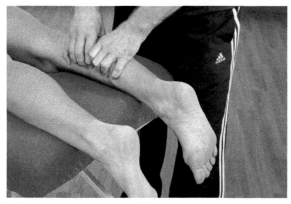

Figure 5.24 Calf squeeze (Thompson) test for Achilles tendon rupture. (A) Hand relaxed on calf, foot hangs over couch end at 90°. (B) Squeezing calf causes foot to plantarflex.

been bridged by haematoma and scar tissue, giving a raised fibrous area unless the tendon ends have retracted.

Without surgery, the tendon will heal, but very slowly. Granulation tissue forms poorly, partly due to repeated use, and partly as a result of the anticoagulant effect of synovial fluid contained by the unruptured paratenon.

Surgical management

Surgical management of Achilles tendon injuries can carry a high rate of complication. Wound dehiscence (bursting), scar hypertrophy, wound infection and nerve irritation have been reported

in about 10 per cent of cases. A meta-analysis of randomized controlled trials of treatment of Achilles tendon rupture concluded that open operative repair reduced the risk of re-rupture by 27 per cent (statistically significant) compared to non-operative management. However, surgery was associated with a higher risk of complications. Use of a functional brace allowed early mobilization and reduced the complication rate (Khan et al. 2005).

A number of repair methods have been described, including direct suture, reinforcement with plantaris or peroneus brevis tendon, and reconstruction using carbon fibre or polypropylene mesh. Following immobilization, the main problem is initially lack of flexibility to the Achilles tendon, ankle and subtaloid joint in particular. Early mobilization in a functional brace has been shown to improve outcome (Huang et al. 2015). Post-operative weightbearing combined with ankle range of motion exercise was associated with a lower complication rate and a quicker and superior functional recovery than conventional immobilization. Using dynamometry and anthropometry measurements to measure outcome following casting compared to functional rehabilitation, McCormack and Bovard (2015) showed better results at six to twelve weeks post-operation for rehabilitation, but by six months post-op the differences were negligible. They argued that early functional rehabilitation is as safe as traditional non-weightbearing immobilization but had a higher patient-satisfaction score. A PEDro synthesis showed better outcome for early weightbearing and ankle motion exercise than casting. Improvements included shorter time to activity return, greater heel-raise ability, superior achievement of normal ankle range of motion, and lower rates of minor complications (Carvalho and Kamper 2016).

Rehabilitation following surgery

Early phase

Following surgery, subjects will typically be given a post-surgical rehabilitation protocol similar to the example shown in Table 5.7 In the first two weeks post-op, the aim is to rest and control pain and swelling. The subject will be immobilized in a rigid cast, 24 hours each day, with the foot in

Table 5.7 Example post-surgical rehabilitation protocol following Achilles tendon repair

Timing	Activity
0–2 weeks	▶ Lower leg immobilized in rigid boot with foot pointing downwards ▶ Non-weightbearing crutch walking ▶ Upper and trunk body exercise ▶ Limb elevated when resting
2–4 weeks	▶ Walking boot with foot pointing downwards, gradually reduced heel height from week 3 ▶ Toe touch crutch walking to begin ▶ Exercise to spine/hip/knee ▶ Remove boot for ROM exercise (limit dorsiflexion range to that of boot) ▶ Isometric plantarflexion ▶ Soft tissue therapy to scar to mobilize and control swelling
4–8 weeks	▶ Walking boot gradually angled back into neutral (plantigrade) position ▶ Resisted plantarflexion, eversion and inversion with resistance band ▶ Active dorsiflexion to boot position ▶ Static cycle in exercise boot ▶ Gait re-education
8–12 weeks	▶ Boot replaced by shoe with heel raise ▶ Active resisted band exercises with increasing resistance ▶ Plantarflex through full range ▶ Increasing dorsiflexion aiming for normal ROM ▶ Proprioceptive rehabilitation including single-leg stand and balance cushion, initially holding wall bar then free
12–20 weeks	▶ Full active ankle range of movement with dorsiflexion as tolerated ▶ Progress muscle strengthening from open to closed chain ▶ Proprioceptive rehabilitation to include single-leg stand, balance cushion and board ▶ Double-leg heel raise progressing to single-leg

Early　Intermediate　Late

ROM – range of motion

plantarflexion to shorten the Achilles for correct healing. Crutches are used and walking is non-weightbearing. Exercise can be used to the upper body and hip/knee and toe movement for the recovering leg. From two to four weeks, easy walking is begun, and the aim is to gradually regain lost calf muscle strength and obtain normal gait, while at the same time reducing the likelihood of re-rupture. The boot is still worn, but from week three approximately, the ankle is gradually changed to reduce plantarflexion.

Intermediate phase

As pain allows, toe-touch walking can be begun and by weeks four to eight we progress to the full walking phase. The boot is gradually angled back to the neutral (plantigrade) position and resisted plantarflexion exercise is begun. Exercise to the rest of the body is used to maintain cardiovascular (CV) health, and CV activities in the pool (assuming good healing of the scar) are useful to encourage full-body movement without loading the tendon. Static cycle riding can increase until the intensity of rehabilitation itself is sufficient to challenge aerobic fitness.

 Activity is gradually increased so that by two to three months (eight to twelve weeks) post-op, normal walking is used and strengthening increased to the affected limb. Load through the tendon is reduced by using low overload and slow movement, and eccentric actions are begun as soon as they are tolerated (often in a pool to limit weightbearing) to mimic the true function of the tendon. The boot has now been removed, but a heel raise or training shoe with a high heel is worn. Dorsiflexion range will increase back to normal with regular walking and the boot is only worn if using a static cycle. A key marker of function is the ability to perform a single-leg heel raise. The aim should be to increase the subject's ability to perform this action, aiming at 8–20 repetitions depending on the activity/sport to be returned to. Varying heel position (toes in/out) and heel height increases the envelope of function.

Proprioceptive work is begun, with double-leg and then single-leg balance on the flat and varying labile surfaces (balance cushion/wobble board/bosu).

Late phase

By three to five months (twelve to twenty weeks), rehabilitation is progressed with both open- and closed-chain work, and resisted exercise gradually moving from static to dynamic actions. When function has improved sufficiently, walking pace is increased and speed walking introduced, followed by on-the-spot and later small-step jogging (in sports shoes with higher heel initially). Straight running, zig-zags and circle running are all introduced gradually, with increasing pace. Thick-heeled training shoes are used, and gradually the heel is lowered. Toe walking progresses to jogging on the toes once the heel-raise capacity of the subject allows. Heel-raise actions move to flat and then declined surfaces (with a block beneath the forefoot) to introduce stretching forces. The final stages of training must include the use of plyometric exercise to develop elastic strength. Poor results can be expected if the rehabilitation programme is stopped at the stage of heavy isotonic exercise and not progressed in terms of speed. Hopping and jumping actions are used on forgiving surfaces, with progression to bounding.

Foot and lower-limb alignment following repair must be checked. A change in rearfoot position, or excessive tibial rotation caused by hyperpronation, will place increased torsional stress on the Achilles, altering blood flow. Viewing the athlete's foot and lower limb from behind, an optimal alignment of the Achilles would be a near vertical appearance, with the medial longitudinal arch present. The gap between the floor and the navicular bone should be approximately one finger breadth, and be maintained on weightbearing (see Navicular drop test, Chapter 7). Excessive pronation (Fig. 5.25B) causes the Achilles to curve and deviate outwards with the medial longitudinal arch flatter (pes planus). Using a medial calcaneal wedge to control pronation at the subtalar joint (Fig. 5.25C)

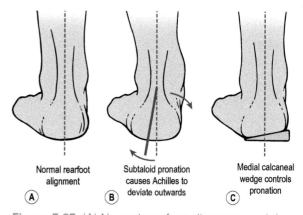

Figure 5.25 (A) Normal rearfoot alignment and the Achilles. (B) Subtaloid pronation causes Achilles to deviate outwards. (C) Medial calcaneal wedge controls pronation.

helps realign the Achilles and may modify any symptoms.

Accessory soleus muscle

Occasionally, athletes may present with an extra soleus muscle (accessory or supernumerary soleus) on one or both sides of the body. The condition occurs in 6 per cent of the population and is more common in males than females, with a ratio of 2:1 (Leswick et al. 2003). It is thought that the accessory muscle originates as a splitting of the embryonic cell cluster (anlage) in early development. The muscle is contained within its own fascial sheath, with its origin typically on the distal posterior aspect of the tibia. Pain and swelling occur with increased tissue tension within the Kager triangle. Typically, symptoms begin with an increase in training volume and are thought to represent a closed compartment ischaemia. Rest, ice and local massage may be used, with advice on training modification. Persistent cases may respond to fasciotomy and debulking. Ultrasound scanning reveals tissue of the same echogenicity as normal muscle, with the appearance of muscle bundles often identified. Differential diagnosis must be made from Achilles tendinopathy, ganglion lipoma, sarcoma and haematoma.

Retrocalcaneal pain

Sever's disease

Calcaneal apophysitis (Sever's disease) may occur in adolescents during the rapid growth spurt, sometimes in association with Achilles tendon pain itself. The condition is more common in boys than girls, and occurs between the ages of 11 and 15 years. The posterior aspect of the calcaneum develops independently of the main body and is separated by an epiphyseal plate. The plate lies vertically and is therefore subjected to shearing stress from the pull of the Achilles tendon and through jarring stress in jumping. Pain frequently occurs during deceleration from running, as well as take-off and landing from a jump. Sever's is inappropriately named as it is not a true disease entity, but rather a traction injury similar in many respects to Osgood–Schlatter's disease in the adolescent knee.

On examination, there is tenderness to medial and lateral heel compression, but no noticeable skin changes. Radiographically, sclerosis and irregularity of the calcaneal apophysis is seen as a result of avascular necrosis. Associated Achilles tendon tightness has been described, with the affected side showing 4 to 5 degrees less passive dorsiflexion than the unaffected side (Mitcheli and Ireland 1987). In addition, excessive foot pronation is also common in this patient group.

Initially, total rest is called for to allow the condition to settle. Later, any sporting activity which exacerbates the pain is avoided, and shock-absorbing heel pads are used in all shoes. Achilles tendon stretching is taught to restore dorsiflexion range, and foot position is corrected.

> **Key point**
>
> In Sever's disease, consider: (i) calf-Achilles stretching, (ii) shock-absorbing heel pads in all footwear and (iii) orthotic prescription.

Retrocalcaneal bursitis

The Achilles has two bursae associated with it. The retrocalcaneal (subtendinous) bursa lies deep to the Achilles, and the subcutaneous bursa lies between the skin and the tendon (Fig. 5.26). The insertion of the Achilles into the calcaneum is called an enthesis organ (see Chapter 1). The tendon tissue gradually changes into calcified fibrocartilage, before merging into the bone. The retrocalcaneal bursa lies between the Achilles and the bone, and a fibrocartilage layer lies between the bursa and the bone beneath, and between the bursa and tendon. The bursa provides two functions. First, it will reduce friction between the tendon and bone, and second it acts as a cam, giving a mechanical advantage to the tendon in the same way as the grater trochanter does for the gluteal tendons, for example. The intimate relationship between tendon, bone and bursa (together forming the enthesis organ) means that dorsiflexion under high load compresses the tendon onto the bone and in so doing loads the bursa, causing adaptation. Over a prolonged period, ossification may occur as part of tissue remodelling to prolonged overload. Traditionally, this was called a Haglands deformity (pump bump) but it may perhaps be better described as a morphology. When the area is painful, it is not the bone which is providing symptoms, but rather the inflamed retrocalcaneal bursa (Cook et al. 2017). Bursal fluid may be visible on MRI, and pain is generally aggravated

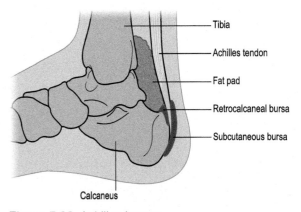

Calcaneus

— Tibia
— Achilles tendon
— Fat pad
— Retrocalcaneal bursa
— Subcutaneous bursa

Figure 5.26 Achilles bursae.

by a dorsiflexed position, even with low loads. Treatment aims at tissue-load management. Initially, rest and the avoidance of dorsiflexed positions is required (heel raise) to reduce compression forces. This is followed by graded loading to give tissue adaptation.

The superficial Achilles bursa lies more proximal between the Achilles and skin. It may be inflamed as a result of friction rather than compression, and as it is lined with synovial cells is can swell. Typically, it presents as a discoloured and swollen region in the area of friction of a tight boot. Treatment is to remove the cause of friction by changing or modifying footwear, and a U-shaped felt pad can often be used to provide deload padding.

References

Alexander, C., McMullan, M., Harrison, P., 2008. What is the effect of taping along or across a muscle on motoneurone excitability? A study using Triceps Surae. *Manual Therapy* **13** (1), 57–62.

Alfredson, H., Pietila, T., Johnsson, P., Lorentzon, R., 1988. Heavy load eccentric calf muscle training for the treatment of chronic Achilles tendonitis. *American Journal of Sports Medicine* **26** (3), 360–366.

Astrom, M., Westlin, N., 1994. Blood flow in the normal Achilles tendon assessed by laser Doppler flowmetry. *Journal of Orthopaedic Research* **12** (2), 246–252.

Batt, M.E., Ugalde, V., Anderson, M.W. (1998) A prospective controlled study of diagnostic imaging for acute shin splints. *Medicine & Science in Sports & Exercise* **30** (11): 1564–71.

Bradshaw, C., Hislop, M., and Hutchinson, M. (2007) Shin Pain. In Brukner, P., and Khan, K (eds) *Clinical sports medicine*. 3rd edition. McGraw Hill.

Carvalho, F.A., Kamper, S.J. (2016) Effects of early rehabilitation following operative repair of Achilles tendon rupture (PEDro synthesis). *British Journal of Sports Medicine* **50** (13): 829–30.

Cheng, V., Screen, H., 2007. The micro-structural strain response of tendon. *Journal of Material Science* **42**, 8957–8965.

Christenson, R.E., 2007. Effectiveness of specific soft tissue mobilizations for the management of Achilles Tendinosis: Single case study – Experimental design. *Manual Therapy* **12**, 63–71.

Cook, J., Silbernagel, K., Griffin S., et al. (2017) Pain in the Achilles region. In Brukner, P., Clarsen, B., Cook, J et al (eds) *Clinical sports medicine* (5th ed) McGraw Hill. Australia.

Cook, J.L., Khan, K.M., Purdam, C., 2002. Achilles tendinopathy. *Manual Therapy* **7** (3), 121–130.

Cook, J., and Purdam, C. (2009) Is tendon pathology a continuum? *British Journal of Sports Medicine* 43(6):409-16.

Detmer, D.E., 1986. Chronic shin splints: classification and management of medial tibial stress syndrome. *Sports Medicine* **3**, 436–446.

Donoghue, O.A., Harrison, A.J., Laxton, P., Jones, R.K. (2008a) Lower limb kinematics of subjects with chronic Achilles tendon injury during running. *Research in Sports Medicine* **16** (1), 23–38.

Donoghue, O.A., Harrison, A.J., Laxton, P., Jones, R.K. (2008b) Orthotic control of rear foot and lower limb motion during running in participants with chronic Achilles tendon injury. *Sports Biomechanics* **7** (2), 194–205.

Griebert, M., Needle, A.R, McConnell, J., Kaminski, T.W. (2016) Lower-leg Kinesio tape reduces rate of loading in participants with medial tibial stress syndrome. *Phys Ther Sport*. 18:62–7.

Grigg, N., Wearing, S., Smeathers, J., 2009. Eccentric calf muscle exercise produces a greater acute reduction in Achilles tendon thickness than concentric exercise. *British Journal of Sports Medicine* **43**, 280–283.

Hamstra-Wright, K.L., Bliven, K.C., Bay, C. (2015) Risk factors for medial tibial stress syndrome in physically active individuals such as runners and military personnel: a systematic review and metaanalysis. *British Journal of Sports Medicine* **49** (6): 362–369.

Hislop, M., and Tierney, P. (2011) Intracompartmental pressure testing: results of an international survey of current clinical practice, highlighting the need for standardised protocols. *British Journal of Sports Medicine* 45:956-958.

Huang, J., Wang, C., Ma, X. et al. (2015) Rehabilitation regimen after surgical treatment of acute Achilles tendon ruptures: a systematic review with meta-analysis. *American Journal of Sports Medicine* (4):1008–16.

Khan, K.M., Maffulli, N., 1998. Tendinopathy: an Achilles heel for athletes and clinicians. *Clinical Journal of Sports Medicine* **8** (3), 151–154.

Khan, R.J., Fick, D., Keogh, A., Crawford, J., Brammar, T., Parker, M. (2005). Treatment of acute Achilles tendon ruptures. A meta-analysis of randomized controlled trials. *Journal of Bone Joint Surgery* **87** (10), 2202–2210.

Kvist, M., 1994. Achilles tendon injuries in athletes. *Sports Medicine* **18**, 173–201.

Kvist, M.H., Lehto, M.U.K., Jozsa, L. et al., 1988. Chronic Achilles paratenonitis. *American Journal of Sports Medicine* **16** (6), 616–622.

Langberg, H., Ellingsgaard, H., Madsen, T., Jansson, J., 2007. Eccentric rehabilitation exercise increases peritendinous type I collagen synthesis in humans with Achilles Tendinosis. *Scandinavian Journal of Medicine Science and Sports* **17** (1), 61–66.

Leswick, D.A., Chow, V., Stoneham, G.W., 2003. Answer to case of the month 94: Accessory soleus muscle. *Canadian Association of Radiologists Journal* **54** (5), 313–315.

Li, G., Zhang, S., Chen, G., et al., 1985. Radiographic and histological analysis of stress fracture in rabbit tibias. *American Journal of Sports Medicine* **13**, 285–294.

Lysholm, J., Wiklander, J., 1987. Injuries in runners. *American Journal of Sports Medicine* **15**, 168–171.

Maffulli, N., Ewen, S.W., Waterston, S., 2000. Tenocytes from ruptured and tendinopathic Achilles tendons produce greater quantities of type III collagen than tenocytes from normal Achilles tendons: an in vitro model of human tendon healing. *American Journal of Sports Medicine* **28**, 499–505.

Malliaras, P., Richards, P.J., Garau, G., Maffulli, N., 2008. Achilles tendon Doppler flow may be associated with mechanical loading among active athletes. *American Journal of Sports Medicine* **36** (11), 2210–2215.

McBryde, A.M., 1985. Stress fractures in runners. *Clinics in Sports Medicine* **4** (4), October, 737–752.

McCormack, R., Bovard, J. (2015) Early functional rehabilitation or cast immobilisation review and meta-analysis of randomised controlled trials. *Br J Sports Med.* 49(20):1329–35.

Mitcheli, L.J., Ireland, M.L., 1987. Prevention and management of calcaneal apophysitis in children: an overuse syndrome. *Journal of Paediatric Orthopaedics* **7**, 34–38.

Ng, G., Richardson, C.A., 1990. The effects of training triceps surae using progressive speed loading. *Physiotherapy Practice* **6**, 77–84.

Niesen-Vertommen, S.L., Taunton, J.E., Clement, D.B., Mosher, R.E., 1992. The effect of eccentric versus concentric exercise in the management of Achilles tendonitis. *Clinical Journal of Sports Medicine* **2** (2), 109–113.

Norris, C.M. 2001. *Acupuncture: treatment of musculoskeletal conditions*. Butterworth-Heinemann, Oxford.

O'Neill, S., Raida, J., Birds, K. et al. (2016) Acute Sensory and Motor Response to 45-Seconds Heavy Isometric Holds for the Plantar Flexors in Patients with Achilles Tendinopathy. International Scientific Tendinopathy Symposium.

Pillai, J., 2008. A current interpretation of popliteal vascular entrapment. *Journal of Vascular Surgery* 61S-64S.

Puddu, G., Cerullo, G., Selvanetti, A., De Paulis, F., 1994. Stress fractures. In: Harries, M., Williams, C., Stanish, W.D., Micheli L.J. (eds), *Oxford Textbook of Sports Medicine*. Oxford University Press, Oxford.

Puffer, J.C., Zachazewski, J.E., 1988. Management of overuse injuries. *American Family Physician* **38** (3), 225–232.

Rajasekaran, S., Kvinlaug, K., Finnoff, J. (2012) Exertional Leg Pain in the Athlete. *Physical Medicine and Rehabilitation* 4:985–1000.

Rio, E., Kidgell, D., Moseley, G.L. et al. (2016) Tendon neuroplastic training: changing the way we think about tendon rehabilitation: a narrative review. *British Journal of Sports Medicine* 50(4):209–15.

Rio, E., Kidgell, D., Purdam, C. et al. (2015) Isometric exercise induces analgesia and reduces inhibition in patellar tendinopathy. *British Journal of Sports Medicine* 49:1277–1283.

Roos, E.M., Engstrom, M., Lagerquist, A., Soderberg, B., 2004. Clinical improvement after 6 weeks of eccentric exercise in patients with mid-portion Achilles tendinopathy – a randomized trial with 1-year follow-up. *Scandinavian Journal of Medicine Science and Sports* **14** (5), 286–295.

Shalabi, A., Kristoffersen-Wilberg, M., Svensson, L. et al., 2007. Eccentric training of the gastrocnemis-soleus complex in chronic Achilles Tendinopathy results in decreased tendon volume and intratendinous signal as evaluated by MRI. *Scandinavian Journal of Medicine Science and Sports* **17** (3), 298–299.

Stager, A., Clement, D., 1999. Popliteal artery entrapment syndrome. *Sports Medicine* **28** (1), 61–70.

Stanish, D.W., Robinovich, R.M., Curwin, S., 1986. Eccentric exercise in chronic tendinitis. *Clinical Orthopedics and Related Research* **208** (7), 65–68.

Steinberg, B.D., 2005. Evaluation of limb compartments with increased interstitial pressure. An improved non-invasive method for determining quantitative hardness. *Journal of Biomechanics* **38**, 1629–1635.

Styf, J., 1989. Chronic exercise-induced pain in the anterior aspect of the lower leg. Sports Medicine 7, 331–339.

Taunton, J.E., Clement, D.B., 1981. Lower extremity stress fractures in athletes. *Physician and Sports Medicine* **9**, 77–86.

Taylor, A., Kerry, R., 2002. Altered haemodynamics. Vascular issues in sport. *Sportex medicine* **12**, 9–13.

Williams, J.G.P., 1986. Achilles tendon lesions in sport. *Sports Medicine* **3**, 114–135.

Warden S., Cook, J., and Purdam, C. (2017) Tendon overuse injury. In Brukner, P., Clarsen, B., Cook, J. et al. *Clinical Sports Medicine*. 5th edition. McGraw Hill.

CHAPTER 6

The ankle

'It's just a sprain' is a phrase used all too commonly when someone twists their ankle. Unfortunately, this relatively familiar injury often leads to unnecessary disability in daily living activity simple because it is taken far too lightly and subjects often accept poor quality movement. In sport, the situation is very similar. Approximately 14 per cent of all sports injuries are sprains to the ankle, representing one ankle injury each season for every 17 participants. In high-risk sports, such as jumping and running, this percentage is even higher, at 25 per cent of all lost-time injuries. Ankle sprain has been shown to be 2.4 times more common in the dominant leg, and to have a high (73.5 per cent) prevalence of recurrence (Yeung et al. 1994). Lateral ankle sprain is the most common musculoskeletal injury in physically active individuals, with the majority of subjects sustaining at least one further sprain (Gribble et al. 2016).

The ankle region consists of three joints: the talocrural joint, the subtar joint and the syndesmosis between the inferior part of the tibia and fibula (inferior tibiofibular joint).

Definition

A *syndesmosis* is a largely immobile joint where two bones are joined by connective tissue.

The ankle joint itself (talocrural joint) is the articulation between the trochlear surface of the talus (top) and the distal ends of the tibia and fibula. The fibula may support 15–20 per cent of the bodyweight, with the fibula moving downwards and laterally during the stance phase of running to deepen the ankle mortise and enhance stability. This fibular motion creates tension in the interosseous membrane and tibiofibular ligament to provide some shock attenuation. Loss of this mechanism through tibiofibular disruption greatly affects the ankle joint, with a 1–2 mm lateral shift of the fibula increasing joint forces by as much as 40 per cent.

Key point

The fibula can support up to a fifth of the bodyweight and moves during the stance phase of running to deepen the ankle mortise and enhance ankle stability.

The ankle is subjected to considerable compression forces during sport (Fig. 6.1). Compression forces as high as five times bodyweight have been calculated during walking, and up to 13 times bodyweight during running (Burdett 1982).

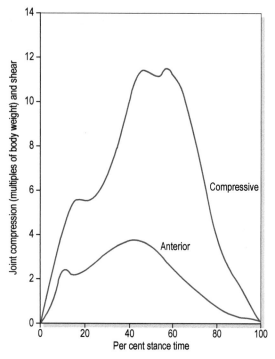

Figure 6.1 Compression forces on the talus during running. From Burdett, R.G. (1982) Forces predicted at the ankle during running. *Medicine and Science in Sports and Exercise*, **14** (4), 308. With permission.

Ankle joint mechanics

The trochlear surface of the talus is wider anteriorly, and so plantarflexion is more free than dorsiflexion, average values being 30–50 degrees and 20–30 degrees, respectively. Marked variations occur, both between individuals and following injury, and normal foot function can be achieved with as little as 20 degrees of plantarflexion and 10 degrees of dorsiflexion. The ankle is essentially a hinge, externally rotated to between 20 and 25 degrees with the malleoli. In the neutral position, with the foot perpendicular to the lower leg, there is very little frontal or transverse plane motion. With dorsiflexion, abduction of the foot is possible, and during plantarflexion, adduction can occur. In dorsiflexion, the broad anterior part of the talus is forced into the narrower mortise between the tibia and fibula. The interosseous and transverse tibiofibular ligaments are stressed, as the bones part slightly, and the joint moves into close-pack position.

Plantarflexion sees the narrow posterior part of the trochlear surface of the talus moving into the broader tibiofibular mortise. Recoil of the above ligaments causes the malleoli to approximate and maintain contact with the talus.

> **Key point**
>
> The trochlea surface of the talus is wider at the front. This wedge shape makes the range of plantarflexion greater than that of dorsiflexion. In addition, injury to the talar surface or swelling within the ankle joint is often seen clinically as a marked reduction in dorsiflexion.

During running, the ankle is dorsiflexed at heel strike, and plantarflexes to bring the forefoot to the ground. Plantarflexion occurs again at push-off, and the foot dorsiflexes throughout the swing phase of running. Joint forces at the ankle at heel strike are three times bodyweight for compression and 80 per cent bodyweight for antero-posterior (AP) shear. At heel lift, muscle force creating the plantarflexion force to lift the body increases compression at the ankle to five times bodyweight. Subjects with ankle pain modify their gait pattern to reduce these forces, but in so doing stress other areas of the kinetic chain.

> **Key point**
>
> Subjects with ankle pain often modify their gait pattern to reduce compression forces within the ankle joint. This change throws stress onto joints further up the leg.

Collateral ligaments

The ankle joint is strengthened by a variety of ligaments, the collaterals being the most important from the point of view of injury. Both medial and lateral collateral ligaments travel from the malleoli,

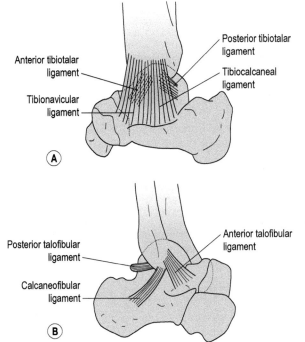

Figure 6.2 The ankle ligaments. (A) Deltoid (medial). (B) Lateral.

The posterior talofibular (PTF) ligament travels almost horizontally from the fossa on the bottom of the lateral malleolus to the posterior surface of the talus. Lying between the ATF and PTF ligaments is the calcaneofibular ligament, arising from the front of the lateral malleolus to pass down and back to attach onto the lateral surface of the calcaneum. The role of the collateral ligaments in maintaining talocrural stability is summarized in Table 6.1.

Table 6.1 Role of the collateral ligaments in ankle stability. Adapted from Palastanga, Field and Soames (2013)

Movement	Controlled by
Abduction of talus	Tibiocalcaneal and tibionavicular bands
Adduction of talus	Calcaneofibular ligament
Plantarflexion	ATF ligament and anterior tibiotalar band
Dorsiflexion	Posterior tibiotalar band and PTF ligament
External rotation of talus	Anterior tibiotalar and tibionavicular bands
Internal rotation of talus	As above with ATF ligament

and have bands attaching to the calcaneus and talus.

The medial (deltoid) ligament (Fig. 6.2A) is triangular in shape. Its deep portion may be divided into anterior and posterior tibiotalar bands. The more superficial part is split into tibionavicular and tibiocalcaneal portions, which attach in turn to the spring ligament. The lateral ligament (Fig. 6.2B) is composed of three separate components, and is somewhat weaker than its medial counterpart, and therefore more commonly injured. The anterior talofibular (ATF) ligament is a flat band 2–5 mm thick and 10–12 mm long which travels from the anterior tip of the lateral malleolus to the neck of the talus, and may be considered the primary stabilizer of the ankle joint.

Key point

The anterior talofibular (ATF) ligament is the primary stabilizer of the ankle joint.

Injury

The most common injury to the ankle is damage to the ATF ligament, with or without involvement of the peroneus brevis. The subtaloid and mid-tarsal joints may be involved, but will be dealt with separately for clarity. The typical history of ankle injury is one of inversion, sometimes coupled with plantarflexion. The athlete 'goes over' on the ankle, usually on an uneven surface. One of three grades of ligament injury may occur.

Key point

The anterior talofibular (ATF) ligament is 2–5 mm thick and 10–12 mm long, approximately the width of the index finger. Its fibres run roughly parallel to the sole of the foot. Injury to the ATF is the most common sports injury affecting the ankle.

Swelling

There is usually an egg-shaped swelling in front of, and around, the lateral malleolus. When viewed from behind, the definition of the Achilles tendon is a good indicator of severity of injury. With more severe injuries (Grade III), the definition of the Achilles tendon is lost due to excessive bleeding into the joint (Fig. 6.3).

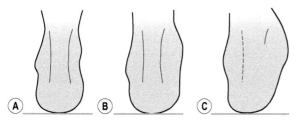

Figure 6.3 Assessing severity of ankle injury from swelling. (A) Normal joint. Contour of Achilles tendon well defined. (B) Grade I/II injury. Clear swelling but Achilles tendon outline still visible. (C) Grade III injury. Profuse swelling obscures outline of Achilles tendon.

Objective measurement of swelling can be made using the figure-of-eight measure, a valid and reliable measure (Rohner-Spengler, Mannion and Babst 2007). For this test, the end of a tape measure is placed on the anterolateral aspect of the ankle, midway between the tibialis anterior tendon and the lateral malleolus. The tape is passed medially over the dorsum of the foot to the tuberosity of navicular and then beneath the plantar aspect proximal to the tubercle of the fifth metatarsal. The tape passes medially once more to rest distal to the medial malleous and is pulled across the Achilles back to the starting point.

Manual evaluation

The lateral malleolus should be gently palpated to assess if bone pain is present; if it is, an X-ray may be required (see below). If palpation reveals tenderness below, rather than over, the lateral malleolus and the athlete is able to bear weight, there is a 97 per cent probability of soft tissue injury alone (Vargish and Clarke 1983). Any fracture that is missed by this type of close palpation is likely to be an avulsion or non-displaced hairline type that should respond favourably to management as a sprain.

Stress tests to the ankle are useful to assess the degree of instability in the subacute phase, and to give a differential diagnosis. Acute injuries may be exacerbated by full-range motion with overpressure. The capsule of the ankle joint itself is assessed by passive dorsiflexion and plantarflexion only, the capsular pattern presenting as a greater limitation of plantarflexion. However, as the ankle ligaments span the subtaloid and mid-tarsal joints, inversion/eversion and adduction/abduction are also included in ankle joint examination.

The ATF ligament is placed on maximum stretch by passive inversion, plantarflexion and adduction. The heel is held with the cupped hand and the subtaloid joint inverted. The opposite hand grasps the forefoot from above and swings it into plantarflexion and adduction. In addition, anterior glide of the talus on the tibia should be assessed with the foot in a neutral position. The heel is again held in the cupped hand, but this time the palm of the opposite hand is over the anterior aspect of the lower tibia. The calcaneus and talus are pulled forward as the tibia is pushed back. Movements are compared with that of the uninjured side for range and quality.

> ### Key point
> The ATF ligament is tested by passive inversion, plantarflexion and adduction. The athlete's heel is held with the cupped hand and the heel is twisted inwards. The opposite hand grasps the forefoot from above and draws down and in.

The calcaneocuboid ligament is stressed by combined supination/adduction and the calcaneofibular ligament by inversion in a neutral position. The medial collateral ligament is stressed by combined plantarflexion/eversion/abduction

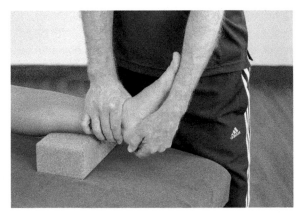

Figure 6.4 Anterior drawer test.

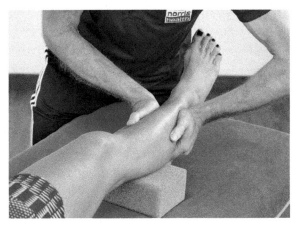

Figure 6.5 Syndesmosis test.

(anterior fibres) or eversion alone (middle fibres). Resisted eversion will not be painful unless the peronei are affected (see below).

Ligamentous laxity may be assessed using the *anterior drawer test* when acute inflammation has subsided. The patient's foot is placed in slight (10–15 degrees) plantarflexion and the heel is gripped with the therapist's cupped hand, while the other hand stabilizes the lower tibia and fibula. The heel is drawn forwards against an opposite force, pressing the tibia backwards, and the amount of anterior movement is noted if the talus moves out of the ankle mortise (Fig. 6.4). The test determines the integrity of both the anterior talofibular ligament and the calcaneofibular ligament, and has been shown to be valid when compared to surgical observation.

> ### Key point
> The anterior drawer test assesses ligamentous laxity, and is most useful when acute inflammation and muscle spasm have subsided.

The syndesmosis must also be evaluated where pain is located higher up between the anterior ankle tendons crossing the joint line. This type of high ankle sprain involving the syndesmosis may be assessed by the squeeze test, providing fracture (and compartment syndromes) have been

ruled out first. For the squeeze test, the patient is positioned in crook (hook), lying with the affected leg closest to the therapist. The test begins by placing the hands over the tibia and fibula, making bone contact with the heel of the hand and keeping the forearms horizontal. The action is to press the hands towards each other to compress the tibia and fibula. Perform the test at several locations from the knee to the ankle to assess pain in comparison to the non-injured limb. The severity of the ankle syndesmosis injury may be indicated by how high up the leg the pain is felt, the condition being more severe if pain travels from the ankle up to the knee (Fig. 6.5)

Following severe ankle sprain or fracture, a bony link may form between the tibia and fibula (tibiofibular synostosis). Typically, pain occurs after an injury, and increases during vigorous activity, mimicking stress fracture. Pain is most severe during the push-off action of running and jumping, and dorsiflexion is often limited to 90 degrees, mimicking impingement pain (see below). The synostosis is revealed by X-ray and removed surgically (Flandry and Sanders 1987).

X-ray

Accurate physical examination will usually give sufficient information to preclude fracture, making X-ray unnecessary in most cases. Only 15 per cent of patients suffering an acute ankle injury may have a fracture, and the Ottawa Ankle Rules provide a highly accurate clinical decision guide in this respect (Stiell et al. 1994). The rules state:

▶ An ankle X-ray is only needed if there is pain in the distal six centimetres of the malleolar region, together with an inability to take four steps and point tenderness of bone at the posterior edge or tip of the lateral malleolus or medial malleolus.

▶ A foot X-ray is only required if there is pain in the midfoot, an inability to take four steps or bone tenderness to the base of the fifth metatarsal or tubercle of navicular.

A poster describing the rules is free to download at www.ohri.ca/emerg/cdr/docs/cdr_ankle_poster.pdf.

In a systematic review of 27 studies (15,581 patients) Bachmann et al. (2003) found the sensitivity of the Ottawa Ankle Rules to be almost 100 per cent and claimed that their application would reduce the number of unnecessary radiographs by 30 to 40 per cent.

Key point
Use of the Ottawa Ankle Rules is essential prior to X-ray following ankle sprain.

Fractures associated with ankle injuries

Several fractures may occur at the time of injury, and can go unnoticed unless a thorough examination is carried out. Often these fractures only become apparent during rehabilitation, when swelling begins to subside. It falls on the astute therapist to question why rehabilitation is not progressing normally and to refer for further investigation, which may include X-ray, MRI or CT scan.

Pott's fracture

This is a fracture affecting either the lateral or medial malleolus. To palpation, pain is located close to the malleolus itself rather than in the ligament tissue. The subject usually finds it difficult to bear weight in the clinic, and will not have been able to bear weight immediately after injury. Where the ankle mortise has been compromised, internal fixation is usually required. Hairline fractures, stable fractures and those affecting the posterior aspect of the malleolus and/or involving less than 25 per cent of the articular surface are normally managed conservatively.

Maisonneuve fracture

This is a spiral fracture of the fibula together with a tear of the distal tibiofibular syndesmosis and the interosseous membrane. The medial malleolus normally fractures and the deltoid ligament ruptures. The injury occurs only in high-impact activities and requires urgent surgical referral.

Osteochondral lesion of talar dome

This fracture is more common in cases where ankle sprain has occurred in the presence of a compression force, such as landing from a single-leg jump. The talar dome is compressed within the ankle mortise and may fracture, at the superomedial corner particularly. The condition is normally not recognized at the time of injury, but presents as a dull persistent ache during rehabilitation. There will be persistent swelling with stiffness. The site can be palpated by plantar flexing the ankle to draw the talar dome forwards of the ankle mortise. Injury may be graded from (I) focal compression of the subchondral bone through to (IV) fully detached bone fragment. Treatment is by reduced weightbearing while maintaining motion to stimulate cartilage healing (Karlsson 2007). Occasionally, arthroscopic removal of the bone fragment may be required.

Avulsion fracture of fifth metatarsal base

The force which causes an acute lateral ligament injury is sometimes severe enough to pull (avulse) the peroneus brevis tendon away from its attachment to the fifth metatarsal. The avulsion fracture is usually treated conservatively.

Fracture of talar process

The lateral aspect of the talus, which normally articulates with the fibula and calcaneus, may fracture. Pain occurs over the bone area, which is palpated anterior and inferior to the tip of the lateral malleolus. If the fracture is not displaced, simple immobilization is required. Where displacement is greater than 2 mm, excision or internal fixation is generally required (Karlsson 2007).

Fracture of calcaneus process

The anterior calcaneal process is palpated anterior to the sinus tarsi. This area is normally not tender in cases of lateral ligament injury, but where fracture has occurred tenderness is exquisite. The fracture may not be revealed by X-ray and can require MRI or CT scan. Again, immobilization is required unless the fragment is displaced, in which case excision may be called for.

Management of an ankle sprain

A recent systematic review and meta-analysis of the treatment of ankle sprain (Doherty et al. 2017) found strong evidence for early mobilization (with non-steroidal anti-inflammatory drugs), and moderate evidence supporting exercise and manual therapy techniques for pain, swelling and function. Exercise therapy and bracing was supported for the prevention of chronic ankle instability (CAI). The immediate management of acute ankle sprain consists of the POLICE protocol (see Chapter 1), following evaluation. Analgesia may be provided by electrotherapy modalities or medication as appropriate. Intermittent pneumatic compression (IPC) used in conjunction with cooling can be effective to reduce pain and limit swelling. In the subacute phase, massage, especially finger kneading around the malleolus, is of value in lessening the development of pitting oedema,

and to modulate pain. Transverse frictions may be used to encourage the development of a mobile scar (before active exercise is tolerated), and may be used as a prelude to joint mobilization or manipulation in chronic injuries. Grade II and III injuries present with marked swelling and are protected non-weightbearing (severe injury) or preferably partial weightbearing with a compression bandage. Where minimal swelling indicates a Grade I injury, an eversion strapping may be applied to protect the ligament from inversion stresses and to shorten it. A felt wedge is used beneath the heel to evert the subtaloid joint, and a U-shaped pad is placed over the submalleolar depressions to prevent pockets of oedema forming and to apply even compression when the ankle is strapped. Adhesive strapping is applied after skin preparation or underwrap, initially to lock the subtaloid joint and then to passively evert the foot. The athlete can then walk partial weightbearing in a well-supporting shoe.

Early mobility is essential to increase ligament strength and restore function. For Grade I and II injuries, early mobilization has been shown to be more effective than immobilization. In a group of 82 patients with these grades of injury, 87 per cent who were immobilized with a plaster cast for ten days still had pain after three weeks. This compared to 57 per cent of those who received early mobilization in the form of an elastic strap for two days followed by a functional brace for eight days (Eiff, Smith and Smith 1994). Even Grade III injuries (rupture) respond better to conservative treatment than surgery. Studies have shown 87 per cent good and excellent results with conservative management compared to 60 per cent for surgery of Grade III injuries. In addition, at six weeks post injury, the surgical group had limited range of motion not seen in the conservative group (Kaikkonen, Kannus and Jarninen 1996).

Non-weightbearing ankle exercise is instigated within the pain-free range, and fitness is maintained by general exercise. Strapping is replaced by a tubular elastic bandage as pain subsides.

Manual therapy for ankle joint stiffness

Joint stiffness is often of concern following injury, and although exercise therapy is normally the treatment of choice, manual therapy has a significant part to play. Both accessory movements and mobilization with movement (MWM) are useful techniques to assist with mobility and modulate pain.

Subtle movement of the talus on the tibiofibular mortise can be achieved with the subject in prone with the knee bent. The therapist places one hand over the front of the talus, using webspace as a contact point, and the other hand on the back of the tibia. The action is to move in an antero-posterior (AP) direction, pressing the talus across the tibial plane. For a posteroanterior (PA) direction, the hand position changes, with the back hand contact on the posterior calcaneus and the front hand over the anterior shaft of the tibia. In both cases, the tibia is vertical and held close into the therapist's body to make the subject feel secure. The therapist's forearms are horizontal, with the force from the shoulders and arms transmitted by (but not created by) the hands (Fig. 6.6).

AP movement in a stiff ankle can require significant strength on the part of the therapist, so the classic mobilization (above) can be modified with the use of a block. For PA movement, the subject is supine and a firm block is placed beneath their heel. The therapist applies pressure over the anterior tibia through their webspace, with their hand close to the ankle joint. For an AP glide, the patient is prone with the block placed over the anterior tibia, with the lower edge of the block across the ankle joint line. The action is to press against the back of the calcaneum.

An MWM is performed with the subject half-kneeling on a treatment couch, with the affected leg forwards, foot flat. The aim is to block the talus from drifting forwards as the subject presses into dorsiflexion (knee moving over toes). The therapist places either their thumbs or webspace over the anterior joint line to contact the talus and pushes

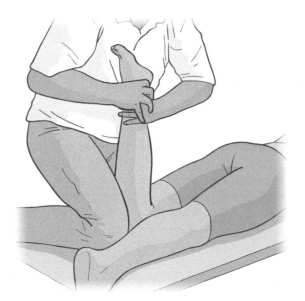

Figure 6.6 Ankle joint mobilizations.

in an AP direction as the patient moves into a lunge. The dorsiflexion force from the subject can be reinforced by the therapist using a webbing belt wrapped around the back of the tibia. A self MWM can be used to follow-up as a home exercise. The subject places a resistance band on stretch (attached to a table leg) over the front of their ankle as they perform the half kneeling lunge (Fig. 6.7).

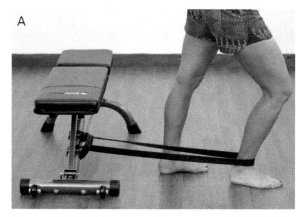

Figure 6.7 Mobilization with movement (MWM) to ankle joint.

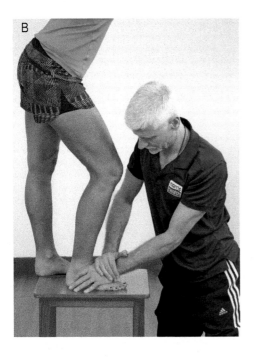

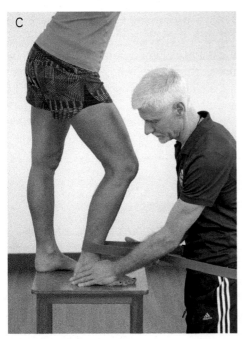

Figure 6.7 Continued

(A) Lunge position with resistance band, (B) hand placement for AP gliding force, (C) AP glide on talus using webbing belt to assist dorsiflexion.

Rehabilitation of the injured ankle

As with any joint, rehabilitation of the ankle aims at restoring mobility, strength and function (Table 6.2). With the ankle, however, of particular concern is the restoration of normal proprioception.

Resisted exercise using rubber powerbands is used for inversion, eversion, dorsiflexion and plantarflexion, together with combinations of these movements. Maximum repetitions are used to restore muscle endurance, while strength is

Table 6.2 Guidelines for rehabilitation of ankle sprain

Immediate post-injury management
POLICE protocol Consider use of intermittent pneumatic compression (IPC) with ice Other modalities to reduce pain and inflammation Careful assessment of possible bony injury Athlete non-weight bearing
Initial rehabilitation (2–5 days after injury)
Massage, especially finger kneading around malleolus Range of motion exercise, inversion to pain tolerance only Tranverse frictions to encourage mobile scar formation Partial weight bearing with eversion taping and felt padding or ankle orthosis Walking re-education Begin resisted exercise (elastic bands) Active stretch into inversion and plantarflexion Begin accessory mobilizations of surrounding joints
Intermediate rehabilitation (6–14 days)
Progress resisted exercise of ankle in all directions Passive stretching into inversion and plantarflexion Proprioceptive work (single-leg standing, eyes closed) Gradually introduce balance board and trampette work Ensure full range dorsiflexion Uphill treadmill work progressing to speed walk and slow run Side step and zig-zag speed walking—building endurance Introduce varied terrain—slopes, rough ground, sand Ensure cuboid mobility
Final rehabilitation (2–6 weeks)
Build to maximum resisted eversion General weight training for lower limb Running drills—figure-of-eight, circle run, zig-zag Introduce low hop and progress to hop and hold, side hop, and hop and twist—building power and speed Sport-specific work including ball kicking and varying terrain

developed using maximal resistance. Eversion movements are performed with the band placed over both forefeet. For other movements, one end of the band is placed around a table leg, and the other over the foot. Various thicknesses of band are used as the exercises are progressed.

Static stretching exercises, if required, include calf and Achilles tendon stretching (see above), and inversion/eversion movements applied manually by the athlete. The starting position for these latter movements is sitting with the injured leg crossed over the contralateral limb. The exercise mimics the stability test for the ligaments outlined above.

Partial, and then full, weightbearing exercises are used to develop strength in a closed kinetic chain position and to restore proprioception. In single-leg standing (wall-bar support), trunk movements are performed to throw stress onto the ankle; in addition, exercises such as heel raising, toe lifts and inversion/eversion are performed. A balance beam (flamingo balance) or balance cushion may be used, and again trunk and hip movements of the contralateral limb throw stress onto the injured ankle. The foot may be placed along the beam, or with the beam travelling transversely and only the toes supported. Intense muscle activity is seen around the ankle as the athlete attempts to maintain his or her balance. By varying the athlete's footwear and performing the exercises in bare feet, the stresses imposed are altered.

A balance board with a single transverse rib is used for sagittal movements, and a longitudinal rib for frontal plane actions. A board with a domed central raise (wobble board or ankle disc) is used to combine movements for circumduction. In addition to trunk movements, actions such as throwing and catching while standing on the balance board are helpful as these take the athlete's attention away from the ankle, and so are a progression in terms of skill. Performing balance board exercises blindfolded, and therefore eliminating visual input, has been shown to be effective at improving proprioception in the ankle. The use of a labile (unstable) surface is more appropriate for those

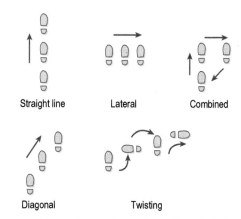

Figure 6.8 Hopping patterns in ankle rehabilitation.

who work or train on a selection of surfaces (field sports, gardeners, farmers for example).

Running, hopping and jumping activities are all used, on an even floor and then on varying surfaces including sand, grass and a mini-trampoline. Hopping direction is varied to alter the stress on the joint. Straight-line hopping places an anteroposterior stress on the joint, while lateral hopping imposes a mediolateral stress. Combined directions, diagonal hopping and twisting when hopping are all used to impose multiple stresses on the joint (Fig. 6.8). Running in a circle, figure-of-eight and on hills/cambers all change the stress on the ankle, and hopping and jumping develop power rather than strength.

Proprioception in the unstable ankle

The importance of proprioceptive training to prevent the development of CAI (giving way in normal usage) is of great importance. In the 1960s, proprioception was first highlighted as important to ankle rehab. Freeman, Dean and Hanham (1965) compared ligament injuries to the foot and ankle treated by immobilization, 'conventional' physiotherapy and proprioceptive training, which consisted of balance board exercises. After treatment, 7 per cent of the proprioceptive group showed instability, compared to 46 per cent of those treated by other means. Balance ability was measured using a modified Rhomberg test, which assesses the ability to maintain single-leg standing while the eyes are closed. Lentell, Katzman and Walters (1990) assessed the strength of the ankle musculature in 33 subjects with instability and found that there was no significant difference between the injured and uninjured sides. However, when balance ability was measured, the majority of subjects exhibited a deficit between the two extremities. Konradsen and Ravn (1990) measured the time taken for peroneal contraction to occur in response to a sudden inversion stress in chronically unstable ankles. Their results showed the peroneal reaction time to be prolonged with injured ankles (82 ms) compared to the uninjured side (65 ms), indicating a proprioceptive deficit. Karlsson and Andersson (1992) found similar results, quoting 84.5 ms and 81.6 ms for peroneus longus and peroneus brevis, respectively, for involved limbs, compared to 68.8 and 69.2 for uninvolved.

Glencross and Thornton (1981) assessed joint position sense to plantarflexion and found significantly greater errors in the replication of the test position for injured ankles compared to uninjured controls. Lentell et al. (1995) measured the threshold of the detection of passive motion and found a significant difference (greater amount of inversion) between injured and uninjured sides.

Definition

Peroneal reaction time is the difference between the onset of a rapid inversion force acting on the ankle (mechanical joint displacement) and the initiation of peroneal muscle contraction to try to resist this force (physiological muscle splinting).

Although reflex control of the ankle through peroneal reaction time may be important, central nervous system (CNS) factors have also been shown to act. Konradsen, Voight and Hojsgaard (1997) showed that inversion stress sufficient to cause ligament damage occurred within 100 ms.

Although the peroneal muscles may begin their contraction rapidly in response to such a stress (within 50–60 ms), it takes time for sufficient tension to build up to overcome the force of bodyweight. Such a force has been shown to require 170–180 ms to build to sufficient intensity, showing that the ankle musculature cannot react fast enough to protect the ankle from injury due to sudden inversion stress (Caulfield 2000).

In the trunk, it has been shown that some patients with chronic lower back pain have lost the ability to anticipate the need for stability (Hodges and Richardson 1996) and it seems that this anticipatory function may also be important in ankle stability. Dyhre-Poulsen, Simonsen and Voight (1991) measured EMG activity in the soleus and tibialis anterior in jumping activities and found that these muscles contracted before landing, and similar results have been found with the peroneal muscles in jumping tasks (Caulfield 2000).

As the ankle ligaments and capsule are torn, articular nerve fibres are also likely to be damaged, leading to a partial deafferentiation of the joint. This, in turn, will decrease the athlete's motor control and inhibit reflex stabilization of the foot and ankle. In addition, joint swelling has been shown to affect muscle control in the knee (Stokes and Young 1984) and ankle (Petrik et al. 1996), and alteration in the motor programme provided by the CNS may occur (Caulfield 2000).

Key point

Following ankle injury, loss of joint sensation and changes in motor control affect movement and stability of the joint.

Proprioceptive training should be incorporated into general rehabilitation training. Where CAI is seen, the modified Rhomberg Test or Star Excursion Balance Test (SEBT) (Table 6.3) may be used to monitor the degree of proprioceptive deficit. The modified Rhomberg test, although simpler to apply in the clinic, measures unidirectional stability,

Table 6.3 Measurement of ankle stability

Modified Rhomberg Test	Star Excursion Balance Test (SEBT)
The subject stands on their injured leg with their eyes open and hands by their sides. If they are able to maintain their balance for 5–10 seconds they are instructed to close their eyes. Body sway and loss of balance are noted.	The subject stands on their injured leg in the centre of a grid (star) marked with tape on the floor. Each arm of the grid extends at 45° increments from the centre. The subject reaches along each line as far as they can with their contralateral leg while maintaining balance. The distance of the reach is recorded for each limb of the grid and any asymmetry noted.

whereas the SEBT measures multidirectional stability. A simpler version of the SEBT is the Y balance test (YBT), where the subject stands on the injured leg and reaches in three directions (anterior, posteromedial and posterolateral) with the other leg (Fig. 6.9). The distance measured for each movement can be summed to produce a composite reach distance, which may be used to assess injury risk.

Progressive stability training has been shown to improve ankle stability measured on the SEBT (Rasool and George 2007), the programme progressing from solid floor to soft mat, with eyes open and then closed. A review of the effect of proprioceptive training on the ankle (Hughes and Rochester 2008) concluded that muscle reaction time, kinaesthetic deficits and postural sway all improve with proprioceptive exercise. A sample ankle stability training protocol is shown in Box 6.1.

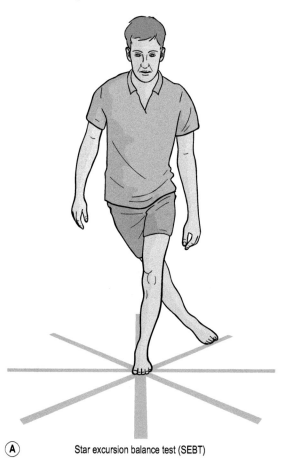

(A)   Star excursion balance test (SEBT)

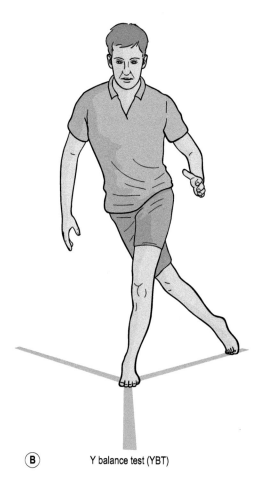

(B)   Y balance test (YBT)

Figure 6.9 Balance tests for ankle stability.

Box 6.1 Example of ankle stability protocol

Single-leg standing (SLS) hard floor eyes open

Single-leg standing hard floor eyes closed

SLS mini dip

Single-leg standing trunk rotation

SLS controlateral leg movement

Modified Rhomberg test (eyes open/closed, hands by sides, SLS)

SEBT star excursion balance test – star with 8 lines at 45 degrees. SLS in centre, reach with other leg

Soft mat

Wobble board

Fitter

Hop forwards back

Hop side to side

Cut

Cut and turn

Chronic ankle instability

Chronic ankle instability (CAI) is a feeling of the ankle 'giving way' or 'feeling unstable', typically in daily living on a regular basis (usually more than two occasions within the last six months) and gives both functional and quality of life (QOL) effects. Typical signs and symptoms are shown in Table 6.4. A number of questionnaires are available to test for the presence of CAI, and the Chronic Ankle Instability Scale (CAIS) is one example which has been tested for validity and reliability (Eechaute et al. 2008). The questionnaire consists of 14 questions concerning daily activities, function and psychosocial factors (Fig. 6.10).

Ankle taping

Ankle taping may be used to reduce excessive inversion–eversion stress in the previously injured individual, or as a preventive measure. Taping itself has traditionally been used, but semi-rigid orthoses are increasingly popular. These allow dorsiflexion–plantarflexion but limit inversion–eversion and so should have a less detrimental effect on overall lower-limb mechanics.

Orthoses have been shown to be as effective as taping at reducing inversion–eversion movement, but have the advantage that this support is more effectively maintained throughout training. Greene and Hillman (1990) compared several ankle orthotics with taping and found that after 20 minutes of exercise the taping revealed maximal losses of restriction while the orthoses demonstrated no mechanical failure. Rovere et al. (1988) showed ankle stabilizers to be more effective than taping at reducing ankle injuries. Surve et al. (1994) showed a lower incidence of ankle sprain and a reduced severity of injury in soccer players with a previous history of ankle injury who wore a semi-rigid ankle orthosis. No change in incidence of injury was seen in those without a previous history of injury.

In addition to support characteristics, the effect on lower-limb mechanics is important. Taping has

Table 6.4 Indications of chronic ankle instability (CAI) (data from Kosik et al 2017)

Signs & symptoms	Mechanical changes	Sensorimotor changes
▶ Recurrent injuries ▶ Perceived ankle instability and/or 'giving-way' ▶ Decreased self-reported function ▶ Structural alterations visible on scanning ▶ Sensorimotor impairments ▶ Participation restrictions ▶ Reduction in the overall health-related quality of life ▶ Increased risk of other chronic diseases	▶ Arthrokinematic restrictions ▶ Ligamentous laxity ▶ Joint degeneration	▶ Altered movement patterns ▶ Reduced static and dynamic postural control ▶ Loss of strength ▶ Altered spinal reflex excitability

THE CHRONIC INSTABILITY SCALE

Please rate every question by checking only one of the possible boxes that best describes your present condition (compared to your pre-injury level)

1. How much fear do you have of respraining your ankle?

☐ none ☐ a little bit ☐ moderate ☐ a lot ☐ extremely much

2. To what extent do you have difficulties/problems with cutting or changing directions (during walking, running or jumping) because of your ankle instability problem?

☐ none ☐ some ☐ moderate ☐ a lot ☐ unable to do

3. How often do you use an external ankle support when performing sports or recreational activities?

☐ never ☐ rarely ☐ sometimes ☐ often ☐ always ☐ N/A

4. To what extent do you avoid performing certain activities (such as walking, running, jumping, cutting) because of your ankle instability problem?

☐ not at all ☐ rarely ☐ sometimes ☐ often ☐ constantly

5. To what extent do you have difficulties/problems with walking on uneven ground because of your ankle instability problem?

☐ none ☐ some ☐ moderate ☐ a lot ☐ unable to do ☐ N/A

6. To what extent has the overall quality of your sports or recreational activities decreased as a result of your ankle instability, when compared to your pre-injury level?

☐ not at all ☐ slightly ☐ moderately ☐ strongly ☐ extremely ☐ N/A

7. How unstable does your ankle feel?

☐ not at all ☐ slightly ☐ moderately ☐ strongly ☐ extremely

8. To what extent do you have difficulties/problems with jumping because of your ankle instability problem?

☐ none ☐ some ☐ moderate ☐ a lot ☐ unable to do ☐ N/A

9. To what extent do you have difficulties/problems with running on even ground because of your ankle instability problem?

☐ none ☐ some ☐ moderate ☐ a lot ☐ unable to do ☐ N/A

10. To what extent do you have difficulties/problems with running on uneven ground because of your ankle instability problem?

☐ none ☐ some ☐ moderate ☐ a lot ☐ unable ☐ N/A

11. How frequently do you still sprain your ankle?

☐ not anymore ☐ rarely ☐ sometimes ☐ often ☐ constantly

12. If you sprain your ankle, how often does it cause symptoms such as pain, stiffness and swelling?

☐ not at all ☐ rarely ☐ sometimes ☐ often ☐ always ☐ N/A

13. To what extent are you concerned about your ankle instability problem?

☐ not at all ☐ slightly ☐ moderately ☐ very ☐ extremely

14. To what extent has your participation in certain sports or recreational activities decreased as a result of your ankle instability, when compared to your pre-injury level?

☐ not at all ☐ slightly ☐ moderately ☐ much ☐ do not participate any more ☐ N/A

Figure 6.10 The Chronic Ankle Instability Scale (Eechaute et al. 2008).

been shown to throw stress onto the forefoot as the foot compensates for the reduction of dorsiflexion in mid-stance in walking subjects. Where an ankle orthosis allows normal dorsiflexion, the forefoot is likely to receive less compensatory stress.

The combination of forefoot stress and loss of restriction capabilities may make the use of ankle orthoses preferable to taping in certain circumstances. The contribution of taping to proprioception, providing an increased skin stimulation to movement, may also be of importance. Restoration of full ankle function with a combination of strength and balance activities must always be the main consideration, with ankle supports used as an interim measure wherever possible. In addition, although taping has been shown to have no significant effect on performance during balance tests (see above), it does increase self-efficacy and perceived confidence in dynamic tasks (Halim-Kertanegara et al. 2017).

Impingement syndromes

Repeated forced dorsiflexion, such as occurs with dismounts in gymnastics, jumps in ballet and especially soccer may cause *anterior impingement* of the talus on the tibia (anterior tibiotalar impingement), a condition described colloquially as 'footballer's ankle'. The synovium may be repeatedly trapped, becoming chronically swollen and hypertrophied. The condition may also occur secondary to a severe lateral ligament sprain if the distal aspect of the ATF ligament impinges on the talus. Pain occurs over the front of the ankle and is exacerbated by dorsiflexion with overpressure. Radiographs may reveal talar osteophytes, but these may not actually contribute to the impingement or be symptomatic.

Forced plantarflexion, for example repeated bag work in kickboxing, may cause *posterior impingement*, giving pain over the back of the ankle without tenderness to the Achilles tendon. The area of impingement this time is the posterior talus and the tibia.

Both conditions show slight swelling and represent a repeated impaction of the joint surfaces, leading to compression of the articular cartilage and subchondral bone. These structures do not show great sensitivity, and will not be the primary source of pain. Instead, pain must come from the periosteum, the joint capsule or, more likely, from chemical irritation and mechanical stress caused by the inflammatory response itself. Impingement syndromes respond to rest, anti-inflammatory modalities and training modification.

If the impingement force persists, an exostosis may form on the back or front of the lower tibia, depending on the type of stress involved.

> **Definition**
>
> An exostosis is a benign (non-harmful) growth of bone which occurs at the edge of a joint. It may occur through mechanical stimulation of the bone membrane (periosteum) through repeated microtrauma.

The exostosis may be up to a centimetre long in some cases, and should it break off, it will float in the joint as a loose body. In cases where the exostosis causes symptoms, it may be surgically removed.

Rapid, forceful dorsiflexion, such as may occur in a fall onto the feet from a height, can force the talus up with enough force to stress the inferior tibiofibular ligament. The joint is tender to palpation within the sulcus between the tibia and fibula, and pain is elicited to passive dorsiflexion, but not inversion or eversion. Treatment involves strapping the foot to limit dorsiflexion, and using a heel raise.

On the posterior aspect of the talus, the flexor hallucis longus travels in a small groove. If the bone lateral to this point is extended, it is called *Stieda's process*. When this piece occurs as a separate bone (ossicle) attached to the talus by fibrous tissue, it is known as the *os trigonum*. Between 8 and 13 per cent of the population have one of these bony configurations (Brodsky and Khalil 1987) (Fig. 6.11). Three mechanisms are generally proposed for the

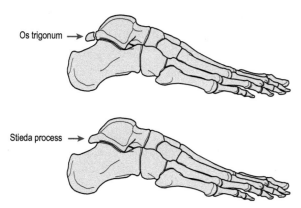

Figure 6.11 Lateral view of the ankle, showing the os trigonum and Stieda's process. From Brodsky, A.E. and Khalil, M.A. (1987) Talar compression syndrome. *Foot and Ankle*, **7**, 338–344. With permission.

development of the os trigonum. The secondary ossification centre in the region may fail to fuse, or repeated trauma (impingement) may cause a stress fracture. An acute fracture may also ensue following forced plantarflexion, with or without avulsion of the posterior band of the lateral ligament.

Repeated plantarflexion may compress the os trigonum and give impingement pain, palpable over the posterolateral talus between the Achilles tendon and the peroneal tendons. If symptoms fail to settle with conservative management, surgical removal of the ossicle may be called for. This is often performed with release of the adjacent tendon sheath of flexor hallucis longus.

Tendinopathy in association with the malleoli

Peroneal muscles

The tendons of peroneus longus and brevis pass around the lateral malleolus, while those of tibialis posterior, flexor digitorum longus and flexor hallucis longus pass around the medial malleolus (Fig. 6.12). Any of the tendons, their sheaths or their retaining retinacula may be inflamed or injured.

One complication of ankle sprain is a strain or avulsion of the peroneus brevis as it attaches to the

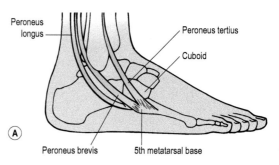

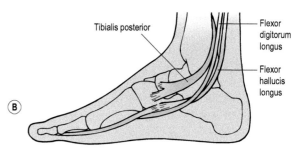

Figure 6.12 Tendons near the malleoli. (A) Lateral view. (B) Medial view.

base of the fifth metatarsal (see above). There may be local bruising, and pain is reproduced by resisted eversion. Point tenderness, proximal to the base of the fifth metatarsal, indicates the tendon, while bone pain may indicate avulsion. Radiographs are required to differentiate avulsion from a fracture to the fifth metatarsal itself (Jones fracture). Treatment of peroneus brevis strain is similar to that of an ankle injury, with frictions performed to the tendon while the foot is inverted and exercises to restore strength and flexibility of the peroneus brevis. Where swelling has occurred over the peroneus brevis insertion, it may spread to the joints formed by the cuboid bone, and mobilization of this bone may be required. Complete avulsion of the tendon may require immobilization for one or two weeks (Karlsson 2007).

> **Key point**
> Following ankle sprain, the peroneus brevis muscle and its attachment to the base of the fifth metatarsal should be examined.

In addition, the mobility of the cuboid bone should be checked, to exclude involvement of either of these structures.

Peroneal tendon dislocation may occur if the tip of the lateral malleolus is fractured with forced dorsiflexion (skiing) or a direct blow (soccer). Occasionally, severe inversion injury may rupture the peroneal retinaculum and allow the tendons to sublux or dislocate forwards over the fibula with resisted dorsiflexion and eversion. Local pain is present, and a 'snapping' sensation is felt as the tendons move over the bone. Surgical management is required, with several procedures being performed to re-establish the anatomy of the region. Re-attachment of the retinaculum, deepening of the peroneal groove, and placing the peroneal tendons under the calcaneofibular ligament have been variously described.

Flexor hallucis longus

The flexor hallucis longus (FHL) passes behind the medial malleolus in a separate tendon sheath, which runs along the anterior aspect of the talus. The sheath passes between the medial and lateral tubercles of the talus, under the sustentaculum tali, and beneath the flexor retinaculum. The fibro-osseous tunnel so formed predisposes the tendon to mechanical irritation.

Pain may occur to resisted hallux flexion, with tenderness lying medial to the Achilles tendon. Pain is usually noticeable during the push-off phase of walking and running. A fusiform swelling and thickening of the tendon may occur in dancers with repeated point work. Eventually, the thickening may interfere with the movement of the tendon within its sheath, giving rise to 'trigger toe' (Sammarco and Miller 1979).

Tibialis posterior

The tibialis posterior tendon passes in a groove around and beneath the medial malleolus, the latter structure acting as a pulley. During pronation, the tendon is pressed onto the underlying bone of the groove, and in athletes who hyperpronate during the stance phase, tendon or tendon-sheath pathology may occur, representing *posterior tibial tendon dysfunction*.

Posterior tibial tendon dysfunction

Posterior tibial tendon dysfunction (PTTD) is a cause of persistent pain around the medial malleolus, and a leading cause of flat foot disorders, especially in seniors. The prevalence rate is 3.3 per cent in the over-forties, which is actually greater than that for Achilles tendinopathy in the non-athletic population (Albers et al. 2014).

Structure and function

The tibialis posterior (TP) is the deepest of the muscles on the back of the shin, lying within the deep posterior compartment. It attaches to the posterior aspect of the tibia and fibula and the interosseous membrane between the two. From here it passes in the groove of the medial malleolus, to enter the foot and insert into the navicular and the medial cuneiform. The navicular is the keystone of the foot arch, and its height is maintained by the pull of the tibialis posterior. As a consequence, the muscle inverts the foot at the subtalar joint, and importantly acts to maintain the height of the medial longitudinal arch. Additionally, the muscle is a plantarflexor of the ankle joint, the combination of these two actions making it the main supinator of the foot in the stance phase of walking.

Injury

The condition may be categorized into one of four stages, depending on the height of the medial foot arch and the available movement (flexible or rigid) of the rearfoot joints as shown in Table 6.5. Early stages (1 and 2) represent a flexible flat-foot deformity (FFD) and are generally managed conservatively. Later stages (3 and 4) may benefit from conservative management in the short term, but may require surgical intervention to

Table 6.5 Posterior tibial tendon dysfunction (PTTD) categorization

Stages	Clinical findings
1	Mild swelling, medical ankle pain, no deformity and minimal pain when rising onto the toes (heel raise action).
2	Flattening of medial arch, abducted midfoot, but hind foot still flexible (can be corrected passively). Calcaneus may event over time. Patient may be unable to perform heel raise action. Tibialis posterior swollen and ineffective.
3	Fixed hind foot deformity, cannot be corrected passively. Lateral abutment over calcanea-fibular articulation possible and X-ray shows degeneration of midfoot joints (talonavicular and calcaneocuboid joints).
4	Stage 3 fixed deformity has progressed to allow the ankle joint (tibiotalar joint) to degenerate.

regain foot function. Tissue changes to the tibialis posterior in PTTD suggest degeneration rather than inflammation, implying tendinopathic changes (see Chapter 1). Disruption of the linear organization of collagen bundles occurs, giving a reduction in tensile strength, with few inflammatory infiltrates found at surgery (Mosier et al. 1999, Kulig et al. 2009).

Assessment

Subjective assessment often reveals a history of slow onset over months or years, with activities such as prolonged standing increasing symptoms. A recent shopping trip or standing at an event is often the trigger. Tenderness is frequently described over the inner ankle, extending to the posterior portion of the inner foot edge. Pain is often dull and aching in nature and affected by choice of footwear in Stages 1 and 2 especially. Soft un-supporting shoes such as ballet pumps, or slippers may make pain worse, while it can be eased when wearing supporting sports shoes or more rigid leather shoes.

Objective assessment should initially be made in standing. The height of the medial longitudinal arch should be assessed and the navicular drop test may be useful. The height of the navicular is assessed using a ruler placed vertically on the inside of the

foot. To begin, the patient stands with their weight on the unaffected leg, and then transfers the weight across to the affected leg to try to stand on one leg. Assess if the navicular height drops, and if so can the patient prevent this by trying to lift the inner edge of the foot upwards.

Definition

The *navicular drop test* assesses the subject's ability to maintain the height of the medial longitudinal arch when moving from non-weightbearing to full weightbearing.

The navicular drop test determines the subject's ability to maintain medial arch height, and the test can be extended with the supination resistance test (SRT). Here the subject is in standing and the therapist places their fingers under the navicular (or talonavicular joint) and attempts to lift the medial arch by applying a longitudinal force along the length of the tibia. The resistance required to form the arch is assessed and scored from 1 (low) to 5 (high). Comparison is made between the affected and unaffected foot. The test has shown good reliability (44 subjects tested by 4 clinicians), with reliability improving with therapist experience (Noakes and Payne 2003). However, greater variability is introduced by changes in bodyweight and alteration in foot position (Bennett et al. 2015).

If the inner arch has flattened (Stage 1), is the deformity correctable by passively lifting the joint up, or is it fixed? Where the arch height has lowered, has the heelbone (calcaneus) also been pulled outwards (subtalar joint valgus)? A final foot position may be forefoot abduction, where the front portion of the foot splays outward. A useful visual check of this, when viewed from behind, is that the patient appears to have too many toes (Davey 2016). Here, when looking from behind past the heel and Achilles, you should normally be able to see the fourth and fifth toes as well. However, if the forefoot has abducted (moved outwards), more of the toes are visible.

The navicular bone may be more prominent as it presses inwards, and sometimes an accessory navicular is present – this is an extra piece of bone or cartilage which is located within the tibialis posterior tendon as it attaches to the navicular proper, and is visible on X-ray.

Commonly with PTTD the calf muscles may be tight, limiting the amount of dorsiflexion (ankle bending forwards) at the end of the stance phase of walking. As dorsiflexion is reduced, the foot compensates by abducting the forefoot and rolling over the inner edge of the foot with each step. Raising up onto the toes (heel raise action) may also be limited or changed. Normally, when a person performs a heel lift the heels swing inwards slightly (varus) but with PTTD the heelbone can begin outwards (valgus or flatfoot appearance) and fail to correct as the patient raises onto their toes. Commonly, the tendon may be painful to palpation behind the malleolus in its groove, or at its insertion into the navicular tuberosity.

The foot posture index (FPI-6) is a useful general assessment of the foot which may be used before and after treatment to assess improvement in any flexible foot disorder (FFD). Using it, the clinician assesses the position of the head of talus, the curves beneath the malleolus, heel (calcaneal) position, prominence of the navicular head, height of the medial longitudinal arch and the presence of forefoot abduction. FFD is said to be present in standing when one or more of the following is shown: calcaneal valgus, medial longitudinal arch depression and forefoot abduction (Bowring and Chockalingam 2009).

Exercise

The aim of conservative management is to reduce pain and inflammation, lessen the strain on the TP tendon and promote healing. Strength and function are enhanced, and foot alignment improved, to prevent the condition progressing. Passive modalities (electrotherapy, acupuncture), manual therapy (massage, soft tissue manipulation) and support (taping, orthotics) all have their place in the management of this condition. Generally, they are used to modify symptoms and especially to modulate pain.

Graded exercise constitutes a major part of the treatment of PTTD, as with other forms of tendinopathy. The tibialis posterior can be exercised using a resistance band into plantarflexion and inversion, and both concentric and eccentric actions are required. This is best achieved with the subject sitting (sports shoes on) with their knee bent, heel in contact with the floor. Loop a resistance band around the foot and perform the action holding the hand out to the side, or with the band attached to a table leg. Where a person has a normal arch height, this action may be performed barefoot. Although this is a non-weightbearing movement and so not functionally specific to walking and running, it has the advantage of taking compression away from the tibialis posterior tendon, and so not exacerbating pain. Once this action is pain-free, dorsiflexion and plantarflexion (heel aligned) may be used against band resistance prior to double-leg and single-leg heel raises, again with correct heel alignment. Where the heel falls outwards (valgus), gripping a foam block between the heels of a double-leg heel lift can be a good cue to aid correction (Fig. 6.13).

Arch lift exercises are also useful. These can begin in sitting, lifting the centre of the medial arch upwards (increasing the dome height) while keeping the ball of the foot pressing down on the floor to avoid forefoot supination (Fig. 6.14).

Once the calf is stretched (leg straight and knee bent), a step-down action may be used (Fig. 6.15). The action is to keep the affected foot on the step facing forwards and to step down with the non-affected foot. The knee should pass over the centre of the foot to avoid forefoot abduction (flattening the foot and rolling over the inner edge).

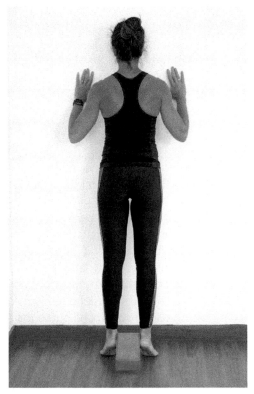

Figure 6.13 Heel raise action gripping block.

The exercise response should be graded over time. The aim is to build resilience in the tissues by overloading them sufficiently to stimulate change but not so much that they are irritated or damaged. As the tissues adapt, the overload (hardness of exercises) should increase to keep pace, with the aim being pain-free full function.

Tarsal tunnel syndrome

The tarsal tunnel is formed by the medial malleolus, calcaneus and talus on one side and the flexor retinaculum and medial collateral (deltoid) ligament on the other (Fig. 6.16). It begins approximately two to three centimetres proximal to the medial malleolus, and through it travels the posterior tibial nerve. The tunnel ends where the medial and lateral plantar nerves enter the abductor hallucis.

The tunnel may be restricted anatomically by tightness in the fascia and retinacula, which normally result from trauma or overuse, and the build-up of scar tissue. Increased pronation and a valgus (outwardly tilted) heel will tighten the flexor

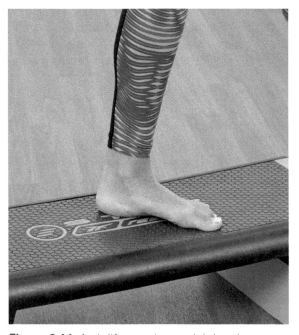

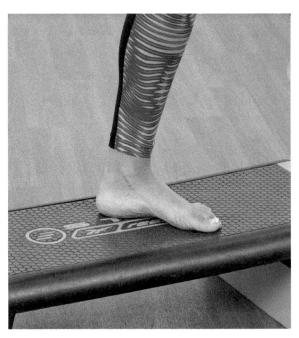

Figure 6.14 Arch lift exercise, weightbearing.

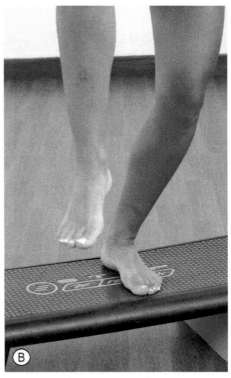

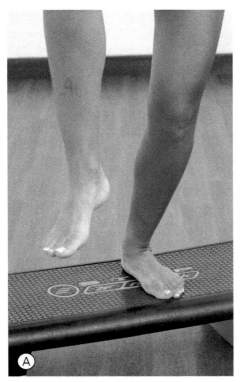

Figure 6.15 Step down maintaining arch height. (A) Correct alignment. (B) Incorrect alignment.

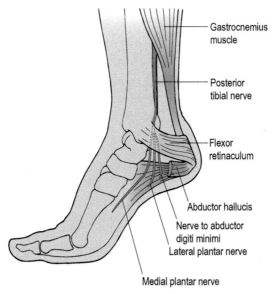

Figure 6.16 The tarsal tunnel. From Magee (2002), with permission.

Gastrocnemius muscle

Posterior tibial nerve

Flexor retinaculum

Abductor hallucis

Nerve to abductor digiti minimi

Lateral plantar nerve

Medial plantar nerve

retinaculum and make the condition more likely. Following fracture of the calcaneum, tarsal tunnel syndrome may occur as a result of either bony impingement or tightness of the cast, and irritation from training shoes may also give a similar clinical picture.

The most common symptom is burning and loss of sensation in the plantar aspect of the foot, which is worse with activity and better with rest. The big toe is the most common area of complaint. Nerve conduction tests to the abductor hallucis (and abductor digiti minimi) confirm the diagnosis.

Treatment is by correction of excessive pronation and rearfoot valgus, together with modification of footwear. Soft tissue mobilization and stretching may also be needed. Resistant cases may require surgical decompression.

313

Subtaloid joint

The subtaloid joint (STJ) (Fig. 6.17) has a thin capsule strengthened by the medial, posterior and lateral talocalcaneal ligaments. The joint cavity is isolated from that of the ankle and mid-tarsal joints, and its stability is largely maintained by the interosseous talocalcanean ligament running from the sinus tarsi to the talus.

Subtaloid mobility is often reduced following ankle sprain or fracture of the calcaneus from a fall onto the heel. Movement may also be reduced by impaction when jumping on a hard surface in inadequate footwear. The lack of mobility sometimes goes unnoticed, unless the patient is assessed by a therapist.

Manual assessment and mobilization of accessory movements may be performed with the patient in a supine-lying position, with the heel over the couch end. Initially, the therapist grips around the distal part of the patient's leg, with one hand pressing the leg onto the couch. The therapist's forefingers

grip the talus and the calcaneum is cupped in the opposite hand (Fig. 6.18A). The calcaneum is then moved on the fixed talus. Releasing the talus, both talus and calcaneum are moved together on the fixed lower leg. Gross subtaloid joint movement may be performed by cupping the heel in both hands and performing forceful inversion/eversion actions (Fig. 6.18B).

Some distraction may be given to the STJ in supine, with one hand cupping the calcaneum laterally and applying a caudal force while the other hand stabilizes the dorsomedial aspect of the mid-foot (Fig. 6.18C). In the prone position, with the patient's foot slightly plantarflexed and the toes over the couch end, a distraction force may be imparted by pushing caudally with the heel of the hand onto the posterior aspect of the calcaneus near the Achilles tendon insertion (Fig. 6.18D). Following injury, rearfoot position should be assessed as posting may be required.

Mid-tarsal joint

The mid-tarsal joint (see Fig. 6.17) is composed of the calcaneal cuboid joint (lateral), and the talocalcaneonavicular joint (medial). Four ligaments are important from the perspective of sports injuries. The *plantar calcaneonavicular* (spring) ligament is a dense fibroelastic structure running from the sustentaculum tali to the navicular behind its tuberosity. The *plantar calcaneocuboid* ligament passes from the anterior inferior aspect of the calcaneus to the plantar surface of the cuboid behind the peroneal groove. The *long plantar* ligament stretches the whole length of the lateral aspect of the foot. It arises from between the tubercles of the calcaneus and passes forwards, giving off a short attachment to the cuboid, and so forming a roof over the tendon of peroneus longus. The ligament then attaches to the bases of the lateral four metatarsal bones. The *bifurcate* ligament is in two parts, and travels from a deep hollow on the upper surface of the calcaneus to the cuboid and navicular.

The calcaneocuboid joint takes the full bodyweight as it forms part of the lateral longitudinal arch

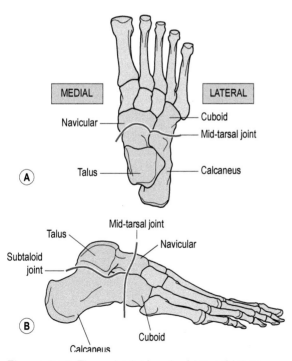

Figure 6.17 The subtaloid and mid-tarsal joints. (A) From above. (B) Lateral view.

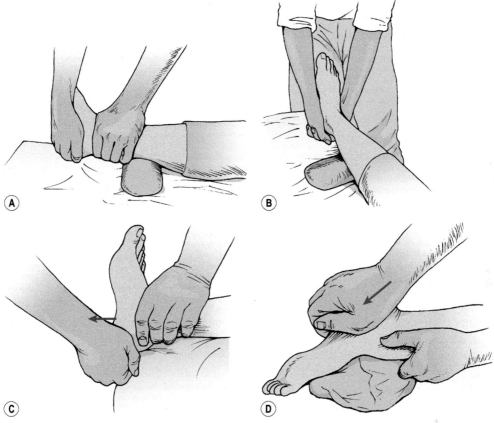

Figure 6.18 Manual therapy of the subtaloid joint. (A) Stabilize lower leg and move talus. (B) Gross subtalar movement. (C, D) Distraction and gliding.

of the foot. Stability is provided by the plantar calcaneocuboid and long plantar ligaments, reinforced by the tendon of peroneus longus. The talocalcaneonavicular joint is stabilized by the plantar calcaneonavicular and bifurcate ligaments, together with the tendon of tibialis posterior.

The calcaneocuboid ligament may be injured at the same time as the ATF. Pain is reproduced by fixing the rearfoot in dorsiflexion and eversion, and inverting and adducting the forefoot. Often the condition goes unnoticed at the time of injury as the AFT sprain is the dominant pain. Chronic pain results, and transverse frictions and scar tissue rupture may be required, with temporary forefoot posting.

References

Albers, S., Zwerver, J. and Akker-Scheek, I., 2014. 7 Incidence and prevalence of lower extremity tendinopathy in the general population. *Br J Sports Med* **48**(Suppl 2), A5.

Bachmann, L., Kold, E., Koller, M. et al., 2003. Accuracy of Ottawa ankle rules to exclude fractures of the ankle and mid-foot: systematic review. *BMJ* **326**, 1–7.

Bennett, P. J., Lentakis, E., & Cuesta-Vargas, A., 2015. Limitations of the manual supination resistance test. *Journal of Foot and Ankle Research* **8** (Suppl 2), O2.

Bowring, B. and Chockalingam, N., 2009. A clinical guideline for the conservative management of tibialis posterior tendon dysfunction. *The Foot* **19** (4), 211–217.

Brodsky, A.E., Khalil, M.A., 1987. Talar compression syndrome. *Foot and Ankle* **7**, 338–344.

Burdett, R.G., 1982. Forces predicted at the ankle during running. *Medicine and Science in Sports and Exercise* **14** (4), 308–316.

Caulfield, B., 2000. Functional instability of the ankle joint. *Physiotherapy*, **86** (8), 401–411.

Davey, N., 2016. Medial ankle pain: how well do you know Tom? *InTouch* magazine. Autumn. **156**, 14–21.

Doherty, C., Bleakley, C., Delahunt, E. et al., 2017. Treatment and prevention of acute and recurrent ankle sprain: an overview of systematic reviews with meta-analysis. *British Journal of Sports Medicine* **51** (2), 113–125.

Dyhre-Poulsen, P., Simonsen, E., Voight, M., 1991. Dynamic control of muscle stiffness and H-reflex modulation during hopping and jumping in man. *Journal of Physiology* **437**, 287–304.

Eechaute, C., Vaes, P., Duquet, W., 2008. The chronic ankle instability scale: clinimetric properties of a multidimensional, patient-assessed instrument. *Physical Therapy in Sport* **9**, 57–66.

Eiff, M.P., Smith, A.T., Smith, G.E., 1994. Early mobilisation versus immobilisation in the treatment of lateral ankle sprains. *American Journal of Sports Medicine* **22**, 83–88.

Flandry, F., Sanders, R.A., 1987. Tibiofibular synostosis: an unusual cause of shin splint-like pain. *American Journal of Sports Medicine* **15**, 280–284.

Freeman, M.A.R., Dean, M.R.E., Hanham, I.W.F., 1965. The etiology and prevention of functional instability of the foot. *Journal of Bone and Joint Surgery* **47B** (4), 678–685.

Glencross, D., Thornton, E., 1981. Position sense following joint injury. *Journal of Sports Medicine* **5**, 241–242.

Greene, T.A., Hillman, S.K., 1990. Comparison of support provided by a semirigid orthosis and adhesive ankle taping before, during, and after exercise. *American Journal of Sports Medicine* **18** (5), 498–506.

Gribble, P.A,, Bleakley, C.M., Caulfield, B.M. et al., 2016. 2016 consensus statement of the International Ankle Consortium: prevalence, impact and long-term consequences of lateral ankle sprains. *British Journal of Sports Medicine* **50** (24), 1493–1495.

Halim-Kertanegara, S., Raymond, J., Hiller, C. et al., 2017. The effect of ankle taping on functional performance in participants with functional ankle instability. *Physical Therapy in Sport* **23**, 162–167.

Hodges, P.W., Richardson, C.A., 1996. Contraction of transversus abdominis invariably precedes movement of the upper and lower limb. In: *Proceedings of the 6th International Conference of the International Federation of Orthopaedic Manipulative Therapists.* Lillehammer, Norway.

Hughes, T., Rochester, P., 2008. The effects of proprioceptive exercise and taping on proprioception in subjects with functional ankle instability: a review of the literature. *Physical Therapy in Sport* **9**, 136–147.

Kaikkonen, A., Kannus, P., Jarninen, M., 1996. Surgery versus functional treatment in ankle ligament tears. *Clinical Orthopaedics* **326**, 194–202.

Karlsson, J., 2007. Acute ankle injuries. In: Brukner, P., Khan, K. (eds), *Clinical Sports Medicine.* 3rd ed. McGraw Hill, Sydney, pp. 612–631.

Karlsson, J., Andersson, G., 1992. The effect of external ankle support in chronic lateral ankle joint instability. *American Journal of Sports Medicine* **20**, 257–261.

Konradsen, L., Ravn, J.B., 1990. Ankle instability caused by prolonged peroneal reaction time. *Acta Orthopaedica Scaninavica* **61** (5), 388–390.

Konradsen, L., Voight, M., Hojsgaard, C., 1997. Ankle inversion injuries: the role of the dynamic defence mechanism. *American Journal of Sports Medicine* **25**, 54–58.

Kosik, K.B., McCann, R.S., Terada, M. et al., 2017. Therapeutic interventions for improving self-reported function in patients with chronic ankle instability: a systematic review. *British Journal of Sports Medicine* **51** (2), 105–112.

Kulig, K., Reischl, S., Pomrantz, A. et al., 2009. Nonsurgical management of posterior tibial tendon dysfunction with orthoses and resistive exercise: a randomized controlled trial. *Physical Therapy* **89** (1), 26–37.

Lentell, G., Bass, B., Lopez, D. et al., 1995. The contributions of proprioceptive deficits, muscle function, and anatomic laxity to functional instability of the ankle joint. *Journal of Orthopedic and Sports Physical Therapy* **21**, 206–215.

Lentell, G.L., Katzman, L.L., Walters, M.R., 1990. The relationship between muscle function and ankle stability. *Journal of Orthopaedic and Sports Physical Therapy* **11** (12), 605–611.

Mosier, S.M., Pomeroy, G., Manoli, A., 1999. II. Pathoanatomy and etiology of posterior tibial tendon dysfunction. *Clin Orthop Relat Res.* **365**, 12–22.

Noakes, H., Payne, C., 2003. The reliability of the manual supination resistance test. *Journal of the American Podiatric Medical Association* **93** (3), 185–189.

Petrik, J., Mabey, M.A., Rampersaud, R.J., Amendola, A., 1996. The effects of isolated ankle effusion on H reflex amplitude, viscoelasticity, and postural control of the ankle. *Proceedings of the American Academy of Orthopedic Surgeons* **12** (2), 81–86.

Rasool, J., George, K., 2007. The impact of single leg dynamic balance training on dynamic stability. *Physical Therapy in Sport* **8**, 177–184.

Rohner-Spengler, M., Mannion, A., Babst, R., 2007. Reliability and minimal detectable change for the figure-of-eight-20 method of measurement of ankle edema. *Journal of Orthopaedic and Sports Physical Therapy* **37**, 199–205.

Rovere, G.D., Clarke, T.J., Yates, C.S., Burley, K., 1988. Retrospective comparison of taping and ankle stabilizers in preventing ankle injuries. *American Journal of Sports Medicine* **16**, 228–233.

Sammarco, G.J., Miller, E.H., 1979. Partial rupture of the flexor hallucis longus in classical ballet dancers. *Journal of Bone and Joint Surgery* **61A**, 440.

Stiell, I.G., McKnight, R., Greenberg, G., et al., 1994. Implementation of the Ottawa Ankle Rules. *JAMA* **271**, 827–832.

Stokes, M., Young, A., 1984. The contribution of reflex inhibition to arthrogenous muscle weakness. *Clinical Science* **67**, 7–14.

Surve, I., Schwellnus, M.P., Noakes, T., Lombard, C., 1994. A fivefold reduction in the incidence of recurrent ankle sprains in soccer players using the sport-stirrup orthosis. *American Journal of Sports Medicine* **22**, 601–606.

Vargish, T., Clarke, W.R., 1983. The ankle injury: indications for the selective use of X-rays. *Injury* **14**, 507–512.

Yeung, M.S., Chan, K-M., MPhil, C.H.S., Yuan, W.Y., 1994. An epidemiological survey on ankle sprain. *British Journal of Sports Medicine* **28**, 112–116.

CHAPTER 7

The foot

The foot is a subject's main contact area with the ground – an obvious point, but one which helps account for the very high number of conditions affecting this area, in sport especially. An athlete's foot may have to withstand forces two or three times greater than body weight, and this may be repeated more than 5,000 times every hour when running. Most sports involve some sort of running or jumping, and so the foot is continually called upon to provide both stability and shock attenuation. Prolonged standing is often part of daily living, and again the foot is placed under considerable stress.

Foot biomechanics

An understanding of the biomechanical factors which affect the foot during gait is important, both to the prevention and management of sports injuries and to foot function in daily life. Abnormal forces placed on the body through alterations in normal walking or running can cause injury. In addition, rehabilitation of lower-limb injuries, if it is to be successful, must involve the restoration of correct gait. We begin with the subtalar joints, the connection between the ankle and foot.

Subtalar joint

The subtalar joint (STJ) lies between the concave undersurface of the talus and the convex posterior portion of the upper surface of the calcaneum. The STJ is in its neutral position when the posterior aspect of the heel lies vertical to the supporting surface of the foot, and parallel to the lower third of the leg.

Determining neutral position of the STJ

Neutral position of the STJ is its optimal alignment and this is often used as a starting point or baseline to determine foot and leg alignment changes. Neutral STJ position may be obtained in standing, supine lying and prone lying. In standing, the practitioner palpates the head of the talus on the dorsal aspect of the foot. The athlete then twists the trunk, forcing the tibia to internally and externally rotate. The neutral position is the point at which the head of the talus appears to bulge equally under each palpating finger. In lying (prone or supine), the practitioner grasps the athlete's foot over the fourth/fifth metatarsal head and presses the foot into dorsiflexion. Again, the practitioner palpates the head of the talus and swings the foot inwards and outwards to stop at the point where the talar head seems not to bulge more on one side.

Key point

Neutral position of the subtalar joint (STJ) is determined by palpating the head of the talus and moving the foot. When the talus appears to bulge equally at each side, the STJ is in neutral.

Biomechanics of the STJ

An essential feature of the STJ is its ability to perform triplane motion. This occurs when movement of one joint is in all three body planes (frontal, sagittal and transverse) because the joint axis is oblique.

Pronation of the foot is a triplane movement of the calcaneum and foot consisting of calcaneal eversion (frontal plane), abduction (transverse plane) and dorsiflexion (sagittal plane). Supination is an opposing movement of calcaneal inversion, adduction and plantarflexion in the same planes. These are both open-chain movements in their pure forms. Functionally, the movements occur in closed-chain formation with the foot on the ground. Abduction and adduction cannot occur owing to friction with the floor, and dorsiflexion and plantarflexion will not occur in their pure form as the joints are no longer free to move. Instead, the talus takes over these movements, with supination consisting of calcaneal inversion with abduction and dorsiflexion of the talus, while pronation combines calcaneal eversion with adduction and plantarflexion of the talus (Fig. 7.1).

Definition

In the weightbearing foot, supination (high-arched foot) consists of calcaneal inversion with abduction and dorsiflexion of the talus, while pronation (flattened foot) combines calcaneal eversion with adduction and plantarflexion of the talus.

The foot has two important functions during the gait cycle. The first is to act as a mobile adaptor, adjusting to alterations in the ground surface and reducing the shock travelling up to the other lower-limb joints. Second, the foot must efficiently transmit force from the muscles of the lower leg to provide propulsion to push off during gait. For this, the foot must change into a rigid lever. These two diametrically opposed functions of mobile adaptor and rigid lever are achieved by changing the bony alignment of the foot joints, and 'locking' or 'unlocking' the foot.

Mid-tarsal joint

The movement of the STJ alters the alignment of the two components of the mid (transverse) tarsal joint (MTJ). These are laterally the calcaneal-cuboid joint, and medially the talocalcaneonavicular joint. The mid-tarsal joint has two axes of motion, one oblique and one longitudinal. The longitudinal axis primarily allows inversion and eversion of the forefoot, while the oblique axis permits

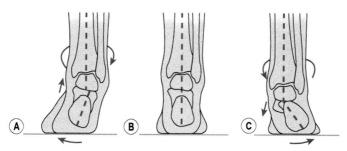

Figure 7.1 Weightbearing motion of the subtaloid joint. (A) Supination. (B) Neutral position. (C) Pronation. From Gould (1990), with permission.

adduction/abduction and plantarflexion/dorsiflexion. The direction of the motions at the mid-tarsal joint causes the dorsiflexion force created by weightbearing to lock the forefoot against the rearfoot.

The position of the STJ alters the neutral alignment of the mid-tarsal joint axes. Supination of the STJ causes the axes to become more oblique and less motion can take place. The foot is said to be locked, and acts as a rigid lever ideal for propulsion. Pronation of the STJ causes the mid-tarsal joint axes to become more parallel and therefore more mobile. Now the foot is unlocked, and acts as a mobile adaptor capable of accommodating to changes in the ground surface.

First ray complex

The first ray is a functional unit consisting of the first metatarsal and the first cuneiform. Its axis is at 45 degrees to the sagittal and frontal planes. The joint does have triplane motion, but little abduction and adduction occur functionally. Dorsiflexion of the first ray is accompanied by inversion, and plantarflexion is combined with eversion.

Definition

The first ray consists of the first metatarsal bone and the first cuneiform.

The gait cycle

The gait cycle can be conveniently divided into two phases. The stance phase occurs when the foot is on the floor, supporting the body weight. Closed-chain motion occurs in the lower limb, as it decelerates. The swing phase takes place as the foot comes off the ground, and open-chain motion follows. This time the limb is accelerating.

Definition

During gait the *stance* phase occurs with the foot on the floor (weightbearing) and

the *swing* phase with the foot off the floor (non-weightbearing).

The foot moves through four positions in three phases during stance. Initially, the heel strikes the ground (contact phase) and as the body weight moves forwards, the foot flattens (mid-stance). Forward movement continues and the heel lifts off the ground; finally the toes push off (propulsion) and the leg moves into the swing phase.

At the start of the swing phase the limb is accelerating. In the mid-swing position the speed is constant, and finally the leg decelerates, and is lowered to the ground where heel strike again occurs and the cycle is repeated (Fig. 7.2).

The stance phase in walking is approximately 60 per cent of the total gait cycle, while the swing phase is 40 per cent. Walking at a normal rate of 120 steps/min, the total cycle takes 1 s, so stance occurs for 0.6 s, while swing takes only 0.4 s. With running, the movements occur more rapidly, and the stance phase occupies less of the total cycle time. A runner with a pace of 6 min/mile has a total cycle time of only 0.6 s. The stance phase would last for 0.2 s, and so events occurring within this phase are performed three times faster.

During the walking gait cycle, overlap of the stance phases of both legs occurs so that, for a short period, both feet are on the ground at the same time (double leg support). As walking speed increases, the double leg support period reduces. When the stance leg 'toes-off' before the swinging leg contacts the ground, double leg support is eliminated and an airborne period is created. Walking has now progressed to running.

Key point

In walking, both legs remain on the ground for a short period (double leg support). As walking speed increases, double leg support time reduces. When the pace has increased to running, double leg support is eliminated.

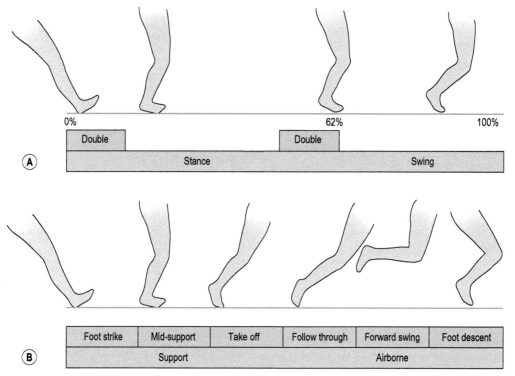

Figure 7.2 (A) The walk cycle and (B) the run cycle. From Subotnick (1989).

Stance phase

During the stance phase, the forces taken by the various areas of the foot will vary, from a peak at the heel during the contact phase to a more gradual and later-occurring force curve at the first metatarsophalangeal region at toe-off (Fig. 7.3).

Contact

With the contact phase, the lateral aspect of the calcaneum strikes the ground. The ankle joint is close to its neutral (90-degree) position, and the subtalar joint is slightly supinated. The hip is flexed to about 30 degrees. The pelvis and the body's centre of gravity are moving laterally over the weightbearing leg, producing closed-chain adduction of the hip.

The STJ starts to pronate, and the mobility of the mid-tarsal joint is increased. The ankle begins to plantarflex to bring the foot flat onto the ground for mid-stance. Pronation causes the tibia to internally

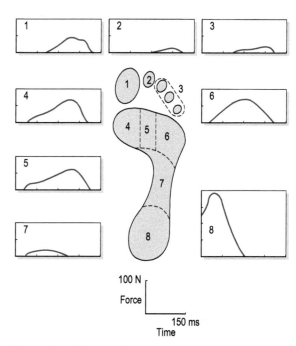

Figure 7.3 Force acting through the foot during walking. From Reid (1992), with permission.

rotate, and this in turn unlocks the knee, allowing it to flex to about 20 degrees, in a movement opposite to the screw home effect (see Chapter 4). The hip begins to extend and internally rotate and this continues until heel raise.

The anterior tibials contract eccentrically to stop the foot slapping at heel strike, and the posterior tibials decelerate pronation. The quadriceps work eccentrically to allow the knee to bend, and the hamstrings prevent trunk flexion at the hip. Later, the hamstrings work concentrically to extend the hip (closed-chain extension). The hamstrings are used in preference to the gluteals here, possibly because they have been pre-stretched. When the knee bends, the hamstrings can no longer produce hip extension, and the gluteals take over.

The hip abductors work eccentrically to control lateral movement over the supporting leg and then concentrically to pull the bodyweight back again in preparation for the next cycle.

Mid-stance

In mid-stance, the transition of the foot from mobile adaptor to rigid lever occurs. The STJ starts to supinate, reducing mid-tarsal mobility and locking the foot. When hip adduction is completed, closed-chain abduction occurs for the rest of the stance phase.

The action of the calf is eccentric to control dorsiflexion and with it forward motion of the body, and the posterior tibials contract concentrically to supinate the foot.

Propulsion

The heel rises with plantarflexion at the ankle and the propulsion phase begins, the knee reaching its point of maximal extension. At toe-off, dorsiflexion again occurs at the ankle to prevent toe drag, and the hip begins to flex. The calf now works concentrically to actively plantarflex the ankle, and the peroneus longus and brevis are eccentric to control supination. The peroneus longus also stabilizes the first ray. The quadriceps work eccentrically to control the knee.

Swing phase

During the swing phase, the maximally supinated STJ moves back to its position of slight supination just before heel strike. The knee continues to flex during the acceleration position of the swing phase, and starts to extend again before heel strike. The hip continues to flex, until it has reached its 30-degree position to begin the cycle again. The quadriceps continue to contract eccentrically to stop the knee 'snapping' back, and the hip flexors are concentric to accelerate the leg forwards. Phasic muscle action during running is summarized in Figure 7.4.

Altered biomechanics of the foot

Excessive pronation/supination

These conditions occur if the normal pronation and supination periods of the gait cycle are extended, or when there is a change in the angulation of the foot segments, and are not always symptomatic. Causes may be extrinsic, such as tight muscles or abnormal lower-leg rotation, or intrinsic, as occurs with fixed deformities of the STJ and MTJ.

Severe pronation causes foot flattening. The range of motion at the STJ is increased, making the mid-tarsal joint axes more parallel and unlocking the foot. The foot can then remain pronated and mobile after the stance phase, hence the terms 'hypermobile' or 'weak' foot.

With excessive supination, the MTJ is locked, the foot is more rigid and the arch higher (cavus). In time the plantar fascia and intrinsic foot muscles become tight, reducing the capacity of the foot to dissipate shock.

Rearfoot varus

The rearfoot and forefoot can both move outward (valgus) or inward (varus), giving the four alignment faults shown in Table 7.1. The first is rearfoot varus. With this condition, the calcaneus appears inverted when the foot is examined in the neutral position. Left uncompensated, the forefoot would

323

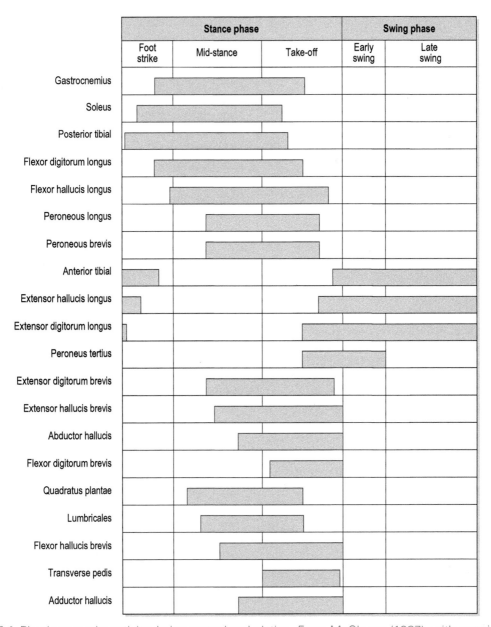

Figure 7.4 Phasic muscular activity during normal ambulation. From McGlamry (1987), with permission.

invert and leave the medial side of the foot off the ground. To compensate, the STJ pronates excessively on ground contact. This deformity has been associated with an increased number of lateral ankle sprains.

Rearfoot varus is usually a result of developmental abnormality. From the eighth to twelfth foetal week

the calcaneum lies at the side of the talus. As the foetus develops, the calcaneum rotates to a more plantar position, so that it lies below the talus. However, the calcaneus may not be completely perpendicular to the ground until the child is six years old, and in some cases the rotation is never complete. In addition to the subtalar

Table 7.1 Biomechanical changes in the rearfoot and forefoot

Deformity	Foot position
With the STJ neutral, compare the calcaneal line with the tibial line	
Rearfoot varus (A)	Tibial line — Calcaneal line — Heel appears inverted
Rearfoot valgus (B)	Heel appears inverted
With the STJ neutral and the midtarsal joint maximally pronated, compare heel with the plane of the metatarsal heads	
Forefoot varus (C)	Plane of metatarsal heads — Medial side of foot raised
Forefoot valgus (D)	Lateral side of foot raised

deformity, the condition is also associated with tibial varum.

Rearfoot valgus

This condition can occur if the calcaneum rotates excessively in its development, or following a Pott's fracture. The posterior surface of the calcaneum will appear everted, and the foot will hyperpronate, giving a severe flatfoot. The condition is associated with genu valgum (knock knees) and the medial longitudinal arch appears flattened.

Forefoot varus

In this deformity the forefoot is inverted in respect to the rearfoot, when the STJ is in a neutral position. To compensate, and bring the forefoot to the ground, the STJ everts and the entire plantar surface of the foot becomes weightbearing, flattening the medial longitudinal arch. The head of the talus bulges proximally to the tuberosity of navicular. Plantar calluses are apparent over the second and third metatarsal heads, and an associated hallux valgus deformity may be present.

If the STJ is unable to pronate sufficiently, the entire plantar surface of the foot will be unable to touch the ground. Weightbearing will therefore be lateral, with callus formation this time over the fourth and fifth metatarsal heads.

Abnormal pronation continues into the propulsive phases of the gait cycle, and the foot tries to push off without becoming a rigid lever. This instability causes shearing forces between the metatarsal heads, giving rise to associated pathologies. Interdigital neuroma, postural fatigue, fasciitis, chondromalacia and shin pain have all been described as resultant to this deformity (McPoil and Brocato 1990).

Forefoot valgus

Here, there is an eversion of the forefoot in relation to the rearfoot, a situation exactly opposite to that above. The medial foot structures are in contact with the ground while the lateral side is suspended. Deformities greater than 6 degrees may require STJ and MTJ compensations. To place the foot flat on the ground, the calcaneus will invert, pulling the talus into an abducted-dorsiflexed position. During the contact phase of gait, the foot will pronate more than normal, and remain pronated and therefore mobile into the propulsive phase. Symptoms associated with hypermobility of the metatarsophalangeal and interphalangeal joints occur.

Plantarflexed first ray

This condition is present when the first metatarsal lies below the level of the other metatarsals in neutral position, causing the forefoot to appear slightly everted relative to the rearfoot. When forefoot eversion continues, a forefoot valgus is present.

Various conditions may give rise to this problem. If the first metatarsal phalangeal (MP) joint is rigid (hallux rigidus) the foot is forced rapidly into supination (a supinatory rock) to allow the lateral side of the foot to bear weight. In so doing, the fifth metatarsal head strikes the ground rapidly. In addition, weakness of the tibialis anterior will allow the peroneus longus to pull the first ray into plantarflexion unopposed. Deformity occurs over time, and is particularly exaggerated in certain neuromuscular diseases.

Biomechanical examination and treatment

Examination of foot biomechanics must include observation of the spine, pelvis, hip and knee as well. Forces acting through the kinetic chain, and referral of pain from other structures, make holistic evaluation of lower-limb function essential. Subjective examination and inspection of the lower limb may act as pointers to further assessment.

Objective examination is made both with the subject weightbearing and non-weightbearing. Positions include standing, sitting, walking and then running. With walking and running, video analysis is often used to slow the motion down and aid in the identification of faults. In each case the examination may be carried out with the athlete in shorts and bare feet, and then while wearing shoes. The wear pattern of the shoes (Fig. 7.5) is often a useful general guide to the existence of underlying biomechanical changes.

In standing, the alignment of the various body segments is assessed. Starting from the top of the body and working down, viewed from behind, the head and shoulder positions are noted, as is the symmetry of the spine. Shoulder and pelvic levels are assessed. Buttock and knee creases are examined for equal level. Knee position gives a clue to the presence of coxa valga/vara and genu vara/valga (Fig. 7.6).

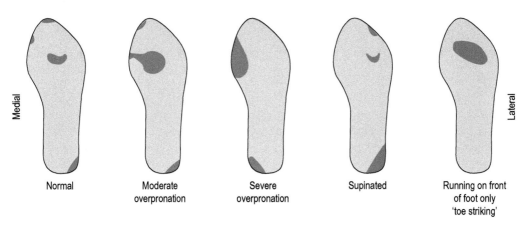

Medial · Lateral

Normal · Moderate overpronation · Severe overpronation · Supinated · Running on front of foot only 'toe striking'

Figure 7.5 Wear pattern on sports shoes. From Reid (1992), with permission.

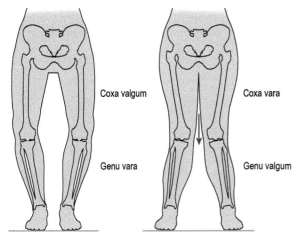

Figure 7.6 Femoral and tibial alignment. From Subotnick (1989).

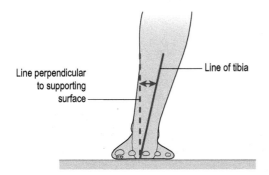

Figure 7.7 Tibia vara measurement made from standing position.

Tibial vara can be measured in standing by comparing the line of the distal third of the leg to a line perpendicular to the supporting surface which passes through the posterior contact point of the calcaneus (Fig. 7.7).

From the front, similar comparisons of shoulder, pelvic, spinal and leg alignments are made. The position of the patella relative to the foot will suggest any tibial torsion. Tibial torsion can be further assessed with the patient in sitting with the knee flexed to 90 degrees over the end of the couch. The examiner places his or her thumbs over the patient's malleoli and compares an imaginary line connecting these two points with the knee axis.

In supine lying, active and passive range of movement at the knee and hip are measured and any asymmetry or alteration in normal end-feel is noted. Resisted strength is measured and limb girths measured. The distribution of any pain or alteration in sensation is mapped. The appearance of the foot is observed and any skin abnormalities noted. In prone lying, range of movement of the foot is measured and compared to normal values.

Calcaneal inversion and eversion are measured by marking a line bisecting the back of the calcaneus (calcaneal line) and comparing this to a line bisecting the calf and Achilles (tibial line).

> **Definition**
>
> The tibial line joins two points on the midline of the lower third of the tibia. The calcaneal line joints the midpoint of the calcaneus at the insertion of the Achilles with a midpoint 1 cm distal to this point.

Forefoot position is assessed by placing the STJ in its neutral position. A goniometer is then placed over the metatarsal heads, and its line compared to one perpendicular to the line of calcaneal bisection. Alternatively, a forefoot measuring device (FMD) may be used. This has a slit which is placed over the line of calcaneal bisection, the plateau on the front of the FMD is placed over the plantar surface of the foot in line with the met heads, and a value for forefoot–rearfoot alignment read from the scale. Using both goniometry and the FMD, the most common forefoot–rearfoot relationship is one of varus, with average values being 7.5 degrees (Garbalosa, Donatelli and Wooden 1989). Significant biomechanical faults of the foot, if symptomatic, may be managed by using a functional orthotic device. These can be either temporary and prefabricated (off the shelf), or custom fabricated (bespoke), made subsequent to foot casting or pressure-plate measurement.

327

The first metatarsophalangeal joint

The first metatarsal bone joins proximally to the first cuneiform to form the first ray complex (above). Distally, the bone forms the first metatarsophalangeal (MP) joint with the proximal phalanx of the hallux. The first MP joint is reinforced over its plantar aspect by an area of fibrocartilage known as the volar plate (plantar accessory ligament). This is formed from the deep transverse metatarsal ligament, and the tendons of flexor hallucis brevis, adductor hallucis and abductor hallucis. It has within it two sesamoid bones, which serve as weightbearing points for the metatarsal head (Fig. 7.8).

Movement of the joint is carried out by flexor hallucis longus, flexor hallucis brevis, extensor hallucis longus, the medial tendon of extensor digitorum brevis, and abductor and adductor hallucis. This fairly complex structure is often taken for granted but does give rise to a number of important conditions.

Turf toe

Turf toe is a sprain involving the plantar aspect of the capsule of the first MP joint. It is most often seen in athletes who play regularly on synthetic surfaces, and results from forced hyperextension (dorsiflexion) of the first MP joint. Forced plantarflexion injury can also occur as a separate entity and is known as sand toe due to its incidence in beach volleyball players. Normally the first MP joint has a dorsiflexion range of 50 to 60 degrees, but with trauma the range may be forced to over 100 degrees. The condition is quite common, with studies of American football players showing that 45 per cent of athletes had suffered from turf toe at some stage (Rodeo et al. 1989a).

Forced hyperextension of the first MP joint causes capsular tearing, collateral ligament damage and damage to the plantar accessory ligament. Sometimes force is so great that disruption of the medial sesamoid occurs (Fig. 7.9). Examination reveals a hyperaemic swollen joint, with tenderness over the plantar surface of the metatarsal head. Local bruising may develop within 24 hours. Differential diagnosis must be made from sesamoid stress fracture (insidious onset) and metatarsal or phalangeal fractures (site of pain and radiograph). Three grades of injury are described. Grade 1 being a capsular strain alone, Grade 2 partial tearing and Grade 3 complete tear with MTP joint instability.

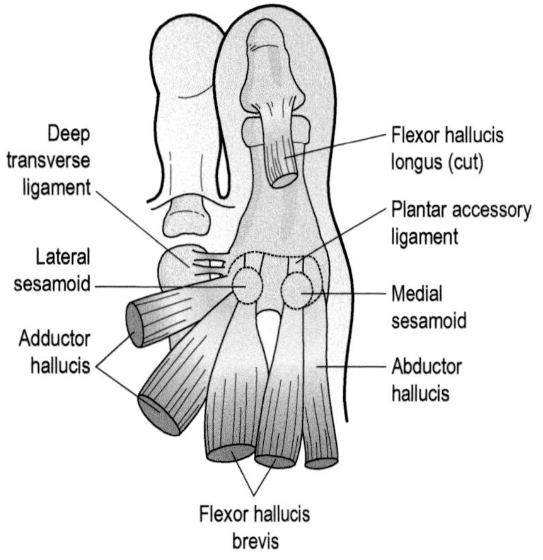

Figure 7.8 Structure of the first metatarsophalangeal joint.

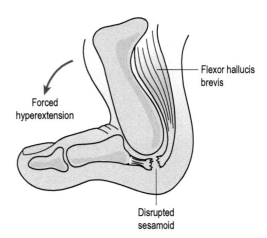

Figure 7.9 Forced hyperextension causes soft tissue damage and possible sesamoid disruption – 'turf toe'.

Key point

Turf toe is a sprain of the plantar capsule and ligament of the first MP joint.

Treatment aims at reducing pain and inflammation and supporting the joint by taping (Fig. 7.10). An oval piece of felt or foam with a hole in the middle is placed beneath the toe, the hole corresponding to the metatarsal head. The first MP joint is held in neutral position and anchors are applied around the first phalanx and mid-foot. Strips of 2.5 cm inelastic tape are applied as stirrups between the anchors on the dorsal and plantar aspects of the toe. In each case the tape starts at the toe and is pulled towards the mid-foot, covering the first MP joint. The mid-foot and phalanx strips are finished with fixing strips.

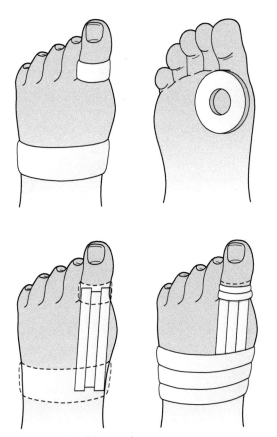

Figure 7.10 Turf toe taping.

A number of factors may predispose the athlete to turf toe. The condition is more common with artificial playing surfaces than with grass. Artificial turf is less shock-absorbing, and so transmits more force directly to the first MP joint. Sports shoes also have an important part to play. Lighter shoes tend to be used with artificial playing surfaces. These shoes are more flexible around the distal forefoot, and allow the MP joint to hyperextend. In addition, shoes which are fitted by length size alone, rather than width, may cause problems for athletes with wider feet. This person must buy shoes which are too long to accommodate his or her foot width. Such a shoe increases the leverage forces acting on the toe joints and allows the foot to slide forwards in the shoe, increasing the speed of movement at the joint.

Preventive measures include wearing shoes with more rigid soles to avoid hyperextension of the injured joint. In addition, semi-rigid (spring steel or heat-sensitive plastic) insoles may be used. Some authors have recommended the use of rigid insoles as a preventive measure when playing on all-weather surfaces, for all athletes with less than 60-degree dorsiflexion at the first MP joint (Clanton, Butler and Eggert 1986).

An increased range of ankle dorsiflexion has been suggested as a risk factor which may predispose an athlete to turf toe (Rodeo et al. 1989b). However, in walking subjects, when the ankle is strapped to reduce dorsiflexion, the heel actually lifts up earlier in the gait cycle, causing the range of motion at the metatarsal heads to increase (Carmines, Nunley and McElhaney 1988). This increased range may once again predispose the athlete to turf toe (George 1989), so the amount of dorsiflexion per se may not be that important. If injury has recently changed the range, the athlete may not have had time to fully adapt to the altered movement pattern, and the altered foot/ankle mechanics in total may be the problem.

As with many soft tissue injuries, if incorrectly managed the condition may predispose the athlete to arthritic changes in later life. In the case of turf toe, this may occur as calcification of the soft tissues around the injury site, presenting as hallux valgus or hallux rigidus.

Hallus valgus

Hallux valgus (hallux abductovalgus or HAV) usually occurs when the first MP joint is hypermobile, and the first ray is shorter than the second (Morton foot structure). When this is the case, the second metatarsal head takes more pressure than in a non-Morton foot (Rodgers and Cavanagh 1989) (Fig. 7.11). In addition, hallux valgus is more common in athletes who hyperpronate. Often the combination of hyperpronation and poorly supporting fashion footwear exacerbates the condition.

Pronation of the subtaloid joint reduces the stabilizing effect of the peroneus longus muscle, allowing the first metatarsal to displace more easily. The increased motion leads to the combined deformity of abduction and external rotation of the first toe (phalanges) and adduction and internal rotation of the first metatarsal. Joint displacement occurs at both the MP joint and the metatarsal/medial cuneiform joint (Lorimer et al. 2002).

As the first MP joint dorsiflexes during the propulsive phase of running, the instability allows the hallux to deviate from its normal plane. Adduction and axial rotation occur, and the long flexors which normally stabilize the joint now themselves become deforming influences, causing

bowstring effect. As the first metatarsal head adducts, the sesamoids sublux and eventually erode the plantar aspect of the first metatarsal head – this is one source of pain. Compensatory stress is placed on the joints proximal and distal to the first MP and further pain arises through synovial inflammation and capsular distraction. Eventually, secondary osteoarthritis occurs in the first MP joint and sesamoids. High-heeled and constrictive footwear may predispose to the condition.

Hallux valgus may occur in one of two types. *Congrous hallux valgus* is an exaggeration of the normal angulation between the metatarsal and the phalanx of the first toe. Importantly, the joint surfaces remain in opposition and the condition does not progress. The normal angulation of the first MPJ (measured between the long axis of the metatarsal and that of the proximal phalanx) is 8 to 20 degrees; in congruous hallux valgus this angle may increase to 20 to 30 degrees (Fig. 7.12A). Once the angle increases above 30 degrees, the joint surfaces move out of congruity and may

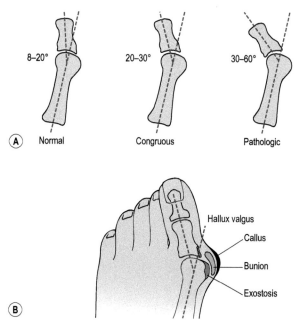

Figure 7.12 Hallux valgus. (A) Metatarsophalangeal angle and (B) appearance. After Magee (2002), with permission.

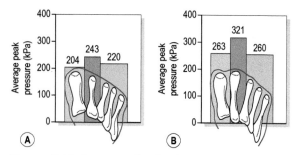

Figure 7.11 Pressure distribution in (A) non-Morton and (B) Morton feet. From Rodgers, M.M. and Cavanagh, P.R. (1989) Pressure distribution in Morton's foot structure. *Medicine and Science in Sports and Exercise*, **21**, 23–28. With permission.

eventually sublux. This condition is now classified as *pathological hallux valgus*, and may progress, with the angulation increasing to as much as 60 degrees (Magee 2002).

Bunion formation to the side of the first metatarsal head is common. The bursa over the medial aspect of the MPJ thickens and a callus develops. In time an exostosis is seen on the metatarsal head and the three structures combined lead to the cosmetic change which is noticeable (Fig. 7.12B). A gel-padded bunion shield can help reduce both abnormal shearing and compressive stress to ease symptoms when walking. At night a bunion regulator which resists the abduction forces acting on the first toe can help to protect the overstretched soft tissues and reduce inflammation and pain.

Definition

A bunion shield is a soft pad placed over the toe joint. A bunion regulator is a firmer splint placed over the forefoot to resist abduction of the first toe.

Management of this condition is initially to stabilize the first MP joint by correcting faulty foot mechanics (especially hyperpronation) and advising on correct athletic footwear. If conservative management fails, surgery may be required. If the deformity is purely soft tissue in nature, the bunion may be removed, and the dynamic structures around the first toe realigned. If bony deformity is present, osteotomy (bone realignment), arthroplasty (forming a new joint) or arthordesis (joint fusion) may be necessary.

Hallux limitus/rigidus

A reduction in movement of the first MP joint, *hallus limitus*, may progress to complete immobility or *hallux rigidus* where the joint is ankylosed. The condition is more common when the first metatarsal is longer than the second. Pain is generally worse during sporting activities, and occurs especially when pushing off. On examination, the joint end feel is usually firm, and limitation of movement is noted to dorsiflexion. To differentiate between a tight flexor hallucis longus and joint structures, the foot is assessed, both with the foot dorsiflexed and everted (tendon on stretch) and then plantarflexed and inverted (tendon relaxed).

Key point

In hallux limitus, movement may be restricted by either a tight flexor hallucis longus (FHL) or joint structures. To differentiate between the two, movement range is assessed both with the tendon on stretch (FHL limits) and with the tendon relaxed (joint limits).

Limitation of motion through muscle tightness can respond well to stretching procedures, while joint limitation which is soft tissue in nature is often treated by joint mobilization. Distal distraction and gliding mobilizations with the metatarsal head stabilized are particularly useful. Where bony deformity is present, surgery may be indicated if the condition limits the subjects mobility.

Taylor's bunion

A Taylor's bunion is seen over the base of the fifth metatarsal. It is normally associated with a wider fourth/fifth inter-metatarsal (IM) angle which in turn leads to an associated varus (towards the centre of the foot) angle of the fifth metatarsophalangeal joint. The condition is more common in athletes who have a cavus foot with splaying toes, and may cause abrasion in unyielding sports footwear such as ski boots, cycling shoes and roller boots. Management is generally conservative, encouraging athletes to select sports shoes with a wide toe box. Severe cases may require surgical intervention.

Definition

The intermetatarsal (IM) angle is the angle between the first and second metatarsal shaft when viewed on an X-ray. Normal values are less than 9 degrees.

Plantar fasciitis

Plantar fasciitis, or more correctly chronic plantar heel pain (CPHP), is pain under the front of the heelbone, and is known by several names (Table 7.2). It is said to account for about 1 per cent of all orthopaedic referrals, and occurs in up to 7 per cent of the adult population in general. In runners, the incidence is slightly higher, with 8 to 10 per cent affected (Stecco et al. 2013, Rathleff et al. 2014).

Function

Functionally the plantar fascia (PF) acts as an important mechanical link between the rearfoot and forefoot. At heel contact, the curved surface of the heel bone (calcaneus) acts as a rocker or roll-over shape (Hansen et al. 2004) to help facilitate forward body motion. Similarly the bodyweight

Table 7.2 Plantar fasciitis nomenclature and differential diagnosis

Alternate names	Differential diagnosis
▶ Chronic Plantar Heel Pain (CPHP) ▶ Painful heel syndrome ▶ Plantar fasciitis ▶ Plantar fasciopathy ▶ Plantar tendinopathy ▶ Plantar enthesiopathy ▶ Subcalcaneal bursitis ▶ Neuritis ▶ Medial arch pain ▶ Stone bruise ▶ Calcaneal periostitis ▶ Heel spur ▶ Subcalcaneal spur ▶ Calcaneodynia	▶ Calcaneal epiphysitis (Sever's disease) ▶ Calcaneal stress fracture or other bone injury ▶ Fat pad syndrome (atrophy, heel bruise) ▶ Inflammatory or reactive arthritis (Reiter syndrome/ankylosing spondylitis/psoriatic arthritis) ▶ Bone pathology (Osteomalacia/Osteomyelitis/Paget disease/bone cyst) ▶ PF rupture/local tissue infection ▶ Tumour (Sarcoma) ▶ PF fibromatosis (Ledderhose's disease) ▶ Calcaneal or retrocalcaneal Bursitis ▶ Neural referral (lumbosacral, local neuritis, tarsal tunnel syndrome)

rolls over the curved ankle (talocrural) joint mortise and ball of the foot (first MTP joint), the combined motion of the three body parts being described as the three-rocker system (Perry 1992). As the bodyweight moves forwards, the foot acts as a mobile adaptor (see above), flattening both the longitudinal and transverse arches to absorb load through tissue extensibility. Further forward motion of the body sees the foot change to a rigid lever to prepare for the propulsive phase of gait and toe-off. The change from tissue lengthening (adaptor) to tissue tension (lever) comes about as a result of the windlass effect, where the PF is wound up around the first MTP joint as the heel lifts and the foot moves into plantarflexion. Tension is seen in both the PF and Achilles tendon, which effectively transmits the contractile force created by the calf musculature.

Definition

The *windlass effect* (mechanism) occurs when the PF is tightened like a cable, running from the calcaneus and the metatarsophalangeal joints. Tightening the PF shortens the distance between the two bone regions to elevate the medial longitudinal arch.

As the fascia tightens through the windlass effect, it shortens the foot by raising the longitudinal arch (Fig. 7.13). The combination of these effects supinates the foot (high arch), making it more rigid to push from the ground. As the foot contacts the ground again at heel strike the arch lowers and the foot pronates (flat arch), becoming more mobile to adapt to the uneven ground. The plantar fascia is relaxed as the foot lengthens, to accommodate to the surface.

The functional linkage between the PF and posterior leg structures is paralleled by pathology. A positive correction between Achilles tendon loading and PF tension has been demonstrated, and chronic stretching and tightness of the Achilles tendon are risk factors for PF (Carlson et al. 2000). Greater tightness in posterior leg muscles is also seen in PF patients (Bolivar et al. 2013).

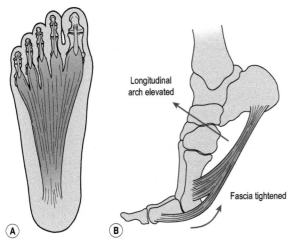

Figure 7.13 Plantar fascia structure and action. (A) Normal tension in fascia. (B) Raising onto the toes tightens the plantar fascia and raises the longitudinal arch.

Differential diagnosis

Pain and tenderness in this condition is usually over the calcaneal attachment of the PF or its medial edge. The feeling may be localized to the heel, as though the subject is 'stepping on a stone', or present as a burning sensation over the inner foot arch.

> ### Key point
> PF pain can be either localized to the heel, as though the subject is 'stepping on a stone', or present as a burning sensation over the inner foot arch.

Imaging may be used to assess the condition, and to rule out other pathologies. Plain radiograph (X-ray) is non-specific, but will often show a calcaneal bone spur, which may be asymptomatic. Bone scan will show increased uptake at the medial calcaneal tubercle and may be used to rule out stress fracture. Ultrasound has the convenience of immediate application, but is far more reliant on the skill of the operator (user dependence). Typically, it shows fascial thickening and fascial regions which appear darker as they reflect less

ultrasound (hypoechoic). MRI can be used to show swelling (oedema) of the fascia and adjacent fat pad, fascial thickening (usually in the proximal PF), bone marrow oedema to the medial calcaneal tuberosity, and altered tissue signal. MRI has an important use in ruling out co-morbidities such as infection or tumour (Medscape 2016). U/S scanning has been shown to be reliable in assessing the progress of treatment, to indicate tissue changes over a time period (Mohseni-Bandpei et al. 2014).

Bilateral or atypical heel pain may require laboratory tests such as rheumatoid factor, uric acid, blood count or ESR to assess systemic causes. See Table 7.1 for differential diagnoses.

Structure

The PF averages 12 cm in length and 2–6 cm in width. Attaching from a point just behind the inner (medial) tubercle of the heel bone, it runs anteriorly as medial, lateral and central portions. The PF is divided into a thicker central portion and thinner medial and lateral bands. The medial band is continuous with the abductor hallucis muscle (big toe abductor), the lateral band with the abductor digiti minimi (little toe abductor) (Fig. 7.14). As it approaches the metatarsal heads, the fascia divides into superficial and deep layers, with the superficial

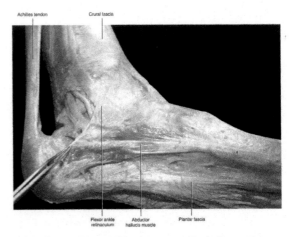

Figure 7.14 Plantar fascia anatomical dissection (From Stecco, C. (2015) Functional atlas of the human fascial system. Churchill Livingstone).

layer attaching beneath the skin, and the deep layer dividing into two portions to surround each of the five flexor tendons. Each of these five portions attaches to the base of a proximal phalanx and to the deep transverse ligament, which runs across the centre of the forefoot.

On dissection, the PF has been found to extend backwards over the calcaneus as a 1–2 mm thick band (continuous with the periosteum) to merge with the paratendon of the Achilles tendon (Stecco et al. 2013). Through this linkage forces within the fascia may be transmitted to and from the myofascia stretching along the length of the posterior leg.

> **Key point**
> A portion of the PF is anatomically continuous with the Achilles tendon, transmitting tension to and from the calf.

Gross attachment of the PF to the calcaneus is via an enthesis (connective tissue junction) formed of fibrocartilage. The fibrocartilaginous layer represents a zone of transition from soft to hard tissue and this region can calcify, a change visible on X-ray.

The PF has structural similarities to ligaments and tendons. Like these structures it consists of a ground matrix with cells (fibrocytes and fibroblasts) embedded in it. These cells produce collagen (connective tissue), which in the case of the plantar fascia is crimped, producing a highly adaptive matrix which may also have a sensory function. The combination of these two features makes it possible that the PF may transmit force passively (like an elastic band) and be able to change its response depending on the stresses imposed upon it.

Type I collagen is found arranged longitudinally throughout the PF, with Type III in the loose connective tissue and within areas where the PF bundles are arranged haphazardly. Type II collagen is found close to the heel, and very few elastic fibres are present. Hyaluronan (HA) is found between fibres, and fibroblast-like cells arranged in the direction of the collagen fibres. The HA may facilitate gliding between the PF fibrous bundles and have an anti-inflammatory nature. It is most likely secreted by fasciacytes. Nerve endings and Ruffini and Pacini corpuscles are found within the PF, more concentrated in the medial, lateral and distal portions where the PF joins onto muscle. The inner surface where the muscles of the sole of the foot attach is more innervated than the outer surface, which is continuous with the skin. The PF innervations have been proposed to give it a proprioceptive role (Stecco et al. 2013). The PF is said to be capable of perceiving both foot position and intrinsic foot muscle contraction.

Pathology

A systematic review of factors associated with CPHP (Irving et al. 2006) concluded that only body mass index (BMI) and calcaneal spur in a non-athletic population had been shown to have a strong association. Increased age, decreased ankle dorsiflexion, decreased first MPJ extension and prolonged standing showed a weak association (Table 7.3).

Calcification of the PF enthesis increases tissue stiffness, a process increased in the elderly, perhaps explaining the greater incidence of PF in these subjects. Traction (tensile loading) at

Table 7.3 Factors associated with the development of CPHP

Strength of association	Factor considered
Strong	Body Mass Index (BMI) in sedentary individuals Presence of Calcaneal spur on X-ray
Weak	Increased bodyweight in sedentary individuals Increased age Reduced ankle dorsiflexion Reduced 1st MTP joint extension Prolonged standing in daily living
Inconclusive	Static foot posture Dynamic foot motion

(Data from Irving et al. 2006)

Table 7.4 Pathological changes seen in plantar fasciitis

> ▷ Degenerative changes at the plantar fascia enthesis
> ▷ Deterioration of collagen fibres
> ▷ Increased secretion of ground substance proteins
> ▷ Focal areas of fibroblast proliferation
> ▷ Increased vascularity

Data from Rathleff et al. (2014)

the enthesis is often considered a causal factor in PF, but shearing and compression stress is likely equally important. Compressive forces are associated with similar conditions such as tendinopathy (Cook and Purdam 2012).

The term plantar fasciitis itself implies an inflammatory reaction to the fascia (-itis being a suffix meaning inflamed in medicine) but there is a question as to whether this is appropriate. Studies have shown degeneration and fragmentation of the fascia, with bone marrow vascular ectasia (expansion) at its insertion, but no inflammatory markers are generally present. Changes have been summarized by Rathleff et al. (2014) (Table 7.4).

Such changes imply that the condition may be more accurately termed a fasciosis (-osis meaning an abnormal state) rather than a fasciitis. This fact is important when treating the condition, as steroid injections (anti-inflammatory) often used to treat plantar pain have a strong association with plantar ruptures (Murphy 2006). In a study of 765 patients with plantar fascial pain Acevedo and Beskin (1998) found 51 patients who had received corticosteroid injection. Of this subgroup, 44 ruptured, with 68 per cent showing sudden onset tearing and 32 per cent gradual onset tearing. At follow-up, 26 subjects still showed symptoms a year after rupture. Rupture as a result of corticosteroid injection can be seen in up to 10 per cent of patients in general (McMillan et al. 2012).

Definition

Medical terms ending in 'itis' mean inflamed, and those ending in 'osis' mean an abnormal state.

As indicated above, normally during mid-stance the foot is flattened, stretching the PF and enabling it to store elastic energy to be released at toe-off. However, a variety of suboptimal foot postures (malalignment) may increase stress on the fascia. Excessive rearfoot pronation (see above) will lower the arch and overstretch the fascia, and a reduction in mobility of the first metatarsal may also contribute to the condition (Creighton and Olson 1987). In addition, weak peronei, often the result of incomplete rehabilitation following ankle sprains, may reduce the support on the arch, thus stressing the plantar fascia. Congenital problems such as pes cavus (high instep) may also leave an athlete more susceptible to CPHP. PF tension through a prolonged windlass effect may exacerbate the condition, and tightness in the Achilles tendon or a plantaflexed foot position (high-heeled shoes) can produce this.

Sports shoes and general footwear may exacerbate symptoms. Inadequate rearfoot control may fail to eliminate hyperpronation, and a poorly fitting heel counter will allow the calcaneal fat pad to spread more at heel strike, transmitting extra impact force to the calcaneus and PF. Degeneration of the fat pad with ageing has been suggested as a risk factor for the condition.

Both static and dynamic foot posture have been examined using Navicular height, calcaneal angle (pitch) using radiographs, and medial longitudinal arch contour using a footprint test. Looking for an association with the development of CPHP, the evidence produced was inconclusive (Irving et al. 2006). Modification of foot position using orthotics or shoe types should be considered (Rogers et al. 2016) if they modify a patient's symptoms, but used with caution as they may build dependence and distract from one of the primary aims of rehabilitation, which should be to build increased tissue capacity.

Passive treatments

Taping

Taping (low dye taping) may give temporary pain relief and allow continuation of daily living activities or low-level sport. A systematic review of six trials (Radford et al. 2006) showed an immediate increase in navicular height (mean 5.9 mm) post application. This was not maintained during exercise, and the authors questioned whether the change was clinically useful. Low dye taping has also been shown to reduce mid-PF strain in a cadaveric study (Bartold et al. 2009).

For the classic low dye method, a strip of zinc oxide tape is placed along the medial edge of the foot, proximal to the first MP joint around the back of the calcaneus (heel lock), to finish proximal to the base of the fifth Metatarsal; a second strip may be used to reinforce if required. Reins are then placed between the longitudinal strips across the sole of the foot, and tension altered to suit requirements. Metatarsal or longitudinal arch padding may be placed on the sole of the foot prior to tape application to give extra support. An X rein may be used to reinforce the taping. It is placed around the back of the calcaneus to the heads of the first and fifth MP joints, beneath the transverse strips (Fig. 7.15).

PF-specific tape may be applied in a similar fashion. With the foot in its neutral position, one anchor surrounds the heel and the other is placed just behind the metatarsal heads. Three strips of tape (medial, lateral and central) are then passed from the anchor over the heel to stop on the posterior aspect of the calcaneum, and tension in each may be varied. A horseshoe-shaped fixing strip secures the tape behind the heel. Additional strips may be placed transversely across the foot from the metatarsal heads to the calcaneal tubercle (Fig. 7.16).

Manual therapy

Manual treatments such as deep-tissue massage, and trigger-point therapy for the plantar muscles (quadratus plantae and flexor hallucis) may give

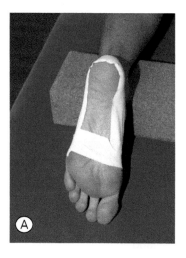

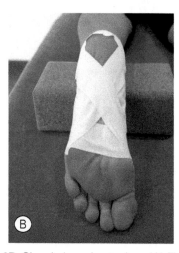

Figure 7.15 Classic low-dye taping. (A) First strip on outside of foot with transverse arch reinforce. (B) X rein to reinforce.

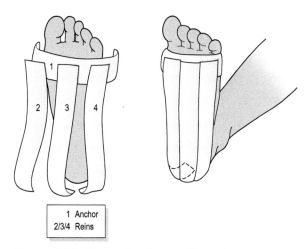

| 1 Anchor |
| 2/3/4 Reins |

Figure 7.16 Plantar fascia specific taping.

some short-term benefit, although the results are likely to be non-specific. Patients can be taught self-pressure techniques using a roller (foam or hard) or ball (tennis or golf ball) placed on the floor with the sole of the foot resting on the object. Self-massage may be applied with the legs crossed to expose the plantar surface of the foot. It is unlikely that passive techniques of this type will structurally affect the PF long term, but they may produce neuro-modulation to relieve pain and reduce the requirement for medication.

Dry needling to the foot and calf musculature has shown some benefit in an RCT (Cotchett et al. 2014) although the statistically significant difference between groups (dry needling versus sham) was less than the clinically important difference. The authors argued that the small benefit obtained may be offset by pain caused by the needling technique itself (32 per cent dry needling compared to 1 per cent sham).

Foot support

Foot supports, including gel heel inserts, longitudinal arch supports, and/or orthotics, may be used to modify weightbearing forces imposed upon the PF or control excessive pronation. Both custom-fit orthotics (CFO) and prefabricated orthotics (PFO) have been shown to produce similar effects in the treatment of PF pain and provide short-term relief and improvement of the foot function index (Lewis et al. 2015), PFO being lower cost and giving immediate access. Gel inserts may be used (strong evidence, Martin et al. 2014) to provide temporary relief in the short to mid-term (2–52 weeks).

Exercise therapy

Exercise approaches to PF pain fall broadly into two categories: stretching and strengthening. Specific stretching is aimed at the PF in isolation. The gastro-soleus complex is assessed and stretched using a generalized programme if the muscles are found to be tighter than the non-injured side or judged to be below what is considered optimal for a patient's daily requirement or sport. Specific PF stretching has been shown to be superior to general calf stretching when measured for worse pain, and first step morning pain on the Foot Function Index (DiGiovanni et al. 2003)

Plantar-specific stretching (DiGiovanni et al. 2006) can be performed by having the patient sit and cross the affected leg over the non-affected (Fig. 7.17A). Placing their fingers distal to the MTP joints, they flex the toes to draw the foot down into

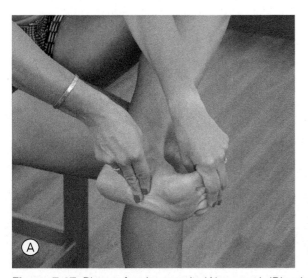
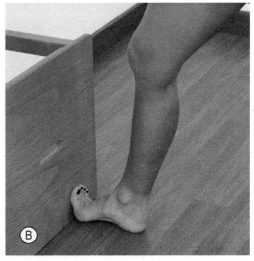

Figure 7.17 Plantar fascia stretch: (A) manual, (B) using vertical surface.

337

ankle plantarflexion, to mimic the windlass effect. The stretch is held for ten seconds and ten reps are performed three times per day. The PF-specific stretch aims to reduce patient symptoms and may be performed prior to taking the first steps in the morning and following prolonged sitting. Where this protocol interferes with daily living, longer stretches of up to 30 to 60 seconds hold may also be used and performed for five reps twice each day. The patient palpates the PF with the opposite hand to ensure that tension is placed on the structure, and foot/toe angle may be varied to increase tension.

Where the first MTP joint motion is very limited, joint mobilization may be used as a passive therapy, and exercise therapy used to maintain the effect between treatment sessions. A combination of first MTP extension and ankle dorsiflexion (Fig. 17.7B) may be performed with the toes extended against a wall, knee pressing over the foot to place the foot into dorsiflexion. Where this relieves symptoms stretching may be of benefit, as limited motion range at the ankle and MTP joint have been shown to have an association with the condition (Irving et al. 2006). However, prolonged or repeated tensile stress to the PF over the longer term may not be useful, as it can produce compression within the tissue, a factor shown to be association with tendinopathy-like pain (Cook and Purdam 2012).

Strengthening may be to the limb in general, or to the plantar foot musculature. High-load strength training has also been shown to be effective when targeting the PF in a similar fashion to that used when treating tendinopathy (Rathleff et al. 2014). High-load training uses the windlass effect and combines flexion of the MP joints with a heel-raise action. The connection between the PF and Achilles paratenon found at dissection (Stecco et al. 2013) implies that load will be transferred between the two structures.

A slim lift (folded towel or slim plank) is placed under the toes to obtain maximal extension. A heel raise action is then performed from this starting position using a slow 3-2-3 count of concentric/

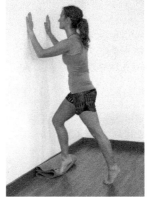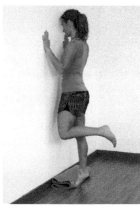

Figure 7.18 High-load training for PF.

isometric/eccentric muscle action (Fig. 7.18). The training volume is increased using 12 reps at maximal load to failure, and then 14 days later this is progressed to 10 reps at maximum load, and again after 14 days to 8 reps at maximum load (Rathleff et al. 2014). Where patients are not strong enough to perform single-leg heel raises or pain limits activity, the exercise is regressed to bilateral heel raises until the necessary strength is obtained. High-load strength training of this type has been shown to be superior to specific stretching using the Foot Function Index (FFI), a 0–230 point scale (0 indicating no pain, disability or limitation of activity). High-load training was superior to specific stretching by 29 points on FFI at 3 months post intervention, and 22 points after 12 months (Rathleff et al. 2014), showing quicker pain reduction and improvement in function.

Key point
High-load training of the PF combines the windlass effect with a heel-raise action against resistance.

Once pain has reduced and daily function returned to pre-injury levels, reconditioning is used to build physical resilience and prepare for competitive sport and daily life challenges (Table 7.5). The tissue-specific rehabilitation described above is augmented and progressed using weightbearing

Table 7.5 Plantar heel pain late-stage rehab

Exercise aim	Action
▸ Balance training	▸ Rocker board, balance board, balance cushion ▸ Line/beam walk
▸ Foot-ankle stability	▸ Single-leg standing ▹ eyes open/closed ▹ arm/trunk movements
▸ Force generation through posterior chain	▸ Squat/deadlift/press actions ▸ Double-/single-leg vertical jump (free & weighted) ▸ In place hop ▹ forward/back ▹ side/side ▹ hop & twisting ▹ as above using line/beam/low hurdle. ▹ Wall/object push (box/prowler)
▸ Force acceptance through lower limb	▸ Barefoot landing straight/lateral/ rotation
▸ Foot as mobile adaptor	▸ Uneven surface walk/run

barefoot actions to work the intrinsic foot musculature. This can include single-leg standing, multidirectional walking and running (forward/back/side-side/rotation), progressing to bilateral and unilateral jumps of varying breadth (standing broad jump) and height (vertical jump). Varying surface (mats, sand, grass), movement complexity (single-leg standing barefoot with/without upper limb or trunk movement), timing (slow, fast) and load (bodyweight, external). Movement variation of this type is likely to enhance function more than the repeated use of the same exercise actions over time.

Heel pad

The calcaneus is covered by elastic adipose tissue in the same way as the fingertips. The fat cells are arranged in columns made from fibrous septa, which lie vertically. As weight is taken, the walls of the columns bulge, and they spring back as the weight is released. With age the septa lose elasticity and the thickness of the heel pad reduces.

Athletes who wear poorly padded sports shoes and those who land heavily on the heel when jumping may bruise this area. In more severe cases rupture of the fibrous septa may occur, causing spillage of the enclosed fat cells. In turn, the loss of the heel pad shock-absorbing mechanism places excessive compression stress onto the calcaneum.

Pain is increased when walking barefoot. Typically, athletes complain of pain first thing in the morning when getting out of bed. The first few steps are exquisitely tender, later subsiding to a dull ache. Pain is brought on by prolonged standing and walking.

The condition must be differentiated from Calcaneal stress fracture and entrapment of the lateral plantar nerve. Calcaneal stress fracture typically gives pain to palpation to the side of the calcaneus rather than the fat pad. X-ray typically shows faint sclerosis, and MRI a high signal either to the upper posterior portion of the calcaneus, or to the area where bone spur forms near the medial tuberosity.

> **Definition**
>
> On X-rays, *bone sclerosis* (increased bone density) shows as a radiopaque or whiter region.

The lateral plantar nerve (Baxter's nerve) is a terminal branch of the posterior tibial nerve. It can become trapped between the abductor hallucis longus muscle and the quadratus plantae, and is often associated with PF pain as part of CPHP (see above).

Management of heel pad pain is by additional padding and preventing the heel pad from spreading. Non-bottoming shock-absorbing materials are useful, and taping to surround the heel and prevent spread of the pad is effective in the short term (Fig. 7.19). Activity modification is required during the acute stage of the condition.

Morton's neuroma

Morton's neuroma (plantar neuroma) affects the plantar interdigital nerve between the third and

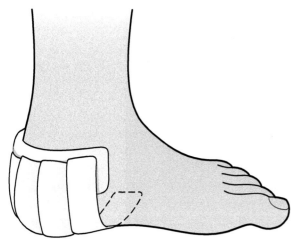

Figure 7.19 Taping for heel pad.

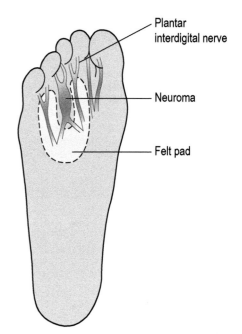

Figure 7.20 Padding for interdigital neuroma.

fourth metatarsal heads. The condition is not a true neuroma (nerve tumour), but simply a localized swelling and scarring of the nerve. Symptoms may occur spontaneously and are often described as feeling like 'electric shocks' along the sensory nerve distribution. The condition is more common with runners (particularly when sprinting and running uphill) and dancers, and is often aggravated by wearing narrow, high-heeled shoes. The sustained dorsiflexed position of these activities stretches the digital nerve, causing inflammation. Once swollen, the nerve is open to entrapment between the metatarsal heads, and eventually the nerve is scarred and permanently enlarged to form a neuroma.

The patient's pain may be reproduced by direct pressure over the neuroma while compressing the forefoot medially and laterally to shorten the transverse arch (Mulder's sign). The condition must be differentiated from Freiberg's disease (see below), which occurs in younger athletes.

Key point

Mulder's sign is a test for Morton's neuroma. The test is positive if pain is reproduced by palpating the neuroma while compressing the forefoot in a medial–lateral direction to shorten the transverse arch.

If the condition is caught in its oedematous stage, alteration of footwear (larger toe box and lower heel), ice application and ultrasound are effective. Injection with corticosteroid and local anaesthetic is also used. Padding the area with orthopaedic felt (Fig. 7.20) to take some of the bodyweight off the neuroma can give temporary relief. The arms of the pad rest on the adjacent metatarsals, leaving the area of the neuroma free.

Once the neuroma has formed and is larger than 5 mm, surgical excision under local anaesthesia may be required, with some studies showing improvement in 80 per cent of patients. There may be a permanent loss of sensation over the plantar aspect of the foot supplied by the digital nerve, but in some cases regeneration can occur between eight and twelve months after surgery. Follow-up after two years (mean 29 months) has shown an 88 per cent reduction in pain with overall satisfaction being excellent or good in 93 per cent of sporting patients (Akermark, Saartok and Zuber 2008). Treatment alternatives include ultrasound-guided corticosteroid injection, radiofrequency ablation (RFA) and cryoneurolysis.

Freiberg's disease

Freiberg's disease (lesion) is an osteochondrosis of the second metatarsal head, most commonly seen in young ballet dancers. Pain occurs over the bony head of the metatarsal (contrast this with Morton's neuroma, which gives pain between the metatarsals) and is aggravated by raising onto the ball of the foot. In longer-standing cases, X-ray reveals flattening of the metatarsal head with damage to the epiphyseal plate. Initially no changes may be apparent on radiographs (Fig. 7.21), with bone scan or MRI being more sensitive. Management is by modification of weightbearing

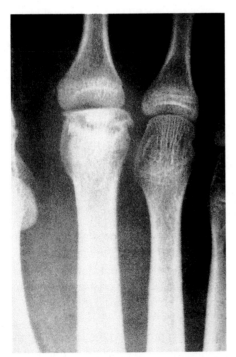

Figure 7.21 Freiberg's disease of the metatarsal head. From Dandy and Edwards (2009).

activities and padding over the metatarsal head to offload the joint and reduce direct pressure over the painful area. Orthotic prescription is often required.

Metatarsalgia

The term 'metatarsalgia' is often used to describe any pain in the forefoot. Such pain may come from a variety of conditions, including those affecting the hallux, a digital neuroma or even stress fractures. However, in this description we will limit the term to 'functional metatarsalgia', where altered foot function causes abnormal mechanical stress in the forefoot, which is symptomatic.

The transverse arch of the foot is supported at the level of the cuneiforms by the peroneus longus, which pulls the medial and lateral edges of the foot together. More distally, the arch is formed by the metatarsal heads, the highest point or 'keystone' being the second metatarsal.

Key point

The transverse arch of the foot is supported by the peroneus longus. Distally, the arch is formed by the metatarsal heads, the highest point or 'keystone' being the second metatarsal.

In mid-stance, the arch flattens and the five metatarsal heads come to lie in the same transverse plane to take the bodyweight. The first metatarsal takes weight through its sesamoid bones, and it and the fifth metatarsal are more mobile than the other three. Stability to the metatarsal heads is provided both passively, by the transverse metatarsal ligament, and actively, by adductor hallucis and, to a lesser extent, the intrinsic muscles. Normally, these structures keep the metatarsals together. However, in cases of hypermobility, such as excessive pronation or hallux valgus, the metatarsal heads may splay apart, effectively increasing the width of the forefoot, and allowing the central metatarsal heads to take too much weight.

Hypermobility may cause abnormal shearing forces, especially in an ill-fitting shoe, giving plantar keratosis. As the metatarsal heads splay, the transverse ligament and intrinsic muscles are subjected to tensile stress, giving pain. Rigidity of the foot may also cause problems. If any of the metatarsals are fixed, or if the toes are 'clawed', plantar compression will occur, again giving keratoma.

Successful management of the condition relies to a large extent on the identification of any underlying biomechanical abnormality in the foot. Short-term relief may be obtained by using anti-inflammatory modalities, and padding and strapping to relieve the stress on the forefoot tissues. An adhesive plantar metatarsal pad (PMP), made from orthopaedic felt, is contoured to cover the heads and upper shafts of the three central metatarsals, lifting them above ground level on weight bearing (Fig. 7.22). The pad is cut around the head of the first metatarsal to avoid excessive pressure at this point. To prevent metatarsal splaying, inelastic strapping is placed around the forefoot, encircling the metatarsals just beneath the first and fifth metatarsal heads. If the metatarsals are immobile, a metatarsal bar may be built into the shoe. This has the effect of transferring the body weight to the metatarsal shafts and away from the painful metatarsal head.

Coupled with strapping and padding, strengthening the intrinsic muscles is essential. Simple exercises,

such as gripping the floor with the toes in bare feet, are effective at building isometric strength and endurance of the intrinsics. Eccentric strength is similarly developed by initially tensing the intrinsic muscles of the foot and increasing the arch with the non-weightbearing leg. The body weight is then taken onto the foot and gradually the arch is allowed to flatten under control.

Cuboid syndrome

Pain over the lateral aspect of the foot may represent subluxation of the cuboid. This is more common in dancers, where 17 per cent of foot and ankle injuries have been found to be cuboid-related (Marshall and Hamilton 1992). The condition is also seen following ankle sprain. At the time of injury, the ligamentous support of the calcaneocuboid joint and the metatarsal cuboid joint may be disrupted. When this occurs in an athlete with a markedly pronated foot, the peroneus longus, travelling through the groove of the cuboid, may pull the medial edge of the cuboid down.

Dull pain is experienced over the lateral aspect of the foot and along the course of the peroneus longus tendon. Pain is increased with prolonged standing and exercise on unforgiving surfaces and/or in poor athletic footwear. Typically, the pain is worse for the first few steps in the morning and is lessened when not weightbearing, and when walking on the toes (foot supinated).

The subluxation may be reduced by manual therapy. Two methods are typically used, with each using passive plantarflexion to reduce the subluxed cuboid:

▶ The patient is supine and the therapist distracts the cuboid and fourth metatarsal joint by placing *traction through the fourth metatarsal shaft*. At the same time the foot is *plantarflexed* and relocation of the cuboid is spontaneous. Where this technique fails, manipulation may succeed.

▶ The patient is prone and the therapist grasps the patient's foot, placing his or her thumbs over the *plantar surface of the cuboid*. A

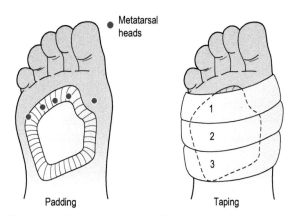

Metatarsal heads

Padding

Taping

1
2
3

Figure 7.22 Metatarsal padding and tape.

high-velocity, low-amplitude thrust is then performed, forcing the foot into *plantarflexion*, while the reduction pressure is maintained over the base of the cuboid. Once reduced, the cuboid position is maintained with a felt pad and tape.

Accessory movements of the foot

In many conditions affecting the foot and ankle, accessory movements of the joints of the mid-foot and forefoot may be reduced. Mobilization procedures require accurate fixation of one segment while mobilization of an adjacent segment is carried out. Examination and manual treatment follow a logical series of movements.

On the lateral side of the foot a number of movements focus on the cuboid. Initially, the cuboid is moved on the fixed calcaneum. The navicular and lateral cuneiform are fixed and the cuboid is then moved upon them. Finally, the cuboid itself is fixed and the fourth and fifth metatarsals are moved.

On the medial side of the foot, movements are around the navicular and cuneiforms. The navicular is fixed and the cuboid and then the cuneiforms are moved. The navicular itself is moved on the talus.

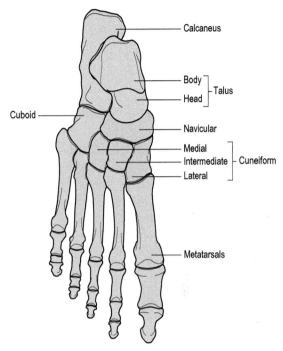

Figure 7.23 The lateral side of the foot is moved around the cuboid, the medial side around the navicular cuneiforms.

Finally, the cuneiforms are fixed and the second and third metatarsals moved (Fig. 7.23). See also Treatment Note 7.1.

Treatment note 7.1   Manual therapy techniques for the foot

Mobilization of the cuboid bone

The cuboid may become stiff due to lateral ligament sprain, where inflammation has been caused to the peroneus brevis tendon connected to the tubercle of the fifth metatarsal. Swelling may then spread onto the cuboid articulations.

To locate the cuboid, find the tubercle on the fifth metatarsal. The cuboid is the flat block-like bone which lies immediately superior to this. Grip the cuboid with the thumb and forefinger of one hand and fix the calcaneous with the other. Move the cuboid on the fixed calcaneus (Fig. 7.24). Then fix

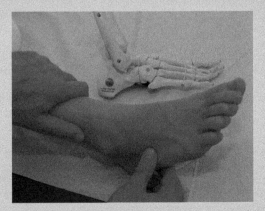

Figure 7.24 Mobilizations of the cuboid bone.

Treatment note 7.1 *continued*

the cuboid with the thumb and forefinger of one hand and move the fourth and fifth metatarsals on this fixed point.

Mobilization of the tarsometatarsal (TM) joint of the first toe

To find the first TM joint, palpate the ball of the large toe and follow the metatarsal along its length, tracing it with the knife edge of the thumb. The thumb comes to rest in a shallow hollow between the base of the first metatarsal and the medial cuneiform bone. Stabilize the metatarsal with the thumb and forefinger of one hand while mobilizing the medial cuneiform with the thumb and forefinger of the opposite hand.

Longitudinal mobilization traction of the first ray

Longitudinal mobilization to the first metatarsal phalangeal (MP) joint and the tarsometatarsal (TM) joint of the first toe can be extremely relieving in cases of halux rigidus. Support the shaft of the first metatarsal with one hand while surrounding the proximal phalanx of the great toe with the fingers of the opposite hand (Fig. 7.25). The movement is a distraction force for the first MP joint. While maintaining the stabilization on the shaft of the first metatarsal bone, abduction and adduction may be imposed on the first MP joint.

Trigger point massage of the quadratus plantae and the flexor digitorum

These muscles (quadratus plantae is also known as flexor accessorius) become tight and painful in cases of plantar fasciitis and respond well to ischaemic compression. Because of the thickness of the sole of the foot it is difficult to provide sufficient pressure using the practitioner's thumb.

For this reason, a plunger is used. Pressure is initially applied with the foot slightly plantarflexed and the toes flexed to release the muscle (Fig. 7.26). As pain eases, the plantar fascia itself is stretched by plantarflexion and flexion of the first toe to use the windlass effect. The patient may be taught this technique, using a small marble or ball on the floor and moving the foot up and down over it. Alternatively, massage into the sole of the foot by crossing one leg over the other and using the ball of the thumb (Fig. 7.27).

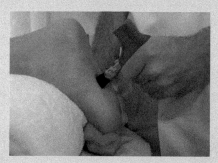

Figure 7.26 Ischaemic pressure using a 'plunger' for the plantar fascia.

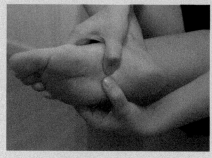

Figure 7.27 Self-treatment in cross-leg sitting using thumbs.

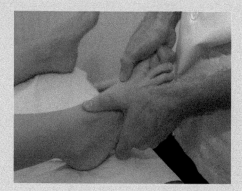

Figure 7.25 Longitudinal mobilization of the first ray.

Skin and nail lesions

Subungual haematoma

In this condition, a haematoma forms directly below the nail plate as a result of direct trauma. Pressure builds up in the space between the nail and the nail bed, causing acute pain and throbbing. In some cases, the pressure may be great enough to loosen the nail from its bed. Subungual haematoma is often referred to as 'black toe' or 'runner's toe'. Ill-fitting shoes are a common cause; if the toe box is too small the nail may rub, especially when running downhill.

If acute, the haematoma may be decompressed using a sterile needle, and the area covered with a sterile dressing. The best treatment for chronic haemorrhage is to remove the cause, and use shoes which allow enough room for the toes to spread on weight bearing and expand with warmth. When standing, a sports shoe should allow one thumb's breadth between the end of the shoe and the athlete's longest toe.

Ingrown toenail (onychocryptosis)

Onychocryptosis, or ingrown toenail, is particularly common in the hallux of athletes, especially males. It may occur secondarily to ill-fitting sports shoes, or to incorrect toenail cutting. Shoes are often too narrow, leading to lateral pressure on the hallux, and athletes often cut the toenails too short, causing the underlying soft tissues to protrude. Cutting across the corners of the nail is another common fault in foot care, allowing the nail to embed itself into the nail grooves. Frequently, excessive sweating (hyperhidrosis) causes skin softening, a condition exacerbated by prolonged hot bathing.

A splinter of nail grows into the subcutaneous tissue, and with time acute inflammation occurs, possibly with infection (paronychia). The skin becomes red, tight and shiny, and the toe swells. There is throbbing pain and acute tenderness to palpation. Normal healing will not take place as long as the nail splinter remains, and so

hypergranulation occurs. The combination of granulation tissue and the swollen nailfold overlaps the nail plate itself.

When the condition occurs without infection, the nail splinter may be removed with a scalpel (size 15), avoiding further damage to the sulcus. The edge of the nail is smoothed and the area washed with saline. The nail edge is then packed with cotton wool, allowing some to rest under the nail plate itself. The area is protected with a sterile dressing, and regularly inspected.

When the condition is accompanied by infection, a local anaesthetic is used, injecting at the base of the toe away from the infected area. Oral antibiotics may be used and/or an antiseptic dressing applied. Hypergranulation tissue is excised. If this procedure is ineffective, nail surgery involving partial or complete nail avulsion is required (Neale and Adams 1989).

Prevention of the problem relies on the use of correctly fitting sports shoes, and on cutting the nails to the shape of the end of the toe while avoiding splintering the nail sides. It is good practice to address basic foot care at the beginning of the season, especially with athletes new to the squad.

Nailbed infection (onychia)

Nailbed infection (onychia) and inflammation of the lateral aspect of the nail (paronychia) is common with the nail of the first toe. The condition occurs through poor foot hygiene and nail management, repetitive trauma, and as a reaction to soaps, nail varnish, and so on. The infection is usually due to staphylococcus or streptococcus, or as a secondary effect of a fungal infection (see below). There is intense pain, redness and pus formation (suppuration), which may also be accompanied by changes in the appearance of the nail itself.

Management is by antiseptic soaks three times a day, with the application of a topical antiseptic cream together with general foot hygiene (clean, breathable socks and disinfected normal footwear which has been worn without socks). Persistent cases may require antibiotics, nail debridement or even nail excision.

Blisters

Blisters occur as a result of compression or shearing on the skin. A narrow toe box may cause blisters over the medial aspect of the fifth toe, and between the first and second toes in the case of hallux valgus. Blisters over the plantar aspect of the foot are common when sports shoes are loose. Shoes should be fitted correctly and friction reduced wherever possible. Petroleum jelly or plastic-backed moist gel squares used between the toes are helpful. Proper foot hygiene, which may include powder or astringents to dry the foot, should be observed.

Acute blisters may be drained through a puncture hole. A sterile needle is used and enters the blister at the side, the needle being held parallel to the skin. This will leave a skin flap intact for protection. The underlying cause of the blister should be addressed.

Athlete's foot

Tinea pedis or 'athlete's foot' is the most common fungal infection of the feet, and is particularly rampant in communal washing areas within sport and where standards of hygiene are poor. Sports shoes create moisture and warmth between the toes, conditions in which the complaint thrives. Three types of tinea pedis are generally seen. First, the lateral toe spaces become macerated due to three organisms: *Trichophyton rubrum*, *Trichophyton interdigitale* and *Epidermophyton floccosum*. Second, the condition may spread to the soles of the feet, where vesiculation occurs as a result of *T. interdigitale* and *E. floccosum*, and finally a diffuse 'moccasin type' scaling appears, usually due to *T. rubrum*. The condition may also spread to the nails and hands in some cases.

Treatment is initially aimed at removing the scaling tissue by the application of surgical spirit. When the scaling has cleared, antifungal dusting powders, such as tolnaftate, are used. Sprays containing clotrimazole and dusting powders are used by the athlete, and socks and footwear should be changed daily and preferably disinfected. Tea tree oil (*Melaleuca alternifolia* essential oil) as a 10 per cent cream has been shown to reduce symptoms of tinea pedis as effectively as tolnaftate (1 per cent) in a study of 104 patients (Tong, Altman and Barnetson 1992). In a randomized controlled double-blind study of 158 patients, Satchell et al. (2002) used a twice daily application of tea tree oil solution (25 per cent and 50 per cent) for 4 weeks and showed a marked clinical response. Mycological cure rate was 64 per cent for the tea tree oil group (50 per cent concentration) compared to 31 per cent for the placebo.

While the infection remains, athletes should not go barefoot in public areas (changing rooms and swimming baths), and should not share towels, socks or footwear.

> ### Key point
> Tea tree oil (as a solution or cream) has been shown to be effective in the treatment of athlete's foot.

Callus formation (hyperkeratosis)

Keratinization is a normal physiological process which turns the stratum corneum of the skin into a hard protective cover. The process becomes overactive if the skin is continually subjected to mechanical stress, for example on the hands of heavy manual workers or the feet of athletes. Hyperaemia occurs, stimulating a proliferation of epidermal cells, and at the same time the rate of desquamation reduces. This type of keratoma or callus on the foot has a protective function, and providing it is asymptomatic it should be left in place. However, when the bulk of such tissues becomes excessive and causes pain or deformity, treatment is required.

The size and shape of the hyperkeratosis is largely dictated by the stress imposed on the skin. A callus is a diffuse area of thickened skin resulting from stress over a fairly wide area, while a corn is a smaller concentrated area which has formed into a nucleus.

Definition

A callus is a diffuse area of thickened skin resulting from stress over a fairly wide area, while a corn is a smaller concentrated area which has formed into a nucleus.

Corns typically seen in sports medicine are either soft or hard, although vascular and neurovascular types do exist. Soft corns are common in the cleft between the fourth and fifth toes, and appear macerated due to sweat retention. The corn nucleus is generally ring-shaped and the centre of the lesion is very thin. Hard corns occur on the plantar aspect of the foot beneath the metatarsal heads, or on the dorsum of the interphalangeal joints. They develop because of concentrated pressure due to body weight and ground reaction forces. The corn nucleus is often associated with surrounding callus due to shearing stress.

The corn or callus may be removed with a scalpel by a therapist and the corn nucleus eradicated. Antiseptic agents such as cetrimide and chlorhexidine are then applied. Moist skin is treated with salicylic acid or aluminium chlorohydrate, and excessively dry skin managed with an emollient containing urea, or soft white paraffin. It is important to remove the underlying cause of the keratoma so that it does not simply return. Examination of foot biomechanics and sports footwear is therefore essential.

Verruca

Verruca pedis is a lesion caused by one of the human papilloma viruses (HPV), of which about 15 have been identified. A benign epithelial tumour which is self-limiting is produced in the plantar skin. The wart is covered by hyperkeratotic tissue, and contains brown or black specks caused by intravascular thromboses within its dilated capillaries. Where the wart is over a weightbearing site, it is forced into the dermis leaving just the hyperkeratotic area on the surface. For this reason, athletes often assume a verruca is simply a corn or callus. However, close inspection will usually reveal the papillary appearance of the verruca. A number of other factors differentiate the two. A wart has a far more rapid onset than an area of callus, and may occur in an area of skin not associated with mechanical stress. In addition, bleeding can occur if the verruca is cut because of capillary dilatation, whereas a callus is avascular.

Key point

Differentiation of a verruca from a corn:
(i) a verruca forms more quickly than corn;
(ii) a verruca is found on skin which is not associated with mechanical stress; (iii) a verruca will bleed if cut, but a corn will not.

The virus normally enters the body through broken skin in the foot, especially if the foot has been wet and the skin macerated. Unfortunately, the virus spreads quickly through a population before the plantar wart becomes obvious. The aim of treatment is to destroy all the cells within the lesion by chemical cautery or cryosurgery. Various preparations are used. The skin surrounding the area is protected, and a liquid or paste of salicylic acid (or monochloroacetic acid) is applied. An aseptic necrosis is produced, and destroyed tissue is removed one week later.

Cryosurgery aims to freeze the verruca with carbon dioxide snow, nitrous oxide or liquid nitrogen applied through a probe. Tissue necrosis with blister formation occurs when the skin is cooled to −20°C and bluish coloration results. The rapid cooling causes ice crystals to form in the body cells and interstitial fluids, which in turn ruptures the cells. Liquid nitrogen is perhaps the most common of the cryosurgery techniques, applied by dipping a cotton-tipped stick into the liquid. This is applied to the verruca for about 30 to 60 seconds. The lesion is protected by a cavity pad if it is over a weightbearing area.

There is evidence of the effectiveness of tea tree essential oil in the treatment of hand warts (Millar and Moore 2008), and this treatment is used by some practitioners to successfully manage verrucae.

If the verruca is not painful, treatment may not be required as the lesion will regress naturally in some months (Neale and Adams 1989). However, cross-infection must still be guarded against by the use of plastic waterproof socks in public areas.

The sports shoe

The design of sports shoes has received a great deal of attention over the last four decades. This interest has to a large extent been market-led due to the massive increase in the number of people jogging. Manufacturers vie with each other to produce a shoe feature which can act as a 'unique selling point' to give them an increased market share.

There is little doubt that shoe design has improved, and that athletes have benefited from this. However, many developments are simply variations on the same theme and give little substantial improvement to overall shoe design. In addition, the mounting cost of sports shoes makes it imperative that athletes receive the right advice concerning the shoe which will best suit their foot and be appropriate to their sport.

Forces acting on the foot

During the stance phase of running, the foot must accommodate to three phases – heel strike, mid-stance and toe-off – during which the biomechanics of the foot change considerably. At heel strike the single force of the foot moving downwards and forwards may be resolved into two components. The first is an impact stress acting vertically, and the second a horizontal shearing force, creating friction. Not all athletes strike the ground with the heel when running. For some 80 per cent, the initial contact point is at the heel, and the ground reaction force curve in this case shows an initial (passive) peak at heel strike of about half bodyweight, occurring 20 to 30 ms after heel strike. A secondary (active) peak occurs approximately 100 ms after heel contact as the centre of pressure moves over the ball of the foot prior to toe-off (Fig. 7.28).

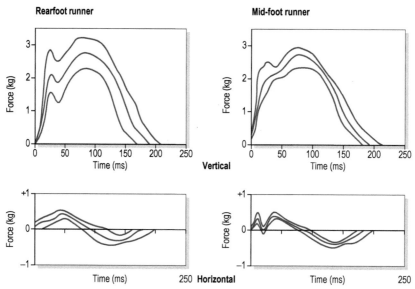

Figure 7.28 Ground reaction forces in rearfoot and mid-foot runners. From Segesser and Pforringer (1989).

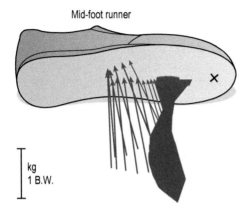

Mid-foot runner

kg
1 B.W.

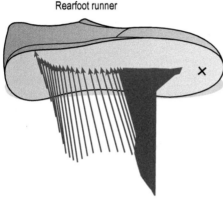

Rearfoot runner

Figure 7.29 Force vector curves for rearfoot and mid-foot runners. From Segesser and Pforringer (1989), with permission.

Other runners show a centre of pressure over the mid-foot or rearfoot (Fig. 7.29). The magnitude of the force acting on the foot can be as much as three times bodyweight.

The rearfoot runner strikes the ground with the knee locked, and consequently will require more shock attenuation from the sports shoe. The mid-foot or forefoot striker has the knee slightly flexed, and so part of the contact shock is absorbed by the elasticity of the knee structures.

Key point

A rearfoot runner strikes the ground with the knee locked, and will require more shock

absorption from a sports shoe. Mid-foot or forefoot strikers have the knees slightly flexed, and so some shock is absorbed by the knee, a point focused on by advocates of minimalist shoes (see below).

In some cases, the heel does not touch the ground at all, leaving the stance phase under the control of the posterior leg muscles. With this type of runner, the shock-absorbing function of a heel wedge will be underutilized.

During mid-stance there can be 5 degrees of abduction of the foot, causing friction between the shoe and the running surface. This creates a torsion force, which tends to rotate the upper part of the shoe in relation to the sole.

Components of a running shoe

Running shoes are manufactured on a model of a foot called a last. Four last shapes are generally used: board, slip, combination and curved.

Key point

The last is a foot-shaped model used to form the shoe in manufacture. Four types are used in sport – slip, board, combination and curved.

▶ *Slip* lasting sees the upper of the shoe formed around the last and stitched together in a line along the centre of the shoe. Removal of the shoe inner will reveal the stitching line (Fig. 7.30). Slip lasted shoes are generally lightweight, but do not offer maximum support. They are traditionally used in racing shoes, for example.
▶ *Board* lasting is a process where the shoe upper is stitched to a rigid or semi-rigid sole-shaped board. Removal of the shoe upper reveals a flat insole shape with no central stitching. This type of shoe is generally heavier, but offers greater stability.

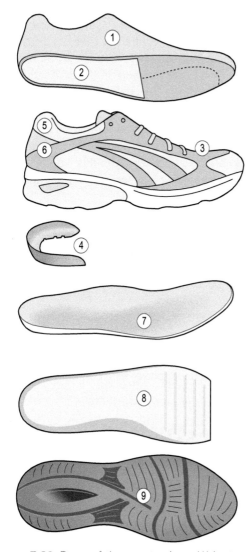

Figure 7.30 Parts of the sports shoe: (1) last; (2) combination last construction; (3) upper – synthetic material and mesh for ventilation; (4) motion control device; (5) Achilles flex notch; (6) heel counter; (7) inner sole – removable; (8) midsole; and (9) outsole. Adapted from Neale and Adams (1989).

▶ A *combination* last is board lasted towards the heel and slip lasted at the front. The combination gives both stability and lighter weight. The last itself will be shaped, either straight, curved or semi-curved depending on

the amount of medial inflare which is given. Drawing an imaginary line from the midpoint of the heel forwards to the toe will reveal the shape of the last. In a straight lasted shoe this line will bisect the toe, dividing the sole into two roughly equal halves. In the curved lasted shoe, the line does not pass through the toe, and the inner half of the sole is different from the outer half.

▶ The *curved* last (Fig. 7.31) has the greatest amount of inflare and gives the least support, but follows the natural curve of the foot. Curved lasted shoes tend to be used for racing. Straight lasted shoes have very little inflare but are more supportive and so are better suited to an overpronating foot.

The *outer sole* (Fig. 7.32) of a shoe is generally a carbon rubber material with treads or studs cut in. The outer sole must provide a combination of four features: grip (traction), durability, flexibility and light weight. Studs provide better cross-country grip, while bars are more durable on hard surfaces and so better suited to road shoes. However, the thicker studs or cleats of a cross-country or fell-running shoe will also add weight, so faster road-racing shoes tend to have thinner, smoother soles.

Beneath the sole is the *mid-sole*, extending the full length of the shoe, and the wedge, which begins behind the metatarsal heads and extends back to the heel. These take the place of the wooden 'shank' of the traditional street shoe. Both the mid-sole and the wedge are designed for cushioning, giving good elastic recoil, but they must also maintain good foot control. They are usually two or three layers of different foam materials, such as ethyl vinyl acetate (EVA), or more expensive polyurethane. Thicker materials tend to give better cushioning, but they will also raise the foot off the ground, creating greater leverage forces if the foot contacts the ground at the side of the sole. The mid-sole may be either single density, with the same material running through its full length, or dual density, where different materials are used for the heel and forefoot sections.

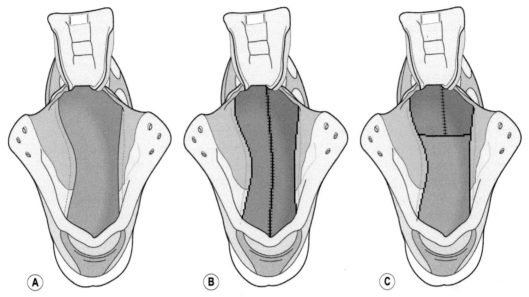

Figure 7.31 Lasts: (A) fully board lasted; (B) slip lasted; and (C) combination lasted. Adapted from Neale and Adams (1989).

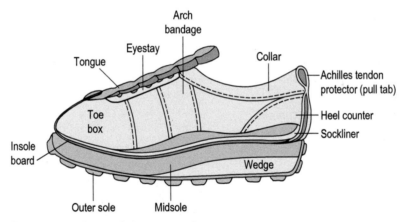

Figure 7.32 Parts of the sports shoe.

On top of the mid-sole is the *insole board*, again running the whole length of the shoe. This semi-rigid board stops the foot from twisting and so provides stability. The edge of the shoe upper is usually fastened below the insole board, and the board itself may be chemically treated to resist deterioration from moisture or micro-organism growth.

The *heel counter* provides rearfoot stability, helping to prevent overpronation, and is usually a hard thermoplastic, which will keep its rigidity. Poorer quality shoes may have cardboard heel counters which will feel stiff when the shoe is new, but quickly soften and allow excessive rearfoot motion. Often the heel counter itself will have an additional support.

The shoe *upper* is contoured to the foot, and made from three sections. The 'vamp' covers the forefoot, and the mid-foot and hindfoot are covered by the medial and lateral quarters, respectively. The nylon upper provides lightness and breathability, and is supported by the eyestay and arch bandage. The eyestay will normally have eyelets for lacing, and the arch bandage is positioned at the highest point of the longitudinal arch of the foot.

The foot rests within the shoe, directly on top of the *sock liner*. This should be removable for washing and can also have further padding, such as gel or air sacks, incorporated into it. The liner is designed primarily to reduce friction and absorb sweat, and may be removed when an orthotic device is placed into the shoe.

The *ankle collar* should be heavily padded and soft, and the heel tab (pull tab) should be notched to prevent friction on the Achilles tendon during toe-off. Some older designs of sports shoes still have so-called 'Achilles tendon protectors'. Unfortunately, the effect of these is usually to injure rather than protect. As the foot is plantarflexed, the Achilles tendon tab will press onto the Achilles tendon, causing friction. Shoes of this type may be modified by cutting a slot down each side of the tab or simply cutting the tab off, providing neither of these solutions interferes with the overall shoe structure.

Many shoes have variable *lacing systems* to accommodate different foot widths and ensure that the shoe fits the foot snugly. With reference to shoe width, it is important to encourage athletes to stand and walk around/jog in sports shoes before they buy them. Obviously the foot spreads with weight bearing, so if the shoe is tried on when sitting it will not give an accurate impression of fit.

Shoe function

Cushioning effects of shoes have been shown to reduce initial impact at heel strike by as much as 50 per cent. The aim is to reduce or 'attenuate' the peak forces to levels which are well tolerated by the human body, and which do not result either in trauma or overuse injury. At the same time, the forces produced at toe-off have to be conserved to maintain running efficiency.

Heel materials which are too soft will compress or 'bottom out', while those which are too hard reduce cushioning. In addition, the construction of the shoe will also affect shock absorption. A stiff insole board, for example, cemented to a soft mid-sole, will give the shoe a functional hardness usually found only with much firmer mid-sole materials.

The overhang or 'flare' of the sole of a running shoe creates leverage force which exaggerates pronation and foot slap (Fig. 7.33). When running barefoot, the subtalar joint axis lies over the ground contact point, as does the ankle joint axis. Wearing a typical running shoe, the leverage force created by the heel flare places the ground contact point further away from the subtalar joint axis, thus increasing the leverage effect by a factor of three. In the sagittal plane, the heel flare moves the ground contact point back, further from the ankle joint, thus increasing the leverage effect. To compensate, the anterior tibial muscles have to work harder. By altering the heel to a more rounded design, and using a shoe with a dual density mid-sole, overpronation can be limited.

The sole of a sports shoe should bend at a point just proximal to the metatarsal heads, to an angle of about 30 degrees. Bending a stiffer sole may increase energy expenditure, and could therefore lead to local muscle fatigue; a lighter shoe is more energy conserving. Fig. 7.34 demonstrates the stresses produced when a sole is bent. The top of the sole is compressed, and the bottom tensioned. To make the sole more flexible, while still maintaining its cushioning effect, a bar of softer material is often placed in the top layer of the sole just behind the metatarsal heads. In addition, grooves are cut in the bottom of the sole at the point of bending.

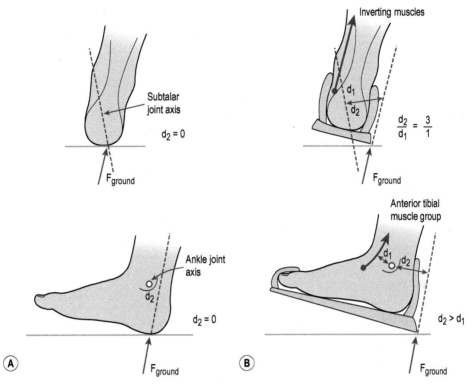

Figure 7.33 Effect of leverage in running shoes. (A) Running barefoot, the subtalar joint axis lies over the ground contact point, as does the ankle joint. (B) The 'overhang' of the shoes moves the ground contact point further from the subtaloid and ankle joints, increasing the leverage effect. Muscle action is required to compensate. From Subotnick (1989).

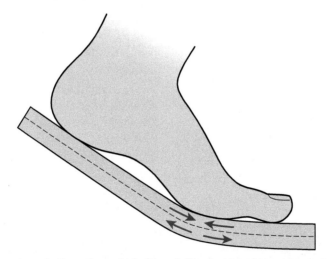

Figure 7.34 Stresses produced when the sole is flexed. The bottom layers are in tension, while the top layers are compressed. From Segesser and Pforringer (1989), with permission.

<table>
<tr><td colspan="2">Treatment note 7.2   Fitting a running shoe</td></tr>
</table>

The correct fit of a running shoe is vital. Most individuals have one foot slightly larger than the other, so both shoes must be tried on. Fit the shoe to the larger foot, and use extra padding for the smaller foot. If the shoe is too narrow, extra stress may be placed on the longitudinal arch and callus formation over the metatarsal heads is more likely. To test for correct shoe width, take all of the body weight through the shoe and ensure that firstly the shoe does not bulge over the sole (too small) and secondly that creases do not form in the shoe upper (too big).

The toe box must be long enough and wide enough to allow the toes to spread and to enable them to fully extend (flatten out). In general, the end of the shoe should be about 1 cm longer than the end of the longest toe. It is often easier simply to take the insole out of the shoe and rest the foot on this to assess correct length.

Palpate the longest toe when the shoe is on the foot, and also palpate the forefoot at its widest part (first MP joint) to ensure that the toe is not being pushed into a valgus position. Ensure that the highest point of the mid-foot fits well into the shoe.

For running, the shoe should flex at the first MP joint, and this can be assessed simply by holding the main shoe in one hand and pressing the sole with the other. Excessive flare of a shoe heel will introduce dangerous leverage forces on the foot and, broadly speaking, the flare should not extend beyond the apex of the malleoli.

The shape of the shoe 'footprint' is called the last, and this may be straight or curved. A straight last is usually more stable and a curved last less stable. Athletes with a very flexible (pronating) foot will need more control in a shoe and should therefore chose a straight lasted shoe.

Minimalist running shoes

In the late 1980s, arguments for minimalist shoes began to emerge. Robbins and Hanna (1987) maintained that habitually unshod humans are not susceptible to chronic overloading of the foot. Locomotion in barefoot-adapted subjects (those who regularly run unshod) differs considerably from that of normal shod subjects. When walking, unshod subjects attempt to grip the ground with their toes, and when running the medial longitudinal arch flattens completely during mid-stance. Foot flattening when running unshod is probably a result of eccentric muscle action and elastic deformation of the intrinsic foot musculature and plantar fascia. Robbins and Gouw (1990) claimed that this response is behaviourally induced in the barefoot-adapted runner. They argued that the subject was attempting to minimize discomfort by transferring forefoot load from the metatarsal phalangeal joints to the distal digits. This process, they claimed, results in hypertrophy of the intrinsic musculature, and relaxes the

plantar fascia (Fig. 7.35). The argument was that the shock-moderating behaviour of the foot is related to plantar sensibility. The subject attempts to minimize discomfort by increasing the activity of the intrinsic muscles. However, a running shoe with a thick soft sole will mask sensation to the plantar surface of the foot, and so the subject will not use the intrinsic muscles to their full extent.

The recommendation was that runners run barefoot, after a progressive period of adaptation. Where a runner is not able to do this each day, or where safety factors prevent it, a less yielding shoe could be used which provides adequate sensory feedback.

When assessing proprioceptive function of the foot, foot position error has been shown to be 107.5 per cent poorer with subjects wearing athletic footwear than those who were barefoot. In addition, those who wore footwear were unable to distinguish between a flat surface and a 20-degree slope when blindfolded (Robbins, Waked and Rappel 1995). These authors argued that the use of

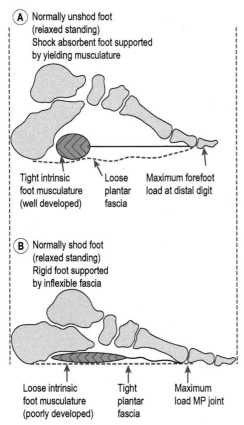

(A) Normally unshod foot
(relaxed standing)
Shock absorbent foot supported
by yielding musculature

Tight intrinsic | Loose | Maximum forefoot
foot musculature | plantar | load at distal digit
(well developed) | fascia |

(B) Normally shod foot
(relaxed standing)
Rigid foot supported
by inflexible fascia

Loose intrinsic | Tight | Maximum
foot musculature | plantar | load MP joint
(poorly developed) | fascia |

Figure 7.35 Function of intrinsic musculature in the (A) unshod and (B) shod foot. From Robbins, S.E. and Gouw, G.J. (1990) Athletic footwear and chronic overloading. *Sports Medicine*, **9** (2), 76–85. With permission.

footwear was largely responsible for ankle injury, in that it reduced the input from plantar cutaneous mechanoreceptors.

Athletic footwear has also been shown to contribute to falling frequency. Using balance beam walking, mid-sole hardness was positively related to stability, while mid-sole thickness was negatively related. The authors above concluded that shoes with thick, soft soles acted to destabilize an individual, whereas thin, hard-soled shoes provided superior stability. Waddington and Adams (2000) compared barefoot conditions, athletic shoes and textured insoles within athletic shoes to determine the effect on ankle movement discrimination.

They found that athletic shoes gave significantly worse movement discrimination scores compared to barefoot levels, confirming the work previously quoted. However, the addition of a textured insole improved movement discrimination back to barefoot levels, through enhanced cutaneous feedback on the sole of the foot.

> **Key point**
>
> The foot itself has active shock-absorbing mechanisms. In addition, sensory feedback from the plantar surface of the foot is vital for movement discrimination. Protected barefoot activities should be encouraged to enhance both of these features.

In popular sports culture, minimalist shoes or barefoot running became popular in the early 2000s, with several manufacturers producing shoes with thin soles or glove-like features, claiming a more natural running experience. Several leading athletes in the 1960s, such as the marathon running Abebe Bikila and European record holder Bruck Tullock, ran barefoot, and in 2004 a paper was published in the leading scientific journal *Nature* arguing that man had evolved to run (Bramble and Lieberman 2004). As barefoot running gained momentum, papers claimed that as a barefoot runner would strike the ground mid-foot with the knee slightly flexed (see above). As this differs from a shod runner who strikes at the heel with the knee straight, smaller impact forces would be generated which may be protective against injury (Lieberman et al. 2010). Researchers from the same group (Daoud et al. 2012) demonstrated increased rates of repetitive stress injuries in subjects with a rearfoot strike compared to those with a forefoot strike. These authors proposed the hypothesis that the absence of an impact peak in the ground reaction force (see above) with forefoot striking runners may have contributed to lower injury rates. However, using video analysis Goss et al. (2015) compared runners with traditional shoes to those with minimalist shoes. They showed, first, that many runners failed to accurately report their

355

foot-strike pattern, and second, that many subjects failed to transition from rearfoot strike to forefoot strike when wearing minimalist shoes. A study by Altman and Davis (2016) showed similar injury rates between shod and barefoot runners. Injury types varied, with descriptive analysis showing barefoot runners had a greater number of plantar surface injuries but fewer cases of plantar fasciitis, and shod runners suffering a greater number of calf, knee and hip injuries.

Clearly the foot is an active body part, possessing the same sensory mechanisms and muscle action as any other part of the body. However, the use of minimalist footwear would seem to be a personal choice. If the intention is to exercise the foot, using minimalist footwear to achieve this, as with any form of overload time for adaptation, must be allowed.

> **Key point**
>
> Minimalist footwear can change the type of injury seen in runners, but is unlikely to change the overall incidence (number of injuries).

The court shoe

In running, foot movements occur cyclically, but in court games such as tennis, squash and badminton the movements are more varied, both in direction and speed. The casual tennis player makes contact mostly with the heel and less often with the ball of the foot. However, when a player is under pressure the situation is reversed. Now contact is more frequently made with the ball of the foot than the heel, and contact with the medial and lateral edges of the foot is increased (Nigg, Luthi and Bahlsen 1989).

Movement most commonly occurs in the forward direction, but when under pressure, the tennis player moves laterally more frequently. This movement is often combined with contact on the forefoot.

A court shoe must allow all of these movements. The same heel–toe mechanism found in a running shoe is required, but in addition, force attenuation from forefoot contact is needed. The frictional characteristics of the shoe to surface are important. Both translational and rotational movements are needed, translation less so in surfaces which permit some degree of sliding, such as indoor courts or sand/granules.

Because the demands placed on the foot when playing court games are so different to those encountered in road running, athletes must be discouraged from wearing the same shoes for both sports unless they use specifically designed 'cross training' footwear. During lateral movements, in particular, the leverage involved with the higher (flared) heel of the running shoe makes injury much more likely. Similarly, tennis shoes do not give adequate rearfoot control or shock attenuation for running.

The soccer boot

In football (soccer), the ball may reach velocities of 140 km/h. This speed, combined with the weight of the ball, especially when wet, leads to deformation of both the boot and foot with kicking. Forces generated may lead to microtrauma to the foot and ankle. Soccer footwear must therefore be as light as possible to minimize any excessive forces created by kicking. At the same time, the shoe must provide both support and protection for the foot.

Combinations of rotation and flexion with the foot fixed to the ground are particularly taxing on the knee structures. Most boots unfortunately compound this problem by the use of cleats or studs, which, although improving grip on a wet surface, will also increase rotation forces by reducing 'give'. Indoor surfaces in some cases offer greater grip with similar problems, and shoes need a sole with a greater number of smaller studs to compensate for this.

Shoes must allow the increased range of movement required in soccer, and be flexible enough to accommodate forefoot rocking. Any studs must be placed to avoid pressure irritation to the plantar aspect of the foot. Studs on the heel are placed towards the outside of the shoe to avoid rocking or buckling on weight bearing.

References

Acevedo, J.I., Beskin, J.L., 1998. Complications of plantar fascia rupture associated with corticosteroid injection. *Foot and Ankle International* **19** (2), 91–97.

Akermark, C., Saartok, T., Zuber, Z., 2008. A prospective 2-year follow up study of plantar incisions in the treatment of primary intermetatarsal neuromas (Morton's neuroma). *Foot and Ankle Surgery* **14**, 67–73.

Altman, A.R., Davis, I.S., 2016. Prospective comparison of running injuries between shod and barefoot runners. *British Journal of Sports Medicine* **50** (8), 476–480.

Bartold, S., Clark, R.A., Franklin-Miller, A. et al., 2009. The effect of taping on plantar fascia strain: a cadaveric ex vivo study. *Footwear Science* **1** (sup1).

Bolivar, Y.A., Munuera, P.V., Padillo, J.P., 2013. Relationship between tightness of the posterior muscles of the lower limb and plantar fasciitis. *Foot Ankle Int* **34**, 42–48.

Bramble, D.M., Lieberman, D.E., 2004. Endurance running and the evolution of Homo. *Nature.* **432** (7015), 345–352.

Carlson, R.E., Fleming, L.L., Hutton, W.C., 2000. The biomechanical relationship between the endoachilles, plantar fascia and metatarsophalangeal joint dorsiflexion angle. *Foot Ankle Int* **21**, 18–25.

Carmines, D.V., Nunley, J.A., McElhaney, J.H., 1988. Effects of ankle taping on the motion and loading pattern of the foot for walking subjects. *Journal of Orthopaedic Research* **6**, 223–229.

Clanton, T.O., Butler, J.E., Eggert, A., 1986. Injuries to the metatarsophalangeal joints in athletes. *Foot and Ankle* **7**, 162–176.

Cook, J.L., and Purdam, C., 2012. Is compressive load a factor in the development of tendinopathy? *British Journal of Sports Medicine* **46** (3), 163–168.

Cotchett, M.P., Munteanu, S.E. and Landorf, K.B., 2014. Effectiveness of trigger point dry needling for plantar heel pain: a randomized controlled trial. *Phys Ther.* **94** (8), 1083–1094.

Creighton, D.S., Olson, V.L., 1987. Evaluation of range of motion of the first metatarsophalangeal joint in runners with plantar fasciitis. *Journal of Orthopaedic and Sports Physical Therapy* **8**, 357–361.

Daoud, A.I., Geissler, G.J., Wang, F., et al., 2012. Foot strike and injury rates in endurance runners: a retrospective study. *Medicine & Science in Sports & Exercise.* **44** (7), 1325–1334.

DiGiovanni. B.F., Nawoczenski, D.A., Lintal, M.E., Moore, E.A., Murray, J.C., Wilding, G.E., Baumhauer, J.F., 2003. Tissue-specific plantar fascia-stretching exercise enhances outcomes in patients with chronic heel pain: a prospective, randomized study. *J Bone Joint Surg Am.* **85–A** (7), 1270–1277.

Digiovanni, B.F., Nawoczenski, D.A., Malay, D.P., Graci, P.A., Williams, T.T., Wilding, G.E., Baumhauer, J.F., 2006. Plantar fascia-specific stretching exercise improves outcomes in patients with chronic plantar fasciitis: a prospective clinical trial with two-year follow-up. *J Bone Joint Surg Am.* **88** (8), 1775–1781.

Garbalosa, J.C., Donatelli, R., Wooden, M.J., 1989. Dysfunction, evaluation and treatment of the foot and ankle. In: Donatelli, R., Wooden, M.J. (eds), *Orthopaedic Physical Therapy.* Churchill Livingstone, London, pp. 533–553.

George, F.J., 1989. In: Shephard, R.J. (ed.), *Year Book of Sports Medicine.* Year Book Medical Publishers, Chicago, pp. 75.

Goss, D.L., Lewek, M., Yu, B. et al., 2015. Lower extremity biomechanics and self-reported foot-strike patterns among runners in traditional and minimalist shoes. *J Athl Train.* **50** (6), 603–611.

Hansen, A.H., Childress, D.S. and Knox, E.H., 2004. Roll-over shapes of human locomotor systems: effects of walking speed. *Clinical Biomechanics* **19** (4), 407–414.

Irving, D.B., Cook, J.L, Menz, H.B., 2006. Factors associated with chronic plantar heel pain: a systematic review. *Journal of Science and Medicine in Sport*, **9** (1), 11–22.

Lewis, R.D., Wright, P. and McCarthy, L.H., 2015. Orthotics compared to conventional therapy and other non-surgical treatments for plantar fasciitis. *The Journal of the Oklahoma State Medical Association*, **108** (12), 596–598.

Lieberman, D.E., Venkadesan, M., Werbel, W.A. et al., 2010. Foot strike patterns and collision forces in habitually barefoot versus shod runners. *Nature*. **463** (7280), 531–535.

Lorimer, D., French, G., O'Donnell, M., Burrow, J., 2002. *Neale's Disorders of the Foot*. 6th ed. Churchill Livingstone, Edinburgh.

Magee, D.J., 2002. *Orthopedic Physical Assessment*. 4th ed. Saunders, Philadelphia.

Marshall, P., Hamilton, W.G., 1992. Cuboid subluxation in ballet dancers. *American Journal of Sports Medicine* **20**, 169–175.

Martin, R.L., Davenport, T.E., Reischl, S.F. et al., 2014. Heel pain-plantar fasciitis: revision 2014. *Journal of Orthopedic and Sports Physical Therapy* **44** (11), A1–A33.

McMillan, Andrew, Landorf, M. et al., 2012. Ultrasound guided corticosteroid injection for plantar fasciitis: randomised controlled trial. *BMJ* **344**, e3260

McPoil, T.G., Brocato, R.S., 1990. The foot and ankle: biomechanical evaluation and treatment. In: Gould, J.A. (ed.), *Orthopaedic and Sports Physical Therapy*, second ed. Mosby, St Louis, pp. 293–321.

Medscape (2016) Plantar fasciitis differential diagnosis. http://emedicine.medscape.com/article/86143-differential. Accessed August 2016.

Millar, B., Moore, J., 2008. Successful topical treatment of hand warts in a paediatric patient with tea tree oil. *Complementary Therapies in Clinical Practice* **14** (4), 225–227.

Mohseni-Bandpei, M.A., Nakhaee, M., Mousavi, M.E., Shakourirad, A., Safari, M.R., Vahab Kashani, R., 2014. Application of ultrasound in the assessment of plantar fascia in patients with plantar fasciitis: a systematic review. *Ultrasound Med Biol*. **40** (8), 1737–1754.

Murphy, C., 2006. Plantar fasciitis. *Sportex Medicine* October 14–17.

Neale, D., Adams, I.M., 1989. *Common Foot Disorders*. Churchill Livingstone, London.

Nigg, B.M., Luthi, S.M., Bahlsen, H.A., 1989. The tennis shoe: biomechanical design criteria. In: Segesser, B., Pforringer, W. (eds), *The Shoe in Sport*. Year Book Medical Publishers, Wolfe, London.

Perry, J., 1992. Gait analysis: normal and pathological function. McGraw-Hill, New York.

Radford, J.A., Burns, J., Buchbinder, R., Landorf, K.B., Cook, C., 2006. The effect of low-dye taping on kinematic, kinetic, and electromyographic variables: a systematic review. *J Orthop Sports Phys Ther*. **36** (4), 232–241.

Rathleff, M.S., Mølgaard, C.M., Fredberg, U. et al., 2014. High-load strength training improves outcome in patients with plantar fasciitis: A randomized controlled trial with 12-month follow-up. *Scand J Med Sci Sport*.

Robbins, S., Waked, E., Rappel, R., 1995. Ankle taping improves proprioception before and after exercise in young men. *British Journal of Sports Medicine* **29** (4), 242–247.

Robbins, S.E., Gouw, G.J., 1990. Athletic footwear and chronic overloading. *Sports Medicine* **9** (2), 76–85.

Robbins, S.E., Hanna, A.M., 1987. Running related injury prevention through barefoot adaptations. *Medicine and Science in Sports and Exercise* **19**, 148–156.

Rodeo, S.A., O'Brian, S.J., Warren, R.F., 1989a. Turf toe: an analysis of metatarsophalangeal joint sprains in professional football players. *American Journal of Sports Medicine* **17** (4), 125–131.

Rodeo, S.A., O'Brian, S.J., Warren, R.F. et al. 1989b. Turf toe: diagnosis and treatment. *Physician and Sports Medicine* **17** (4), 132–147.

Rodgers, M.M., Cavanagh, P.R., 1989. Pressure distribution in Morton's foot structure. *Medicine and Science in Sports and Exercise* **21**, 23–28.

Rogers, J.A., Wilson, A., Laslett, L.L., Winzenberg, T.M., 2016. Physical interventions (orthoses, splints, exercise and manual therapy) for treating plantar heel pain. *Cochrane Database of Systematic Reviews* **8**, CD012304.

Satchell, A., Sauragen, A., Bell, C., Barnetson, R., 2002. Treatment of interdigital tinea pedis with 25% and 50% tea tree oil solution: a randomized placebo controlled blinded study. *Australasian Journal of Dermatology.* **43** (3), 175–178.

Stecco, C. (2015) *Functional atlas of the human fascial system.* Churchill Livingstone.

Stecco,C., Corradin, M. et al. (2013) Plantar fascia anatomy and its relationship with Achilles tendon and paratenon. *J. Anat.* **223**: 665–676.

Tong, M., Altman, P., Barnetson, R., 1992. Tea tree oil in the treatment of tinea pedis. *Australasian Journal of Dermatology* **33** (3), 145–149.

Waddington, G., Adams, R., 2000. Textured insole effects on ankle movement discrimination while wearing athletic shoes. *Physical Therapy in Sport* **1** (4), 119–128.

CHAPTER 8

The lumbar spine

Spinal problems are among the most common conditions encountered in physical medicine. More working days are lost because of back pain than any other single condition, and sport does not escape this epidemic. Table 8.1 lays out the cost to the individual and to society as a whole.

In sport, the frequency of back pain suffering presents a similar challenge. Exercise itself has a positive effect on the lower back, both in terms of injury prevention and rehabilitation. Those with an activity level of at least three hours per week have a generally lower lifetime risk of lower back pain (Harreby et al. 1997). After an injury has occurred, exercise therapy has been shown to be effective at returning patients to their daily activities and to work (Mercer et al. 2006), and has been recommended as the mainstay of treatment for this region (Waddell, Feder and Lewis 1997, NICE 2016).

Although exercise is beneficial to the lower back, the varied activities within sport subject the spine to significant stress, which often results in injury. In terms of percentages, 10–20 per cent of all sports injuries involve the spine (Thompson 2002), but this percentage differs between sports (Table 8.2).

A detailed study of back pain is outside the scope of this book, but it is necessary to look at a number of features of spinal injury which are important within the context of sport.

Table 8.1 Low back pain: the scope of the problem

> ▶ 85% of individuals suffer one disabling episode of LBP during their life
> ▶ In the UK 6 out of 10 individuals (aged 18–49) and 7 out of 10 (aged over 50) suffered from LBP in the last year
> ▶ Prevalence in schoolchildren now approaching that of adults
> ▶ At any one time 35% of population is suffering from some form of LBP
> ▶ £481 million cost annually to NHS
> ▶ £1.4 billion paid in benefits annually
> ▶ £3.8 billion lost in production annually
> ▶ 7% of workload of GPs due to LBP
> ▶ 20% of individuals do not recover within 6 weeks.
> ▶ 60% of sufferers will experience a second bout of LBP within 1 year
> ▶ Secondary work absence seen in 33% of individuals
> ▶ Rate of return to work following LBP: 50% after 6/12, 25% after 12/12, 10% after 24/12.

GP—general practitioner; LBP—low back pain; NHS—National Health Service. Compiled from Fryomoyer and Cats-Baril (1991), Clinical Standards Advisory Group (1994), CSP (2004); reprinted from Airaksinen et al. (2005).

Structure

The spinal disc

There are 24 intervertebral discs lying between successive vertebrae, making the spine an alternately rigid then elastic column. The amount

Table 8.2 Back pain in specific sports

Sport	Effect
Canoeing	22.5% suffer from lumbago
Cross-country skiing	64% suffer from back pain
Cycling	Incidence of back pain as high at 73.2%
Golf	Lifetime incidence as high at 63%
Gymnastics	86% of rhythmic gymnasts report low back pain. 63% of Olympic female gymnasts have MRI abnormalities
Rowing	Mechanical back pain most common type
Squash	51.8% of competitive players report back injury
Swimming	37% suffer back pain especially with breaststroke and butterfly
Triathlon	32% suffer low back pain
Windsurfing	Low back pain most common ailment
Yachting	Lumbosacral sprain most common injury (29%)

From Thompson, B. (2002) How should athletes with chronic low back pain be managed in primary care? In *Evidence Based Sports Medicine* (eds D. MacAuley and T. Best). BMJ Books, London. With permission.

of flexibility present in a particular spinal segment will be determined by the size and shape of the disc, and the resistance to motion of the soft tissue support to the spinal joints. The discs increase in size as they descend the column, the lumbar discs having an average thickness of 10 mm, twice that of the cervical discs. The disc shapes are accommodated to the curvatures of the spine, and the shapes of the vertebrae. The greater anterior widths of the discs in the cervical and lumbar regions reflect the curvatures of these areas. Each disc is made up of three closely related components: the annulus fibrosis, nucleus pulposus and cartilage end plates.

> **Key point**
> Discs increase in size going down the spine, with the lumbar (lower back) discs having a thickness of about one centimetre, twice that of the cervical discs. In the cervical and lumbar areas, discs are wider anteriorly, creating the spinal curves.

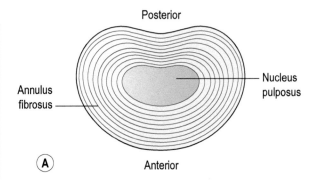

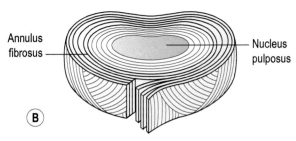

Figure 8.1 (A) Concentric band of annular fibres. (B) Horizontal section through a disc. From Oliver and Middleditch (1991) with permission.

The annulus is composed of layers of fibrous tissue arranged in concentric bands (Fig. 8.1). Each band has fibres arranged in parallel, and the various bands are in turn angled at 45 degrees to each other. The bands are more closely packed anteriorly and posteriorly than they are laterally, and those innermost are the thinnest. Each disc has about 20 bands in all, and fibre orientation, although partially determined at birth, is influenced by torsional stresses in the adult. The posterolateral regions have a more irregular make-up, and this may be one reason why they become weaker with age, predisposing them to injury.

The annular fibres pass over the edge of the cartilage end plate of the disc, and are anchored to the bony rim of the vertebra and to its periosteum and body. The attaching fibres are actually interwoven with the fibres of the bony trabeculae of the vertebral body. The outer layer of fibres blend with the posterior longitudinal ligament, but the anterior longitudinal ligament has no such attachment.

The hyaline cartilage end plate rests on the surface of the vertebra. This is approximately one millimetre thick at its outer edge and becomes thinner towards its centre. The central portion of the end plate acts as a semi-permeable membrane to facilitate fluid exchange between the vertebral body and disc. In addition, it protects the body from excessive pressure. In early life, the end plate is penetrated by canals from the vertebral body, but these disappear after the age of 20 to 30 years. After this period, the end plate starts to ossify and become more brittle, the central portion thinning and in some cases being completely destroyed.

The nucleus pulposus is a soft hydrophilic (water-attracting) substance, taking up about 25 per cent of the total disc area. It is continuous with the annulus, but the nuclear fibres are far less dense. The spaces between the collagen fibres are filled with proteoglycan, giving the nucleus its water-retaining capacity, and making it a mechanically plastic material. The area between the nucleus and annulus is metabolically very active and sensitive to physical force and chemical and hormonal influence. The proteoglycan content of the nucleus decreases with age, but the collagen volume remains unchanged. As a consequence, the water content of the nucleus reduces. In early life, the water content may be as high as 80 to 90 per cent, but this decreases to about 70 per cent by middle age.

> **Key point**
>
> With age: (i) the back wall of the disc becomes weaker, (ii) the end plate at the top and bottom of the disc becomes brittle, and (iii) the disc dries up, reducing its water content from 90 per cent (child) to 70 per cent (middle age).

The lumbar discs are the largest avascular structures in the body. The nucleus itself is dependent upon fluid exchange by passive diffusion from the margins of the vertebral body and across the cartilage end plate. Diffusion takes place particularly across the centre of the cartilage end plate, which is more permeable than the periphery. There is intense anaerobic activity within the nucleus (Holm et al. 1981), which could lead to lactate build-up and a low oxygen tension, placing the nuclear cells at risk. Inadequate adenosine triphosphate (ATP) supplies could lead to cell death.

The facet joint

The facet (zygapophyseal) joints are synovial joints formed between the inferior articular process of one vertebra and the superior articular process of its neighbour. As with all typical synovial joints, they have articular cartilage, a synovial membrane and a joint capsule. However, the zygapophyseal joints do have a number of unique features (Bogduk and Twomey 1991).

The capsule is a lax structure which enables the joint to hold about 2 ml of fluid. It is replaced anteriorly by the ligamentum flavum, and posteriorly it is reinforced by the deep fibres of multifidus. The joint leaves a small gap at its superior and inferior poles, creating the subscapular pockets. These are filled with fat, contained within the synovial membrane. Within the subscapular pocket lies a small foramen for passage of the fat in and out of the joint as the spine moves.

> **Key point**
>
> The facet joint has a loose capsule reinforced by the ligamentum flavum at the front and the multifidus muscle at the back. The capsule has small pockets at its top and bottom which contain fat globules which travel in and out of the joint as it moves.

Intracapsularly, there are three structures of interest (Fig. 8.2). The first is the connective tissue rim, a thickened wedge-shaped area which makes up for the curved shape of the articular cartilage in much the same way as the menisci of the knee do. The second structure is an adipose tissue pad, a 2 mm fold of synovium filled with fat and blood vessels. The third structure is the fibroadipose

363

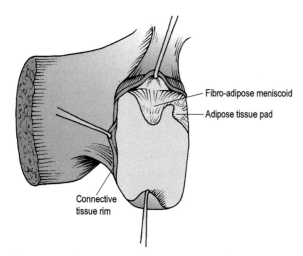

Figure 8.2 Intra-articular structures of the lumbar zygapophyseal joints. From Bogduk and Twomey (1991), with permission.

meniscoid, a 5 mm leaf-like fold which projects from the inner surfaces of the superior and inferior capsules. These latter two structures have a protective function. During flexion, the movement of the articular facets leaves some of their cartilage exposed. Both the adipose tissue pad and the fibroadipose meniscoid are able to cover these exposed regions (Bogduk and Engel 1984).

With ageing, the cartilage of the zygapophyseal joint can split parallel to the joint surface, pulling a portion of joint capsule with it. The split of cartilage with its attached piece of capsule forms a false intra-articular meniscoid (Taylor and Twomey 1986). Normally, the fibroadipose meniscus itself is drawn out from the joint on flexion, and should move back in with extension. However, if the meniscoid fails to move back, it will buckle and remain under the capsule, causing pain and acute locking (Bogduk and Jull 1985). A mobilization or manipulation which combines flexion and rotation may allow the meniscoid to reduce and so relieve pain.

The facet has an overlapping neural supply, with ascending, local and descending facet branches coming from the posterior primary ramus. The nerve endings in the facet joint capsules are similar to those in the annulus of the disc, and although the disc is more sensitive, the facet joints can be a source of referred pain to the lower limb but not neurological deficit (Mooney and Robertson 1976).

> **Key point**
>
> A facet joint can be a source of referred pain, but not neurological deficit (weakness, paraesthesia, or altered reflexes).

Spinal loading

Vertebral body

Within the vertebra itself, compressive force is transmitted by both the cancellous bone of the vertebral body and the cortical bone shell. Up to the age of 40, the cancellous bone contributes between 25 per cent and 55 per cent of the strength of the vertebra. After this age, the cortical bone shell carries a greater proportion of load as the strength and stiffness of the cancellous bone reduces with decreasing bone density due to ageing. As the vertebral body is compressed, blood flows from it into the subchondral post-capillary venous network. This process reduces the bone volume and dissipates energy. The blood returns slowly as the force is reduced, leaving a latent period after the initial compression, during which the shock-absorbing properties of the bone will be less effective. Exercises which involve prolonged periods of repeated shock to the spine, such as jumping on a hard surface, are therefore more likely to damage the vertebrae than those which load the spine for short periods and allow recovery of the vertebral blood-flow before repeating a movement.

> **Key point**
>
> As the spine is compressed, 'spring' is provided by blood flowing out of the spinal bone. As the compression is released, the blood flows back in again. If the spine is not allowed to recover from a single compression force before another is imposed, the spinal bone will be excessively stressed.

Intervertebral disc

Weight is transmitted between adjacent vertebrae by the lumbar intervertebral disc. The annulus fibrosis of a disc, when healthy, has a certain bulk and will resist buckling. When loads are applied briefly to the spine, even if the nucleus pulposus of a disc has been removed, the annulus alone exhibits a similar load-bearing capacity to that of the fully intact disc (Markolf and Morris 1974). When exposed to prolonged loading, however, the collagen lamellae of the annulus will eventually buckle.

The application of an axial load will compress the fluid nucleus of the disc, causing it to expand laterally. This lateral expansion stretches the annular fibres, preventing them from buckling. A 100 kg axial load has been shown to compress the disc by 1.4 mm and cause a lateral expansion of 0.75 mm (Hirsch and Nachemson 1954). The stretch in the annular fibres will store energy, which is released when the compression stress is removed. The stored energy gives the disc a certain springiness, which helps to offset any deformation which occurred in the nucleus. A force applied rapidly will not be lessened by this mechanism, but its rate of application will be slowed, giving the spinal tissues time to adapt.

Deformation of the disc occurs more rapidly at the onset of axial load application. Within 10 minutes of applying an axial load the disc may deform by 1.5 mm. Following this, deformation slows to a rate of 1 mm per hour, accounting for a subject's loss of height throughout the day. Reduction in disc height slackens the collagen fibres in both the annulus and the spinal ligaments. A two-hour compressive force which reduces the disc height by 1.1 mm has been shown to reduce resistance to flexion by 41 per cent and increase flexion range by 12 per cent (Adams et al. 2002). The range of flexion increases gradually throughout the day as tissues slacken and resistance is reduced. The greatest increase is seen in the first hours of rising.

Under constant loading, the discs exhibit creep, meaning that they continue to deform, even though the load they are exposed to is not increasing. Compression causes a pressure rise, leading to fluid loss from both the nucleus and annulus. About 10 per cent of the water within the disc can be squeezed out by this method (Kraemer, Kolditz and Gowin 1985), the exact amount being dependent on the size of the applied force and the duration of its application. The fluid is absorbed back through pores in the cartilage end plates of the vertebra when the compressive force is reduced.

> **Key point**
>
> The disc will compress and deform most within the first 10 minutes of a force being applied. Deformation may be as much as 1.5 mm loss in height initially, and then slows until 10 per cent of the total water content of the disc has been lost.

Exercises which axially load the spine have been shown to result in a reduction in subject height through discal compression. Compression loads of 6–10 times bodyweight have been shown to occur in the L3–L4 segment during a squat exercise in weight training, for example (Cappozzo et al. 1985). Average height losses of 5.4 mm over a 25-minute period of general weight training, and 3.25 mm after a 6 km run have also been shown (Leatt, Reilly and Troup 1986). Static axial loading of the spine with a 40 kg barbell over a 20-minute period can reduce subject height by as much as 11.2 mm. Exercises which involve this degree of spinal loading may be unsuitable for individuals with discal pathology early on in the rehabilitation process (Table 8.3).

Table 8.3 Effect of exercise on the spinal disc

Disc deforms by 1.5 mm within 10 min of compression
10% of water squeezed out of disc when loaded
Forces 6–10 times bodyweight produced in discs by a squat exercise
Height loss of 5.4 mm after 25 min of weight training
Height loss of 3.25 mm after 6 km run
Holding 40 kg barbell for 20 min reduces height by 11.2 mm

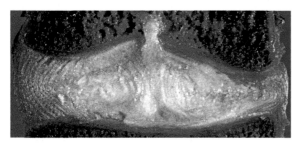

Figure 8.3 Schmorl's node: herniation of nuclear material through the disc end plate. Reproduced from Adams et al. (2002).

The vertebral end plates of the discs are compressed centrally, and are able to undergo less deformation than either the annulus or the cancellous bone. The end plates are, therefore, likely to fail (fracture) under high compression. Discs subjected to very high compressive loads show permanent deformation but not herniation. However, such compression forces may lead to herniation of nuclear material through the disc end plate known as a Schmorl's node (Fig. 8.3; Adams et al. 2002).

Key point

A Schmorl's node is the herniation of discal material through the disc end plate and into the vertebral body.

MRI signal change in the bone marrow adjacent to the disc end plate (Modic changes) may occur as a result of mechanical changes or bacterial infection (Albert et al. 2008). Following disc degeneration, with loss of disc body height and nuclear pressure, shearing forces may occur across the end plate, leading to microfracture and a local inflammatory response. In addition, injury to the disc annulus will lead to neovascularization of material outside the discal rim, with a subsequent inflammatory response. Bacteria may then enter the disc, causing a low-grade infection. Formation of fibrovascular tissue (Modic Type 1), yellow fat (Type II) or sclerotic bone (Type III) may all be visible adjacent to the end plate.

Definition

A *Modic change* is a degenerative change in the spinal disc end plate visible on MRI scan.

Bending and torsional stresses on the spine, when combined with compression, are more damaging than compression alone, and degenerated discs are particularly at risk. Average failure torques for normal discs are 25 per cent higher than for degenerative discs (Farfan et al. 1970). Degenerative discs also demonstrate poorer viscoelastic properties and therefore a reduced ability to attenuate shock.

Age-related changes

We have seen that with age the back wall of the disc weakens, the end plates become brittle and the disk reduces its water content from 90 per cent in childhood to 70 per cent in middle age. In addition, the disc's reaction to a compressive stress changes with age, because the ability of the nucleus to transmit load relies on its high water content. The hydrophilic nature of the nucleus is the result of the proteoglycan it contains, and as this changes from about 65 per cent in early life to 30 per cent by middle age (Bogduk and Twomey 1987), the nuclear load-bearing capacity of the disc reduces. When the proteoglycan content of the disc is high, up to the age of 30 years in most subjects, the nucleus pulposus acts as a gelatinous mass, producing a uniform fluid pressure. After this age, the lower water content of the disc means that the nucleus is unable to build as much fluid pressure. As a result, less central pressure is produced and the load is distributed more peripherally, eventually causing the annular fibres to become fibrillated and to crack.

Brown pigmentation is seen, which is an indication of change in the collagenous tissue (Adams et al. 2002), and the nucleus becomes dry and fibrous. As the disc dries, the annulus takes more of the compressive strain of weightbearing.

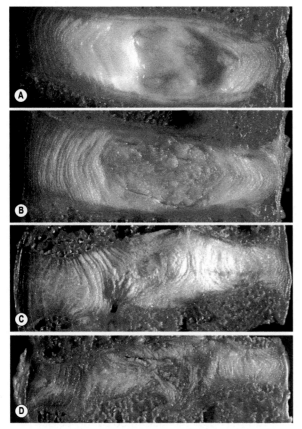

Figure 8.4 Discal degeneration. (A) healthy disc. (B) early shrinkage. (C) Disc thinning with smorls node formation. (D) Gross discal thinning and loss of disc height. Reproduced from Adams et al. (2002).

However, the annulus itself weakens through the accumulation of defects and fissures over time (Fig. 8.4).

As a result of these age-related changes the disc is more susceptible to injury later in life. This, combined with the reduction in general fitness of an individual and changes in movement patterns of the trunk related to the activities of daily living, greatly increases the risk of injury to this population. Individuals over the age of 40, if previously inactive, should therefore be encouraged to exercise the trunk under the supervision of a physiotherapist before attending fitness classes run for the general public.

Movements of the spine

Flexion

During flexion movements, the anterior annulus of the lumbar discs will be compressed while the posterior fibres are stretched. Similarly, the nucleus pulposus of the disc will be compressed anteriorly while pressure is relieved over its posterior surface. As the total volume of the disc remains unchanged, its pressure should not increase. The increases in pressure seen with alteration of posture are therefore due not to the bending motion of the bones within the vertebral joint itself but to the soft tissue tension created to control the bending.

Discal pressure changes

If the pressure at the isolated L3 disc for a 70 kg standing subject is said to be 100 per cent, supine lying reduces this pressure to 25 per cent. The pressure variations increase dramatically as soon

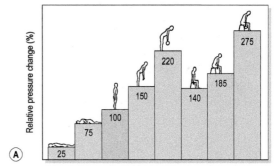

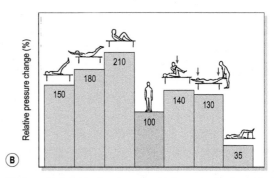

Figure 8.5 Relative pressure changes in the third lumbar disc. (A) In various positions. (B) In various muscle strengthening exercises. From Nachemson (1976).

367

as the lumbar spine is flexed and tissue tension increases (Fig. 8.5). The sitting posture increases intradiscal pressure to 140 per cent, while sitting and leaning forward with a 10 kg weight in each hand increases pressure to 275 per cent (Nachemson 1987).

The selection of an appropriate starting position for trunk exercise may be important following discal surgery. Superimposing spinal movements from a slumped sitting posture, for example, would place considerably more stress on the spinal discs than the same movement beginning from crook lying. Importantly, these studies are of the passive spinal elements (see below) in relative isolation. Subjects may compensate considerably using active (strength) and control (motor) elements, meaning that any pressure changes may not necessarily be clinically significant.

> **Key point**
>
> The highest discal pressures are seen in loaded slumped sitting, that is sitting with the lumbar lordosis reversed (flexed) while holding a weighted object. This type of posture should be avoided unless a subject's body has adapted sufficiently to compensate for this loading.

During flexion, the posterior annulus is stretched and the nucleus is compressed onto the posterior wall. The posterior portion of the annulus is the thinnest part, and the combination of stretch and pressure to this area may result in discal bulging or herniation.

As the lumbar spine flexes, the lordosis flattens and then reverses at its upper levels. Reversal of lordosis does not occur at L5–S1. Flexion of the lumbar spine involves a combination of anterior sagittal rotation and anterior translation. As sagittal rotation occurs, the articular facets move apart, permitting the translation movement to occur. Translation is limited by impaction of the inferior facet of one vertebra on the superior facet of the vertebra below (Fig. 8.6). As flexion increases, or if the spine is angled forward on the hip, the surface

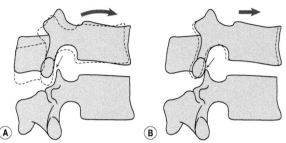

Figure 8.6 Vertebral movement during flexion. Flexion of the lumbar spine involves a combination of anterior sagittal rotation and anterior translation. As sagittal rotation occurs, the articular facets move apart (A), permitting the translation movement to occur (B). Translation is limited by impaction of the inferior facet of one vertebra on the superior facet of the vertebra below. From Bogduk and Twomey (1991), with permission.

of the vertebral body will face more vertically, increasing the shearing force due to gravity. The forces involved in facet impaction will therefore increase to limit translation of the vertebra and stabilize the lumbar spine. Because the zygapophyseal joint has a curved articular facet, the load will not be concentrated evenly across the whole surface, but will be focused on the anteromedial portion of the facets.

The sagittal rotation movement of the zygapophyseal joint causes the joint to open and is therefore limited by the stretch of the joint capsule. Additionally, the posteriorly placed spinal ligaments will also be tightened. Analysis of the contribution to limitation of sagittal rotation within the lumbar spine, through mathematical modelling, has shown that the disc limits movement by 29 per cent, the supraspinous and interspinous ligaments by 19 per cent and the zygapophyseal joint capsules by 39 per cent (Adams, Hutton and Stott 1980).

> **Key point**
>
> The zygopophyseal joint capsule gives the greatest soft tissue limitation to sagittal rotation which occurs between a pair of vertebrae.

Extension

During extension, the anterior structures are under tension while the posterior structures are first unloaded and then compressed, depending on the range of motion. With extension movements, the vertebral bodies will be subjected to posterior sagittal rotation. The inferior articular processes move downwards, causing them to impact against the lamina of the vertebra below. Once the bony block has occurred, if further load is applied, the upper vertebra will axially rotate by pivoting on the impacted inferior articular process. The inferior articular process will move backwards, overstretching, and possibly damaging, the joint capsule (Yang and King 1984). With repeated movements of this type, eventual erosion of the laminal periosteum may occur (Oliver and Middleditch 1991). At the site of impaction, the joint capsule may catch between the opposing bones, giving another cause of pain (Adams and Hutton 1983). Structural abnormalities can alter the axis or rotation of the vertebra, so considerable variation between subjects exists (Klein and Hukins 1983).

Rotation

During rotation, torsional stiffness is provided by the outer layers of the annulus, by the orientation of the zygapophyseal joints, and by the cortical bone shell of the vertebral bodies themselves. In rotation movements, the annular fibres of the disc will be stretched according to their direction. As the two alternating sets of fibres are angled obliquely to each other, some of the fibres will be stretched while others relax. A maximum range of 3 degrees of rotation can occur before the annular fibres will be microscopically damaged, and a maximum of 12 degrees before tissue failure. As rotation occurs, the spinous processes separate, stretching the supraspinous and interspinous ligaments. Impaction occurs between the opposing articular facets on one side, causing the articular cartilage to compress by 0.5 mm for each 1 degree of rotation, providing a substantial buffer mechanism (Bogduk and Twomey 1987). If rotation continues

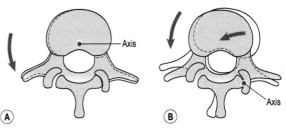

Figure 8.7 Vertebral movement during rotation. (A) Initially rotation occurs around an axis within the vertebral body. (B) The zygapophyseal joints impact and further rotation causes the vertebra to pivot around a new axis at the point of impaction. From Bogduk and Twomey (1987), with permission.

beyond this point, the vertebra pivots around the impacted zygapophyseal joint, causing posterior and lateral movement (Fig. 8.7). The combination of movements and forces which occur will stress the impacted zygapophyseal joint by compression, the spinal disc by torsion and shear, and the capsule of the opposite zygapophyseal joint by traction. The disc provides only 35 per cent of the total resistance (Farfan et al. 1970).

Lateral flexion

When the lumbar spine is laterally flexed, the annular fibres towards the concavity of the curve are compressed and will bulge, while those on the convexity of the curve will be stretched. The contralateral fibres of the outer annulus and the contralateral intertransverse ligaments help to resist extremes of motion. Lateral flexion and rotation occur as coupled movements. Rotation of the upper four lumbar segments is accompanied by lateral flexion to the opposite site. Rotation of the L5–S1 joint occurs with lateral flexion to the same side.

Movement of the zygapophyseal joints on the concavity of lateral flexion is by the inferior facet of the upper vertebra sliding downwards on the superior facet of the vertebra below. The area of the intervertebral foramen on this side is therefore reduced. On the convexity of the laterally flexed spine the inferior facet slides upwards on the superior facet of the vertebra below, increasing the diameter of the intervertebral foramen.

End-range spinal stress in sport

If the trunk is moving slowly, tissue tension will be felt at end-range and a subject is able to stop a movement short of full end-range and protect the spinal tissues from overstretch. However, rapid movements of the trunk will build up large amounts of momentum. When the subject reaches near end-range and tissue tension builds up, the momentum of the rapidly moving trunk will push the spine to full end-range, stressing the spinal tissues. In many popular sports, exercises often used in a warm-up are rapid and ballistic in nature and performed for a high number of repetitions. Unless the tissues have time to adapt, this can lead to excessive flexibility and a reduction in passive stability of the spine.

In addition, end-range stress can be experienced with postural changes and an alteration in the control of movement within the lumbar spine. Clinically, a number of directional patterns have been described (O'Sullivan 2000). Flexion of the lumbar spine is seen, with a gross reduction in the depth of the lumbar lordosis (Fig. 8.8). The subject suffers pain when semi-flexed postures are maintained, and with prolonged sitting activities. When put in a four-point kneeling position, the lumbar spine remains flexed. Extension of the lumbar spine is seen in the lordotic posture with the pelvis anteriorly tilted. In standing, and especially during extension movements of the whole spine or hip, the lumbar spine appears to 'hinge' as a single level rather than extend through its whole length. Lateral flexion movements are seen with tightness to the lateral flexors (quadratus lumborum and lateral external oblique). This is brought to the fore with single-leg standing

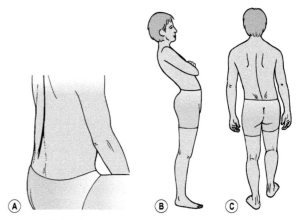

Figure 8.8 Directional patterns of end-range stress in the lumbar spine. (A) Flexion. (B) Extension. (C) Lateral shifting. After O'Sullivan (2000), with permission.

activities. Here, the patient, instead of transferring bodyweight with the pelvis, laterally flexes the spine and a noticeable scoliosis is apparent.

Discal injury

Many studies have examined mechanical changes within the disc during movement. Although of interest, it must be remembered that functionally the disc may be offloaded by muscle action and over time subjects can adapt other elements of their body to compensate for changes in the passive systems (see below). Additionally, morphological changes are not necessarily related to pathology, and pathology to pain. Many subjects may demonstrate structural changes to the disc which are unrelated to their symptoms.

During flexion, extension and lateral flexion, one side of the disc is compressed and the other stretched. In flexion, the axis of motion passes through the nucleus, but with extension the axis moves forwards (Klein and Hukins 1981). This fact, coupled with the increased range of motion during flexion, makes it the more dangerous movement. Combinations of torsion and flexion place the disc at particular risk from plastic deformation, which stretches the annular fibres irreversibly, and may cause fibre damage.

A single movement of flexion will stretch and thin the posterior annulus, but it is repeated flexion, especially under load, which is likely to give the most serious pathological consequences. Discal injury occurs frequently through repeated flexion movements, and when a flexion/rotation strain is placed on the spine during lifting.

When hyperflexion takes place, the supraspinous and interspinous ligaments will overstretch, reducing the support to the lumbar spine. Circumferential tearing will occur to the disc annulus posterolaterally, usually at the junction between the disc lamina and end plate. The outer annular fibres are innervated, a possible cause of the 'dull ache' in the lumbar spine which often precedes disc prolapse. Rotation strain will increase the likelihood of these injuries. Although rotation is limited in the lumbar spine, it is increased significantly as a result of facet joint degeneration and during flexion as the facets are separated.

Posterolateral radial fissuring occurs later, and connects the disc nucleus to the circumferential tear, allowing the passage of nuclear material towards the outer edge of the disc. This type of injury has been produced experimentally during discal compression in a combined flexed and laterally flexed posture (Adams and Hutton 1983). An annular protrusion can occur when the pressure of the displaced nuclear material causes the annulus to bulge. Eventually, nuclear material is extruded (herniated) through the ruptured annular wall (Fig. 8.9).

The discal injury may occur gradually as a result of repeated bending, giving symptoms of gradually worsening pain. Pain occurs initially in the lower back, and with time the symptoms are peripheralized into the buttock and lower limbs.

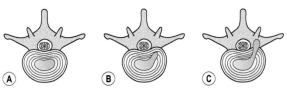

Figure 8.9 Stages of disc herniation. (A) Normal disc. (B) Nuclear bulge with annulus intact. (C) Ruptured annulus, nuclear protrusion onto nerve root.

Key point

Repeated bending can be associated with gradually worsening lower back pain. With time the symptoms peripheralize (travel outwards) into the buttocks and legs.

Sudden pain may occur from a seemingly trivial injury which acts as the 'last straw' to cause the disc herniation. Loads of sufficient intensity may give rise to an abrupt massive disc herniation. The stress is usually one of weight combined with leverage during a lifting action. Hyperflexion of the spine occurs, due in part to overstretching of the posterior lumbar ligaments.

Radiographic investigations of discal movement have been made by inserting metal pins into the lumbar nucleus pulposus and asymmetrically loading the disc, and through the use of MRI scanning (see below). These have shown that the disc may migrate towards the area of least load. When the asymmetrical load was removed, the nucleus remained displaced, but its relocation was accelerated by compression in the opposite direction, or by traction.

A number of studies have investigated the phenomenon of discal nuclear movement within the lumbar discs. Beattie, Brooks and Rothstein (1994) showed movement during extension with healthy discs but not with degenerative discs, and Edmondston, Song and Bricknell (2000) demonstrated 6.7 per cent anterior displacement between flexion and extension in L1/2, L2/3 and L5/S1. Fennell, Jones and Hukins (1996) used MRI scanning to demonstrate anterior movement

371

during extension, while movement of the nucleus in loaded postures has also been demonstrated (Alexander et al. 2007).

Spinal ligaments

A number of spinal ligaments are of concern to the biomechanics of the lumbar spinal segment: the anterior and posterior longitudinal ligaments, the intertransverse ligament, the ligamentum flavum, the interspinous and supraspinous ligaments and the capsular ligaments of the facet joint (Fig. 8.10). A general reduction in energy absorption of all the ligaments has been found with age (Tkaczuk 1968). The stiffest is the posterior longitudinal ligament and the most flexible the supraspinous (Panjabi, Jorneus and Greenstein 1984). The ligamentum

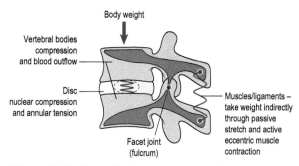

Figure 8.11 The spinal segment as a leverage system. From Kapandji (1974), with permission.

flavum in the lumbar spine is pre-tensioned (resting tension) when the spine is in its neutral position, a situation which compresses the disc. This ligament has the highest percentage of elastic fibres of any tissue in the body (Nachemson and Evans 1968), and contains nearly twice as much elastin as collagen. With age and degeneration there is a reduction of the elastin content of the ligamentum flavum, and calcification is sometimes apparent (Adams et al. 2002). The anterior longitudinal ligament and joint capsules have been found to be the strongest, while the interspinous and posterior longitudinal ligaments are the weakest (Panjabi, Hult and White 1987).

The ligaments act rather like rubber bands, resisting tensile forces but buckling under compressive loads (Fig. 8.11). They must allow adequate motion and fixed postures between vertebrae, enabling a minimum amount of muscle energy to be used. In addition, they protect the spine by restricting motion, and in particular protect the spinal cord in traumatic situations, where high loads are applied at rapid speeds. In this situation, the ligaments absorb large amounts of energy.

The longitudinal ligaments are viscoelastic, being stiffer when loaded rapidly, and they exhibit hysteresis as they do not store the energy used to stretch them.

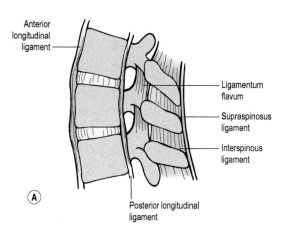

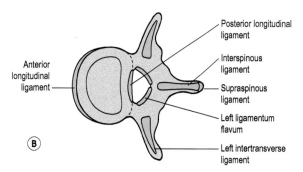

Figure 8.10 Ligaments of the spinal segment. (A) Side view. (B) Superior view. Reprinted by permission from Norris, C.M. (2008) *Back Stability*. Human Kinetics, Champaign, Illinois.

> **Definition**
> Viscoelasticity is the ability of a material to store and dissipate energy during mechanical

deformation. The deformation is dependent on the rate of loading. Hysteresis occurs when a material is stressed and does not immediately return to its previous shape when the stress is released.

When loaded repeatedly, they become stiffer, and the hysteresis is less marked, making the longitudinal ligaments more prone to fatigue failure (Hukins 1987). The supraspinous and interspinous ligaments are further from the flexion axis, and therefore need to stretch more than the posterior longitudinal ligament when they resist flexion.

Lower back pain

Non-specific lower back pain

The management of lower back pain has changed considerably over the last fifty years. Once, the patient with severe lower back pain may have expected to spend up to six weeks in a hospital bed on traction. The 'rest to heal' approach changed to encourage activity, and back rehabilitation programmes were encouraged. This change gave rise to a number of 'back school' and 'back stabilization' approaches to strengthen the spine in the belief that it was fragile and vulnerable to injury. Recently, this belief has been challenged in both the therapy and exercise worlds with several common 'myths' identified (Darlow and O'Sullivan 2016), as outlined in Table 8.4. The Chartered Society of Physiotherapy addressed this problem with the launch of the evidence-based

Table 8.4 Common myths in the management of back pain in sport

Myth 1. Back pain is caused by tissue damage.
Myth 2. The back is vulnerable to injury and needs protection, especially when symptomatic.
Myth 3. Directing treatment at specific tissues or structures will result in symptom resolution.

After Darlow B., and O'Sullivan PB (2016) Why are back pain guidelines left on the sidelines? Three myths appear to be guiding management of back pain in sport *Br J Sports Med* 50(21): 1294–1295

'Backpain Mythbusters' campaign in 2016 (CSP 2016). Although it is important to screen out severe pathologies such as bony injury, carcinoma, cauda equina compromise or progressive neurological deficit, which represent red flags, evidence suggests that there is little correlation between tissue damage and the severity of symptoms. In subjects with LBP, scans are poorly correlated with symptoms (Cheung et al. 2009) and morphological changes are visible on scans and X-rays equally in those without pain (Teraguchi et al. 2014). In some cases, the treatment outcome can be expected to be worse in those who have been scanned, with iatrogenic effects occurring, including increased disability, medical costs, and surgery (Webster et al. 2010).

Movement and exercise may sometimes exacerbate a condition in the acute phase of inflammation, but subsequent to this they have been shown to be beneficial to symptom resolution and to facilitate earlier return to function (Wynne-Jones et al. 2014). Additionally, avoiding movement may result in hypervigilance and the development of fragility beliefs (see Chapter 1), making rehabilitation more challenging later.

Definition

An *iatrogenic effect* is an unwanted effect caused by a therapeutic intervention.

The concept that tissue damage is reflected by the amount of pain that a subject experiences was challenged in Chapter 1. The pain level a subject experiences is often a reflection of how threatened they feel by their condition. The threat response is multifactorial, with items such as past experiences, beliefs, stress levels, sleep, and peer-group pressure all being relevant to a subject's pain experience.

Mechanical pain

The experience of back pain, then, does not necessarily reflect tissue damage. However, within a biopsychosocial approach, tissue is equally important to psychological and social factors and so should not be sidelined or ignored. The exact structure which is affected in lower back pain is open to discussion, and often it is virtually impossible to identify precisely which tissue is related to a patient's symptoms (Spitzer, LeBlanc and Dupuis 1987), and, as we have seen, the tissue is only one of many factors to consider. Diagnostic labels may often be misleading, with pathology identified which does not necessarily relate to the patient's symptoms. In many cases, rather than a structural diagnosis, a functional diagnosis may be more appropriate, with identification of the movement dysfunction or movement impairment (Sahrmann 2002) a better guide to effective rehabilitation.

To this end, the approach taken by McKenzie (1981) may be useful. Here, back pain is classified as *mechanical* or *chemical* (non-mechanical) in nature. Mechanical pain is produced by deformation of structures containing nociceptive nerve endings, and there is a clear correlation between certain body positions and the patient's symptoms.

Non-mechanical pain, on the other hand, is of a constant nature. This may be exacerbated by movement or position, but importantly, no position will be found which completely relieves the symptoms. This category encompasses both inflammatory and infective processes.

> **Key point**
> Mechanical pain is produced by deformation of sensitive structures. There is a definite correlation between body positions and the patient's symptoms. Non-mechanical pain is constant, and no position can be found which completely relieves the symptoms.

Inflammation will occur following trauma, and the accumulation of chemical irritant substances will affect the nociceptive fibres and may give pain. Within this model, pain may continue for as long as the nociceptor irritation continues –

although, as we have seen above, pain may occur in the absence of tissue change, so non-tissue explanations should also be considered. With rest, irritation will settle and healing progresses. Part of this healing process may be the formation of granulation tissue, so the type of pain may change from a constant chemical pain to a mechanical pain developed through adaptive shortening of the affected tissues. Non-mechanical conditions also include those which refer pain to the spine, such as vascular or visceral damage and carcinoma, which represent red flags. Clearly, it is essential to differentiate between mechanical and non-mechanical pain in the lower back. When no movement can be found which reduces the patient's symptoms, and if a period of rest does not allow the symptoms to subside, the patient requires further/medical investigation.

Examination of the back

Screening examination

Examination of the lumbar spine can be either very complex or relatively simple, depending on the approach taken. The reliability and reproducibility of tests for the spine increases when the information to be gained from the tests is kept to a minimum (Nelson et al. 1979). For this reason, the work of Cyriax (1982) and McKenzie (1981) is valuable as it provides enough information to treat the majority of patients. In addition, the tests tell the practitioner when further investigation may be necessary. However, a limitation of this type of assessment is that on the whole the focus is on the mechanical aspects of the condition and does not take into account other factors within a biopsychosocial approach. Additionally, this type of structured assessment often involves direct questioning, which is limited to a small aspect of the subject's whole experience, and fails to take in the patient's story (narrative); that is, their experience of how the condition effects them throughout all aspects of life.

Definition

The patient's story or narrative is a non-structured form of discussion with the patient around their experiences related to their condition.

Observation deals initially with posture while standing and sitting, and the appearance of the spine at rest. Assessment of the patient's movements provides essential information to guide rehabilitation. Scoliosis and loss of normal lordosis can be of particular note, as is the level of the iliac crests. Flexion, extension (standing on both legs and then single-leg standing) and lateral flexion are tested initially as single movements to obtain information about range of motion, end feel and presence of a painful arc. Flexion and extension are then repeated to see if these movements change the intensity or site of pain, bearing in mind the centralization phenomenon and dysfunction stretch. Side-gliding movements are also tested to repetition. Flexion and extension may be further assessed in a lying position to obtain information about nerve root adhesion (flexion) and greater range of extension. This initial examination then indicates whether neurological testing of sensation, power, reflexes and further nerve stretch is required. In addition, the history, signs and symptoms will indicate whether the pelvis and sacroiliac joints warrant further attention, or if resisted tests should be included.

Key point

Observation of the patient stationary (posture) and during motion (movement dysfunction) provides vital information prior to treatment.

Diagnostic triage

Diagnostic triage extends the screening examination by categorizing lower back pain into three types: simple backache (90 per cent), nerve-root pain (5–10 per cent) and serious pathology (1–2 per cent), with the likelihood of seeing each

Table 8.5 Diagnostic triage

Simple backache: specialist referral not required
Patient aged 20–55 years
Pain restricted to lumbosacral region, buttocks or thighs
Pain is 'mechanical' (i.e. pain changes with, and can be relieved by, movement)
Patient otherwise in good health (no temperature, nausea/dizziness, weight loss, etc.)
Nerve root pain: specialist referral not generally required within first 4 weeks, if the pain is resolving
Unilateral (one side of the body) leg pain that is worse than low back pain
Pain radiates into the foot or toes
Numbness and paraesthesia (altered feeling) in the same area as pain
Localized neurological signs (such as reduced tendon jerk and positive nerve tests)
Red flags (caution) for possibly serious spinal pathology: refer promptly to specialist
Patient under 20 or over 55 years of age
Non-mechanical pain (i.e. pain does not improve with movement)
Thoracic pain
Past history of carcinoma, steroid drugs or HIV
Patient unwell or has lost weight
Widespread neurological signs
Obvious structural deformity (such as bone displacement after an accident, or a lump which has appeared recently)
Sphincter disturbance (unable to pass water or incontinent)
Gait disturbance (unable to walk correctly)
Saddle anaesthesia (no feeling in crotch area between legs)
Cauda equina syndrome (bladder and bowel paralysis in addition to saddle anaesthesia)—refer to specialist immediately

After Waddell, G., Feder, G. and Lewis, M. (1997) Systematic reviews of bed rest and advice to stay active for acute low back pain. *British Journal of General Practice*, **47**, 647–652, and Norris (2000).

represented as a percentage (per cent) of the total case load (Table 8.5).

Definition

Triage is the process of assessing a patient to *prioritize* treatment options.

With simple backache (also called non-specific lower back pain, or NSLBP) the patient is generally

375

young to middle-aged (20–55 years), and the pain is restricted to the lower back and buttocks or thighs. The pain is mechanical in nature because it changes with movement, being eased or aggravated by specific actions which are repeatable. The patient is generally in good health and there is no history of weight loss, nausea or fever. Often there is a history of injury or overuse. This is the most common type, and a multidimensional assessment is required to identify psychosocial factors which may influence the condition. The STarT back tool is a simple nine-item validated questionnaire (Hill et al. 2008) which helps therapists identify modifiable risk factors (biomedical, psychological and social) for back pain disability. It is available at https://www.keele.ac.uk/sbst/startbacktool. The score obtained from the tool stratifies patients into low-, medium- and high-risk categories, and can be used to guide subsequent treatment.

Nerve root pain (radicular syndrome) is normally unilateral, with pain referred into the leg, which may be worse than any pain in the lower back. Pain may radiate into the foot, and numbness or paraesthesia (altered sensation) may be present. This type of pain may require further investigation if it does not show signs of significant improvement within four weeks of onset.

Radicular syndrome may be subdivided into three further categories (Bardin et al. 2017). *Radicular pain* occurs normally with nerve irritation and presents as leg pain which can increase with coughing or straining. *Radiculopathy* involves nerve compression and in addition to pain may give numbness or paraesthesia and muscle weakness. *Spinal stenosis* typically gives bilateral symptoms, which often ease with spinal flexion. There may also be *neurogenic claudication*, where walking distance is limited by leg pain.

Definition

Spinal stenosis is narrowing of the spinal canal which compresses the spinal cord or nerve roots. *Claudication* is limping which may result from compromise to nerves

(neurogenic claudication) or blood vessels (vascular claudication).

Where examination reveals non-mechanical pain in a young (under-20) or older (over-55) athlete, specialist investigation may be required. This is especially the case where there is a previous history of an associated medical condition, or if the patient has been unwell, shows an obvious structural deformity of the spine or demonstrates gait disturbance. Where altered sensation is present in the 'saddle' area (perineum and genitals), further investigation is required as this indicates possible disc protrusion of the lower sacral nerve roots. Where this is present with difficulty in passing urine, an inability to retain urine and/or a lack of sensation when the bowels are opened, there is a possibility of compression of the cauda equina and immediate emergency referral is required.

Definition

The *cauda equina* is a bundle of lumbar and sacral nerve roots at the end of the spine. The spinal cord finishes at the level of the first lumbar vertebra (L1) and the cauda equina nerves extend from this point down to the sacrum.

The straight-leg raise

The straight-leg raise (SLR) or Lasegue's sign is a widely used test to assess the sciatic nerve in cases of back pain. Although widely used, the test has limited diagnostic accuracy when evaluating herniated discs. In a systematic review of 11 studies assessing the accuracy of SLR against surgery as a reference standard, Deville et al. (2000) found a low specificity of 0.26 and a sensitivity of 0.91.

Key point

Specificity (true negative) of a test indicates its ability to detect those who do not have a condition, while sensitivity (true positive) indicates how good a test is at detecting patients who have a condition. Both are measures of diagnostic accuracy, which is the measure of agreement between a clinical test and a reference standard.

In addition to its effect on the sciatic nerve, the SLR test also places stretch on the hamstrings, buttock tissues, sacroiliac joint, posterior lumbar ligaments and facet joints, as well as lengthening the spinal canal (Urban 1986). Confirmation that the nerve root is the source of pain may be improved by raising the leg to the point of pain and then lowering it a few degrees. The neuromeningeal structures are then further stretched, either from below by dorsiflexing the foot, or by applying firm pressure to the popliteal fossa over the posterior tibial nerve. Pressure from above is produced by flexing the cervical spine. When performing the SLR, as the leg is raised the knee should not be allowed to bend and the pelvis should stay on the couch.

The dura within the spinal canal is firmly attached to the foramen magnum above and the filum terminale below. Trunk flexion causes the spinal canal to lengthen and therefore stretches the dura, whereas extension, by shortening the canal, induces dural relaxation, allowing the sheath to fold. The neuromeningeal pathway is elastic, so tension imparted at one point will spread throughout the whole length of the spine. As the SLR is performed, the initial motion is of the nerve at the greater sciatic notch. As hip flexion goes through 35 degrees, movement occurs proximal to the ala of the sacrum, and during the next 35 degrees the movement is at the intervertebral foramen itself. The last degrees of the SLR do not produce further nerve movement, but simply increase the tension over the whole course of the nerve (Grieve 1970) (Fig. 8.12).

Testing the unaffected leg (crossed SLR or 'well-leg' test) may also give symptoms. This manoeuvre pulls the nerve root and dura distally and medially, but increases the pressure on the nerve complex

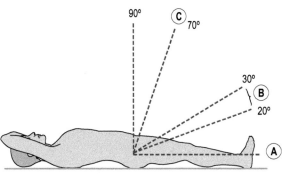

Figure 8.12 Effects of straight-leg raising. (A) Movement of sciatic nerve begins at the greater sciatic notch. (B) Movement of roots begins at the intervertebral foramen. (C) Minimal movement only, but increase in tension. From Middleditch et al. (2005), with permission.

by less than half that of the standard SLR test. When the ipsilateral SLR causes pain, it simply means that one of the tissues connected to the nerve pathway is sensitised. Because the crossed SLR stretches the neural structures less, the resting tension of these tissues must be higher to cause pain. The crossed SLR may therefore be a more reliable predictor of large disc protrusions than the ipsilateral SLR.

> **Key point**
> The well-leg test is a more reliable predictor of a large disc protrusion than the standard straight-leg raise (SLR).

Slump test

The slump is a neurodynamic test used to assess tension in the pain-sensitive structures around the vertebral canal or intervertebral foramen, and to ensure that these structures are able to stretch properly. To perform the manoeuvre, the patient sits unsupported over the couch side with the knees together and flexed to 90 degrees. The posterior thigh is in contact with the couch. The patient is then instructed to relax the spine completely and 'slump' forward, keeping the cervical spine in its neutral position ('look forwards,

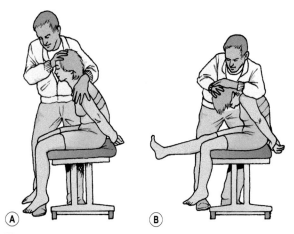

Figure 8.13 The slump test.

not down'). The therapist (standing at the side of the patient) places overpressure onto the patient's shoulders to increase the movement, attempting to bow the spine rather than increase hip flexion (Fig. 8.13A).

From this position, the patient is asked to flex the neck ('chin to chest') and then straighten the leg on the unaffected side first (Fig. 8.13B). In each case, the examiner places overpressure on the area and assesses the result. The athlete is then asked to dorsiflex the ankle ('pull your toes up'). Neck flexion is slowly released, and the response monitored. The opposite leg is then tested. A normal test result is one where there is a pain-free lack of knee extension by about 30 degrees and slight central pain over T9/10.

Mechanical therapy

Three mechanical conditions are recognized in the lower back: the postural syndrome, dysfunction and derangement (McKenzie 1981), and these can be a useful starting point for exercise therapy.

Postural syndrome

The postural syndrome occurs when certain postures or body positions place pain-sensitive soft tissues around the lumbar spine under prolonged stress. Pain is intermittent, only occurs when the

particular posture is taken up and ceases when the offending posture is changed, time in the posture position, rather than the position itself, being key. This can be frustrating for the patient because they can find nothing wrong. There is no deformity and vigorous activity is frequently painless as the stresses it imposes on the tissues are continually changing. The fault usually lies with poor sitting posture, which places the lumbar spine in flexion. After sport, the patient is warm and relaxed and so sits in a slumped position, perhaps in the bar after a game of squash. Discomfort occurs after some time and this gradually changes to pain. The patient often has the idea that sport makes the pain worse, but this is not the case. The poor sitting posture used when relaxing after sport is the true problem.

> **Key point**
>
> With the postural syndrome, pain occurs through tension on pain-sensitive soft tissues in the back. Particular body positions cause pain, and when these are released the pain subsides.

Pain may also occur in sport from extreme positions. Hyperflexion when lifting a weight from the ground or performing stretching exercises, hyperextension when pressing a weight overhead, or performing a back walkover in gymnastics, are common examples.

The most important part of management with the postural syndrome is patient education. To this end, the slouch-overcorrect procedure for correcting sitting posture is useful. The patient sits on a stool, and is allowed to slouch into an incorrect sitting posture for some time until back pain ensues. He or she is then taught a position of maximum lordosis, and learns how to change rapidly and at will, from the incorrect slouch to this overcorrect maximum lordosis. Once the patient has seen the relationship between poor sitting posture and pain, he or she is taught a correct sitting posture mid-way between the two extreme movement ranges. The use of a lumbar pad or roll is helpful to maintain the lordosis in sitting.

Where hyperflexion or hyperextension is the cause of postural pain, video is particularly useful in enabling athletes to appreciate the strain they are placing on the lumbar spine. Re-education of movement and skill training, with emphasis on the position of the spine and hips, are helped by video playback. Body landmarks over the pelvis and spine are marked, first using white adhesive dots. Biofeedback is also useful, especially when trying to correct hyperflexion. In its simplest form, strips of pre-stretched elastic tape are placed at either side of the lumbar spine. When the athlete flexes, the tape 'drags' on the skin and acts as a reminder to avoid the flexed position.

Importantly, part of the educational process with the patient must include an explanation about tissue loading and capacity (Chapter 1). The flexed position has exceeded the capacity of the posterior spinal tissues, and so pain has occurred as a warning. Increasing tissue capacity or reducing tissue loading will both be effective at managing the position. Clearly, increasing capacity requires tissue adaptation, which takes more time than offloading the tissues. However, if the explanation is that flexed sitting is 'wrong' because the back is 'fragile' to this position, hypervigilance may occur.

Dysfunction

Dysfunction pain is caused by overstretching adaptively shortened structures within the lumbar spine. The previously damaged structures have shortened due to prolonged disuse, or granulation (scar) tissue formation. When the normal range of motion is attempted at the affected segment, the shortened soft tissues are stretched prematurely. The essential feature with dysfunction is pain at the end of movement range which disappears as soon as the end-range stretch is released. The position is self-perpetuating because the pain which occurs with stretching causes the patient to avoid the full-range motion and so the adaptive shortening is compounded.

Dysfunction may occur secondary to trauma, or as a result of the postural syndrome. Typically, the patient is stiff first thing in the morning and the back 'works loose' through the day, so the patient is generally better with activity. Loss of extension leads to a reduced lordosis, and loss of flexion becomes apparent when the patient tries to touch the toes. Frequently, the patient will deviate to the side of the dysfunction. Once dysfunction has been detected, (static) stretching is required and/or joint mobilization procedures. Although mobilizations at Grades III and IV are useful to help restore range of movement, this passive treatment must be coupled with active stretching procedures, which the patient can practise at home, to help regain lost physiological range.

Accessory movements cannot usually be practised by the patient, and are perhaps a more appropriate form of manual therapy where physiological stretching causes excessive pain. It is important that stretching be practised little and often, to allow the patient to recover from the soreness which follows the lengthening of contracted tissues. The patient must be instructed to press gently into the painful end-range point in an attempt to increase the range of motion. There is always a tendency to try and avoid the painful position with back pain, but with dysfunction this is precisely the position we want to work in.

Key point

Dysfunction pain is caused by overstretching adaptively shortened structures within the lumbar spine. The most common form is an extension dysfunction, where the lumbar curve (lordosis) appears flat and lumbar extension range is limited.

The most common dysfunction following lower back pain is loss of extension. The extension loss may be regained by a combination of mobilization/manipulation, mechanical therapy and exercise. The classic mechanical therapy procedure is extension in lying (EIL), either with

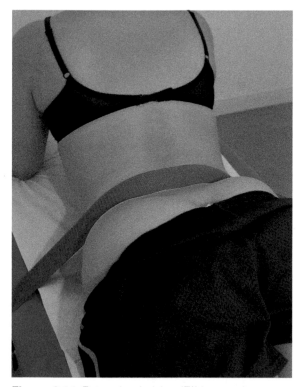

Figure 8.14 Extension in lying (EIL) procedure.

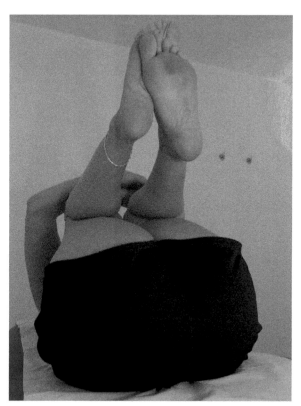

Figure 8.15 Flexion in lying (FIL) procedure.

or without belt fixation. The patient lies prone on the treatment table, with the lumbar spine held by a webbing fixation belt. This is placed around both the lower spine and treatment table at a point just below the spinal segment which is blocked to extension. From this position, the patient performs a modified press-up exercise, trying to fully extend the arms while keeping the hips in contact with the couch surface (Fig. 8.14). At home, the patient should continue the exercise at regular intervals throughout the day. Various modifications may be used to apply the pressure – EIL, with the patient lying on a plank or ironing board using a thick belt, or positioning the spine under a low piece of furniture, or manual pressure from a spouse or the weight of a small child.

Loss of flexion may be similarly regained, but this time the mechanical therapy technique is flexion in lying (FIL), or flexion in standing (FIS). Initially, the patient uses FIL. The movement begins in a crook-lying position. From this position, the patient pulls the knees to the chest. As maximum hip flexion is reached, further movement occurs, initially by flexion of the lower lumbar and lumbosacral segments, and then the upper lumbar area (Fig. 8.15). FIS is simply a toe-touching exercise performed very slowly. Gravitation effects place greater stress on the lumbar discs, so the exercise must proceed with caution. The differences between FIS and FIL are twofold. First, with FIS the legs are straight, and so the nerve roots are stretched, a particularly useful effect when dealing with nerve-root adhesion. Second, the sequence of flexion is reversed, with the upper lumbar areas moving before the lower lumbar and lumbosacral areas. Where there was a deviation in flexion at the initial examination, flexion in step standing may be used (Fig. 8.16). Here, one leg is placed on a stool and the patient pulls the chest downwards onto the

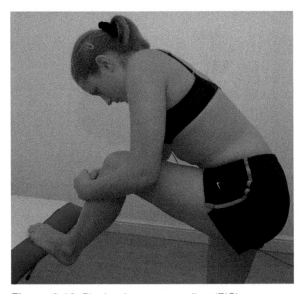

Figure 8.16 Flexion in step standing (FIS).

flexed knee. In so doing, flexion is combined with slight lateral bending. Other dysfunctions, such as loss of lateral flexion, side-gliding, or rotation, may occur, but they are less common. In addition, it must be remembered when assessing symmetry of bilateral movements that most people are slightly asymmetrical anyway. We must be certain that any asymmetry that exists is relevant to the patient's present symptoms before we spend time correcting it.

Derangement

Derangement occurs when the nucleus or annulus of the disc is distorted or damaged, altering the normal resting position of two adjacent vertebrae. Movement of the nucleus palposis in loaded postures has been demonstrated on MRI scan, with sagittal migration of the nucleus measured as the distance from the disc boundary. Extension in prone-lying showed significantly less posterior nuclear migration than sitting, while sitting (flexed and upright) showed more migration than standing (Alexander et al. 2007).

Pain may be constant and movement loss is apparent. Traditionally, disc prolapses have been classified by direction of nuclear material seen on MRI or surgically. The simplest classification (McKenzie and May 2003), is as either central (symmetrical) or unilateral (asymmetrical), with or without pain to the knee.

Deformities of scoliosis and kyphosis are common with this presentation, with local or referred pain over the lumbar and sacral dermatomes, depending on the severity of injury. Initial management may be by manual and/or mechanical therapy, or simply rest to allow the normal healing process to progress. Spontaneous regression of disc prolapse does occur, with the prolapsed material moving back into the parent disc, dehydrating, or moving into the epidural space, where inflammation and neovascularization result in absorption of the nuclear material by phagocytosis and enzyme action (Chiu et al. 2014).

Mechanical therapy aims at centralizing the pain and reversing the sequence of pain development which occurred as the disc lesion progressed. Although changes to the disc may occur, with increased water diffusion into the central disc reported in subjects who respond (Beattie et al. 2010), we have seen that the perception of pain may not necessarily be directly related to tissue damage. The aim is therefore symptom modification by transferring pain which is felt laterally in the spine or in the leg to a more central position. In this approach, it is perfectly acceptable for the intensity of the pain to increase, providing its position is altered to a more central one.

> **Key point**
> Derangement occurs when a spinal disc is distorted, altering the resting position of the vertebrae. Pain is usually constant and movement loss is seen. The aim is to centralize the pain, taking it from the leg or buttock back into the spine, and finally reducing it altogether.

The movements used are those which reduce the patient's symptoms in the initial examination. Where a scoliosis exists, initially

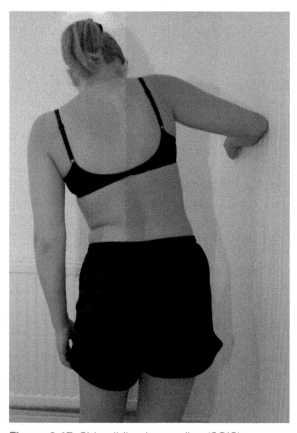

Figure 8.17 Side gliding in standing (SGIS).

the most effective movement is usually side-gliding in standing (SGIS). The therapist stands at the side of the patient holding the patient's hips. The therapist then gently presses the patient's shoulders towards the convexity of the scoliosis aiming to obtain a sliding rather than laterally flexing movement. The patient may continue this by placing the hand on a wall (arm abducted to 90 degrees) and shifting the hips towards the wall (Fig. 8.17). Once the pain moves into a more central position, the EIL exercise begins, with the aim of centralizing the pain further. Although these movements are frequently very effective for posterolateral protrusions, it must be emphasized that it is the movement which reduces the symptoms which is practised, and this may vary tremendously between patients.

Manual therapy of the lumbar spine

Manual therapy is a general term which describes hands-on procedures used to treat the joints and soft tissues. The most common subdivisions are *mobilization* and *manipulation*. Mobilization is a graded form of passive movement used repeatedly (oscillation), while manipulation is a term usually confined to single high-velocity, low-amplitude techniques (thrust). However, the terms are frequently profession-specific and may be used to define scope of practice. Procedures such as fascial manipulation, specific soft tissue mobilization and neural mobilization describe a hands-on technique specific to a target tissue.

The point at which manual therapy is used in sport will vary depending on both the condition and the practitioner using the therapy. Some practitioners rarely use manual therapy, claiming that to do so could make a patient dependent upon this type of care, while others use only mobilization and manipulation, claiming that it gives a more rapid response. The true picture probably lies somewhere between the two extremes. There are certainly patients for whom mechanical therapy or exercise is too painful initially. These patients usually respond to mobilization to relieve pain and then to increase mobility, and this treatment may be followed by mechanical therapy and exercise therapy at a later date. Equally, there are patients who look upon manual treatment as a panacea which will always cure them, and so they feel they have no need to care for their own spine. For these patients, clearly education and exercise therapy must be emphasized.

Mobilization and manipulation techniques for the lumbar spine

For the lumbar spine, there are two techniques (of literally thousands) which are especially valuable and will be briefly described. The first is the rotation movement (Fig. 8.18A). This is performed in the side-lying starting position, with the painful side uppermost generally, so that the pelvis is rotated away from the painful side. Both knees

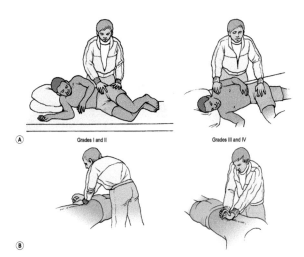

Figure 8.18 Lumbar mobilization. (A) Rotation. (B) Extension.

and hips and bent (crook-side lying), with the upper leg bending slightly more than the lower. The therapist stands behind the patient and imparts a Grade I or II mobilization by rhythmically pushing on the patient's pelvis, allowing the thorax to rock freely. With Grades III and IV, the patient's underneath arm is pulled through to rotate the thorax so that the chest faces more towards the ceiling. The upper leg bends slightly further so that the knee clears the couch side, and the lower leg is straighter to act as a pivot (increasing the flexion of the lower leg will flex the lumbar spine further). Therapist pressure is now over the pelvis and humeral head. This movement may be taken further to apply a manipulation. A lower couch position is used, and the end-range point of spinal rotation is maintained by the therapist pushing down on the patient's pelvis and shoulder through straight arms, and in so doing applying slight traction. As the patient exhales, a high-velocity, low-amplitude thrust is applied. A tremendous number of variations exist to allow for alterations in range of motion, direction of rotation and combined movements.

Extension movements in their simplest form may be produced by using posteroanterior pressures and derivatives of this technique (Fig. 8.18B). Posteroanterior central vertebral pressure (Maitland

1986) may be performed with the patient prone. The pressure may be imparted with the pads of the thumbs, or the ulnar border of the hand (pisiform/hamate), pressing over the spinous processes. Soft tissue compression is gradually taken up as the therapist moves his or her weight directly over the patient's spine and an oscillation is begun. Variations include combined movements, unilateral pressures, bilateral pressure over the transverse processes, and the addition of hip extension, among others.

Where the mobilization is taken to a Grade V, joint manipulation occurs. Mobilization can be differentiated from manipulation in that the former is an oscillatory technique (typically at around 2 Hz) while the latter is a thrust. Usually an audible click or pop is heard (cavitation) with manipulation, whatever velocity is used, and the cavitation effect has been said to be the only characteristic to distinguish manipulation from other spinal techniques (Evans and Breen 2006).

Typically, manipulation is carried out in three or four phases (Herzog and Symons 2001, Evans and Breen 2006): pre-thrust, thrust and resolution (Fig. 8.19). During the orientation phase, the patient is positioned for comfort, safety and joint specificity

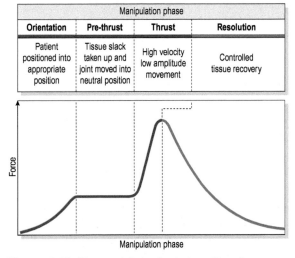

Manipulation phase			
Orientation	**Pre-thrust**	**Thrust**	**Resolution**
Patient positioned into appropriate position	Tissue slack taken up and joint moved into neutral position	High velocity low amplitude movement	Controlled tissue recovery

Figure 8.19 Phases of manipulation. Data from Evans and Breen (2006), Herzog (2010).

383

of the manipulation force. The pre-thrust phase takes up tissue slack prior to the thrust procedure itself. Once cavitation has occurred, the tissues are released in a controlled fashion to prevent painful recoil of elastic soft tissue.

Manipulation effects

Manipulation is thought to have effects in four areas (Evans 2002). The first is the release of trapped intra-articular material such as meniscoids in the spine or synovial folds in peripheral joints. These synovial folds have been shown to contain nociceptive nerve fibres (Giles and Taylor 1987) and can therefore be a source of pain. Thrust manipulation may gap the facet joint (Cramer et al. 2000), reducing impaction and synovial trapping. The second effect is the relaxation of hypertonic muscle through sudden stretching. Thrust manipulation involving a sudden stretch has been shown to excite the motor pool (Herzog, Scheele and Conway 1999). However, clinically, reduction in spasm is seen and it has been suggested that this is a reduction of hypoalgesia of the dorsal horn in the spinal segment targeted by the manipulation (Vernon 2000). Third, it is claimed that articular or peri-articular adhesions may be ruptured. It has been shown that the increased range of motion seen following thrust manipulation is independent of muscle tone. Using anaesthesia and muscle relaxants during surgery, Lewit (1985) demonstrated that cervical range of motion remained unchanged as muscle tone reduced, and suggested that this demonstrated an articular phenomenon in motion change following manipulative thrust.

The fourth area of manipulation effect is perhaps the most traditional, and that is an alteration or relocation of a displaced or subluxed joint. Biomechanical studies of vertebral motion following thrust manipulation demonstrate transient positional changes only (Gal et al. 1997) combined with a cavitation effect. Cavitation occurs in any synovial joint (Unsworth, Dowson and Wright 1971), and is due to suction acting upon the synovial fluid. As the joint surfaces (in this case,

the facet joints of the lumbar spine) are separated, the contact area of the fluid changes, forming a bubble which breaks as suction is continued. As the bubble collapses, it forms a cloud of smaller bubbles and eventually vaporizes, causing the familiar crack. Gas remains in solution for approximately 20 minutes following cavitation, and during this time a second crack cannot be obtained from the same joint. This phase is known as the refractory period.

> **Key point**
>
> Cavitation produces a click or pop during manipulation. The effect occurs as the contact area of the joint fluid changes, forming a bubble which then collapses.

NAGs and SNAGs

Many patients who have disc lesions seem to respond well to techniques which combine a mobilization technique with movement (MWM). The effect is both biomechanical and neurophysiological in nature (Vicenzino et al. 2011). Transient change in bone position may alter CNS input to trigger mechanical hypoalgesia and pain modulation. Psychological effects are also likely to occur, with habitual non-associative learning enabling the subject to repeat a previously painful/restricted action with less pain or increased range to alter motor learning.

> **Definition**
>
> *Non-associative learning* is a change in a response to a stimulus that does not involve associating the stimulus with a familiar pattern.

Mulligan (1989) described a number of procedures which take into account the planes of movement at the facet joints. In the lumbar spine, movement may be assisted using a *sustained natural apophyseal glide* (SNAG procedure) by applying therapist pressure over the spinous processes or articular pillars of the lumbar spine as the patient moves. SNAGs are weightbearing mobilizations, which are applied at end of range. They are applied simultaneously with movement, in line with the treatment plane (orientation of the articular surfaces) of the facet joint. Flexion, extension or lateral flexion may be used either in sitting or standing. Either pisiform or thumb contact is used, and the direction of pressure is vertical.

The starting position is with the patient sitting over the couch side (or standing) with the therapist behind. A belt is placed around the patient's waist over the anterior superior iliac spines (this area may be padded with a towel if necessary). The patient is asked to flex forwards to the point of pain. They then back off slightly and the therapist applies the SNAG as the patient flexes again (Fig. 8.20A). If the correct level has been identified, the movement should be pain-free and of greater range. If pain persists, the level to be treated is changed, or a unilateral SNAG is performed over the articular pillar of the more painful side.

Key point

The movement should be less painful and of greater range when the SNAG is applied. If no change in pain or movement range occurs (symptom modification), change the vertebral level of application.

For extension, the patient is in the same starting position, but the couch is raised to afford the therapist a better mechanical advantage. The therapist stands slightly to one side, in order to be clear of the patient as he or she extends back. The action must be lumbar extension, with the patient extending over the therapist's hand, rather than extension of the whole spine on the hip, with the patient pressing the whole bodyweight against the therapist's hand (Fig. 8.20B). Rotation is performed with the patient stride-sitting over the couch to fix the pelvis. The therapist grips around the patient's trunk just above the painful level. Again, the overpressure is given with the ulnar border of the hand in the treatment plane (Fig. 8.20C).

The direction of motion and level of pressure application is decided both by the movement which is limited and the action which relieves the patient's symptoms. As the patient moves, the vertical pressure is applied until end-range is obtained. Pressure is continued until the patient resumes the neutral position once more.

The sacroiliac joint

Structure

The three bones of the pelvis, the two innominates and the sacrum, form a closed ring. Anteriorly, the innominates join together at the pubic

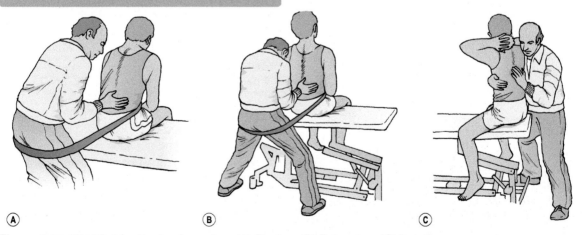

Figure 8.20 'SNAGs' for the lumbar spine. (A) Flexion. (B) Extension. (C) Rotation.

symphysis and posteriorly they join the sacrum via the sacroiliac joints (SIJ). Disorders of the pubic symphysis will often have repercussions on the SIJ, so examination should take place in both joints.

The sacral articular surface is shaped like a letter 'L' lying on its side, and is covered by hyaline cartilage, while the corresponding surface on the ilium is covered by fibrocartilage. The SIJ is a synovial joint, but its posterior surface is firmly secured by the interosseous ligament, so the joint may be considered as fibrous. There is great variation between individuals, in terms of the size, shape and number of articular surfaces, with 30 per cent of subjects having accessory articulations between the sacrum and ilium. With increasing age, the joint becomes fibrosed and may eventually show partial bony fusion.

Movement

The normal SIJ does move, albeit minimally. As the trunk is flexed, the sacral base moves forwards between the ilia and, with trunk extension in standing, the sacrum moves back again. The movement is usually only about 5 mm, but ranges up to 26 mm have been recorded (Frigerio, Stowe and Howe 1974). Roentgen stereophotogrammetric analysis (RSA) has been used to assess SIJ motion. In this technique, small metal (tantalum) balls less than 1 mm in diameter are implanted into the pelvic bones. Two synchronized X-ray tubes are then used to track free movement (Sturesson, Selvik and Uden 1989, Sturesson 2007), a technique considered the gold standard for orthopaedic research investigating small movements around joints. The SIJ research has shown that bone motion is not related to symptoms and that manipulation does not change bone motion, leading researchers to conclude that pain is inflammatory in nature.

Key point:

Motion of the SIJ is not usually directly related to symptoms. It can, however, cause an inflammatory response, creating a nociceptive stimulus.

Table 8.6 Movement of the sacroiliac joint (SIJ)

Nutation	Counter-nutation
▶ Anterior tilting of sacrum	▶ Posterior tilting of sacrum
▶ Sacral base moves down and forward, apex moves up	▶ Sacral base moves up and back, apex moves down
▶ Size of pelvic outlet increased, pelvic inlet decreased	▶ Pelvic inlet increased, outlet reduced
▶ Occurs in standing	▶ Occurs in non-weight bearing position such as lying
▶ Increased as lumbar lordosis increased	▶ Increased as lumbar lordosis decreased (flatback posture)
▶ Iliac bones pulled together, SIJ impacted	▶ Iliac bones move apart, SIJ distracted
▶ Superior aspect of pubis compressed	▶ Inferior aspect of pubis compressed

From Norris (2007), with permission.

SIJ mobility in women is generally 30–40 per cent greater than in men, but hypo- and hypermobility was not found. As the SIJ is loaded, motion is reduced and single-leg standing coupled with spine extension maximally loads the joint through bodyweight and muscle action, perhaps making this a useful screening test during examination of back pain in sport.

Sacral motion is described as *nutation* and *counter-nutation* (Table 8.6). Nutation of the SIJ is an anterior tilting of the sacrum on the fixed pelvic (innominate or iliac) bones. The sacral base (top, flat area) moves down and forwards and the apex (point) moves up, increasing the pelvic outlet. Nutation occurs as the lumbar lordosis increases and the iliac bones are pulled together, impacting the SIJ. With counter-nutation, the opposite movement occurs. It is a posterior tilting of the sacrum, with the base moving back and the apex (normally facing backwards) moving forwards and down. The pelvic outlet reduces and the pelvic bones move apart, distracting the SIJ. Counter-nutation occurs in non-weightbearing position and as the lumbar lordosis flattens.

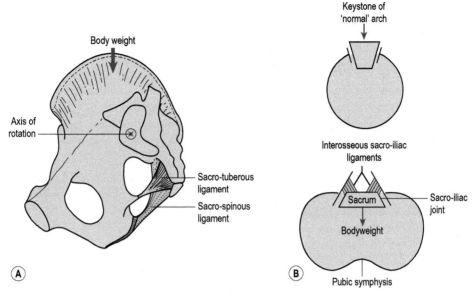

Figure 8.21 The sacroiliac joint. (A) Position. (B) Action in pelvic arch. After Taylor and Twomey (1994), with permission.

Definition

As the sacrum is a triangle pointed downwards, the sacral base is the large flat upper surface and the sacral apex the pointed lower portion. The sacrum and pelvic bones are joined together in a circle. The pelvic inlet is the space between the upper part of the bones and the pelvic outlet the space between the lower parts.

Postural asymmetry of the pelvis is common, and is evident when there is torsion of one ilium in relation to the other. On examination, one anterior superior iliac spine may appear higher and one posterior superior iliac spine lower, for example. Unequal leg lengths, although normally asymptomatic, may in some circumstances alter SIJ, changing gluteal muscle tone. When shortening is more than 1–2 cm, torsion of the pelvis occurs, with the ilium and sacral base on the side of the longer leg moving backwards and the pubis moving upwards. The degree of postural compensation between individuals will differ, so the pelvic position in reaction to altered leg length is variable, and may not be clinically significant.

Hormonal changes in pregnancy and, to a lesser extent, menstruation and menopause will also influence the SIJ. The general softening and relaxation of the pelvis leads to an increased range of motion, which may remain for up to 12 weeks following childbirth. Local irritation of the SIJ leads to pain on gapping tests and limited hip abduction on the painful side.

Stability

The sacrum is inserted like the keystone of an arch, but seemingly the wrong way round, tending to be displaced rather than forced inwards with pressure. However, as the bodyweight is taken, the tension developed in the interosseous sacroiliac ligaments pulls the two halves of the pelvic ring together, producing *form closure* (Fig. 8.21). In the sagittal plane, the bodyweight falls ventral to the axis of rotation of the SIJ. This alignment would tend to rotate the sacrum forwards into a nutated position. During nutation, the sacrotuberous ligament and the large interosseous ligament of

387

the SIJ are tensioned, drawing the posterior part of the innominate bones together in a mechanism called self-locking. Counter-nutation disengages self-locking and so may lead to SIJ instability. Interestingly, because self-locking is disengaged during forward flexion of the trunk without a pelvic tilt (Lee 1994), a stoop lift may dislodge the joint and is often a mechanism in SIJ pathology.

Although no strong muscles cross the SIJ, the joint may be actively stabilized by a combination of forces acting over the joint, a process called *force closure*. The sacrotuberous ligament (sacrum to ischial tuberosity) and the long dorsal sacroiliac ligament (sacral segments 4/5 to posterior inferior iliac spine) blend to form an expansion measuring 20 mm wide by 60 mm long. This expansion attaches to the posterior layer of the thoracolumbar fascia (TLF) and to the aponeurosis of the erector spinae, and a number of other muscles have important tensioning effects in this area (Vleeming et al. 1997). Five stabilizing systems are described involving trunk and lower-limb muscles coupling with lumbosacral fascia and ligaments (Fig. 8.22). These muscle–fascial couplings give the therapist the opportunity to use muscle re-education to stabilize the SIJ during rehabilitation (Treatment Note 8.1).

> **Key point**
> The sacroiliac joint (SIJ) is stabilized by both form closure (passive) and force closure (active).

Examination

Subjective examination usually reveals a unilateral distribution of symptoms, perhaps spreading to the buttock, lower abdomen, groin or thigh, although pain may be referred to the foot. The traumatic history is frequently one of a fall, landing on the ischial tuberosity, with patients unable to walk distances without marked pain. The footballer in a mistimed sliding tackle or the youngster who falls while ice-skating are prime examples. In any sport where the range of motion required at the hip is great, or repetitive unilateral leg movements are performed, SIJ irritation may be encountered. Tensile forces are increased with jumping activities onto both legs, while shear forces are raised with single-leg activities such as running and hopping. Dancers, gymnasts and high-jumpers are particularly prone to SIJ involvement, but any athlete may suffer trauma to the joint, leading to local inflammation or mechanical disturbance.

Objective examination of the pelvis and SIJ is made, initially with the patient standing. The general bony alignment and muscle contour is noted. The patient may be reluctant to take weight through the affected leg, and may walk with a limp. The gluteal bulk, together with the level of the gluteal folds and gluteal cleft, is noted, as is that of the iliac crests and iliac spines.

Motion (kinetic) tests

Motion tests of the SIJ may be used to assess the side of the body with the predominant dysfunction, and therefore the side to treat (Turner 2002). They assess the contribution of the SIJ to general pelvic motion and are used before and after a treatment technique to determine effectiveness. Importantly, motion tests cannot accurately by themselves be used to determine the nature of a dysfunction or to imply that an altered motion test is a cause of pain. In addition, they cannot indicate whether a joint is 'stiff' or 'locked', but may be used to assess patient symptoms and response to treatment.

Two motion tests for the SIJ are typically used in sport: *hip flexion in standing* and *forward flexion in standing*.

▶ For *hip flexion in standing*, the examiner places his or her thumbs over S2/3 and the PSIS. From the standing position, the patient flexes one hip, and movement of the PSIS is noted. Normally, with hip flexion the PSIS moves caudally (drops) and as the leg is brought back to the ground it moves cephalically (lifts).

▶ With *forward flexion in standing*, both PSIS are palpated as the patient flexes the spine.

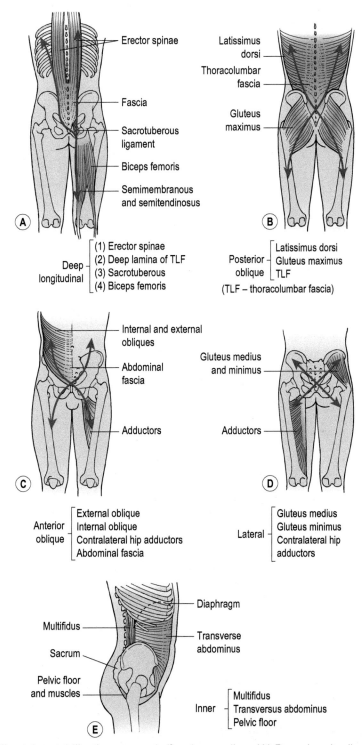

Figure 8.22 'Sacroiliac joint stabilization—muscle/fascia coupling. (A) Deep longitudinal muscle system, (B) posterior oblique, (C) anterior oblique, (D) lateral, (E) inner. From Magee (2002), with permission.

Treatment note 8.1   Lumbar stabilization starting positions

Muscle isolation

Traditional lumbar stability programmes often begin with muscle isolation. The aim initially is to teach the correct abdominal hollowing (AH) action, avoiding substitution strategies such as breath holding, rectus abdominis and

Table 8.7 Starting positions for abdominal hollowing

Starting position	Advantage	Disadvantage
Kneeling (4 point)	Abdominal wall placed on stretch to facilitate AH action Unfamiliar pattern to athletes so avoids 'sit-up' motor programme Comfortable for LBP patient and during pregnancy	Stress on wrists and knees Difficult for obese subject
Prone lying	Easier to avoid spine movement Good cueing to pull abdominal wall away from table AH can be measured using pressure biofeedback	Inappropriate for obese or pregnant subject due to abdominal compression
Supine lying	Good for self palpation Surface EMG (sEMG) and pressure biofeedback used easily Link to PF contraction easier as patients often learn PF work in this position	Position may lead to sit-up muscle strategies in athletes (rectus dominance)
Standing (wall support)	Cueing to pull abdominal wall away from waistband of trousers useful for home exercise Appropriate for obese and pregnant patients Functional for daily activities	Weight bearing may not be suitable for disc patients Those with extreme postural abnormalities may find position uncomfortable

AH = abdominal hollowing
LBP = low back pain
PF = pelvic floor

From Norris, C.M. (2008) *Back Stability*. Human Kinetics, Champaign Illinois. With permission.

Treatment note 8.1 continued

external oblique dominance, and obvious ribcage movement. Four starting positions may be used, and the one which is most suitable for the patient forms the basis of the programme progression (see Table 8.7).

The four-point (prone) kneeling position has the advantage that it is comfortable on the spine and is particularly suitable after lower back pain or following/during childbirth. In addition, as it is an unfamiliar position for abdominal exercises, the position will not encourage a 'sit-up motor programme' – that is, dominance of the rectus abdominis. This makes the position suitable for use with athletes where the aim is to reduce the reliance on the rectus. As abdominal hollowing is performed, the abdominal wall is pulled upwards and a belt may be used to cue this movement, enabling the patient to pull away from the belt. This action is likely to be difficult for obese individuals, simply because they have a greater tissue mass to lift, so another starting position may be more appropriate.

Prone lying (lying on the front) supports the back completely and avoids the 'rocking' action which some patients find it difficult to control in kneeling. In addition, as the abdominal wall is pulled away from the floor, cueing is provided,

and a pressure biofeedback unit may be used to monitor the effect. Again, the starting position may not be suitable for an obese subject as tissue mass makes movement initiation difficult.

Supine lying (lying on the back) enables the subject to self-palpate, and the use of sEMG also adds to self-measurement. In addition, supine lying is the position often used for retraining pelvic floor (PF) muscle action, and linking abdominal hollowing to PF muscle work is a useful method of initiating deep abdominal action. In athletes, however, close supervision will be required as there is a tendency to recruit the rectus abdominis, and even to lift the head, in this position.

Standing against a wall is most suitable for obese subjects as they can pull the abdominal wall away from a belt (or waistband of the trousers) with minimal muscle work, which becomes very motivating. In addition, for those unfamiliar with exercise, standing activities are often better tolerated. Because the position is weightbearing, however, those with acute lower back pain may not be able to tolerate prolonged standing, and a lying starting position may be more suitable for them.

Ideally both PSIS should move equally. If dysfunctional, one joint may move earlier or further up as the patient flexes (Piedallu's sign). It is as though the PSIS is being dragged along by the sacrum.

These tests may be used to guide manual therapy techniques, but should not be used in isolation diagnostically (see below).

Palpation

Motion tests of the SIJ which rely on palpation have been shown to be unreliable (Laslett 1997) and are only of real clinical use when used in

parallel with other forms of objective examination. In a study of 45 patients using experienced manual therapists to assess six commonly used palpation tests, the maximum reliability was only fair, and in some tests the reliability was worse than that obtained through chance (van Duersen et al. 1990). Dreyfuss et al. (1992) found that as many as 20 per cent of asymptomatic individuals gave a false positive on the standing or seated flexion tests, and Potter and Rothstein (1985) used experienced manual therapists to test 13 palpatory tests and found that simple agreement on the tests was less than 70 per cent on most of the procedures.

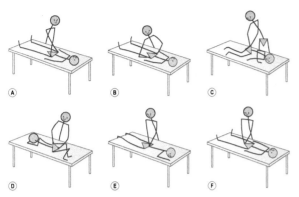

Figure 8.23 Sacroiliac joint pain provocation tests.

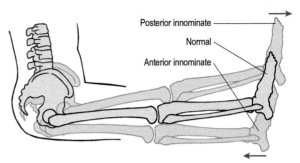

Figure 8.24 Leg-length assessment of sacroiliac joint. From Magee (2002), with permission.

Pain provocation tests are, however, more reliable. Laslett and Williams (1994) assessed 51 patients with six SIJ tests and found that interexaminer agreement was over 94 per cent for the femoral thrust, and 88 per cent for pelvic torsion (Gaenslen's test), distraction and compression tests. These four tests are shown in Fig. 8.23.

With persistent bilateral SIJ pain, the possibility of ankylosing spondylitis should be considered. The range of motion, especially lateral flexion, of the lumbar spine is limited, and muscle spasm may be evident. Where costovertebral involvement is present, chest expansion will be affected – often an early sign. The use of radiographs, erythrocyte sedimentation rate (ESR), and the presence of the antigen HLA B27 aid the diagnosis.

Change in leg length as SIJ assessment

A change in leg length has been used as an assessment of SIJ dysfunction (Don Tigny 1985). The leg length change is claimed to occur because altered position of the innominate bones will also change the resting position of the acetabulum, placing it more proximal or distal, and consequently altering leg length. The tests are used to identify a reduction in self-locking of the SIJ through nutation (anterior rotation) of the sacrum on the innominates.

Initially patients are positioned in crook lying and they are instructed to form a bridge and to place

the hips back onto the couch. The therapist then passively extends the legs and compares leg length by palpating the undersurface, the malleoli, with the edge of the thumbs. The patient then performs a straight-leg sit-up action (they may assist themselves by pulling on the couch with their hands) and the leg length is again assessed. If the leg gets longer (lying to sitting) it is claimed to indicate a posterior innominate on the side of the longer leg, and if the leg gets shorter the indication is of an anterior innominate (Fig. 8.24).

Positional change in the innominates

Three main positional changes are claimed to occur in the SIJ: *anterior innominate* (common), *upslip* (common) and *posterior innominate* (less common) (Fig. 8.25). A variety of other appearances occur but

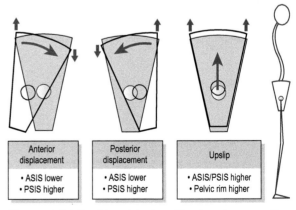

Figure 8.25 Positional faults affecting the sacroiliac joint.

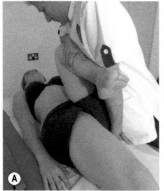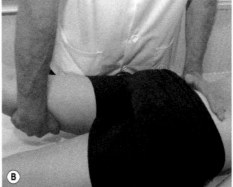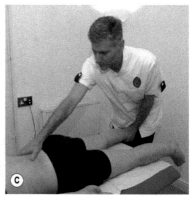

Figure 8.26 Muscle energy techniques (MET) for the sacroiliac joint. (A) Anterior innominate. (B) Posterior innominate. (C) Upslip.

they are not as frequently seen in day-to-day clinical practice. The reader is referred to Lee (1994) for further information.

▶ With an *anterior innominate*, the anterior superior iliac spine (ASIS) appears higher and the posterior superior iliac spine (PSIS) lower. With a posterior innominate, the reverse occurs, with the ASIS higher and the PSIS lower. An upslip sees the whole innominate bone higher on that side, with both the ASIS and PSIS higher and the pelvic rim itself appearing higher on the affected side. A variety of muscle energy techniques (MET) may be used to treat positional faults. An anterior innominate is treated with passive hip flexion. The patient is supine and the therapist places one hand beneath the ischial tuberosity of the near leg. The other arm grips the femur of the near leg. The action is to resist hip extension and as the muscles relax, to impart a posterior pelvic tilting force by rocking the arms and pulling the ischial tuberosity upwards (Fig. 8.26).

Definition

Muscle energy technique (MET) uses the patient's muscle contraction force (energy) to assist in joint mobilization. MET generally involves gentle isometric contraction followed by relaxation to reduce muscle tone. During this relaxed phase the joint is mobilized.

▶ A *posterior innominate* is treated with a posteroanterior (PA) mobilization on the PSIS. The patient lies prone and the therapist grasps the inside of the near knee. Resisted hip flexion is used and, as the muscles relax, downward pressure is imposed through the other arm.
▶ An *upslip* may be treated with leg traction. The patient lies supine and the therapist holds the leg in slight internal rotation to protect the hip joint. The action is initially leg-shortening (contraction of ipsilateral trunk side flexors), followed by leg traction as the muscles are relaxed.

Assessment of SIJ stability

The SIJ is stabilized both passively (form closure) and actively (force closure), as detailed above. Failure of the stabilizing mechanisms may be assessed using the active straight-leg raise (ASLR) test (Mens et al. 1997). The test first identifies SIJ stability, but, importantly, can also be used to highlight the most appropriate way to stabilize the joint and provides a valuable tool for the reassessment of the treatment intervention. It is, therefore, the assessment of choice for functional rehabilitation of SIJ dysfunction.

> **Key point**
>
> The active straight-leg raise (ASLR) test is the assessment of choice for functional rehabilitation of SIJ dysfunction.

The patient is asked to actively lift the leg by 5 cm, keeping it straight, by engaging the hip flexor muscles. Weakness and/or pain on this movement on one side of the body indicates poor dynamic stability of the SIJ (force closure). The test is then performed again while the therapist assists form closure by: (i) compressing the pelvic rims, and (ii) using minimal posterior pelvic tilt (innominate rotation) on the ipsilateral side. Where these techniques reduce pain and increase strength, an SIJ belt should be used initially until force closure has been enhanced. To assess force closure, the ASLR test is repeated while engaging the muscle–fascial systems shown in Fig. 8.22. For the inner system, the transversus abdominis is contracted (abdominal hollowing); for the posterior oblique system, the latissimus dorsi is engaged (resisted shoulder adduction).

The ASLR test has been demonstrated radiographically to alter alignment of the pelvic ring using pubic malalignment as a measure. ASLR of the normal limb shows no step deformity across the pubic ramus, but with the symptomatic limb, step deformity of 5 mm, together with anterior innominate rotation, has been recorded (Mens et al. 1997). In addition, the same study demonstrated that over 70 per cent of symptomatic patients showed less strength in the ASLR, and 80 per cent of these showed strength improvement with a SIJ belt. In addition, in all but one patient, the ASLR was more powerful, with posterior rotation pressure over the ipsilateral ASIS.

The posterior pelvic pain provocation or 'P4' test (also called the thigh thrust) is used in SIJ region pain, especially in pregnancy, to distinguish between pelvic or lumber spine involvement. It has been shown to be negative in those with confirmed lumbar disc herniation (Gutke et al. 2009), and demonstrated a high positive prediction value for

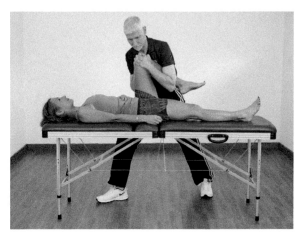

Figure 8.27 Posterior pelvic pain provocation (P4) test.

posterior pelvic pain, together with a high negative prediction value for lower back pain in a population of pregnant women (Ostgaard, Zetherström, and Roos-Hansson 1994). The test is performed by flexing the subject's hip and knee to 90 degrees. The therapist places one hand (flat) between the subject's sacrum and the couch to stabilize the area and the other hand wraps around the subject's thigh, with their knee on the therapist's chest (Fig 8.27). The action is to apply an axial force along the length of the femur, which would tend to displace the ilium on the side of the tested leg. Adding slight adduction (within the subject's comfort zone) may increase stress to the region and refine the test.

Management of sacroiliac pain

In sport, three treatment techniques for SIJ pain are particularly useful: manual therapy, exercise therapy and, in some cases, dry needling. As we have seen, manipulation does not cause movement at the SIJ, but both manipulation and mobilization are effective techniques for SIJ and pelvic pain, giving symptom relief. Lumbar rotator mobilization may be modified to affect the SIJ into the classic 'gapping' technique (Fig. 8.28A). The patient is positioned with the painful side uppermost, and the trunk rotated so that

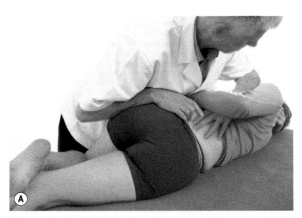 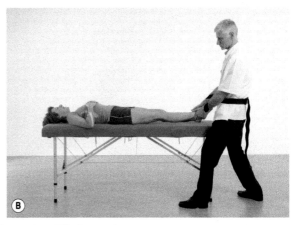

Figure 8.28 Mobilization of the sacroiliac joint (SIJ) (A) gapping (B) distraction.

the shoulders rest close to the couch. The upper knee is drawn over the couch edge and fixed into position using the therapist's body. The therapist uses their forearms as contact points, pressing the cephalic arm onto the lower ribs to fix body position and the caudal arm onto the iliac crest to apply the oscillatory mobilization or manipulative thrust. The direction of pressure is downwards and slightly forwards, aiming the line of force to the near couch edge.

Distraction of the pelvic region is achieved using leg traction applied through a belt (Fig. 8.28B), in the 'leg tug' or longitudinal mobilization procedure. The patient lies supine with their feet at the end of the couch. The therapist fixes the patient's foot of the unaffected side with their knee to stop the patient sliding down the couch. The ankle of the affected side is grasped using a figure-of-eight belt grip. Traction is applied as the therapist leans back, which may be sustained, oscillatory or converted into a thrust.

Dry needling into the interosseous ligament, periosteal needling (pecking) over the posterior superior iliac spine and prolotherapy are all used successfully for SIJ treatment. Cusi et al. (2010) reported positive clinical outcomes in 76 per cent of patients, using three injections of hypertonic dextrose into the dorsal interosseous ligament, assessing outcomes using standard questionnaires,

ASLR, single-leg standing and the posterior pelvic pain provocation test.

Stability exercise is used extensively in management of the SIJ and the muscle-fascia slings may be worked using variations of the hip-hinge action with the legs straight (good morning exercise) or bent (deadlift exercise) shown in Fig. 8.29A & B.

Spondylolysis

Spondylolysis is a defect in the neural arch (pars interarticularis) which may extend to the neighboring lamina or pedicle. In 90 per cent of cases, changes are to the fifth lumbar vertebra (Fig. 8.30). It is a fracture of the pars without slippage, and by the age of 7 years may be present in 5 per cent of the population. In athletes, however, the incidence may be as high as 20 per cent, and it is often associated with other lumbar anomalies (Hoshina 1980). Sports which subject the lumbar spine to repeated loaded extension (gymnastics, ballet, volleyball) typically have a higher incidence, with the highest seen in cricket fast bowlers (Ranson et al. 2010). The condition typically progresses from bone stress (asymptomatic but visible on X-ray screening) to stress reaction and stress fracture (both symptomatic), with a visible fracture line defining the latter.

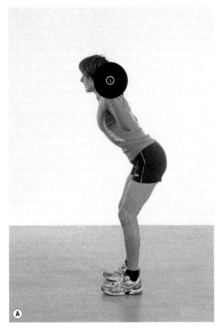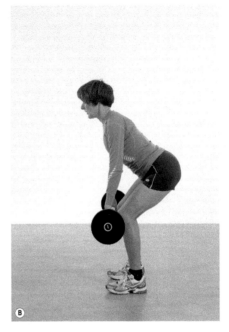

Figure 8.29 (A) Good morning exercise, (B) Deadlift.

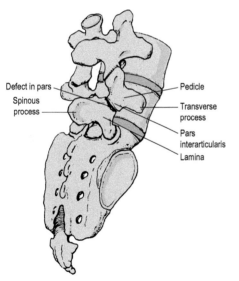

Defect in pars
Spinous
process

Pedicle

Transverse
process

Pars
interarticularis

Lamina

Figure 8.30 Site of defect in spondylolysis. From Gould (1990), with permission.

Diagnosis is by bone scintigraphy, often combined with MRI. In the clinic, the single-leg extension test may be used to recreate symptoms, but is not sensitive or specific for the detection of the active condition (Masci et al. 2006).

> **Key point**
> Bone scintigraphy is a method of assessing blood flow and metabolism of bone. A radioactive tracer is given to the patients and taken up by the bone. The rate and distribution of the tracer indicates affected bone areas.

The single-leg extension test (stork extension) is performed by having the patient stand on one leg (the affected side) and extend the spine to arch backwards. Compression and extension is imparted to the lumbar region. This may be combined with a quadrant test combining extension, lateral flexion and rotation of the lumbar spine to the painful side to maximally stress the region to reproduce the patient symptoms. This test is in no way diagnostic of the condition, but may raise suspicions – and imply that further investigation may be required if symptoms continue.

Where symptoms are present but no deformity is detectable on X-ray or bone scan, a pars interarticularis stress reaction has occurred without cortical interruption (Weber and Woodall 1991). At one stage, a congenital defect was thought to be present. However, the condition is not present from birth and increases in incidence with age. Furthermore, the ossification centres of the vertebra do not correspond to the position of the defect. Familial tendencies do exist, and racial differences have been described.

The most important consideration from the point of view of sport is that of trauma. Direct trauma may result in a non-union of the area or, more likely, a stress fracture forms over a prolonged period, especially as a result of repeated flexion overload, hyperextension or shearing stress to the lumbar spine. Athletes with hypolordosis in the lumbar spine are at risk from flexion overload, whereas those demonstrating hyperlordosis may suffer the condition as a result of forced rotation causing torsion overload. The pars interarticularis is positioned as a pivot between the disc and facet joints, and so is subjected to considerable stress.

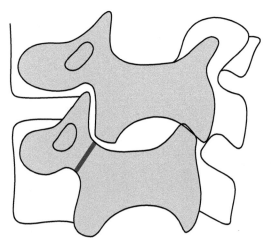

Figure 8.31 An oblique X-ray of the lumbar spine, which has the appearance of a terrier dog. In the lower segment a spondylolysis through the pars interarticularis appears as a collar around the dog's neck. From Corrigan and Maitland (1983), with permission.

> **Key point**
>
> Spondylolysis can form over a prolonged period, usually as a result of repeated flexion, hyperextension or shearing stresses imposed on the lumbar spine.

Repeated stress can lead to microfractures, especially if overtraining has occurred. As these heal they produce an elongated appearance of the bone. Lumbar pain is apparent; this may be unilateral or bilateral but is rarely associated with nerve root compression. Pain is experienced first with hyperextension, such as walk-over movements in gymnastics, and increases in intensity. Pain is aggravated by hyperextension or rotation, and may present with paraspinal muscle spasm. Unilateral pain may be reproduced using the single-leg extension test and quadrant test described above, as these movements compress the pars interarticularis and may reproduce the stress encountered in sport. Flexion is normally painless, although pain may occur as the athlete returns to standing. Oblique X-rays give the classic 'terrier dog' appearance (Fig. 8.31), with the dog's collar represented by the pars interarticularis defect, which is bridged by fibrous tissue rather than bone. A negative X-ray does not rule out spondylogenic conditions, and a bone scan may be required. Increased tracer update on CT or visible bone oedema on MRI indicate an active healing process.

Spondylolisthesis

Spondylolisthesis is an anterior shift of one vertebra on the other, usually L5 on S1, and is normally associated with a bilateral pars defect, typically in early adolescents. The condition can be a progression from spondylolysis, but this is unusual in sport if the original injury is a unilateral pars stress fracture. The condition may also occur in the elderly as a result of degeneration, or congenitally in association with spina bifida. The first-degree injury involves slippage to a distance of one quarter of the vertebral diameter, but further movement may occur up to a fourth-degree injury which

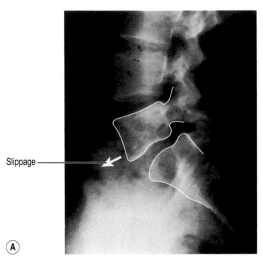
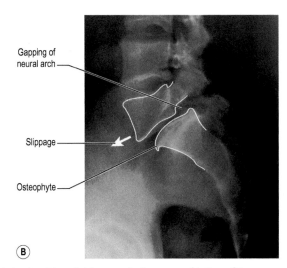

Gapping of neural arch

Slippage

Osteophyte

Slippage

Figure 8.32 Spondylolisthesis of L5 and S1. (A) Grade I defect with mild forward slippage of L5 on S1. (B) Grade III defect showing greater slippage, gapping of the neural arch and osteophyte formation. Reproduced from Magee, D.J. (2002) Orthopedic Physical Assessment, 4th edition, Saunders, Philadelphia.

involves a full diameter displacement. The major symptom is of back pain referred to the buttocks, which is aggravated by movement or exercise. Sciatica may be present as the condition can be associated with disc protrusion. The alteration in spinal alignment may present as dimpling of the skin and extra skin folds above the level of injury. A step deformity to the spinous process at the lower level is normally apparent to palpation. The lordosis may be increased, and severe spasm of the erector spinae may be present. Lumbar extension is often severely limited, and passive intervertebral pressure over the spinous process at the affected level is painful.

Figure 8.32 shows X-rays of spondylolisthesis. Figure 8.32A shows a Grade I defect with mild forward slippage of L5 on S1. Figure 8.32B shows a Grade III lesion with greater slippage, gapping of the neural arch and osteophyte formation on the vertebral body. To palpation, a step deformity may be apparent, with changes to skin folds in the area.

Management of spondylogenic disorders

Treatment aims mainly to eliminate the symptoms of the condition rather than to obtain bony union.

Initially, rest is required. This varies from 'active rest', by avoiding painful movements, with mild conditions, to total bed rest, with very severe lesions. Occasionally, braces and casts are used to protect the spine until the acute pain subsides, but the most important component of management is closely supervised exercise therapy. Thorough functional assessment is carried out to investigate strength and flexibility. In addition to absolute values in comparison to norms for a particular athlete population, muscle imbalance is important. Transmission of ground forces to the spine is governed to a large extent by hip and spine musculature, and weakness or asymmetry here must be corrected. Anterior shear forces are compensated by an extension moment created by the abdominal muscles (especially the internal obliques and transversus) and the latissimus dorsi pulling on the thoracolumbar fascia. In addition, the paraspinals counteract shear forces in the lumbar spine (Farfan, Osteria and Lamy 1976).

Correction of muscle imbalance which results from asymmetry in sport is important in the management of this condition. For example, in cricket, fast bowlers have a high incidence of lumbar spondylolysis (1.65/1000 balls bowled) (Gregory, Batt and Wallace 2002). Forces through the front leg may be up to nine times bodyweight vertically and two times bodyweight horizontally, and this may be repeated for up to 10 overs, each of 6 balls (Becker 2006). Asymmetry of the quadratus lumborum (QL), an important stabilizing muscle, has been shown in bowlers, with the QL being larger on the ipsilateral side to the bowling arm. This correlates with injury, where 80 per cent of unilateral spondylolyses have been shown to occur on the contralateral side to the bowling arm, perhaps reflecting poor stability due to a weaker QL (Becker 2006).

The use of a stability programme based on motor control has been shown to be effective in the management of this disorder (O'Sullivan et al. 1997). A ten-week specific stability programme was shown to be more effective than conventional exercise programmes involving gym work, sit-ups and swimming using measures of pain intensity, pain description and functional ability. In addition, the benefits of specific stabilization training were maintained at a 30-month follow-up.

Rehabilitation for lower back pain

There are many approaches to the conservative treatment of non-specific lower back pain (NSLBP), and the variation in approaches is important for both patient choice and patient specificity. However, current evidence shows that while exercise is effective for the management of NSLBP, one exercise approach is no better than another (Smith, Littlewood and May 2014). Short-term benefits of stability training over general exercise are not maintained in the long term (Wang et al. 2012), and stabilization exercise is no more effective than manual therapy (Gomes-Neto et al. 2017). The 2016 NICE guidelines for the treatment of lower back pain recommend exercise, but no one type over another, and the European guidelines (2006) recommend supervised exercise with adjunctive therapies such as manipulation to be considered in the short term, but electrotherapy is not recommended. The Cochrane database review for motor control exercise in the management of NSLBP recommends exercise, with the choice of exercise to depend on patient or therapist preferences, training, costs and safety (Saragiotto et al. 2015).

Spinal stability

Evaluation

When the lumbar spine demonstrates instability, there is an alteration of both the quality and quantity of movement available within a vertebral segment. The unstable segment shows decreased stiffness (resistance to bending) and as a consequence movement is increased even under minor loads. Clinical assessment may reveal a number of classical physical signs, as outlined in Table 8.8.

Further examination is required to determine the level of loss of motion control, and tests

Table 8.8 Evaluating lumbar instability

Classical physical signs	Evaluation based on movement dysfunction
Step deformity	Younger age (<40 years)
Muscle spasm (transverse band) which reduces on lying	Greater general flexibility (SLR >90°)
Juddering/shaking on forward bend	Aberrant movement raising from a flexed position
Excessive sagittal motion to passive intervertebral motion testing	Positive prone instability test
	Positive P4 test post partum
	Positive ASLR post partum
	Failure to maintain lumbar alignment measured on PBU

Paris (1985), Maitland (1986), Fritz et al (2007); reprinted from Norris (2008).

ASLR—active straight leg raise; PBU—pressure biofeedback unit; P4 – posterior pelvic pain provocation.

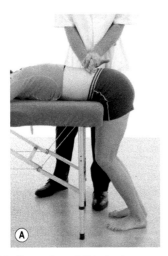
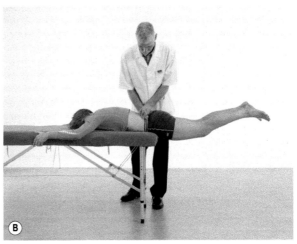

Figure 8.33 Prone instability test.

focus on the reduction of symptoms when the spine is actively stabilized. The ability to maintain a set posture (typically a neutral position, see below) is only relevant where it is considered a driver of the patient's symptoms. Symptom reduction may be assessed using the *prone instability test*, while neutral position maintenance is traditionally assessed using *pressure biofeedback*. Where the patient has recently had a child (post-partum), the posterior pelvic pain provocation (P4) test and active straight-leg raise (ASLR) may also be used to assess instability of the lumbo-pelvic region in general (see above).

For the prone instability test (Fig. 8.33A, B) the patient lies prone, with their chest supported on a treatment couch and legs resting on the floor. The patient's pain is provoked using a posteroanterior (PA) pressure upon the spinous processes of the lumbar spine. They are then asked to lift the legs clear off the ground, and the test is positive if the muscle work of this action (hip extensors and spinal extensors) reduces their lumbar pain. The pressure biofeedback test is described below.

General principles

To maintain spinal stability, three interrelated systems have been proposed (Fig. 8.34). Passive

support is provided by inert (non-contractile) tissues, while active support is from contractile tissues. Sensory feedback from both systems provides coordination via the neural control centres (Panjabi 1992). Importantly, where the stability provided by one system reduces, the other systems may compensate. Thus, the

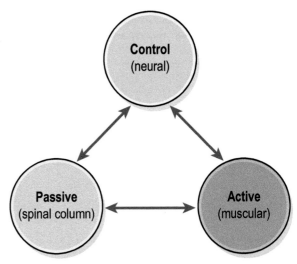

Figure 8.34 The spinal stabilizing system consists of three interrelating subsystems. From Panjabi, M.M. (1992) The stabilizing system of the spine. Part 1. Function, dysfunction, adaptation and enhancement. *Journal of Spinal Disorders*, 5(4), 383–389. With permission.

proportion of load taken by the active system may increase to minimize stress on the passive system through load-sharing. When this happens, we can view stability as a continuously varying process (Bergmark 1989). This process is dynamic and quite different to the traditional view of clinical stability being a static mechanical state (stable or unstable).

opportunity to reduce pain and improve function by rehabilitating active or functional lumbar stabilization. Such improvement may be accomplished by augmenting both the active and neural control systems. Simply developing muscle strength in isolation may be insufficient in some cases.

Key point

Instability of the lumbar spine occurs when there is a decreased stiffness (resistance to bending) of a spinal segment. As a result, excessive movement occurs, even under minor loads.

The concept of a dynamic interrelating system gives the physiotherapist the

Trunk muscle changes in subjects with non-specific lower back pain have traditionally focused on key stabilizing muscles of the spine (Treatment Note 8.2), but this area is less popular as research has indicated that effect sizes are small, the techniques are often difficult for subjects to perform, and the results are similar to those obtained with general exercise (see below).

Treatment note 8.2   Trunk muscle changes in lower back pain

Multifidus

The cross-sectional area (CSA) of the multifidus has been shown to be substantially reduced at the level of lumbar lesion (Hides et al. 1994). The authors suggested that the mechanism for the CSA reduction was inhibition through perceived pain via a long loop reflex. In addition to changes in muscle bulk, alteration in fibre type has been shown in the multifidus in patients with lower back pain (LBP) (Biedermann et al. 1991). A reduced ratio of slow twitch to fast twitch muscle fibres was shown, possibly as an adaptive response by the muscle to changes in functional demand placed upon it. Furthermore, injury may have caused a shift in the recruitment patterns of the motor units of the paraspinal muscles, with the fast-twitch motor units being recruited before the slow-twitch units.

Posture has also been shown to affect the multifidus. Prolonged flexion activities initially result in a reflex spasm of the multifidus, which reduces substantially if the posture is maintained. Williams et al. (2000) used a cat model to investigate sustained moderate flexion

stress on seven preparations. They showed a reduction to 5 per cent of this initial value within 3 minutes of taking up the posture, leading to tissue laxity and a loss of reflex protective muscle activity. Prolonged flexion (20 minutes, using cat preparation) has also been shown to result in multifidus spasm (Jackson et al. 2001), with full recovery not seen for 7 hours after initiation of rest.

Injection of hypertonic saline (a chemical irritant that has an effect similar to swelling) into the multifidus has shown that the muscle can be a source of both local and referred pain (Cornwall, John-Harris and Mercer 2006).

Assessing cross-sectional area (CSA) and muscle-fat infiltration index (MFI) to differentiate between muscle size and intramuscular fat composition, Sions et al. (2017) showed multifidus muscle composition, but not size, to be related to subjects with CLBP. Corticomotor control of the lumbar multifidus has been shown to change in subjects with chronic lower back pain (CLBP) using ultrasound imaging and transcranial magnetic stimulation, demonstrating plasticity of

401

Treatment note 8.2 *continued*

cortical maps controlling the paraspinal muscles (Massé-Alarie et al. 2016).

Although retraining of the muscle may be through isolated contraction initially, successful rehabilitation involves use of the muscle during gross movement (Danneels, Vanderstraeten and Cambier 2003). Changes to the multifidus may not necessarily relate to symptoms. In a systematic review of 15 papers, Wong et al. (2014) showed that temporal changes in multifidus and transversus abdominis morphology or activation were not associated with clinical improvement.

Transversus abdominis

The transversus abdominis shows a similar response in the chronic LBP patient. It is active in both flexion and extension of the lumbar spine (Cresswell, Grundstrom and Thorstensson 1992) and during action of the upper limb and lower limb in multiple directions (Hodges, Richardson and Jull 1996). In addition, contraction of transversus abdominis precedes that of the other abdominal and lumbar extensor muscles (Cresswell, Oddsson and Thorstensson 1994, Hodges, Richardson and Jull 1996). Its primary function would seem to be to contract in response to forces applied to the trunk. In this way, it is anticipating the requirement of stability and providing it.

Following LBP, transversus abdominis function changes (Hodges, Richardson and Jull 1996). Timing of onset of transversus contraction is delayed by a mean of 129 ms, while the action of the other abdominals is largely unchanged. When assessed in a hollowing action, the transversus muscle shows a smaller increase in thickness measured by real-time ultrasound (between rest and contraction) in patients with lower back pain than in normal subjects. Normal subjects showed a mean thickness increase of 49.7 per cent while lower-back patients showed mean values of 19.15 per cent (Critchley and Coutts 2002). Re-education of transversus contraction can be an important

component in lower back pain rehabilitation, but reliance on muscle isolation has been shown to be ineffective when compared to more general back stability programmes (see above).

References

Biedermann, H.J., Shanks, G.L., Forrest, W.J., Inglis, J., 1991. Power spectrum analyses of electromyographic activity. *Spine* **16** (10), 1179–1184.

Cornwall J., John-Harris A., Mercer S.R., 2006. The lumbar multifidus muscle and patterns of pain. *Manual Therapy* **11**, 40–45.

Cresswell, A.G., Grundstrom, H., Thorstensson, A., 1992. Observations on intra-abdominal pressure and patterns of abdominal intra-muscular activity in man. *Acta Physiologica Scandinavica* **144** (4), 409–418.

Cresswell, A.G., Oddsson, L., Thorstensson, A., 1994. The influence of sudden perturbations on trunk muscle activity and intra abdominal pressure while standing. *Experimental Brain Research* **98**, 336–341.

Critchley, D.J., Coutts, F.J., 2002. Abdominal muscle function in chronic lower back pain patients. *Physiotherapy* **88** (6), 322–332.

Danneels L., Vanderstraeten G., Cambier D., 2003. Effects of three different training modalities on the cross-sectional area of the lumbar multifidus in patients with chronic lower back pain. *British Journal of Sports Medicine* **37** (1), 91.

Hides, J.A., Stokes, M.J., Saide, M., et al. 1994. Evidence of lumbar multifidus muscle wasting ipsilateral to symptoms in patients with acute/subacute lower back pain. *Spine* **19** (2), 165–172.

Hodges, P., Richardson, C., Jull, G., 1996. Evaluation of the relationship between laboratory and clinical tests of transversus abdominis function. *Physiotherapy Research International* **1** (1), 30–40.

Jackson, M., Solomonow, M., Zhou, B., et al. 2001. Multifidus EMG and tension-relaxation recovery after prolonged static lumbar flexion. *Spine* **26** (7), 715–723.

Treatment note 8.2 *continued*

Massé-Alarie, H Beaulieu, L., Preuss D et al. (2016) Influence of chronic lower back pain and fear of movement on the activation of the transversely oriented abdominal muscles during forward bending. *Journal of Electromyography and Kinesiology*, **27**, 87–94.

Sions, J. M. et al. 2017. "Multifidus muscle characteristics and physical function among older adults with and without chronic lower back pain. *Archives of Physical Medicine and Rehabilitation* **98** (1), 51–57.

Williams, M., Solomonow, M., Zhou, B.H., Baratta, R.V., Harris, M., 2000. Multifidus spasms elicited by prolonged lumbar flexion. *Spine* **25** (22), 2916–2924.

Wong, A.Y., Parent, E.C., Funabashi, M. et al. 2014. Do changes in transversus abdominis and lumbar multifidus during conservative treatment explain changes in clinical outcomes related to nonspecific lower back pain? A systematic review. *J Pain.* **15** (4), 377.e1–35.

Sensorimotor rehabilitation

Sensorimotor control involves elements of both the sensory and motor systems. Pain and/or injury may be both a cause of changes to sensorimotor control or a consequence of it. Hodges and Falla (2015) give a succinct explanation of the key principles involved in sensorimotor control, and the implications that these have for sensorimotor rehabilitation of functional movement (Table 8.9)

Key point

Changes in sensorimotor control may be a cause or consequence of pain and/or injury.

Movements involve aspects which are both *postural* in nature and *task*-related, and the

emphasis based on each of these two components will vary with the task being performed. In a throwing action, for example, the arm will move rapidly, but requires a stable base upon which to act. The ballistic action of the shoulder muscles requires a 'postural set' in the scapula and thorax to provide its foundation. Clinically, impingement pain can occur as a result of changes in either of these body regions, with supraspinatus tendinopathy associated with alterations in scapula-thoracic stability. In addition, there is no firm distinction between these two elements, with muscles often performing a task or postural function at different times.

Task actions may require motion (*movement*), while postural actions often require stability or lack of motion (*stiffness*). The ratio of movement to stiffness varies between tasks. Muscles acting on the lumbar spine, for example, will need to increase stiffness when performing a heavy deadlift action but increase mobility during running and jumping. Equally, when landing from a jump, the lower-limb muscles must act to absorb shock. If they stiffen the limb, the rigidity introduced may make injury more likely,

The interaction between active (contractile), passive (non-contractile) and control (neural) elements (see above) is important for the control of both movement and stiffness, and changes to any one element will have consequent effects on the others. Alteration in joint stiffness following injury

Table 8.9 Key principles of sensorimotor control

- ▶ Functional movement involves *task*- and *posture*-related components
- ▶ Function requires a balance between *movement* and *stiffness*
- ▶ Function requires a balance between *passive*, *active* and *control* systems
- ▶ Motor control is inherently *variable*
- ▶ *Multiple sources* of sensory information are available
- ▶ Sensorimotor control *varies between individuals*

(Data from Hodges and Falla 2015)

can be compensated by motor changes. A common example is lack of dorsiflexion range (stiffness) following an ankle injury changing gait to allow a subject to roll over the medial border of their foot (motor control). With time, this motor change, if it becomes habitual, may lead to excessive stress on the medial aspect of the knee with stress and pain building in the non-contractile elements within this region.

The variability of motor control means that there are an infinite number of ways to perform a task. Variety in this case shares load between structures and may prevent overuse. Changes to this variability may lead to pain, however. Where variability is reduced, the same tissues are placed under load and overuse may occur. Equally, excessive variability may lead to a reduction in control and less effective methods of performing a task.

Sensory information is available from multiple sources, and the interaction between these can lead to compensation. Swelling may mask joint proprioception, for example, which may be compensated by using a neoprene knee sleeve to increase feedback from the skin as a consequence from movement.

Finally, and in many ways most importantly, motor control is variable between individuals, so there are no correct or incorrect methods of achieving a movement goal. The movement selected will depend not just on a subject's structure (anatomy) but on their experience and psychosocial influences.

> **Key point**
>
> Variability and individuality are essential parts of movement

Motor control training for lower back pain

The use of sensorimotor training in some form for the rehabilitation of the lumbar spine has formed part of therapy for many years. In the 1990s this came to the fore with approaches which built on

Table 8.10 The role of motor control training in the rehabilitation of the Lumbar spine

▶ The manner in which a subject moves, maintains posture / alignment or activates muscle is relevant to the patient's pain presentation
▶ Both peripheral and central elements are involves in this presentation
▶ Tissue loading related to the way in which a subject uses their body
▶ Assessment of movement can identify suboptimal strategies
▶ Sensorimotor rehabilitation used to modify loading to affect subject's symptoms
▶ Movement modification may have positive effects on pain experience even in the absence of peripheral nociceptive input.

(Data from Hodges 2015)

the work of Vladamir Janda (Janda and Schmid 1980) and the concept of muscle imbalance and movement dysfunction. Work by a number of clinicians and researchers focused initially on identification and retraining of dysfunction to 'core stabilizing' muscles of the trunk, especially lumbar multifidus and transversus abdominis. As research developed, the approach has progressed and been modified, and Hodges (2015) summarized the current situation with respect to the use of motor control training for lumbar rehabilitation (Table 8.10).

Motor control training involves an assessment of alignment, movement and muscle activation, and uses a clinical reasoning approach to determine if any or all of these elements relates to the subject's presentation. The term 'control' is often taken to imply the clinical need to reduce or restrict movement, and the original description of 'spinal stabilization' or 'core stability' perhaps reflects this. However, control may be excessive, deficient or irrelevant to symptoms, so assessment throughout treatment is vital to make treatment patient-specific. The aim of sensorimotor training is to optimize control by finding a balance between movement and stiffness required for optimal subject function. Additionally, sensorimotor rehabilitation must be viewed within the context of a biopsychosocial approach to healthcare which recognizes that psychosocial drivers affect motor control. Beliefs and attitudes such as hypervigilance, fragility and catastrophizing (see Chapter 1), together with anxiety and depression, impact a subject's clinical condition and response to treatment. Movement and/or exercise can be strong influencers on psychosocial traits, independent of peripheral effects.

> **Key point**
> Psychosocial factors are important influencers of motor control.

The sensorimotor rehabilitation process focuses on three key features: muscle morphology and behaviour, movement and sensory function (Hodges 2015), which must be individualized to each subject. Progression through the rehabilitation process builds from static to dynamic control and then to functional re-education (Norris 1995), and an integrated approach has been recommended (Norris 2000, Norris 2008, Norris and Mathews 2008).

Developing active lumbar stability

The original approach to lumbar stabilization was to focus on muscle isolation. However, this approach has been shown in many cases not to be effective (Koumantakis et al. 2005) leading to the development of an integrated approach (Norris 2008, Norris and Mathews 2008), which draws on evidence from several sources. The integrated back stability approach is used in three overlapping phases (Fig. 8.35). During Phase I, *movement dysfunction* is addressed, prior to building *back fitness* in Phase II. The final phase is *functional restoration*.

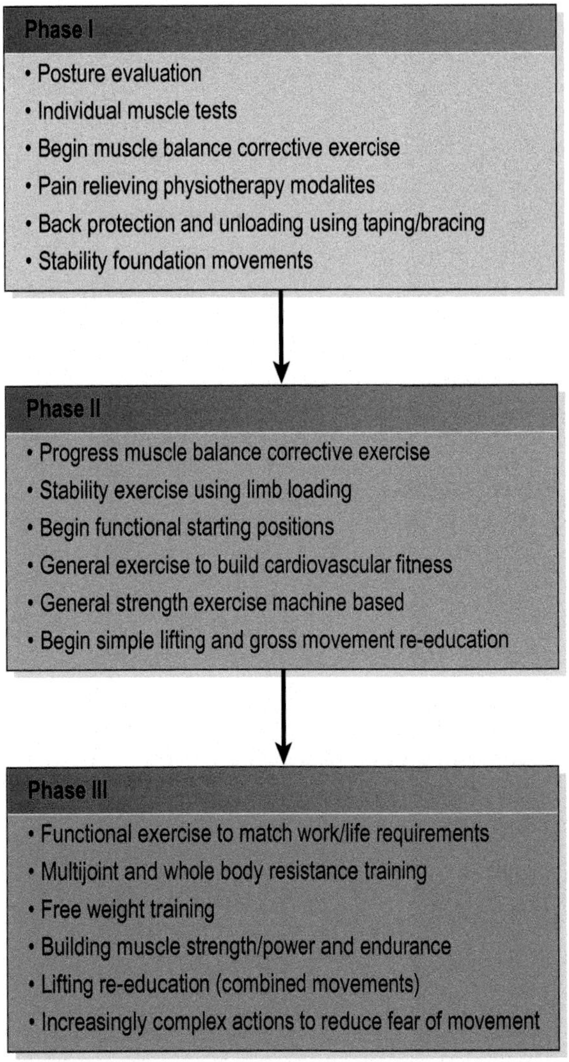

Phase I

Phase I initially focuses on pain relief, using patient education, manual therapy and physiotherapy modalities if required. This is because patients will find it difficult to perform exercise in the presence of pain inhibition. Posture evaluation and muscle-balance tests are used to determine exercises

Phase I
- Posture evaluation
- Individual muscle tests
- Begin muscle balance corrective exercise
- Pain relieving physiotherapy modalites
- Back protection and unloading using taping/bracing
- Stability foundation movements

Phase II
- Progress muscle balance corrective exercise
- Stability exercise using limb loading
- Begin functional starting positions
- General exercise to build cardiovascular fitness
- General strength exercise machine based
- Begin simple lifting and gross movement re-education

Phase III
- Functional exercise to match work/life requirements
- Multijoint and whole body resistance training
- Free weight training
- Building muscle strength/power and endurance
- Lifting re-education (combined movements)
- Increasingly complex actions to reduce fear of movement

Figure 8.35 Norris, C.M and Matthew, M. (2008) The role of an integrated back stability program in patients with chronic low back pain. *Complementary Therapies in Clinical Practice*, **14**, 255–263.

which target postural changes only if these are relative to the patient's symptoms. For example, where a patient has a flat back (reduced lordosis), lumbar extension is used if it modifies symptoms, and for a patient with a more hollow back, lumbar flexion is the exercise of choice. At this stage, management of muscle imbalance can be used if it alters symptoms (see Chapter 2). In the classic lordotic posture, for example, the iliopsoas muscle may be found to be tight. Where this limits the patient's ability to correct their lordotic posture and facet joint impaction is considered a potential source of pain, the iliopsoas may be stretched to enable the patient to posteriorly tilt their pelvis and disengage the lumbar facets. Importantly, postural work is used here to modify symptoms temporarily, so that the subject can progress to the next stage of rehabilitation, and not in an attempt to modify the patient's alignment towards an arbitrary ideal.

> **Key point**
> Postural modification is used only as a temporary means to modify a subject's symptoms.

Where traditional stability training is chosen, foundation movements are begun using isolation of the lumbar stabilizing muscles, with the aim of gaining voluntary control over these muscles. The muscles we target are the deep abdominals, the gluteals and the intersegmental muscles of the spine, especially multifidus. These muscles can function poorly after injury, and may be differently recruited as a result of intense training activities. When this happens, the mobilizer muscles of the lumbo-pelvic region (rectus abdominis, hip flexors and hamstrings) often dominate movements, with the stabilizers being poorly recruited. The focus of the classical back stability programme, therefore, is to reduce the dominance of the mobilizer muscles and enhance the function of the stabilizers, in so far as this modifies a subject's symptoms. This procedure is shown in Treatment Note 8.3.

Phase II

The second phase of the integrated stability programme is to build back fitness. Once the relatively stable base has been established in Phase I, movements of the arms and legs are superimposed. For example, following abdominal hollowing in crook lying, the next exercise progression would be the heel slide (Fig. 8.36A). Initially, the patient may perform the hollowing action, and while maintaining the neutral lumbar position, one leg is straightened, sliding the heel along the ground. The action of the hip flexors in this case tries to tilt the pelvis forwards (iliacus) and increase the lordosis (psoas). The abdominal muscles must work hard to stabilize the pelvis and lumbar spine against this pull. A number of other movements may be used, including the bent-knee fallout (Fig. 8.36B), which works for rotary stability, and bridging actions (Fig. 8.36C, D and E), which combine abdominal work with gluteal actions.

During Phase II, dynamic movements of the spine are also used. Now the aim is to maintain both static (neutral position) and dynamic (lumbo-pelvic rhythm) alignment. Actions such as the trunk curl and hip hinge are useful, as are more traditional lumbar exercises involving rotation. A variety of additional movements may be used, with the aim in each case of maintaining correct alignment of the spine through range and building holding capacity.

Side-support movements (Fig. 8.36F) work the quadratus lumborum and trunk side flexors, which are important stabilizers, in single-handed carrying tasks especially.

The emphasis on maintenance of neutral position and fixed alignment of the lumbar region is only continued while symptoms are present. As we have seen, overprotection builds hypervigilance, and increased muscle tone may be associated with poorer outcome. As symptoms subside, movement is reintroduced, with the aim of building resilience to this body region in Phase III.

In Phase II, general cardiovascular (CV) fitness is also built up and general strength exercises for the upper and lower limbs used. Strength in the limb muscles is vital for spinal health as the power of lifting should come from the legs rather than the spine. Upper limb strength is used for object positioning during manual handling and to bring the object close to the body to reduce leverage effects imposed upon the spine.

Treatment note 8.3 Stability training emphasizing muscle isolation

The process starts with abdominal hollowing, taught traditionally in a prone kneeling position with the spine in its neutral (mid-range) position (slight lordosis). As the transversus abdominis has horizontally aligned fibres, this action allows the abdominal muscles to sag, giving stretch facilitation. The patient focuses attention on the umbilicus and is instructed to pull the umbilicus 'in and up' while breathing normally. This action has been shown to dissociate activity in the internal obliques and transversus from that of the rectus abdominis (Richardson 1992), making the exercise especially useful for re-educating the stability where rectus abdominis has become dominant.

To facilitate learning, multisensory cueing is used (Miller and Medeiros 1987) to increase the sensory input to the patient. Auditory cues can be provided by the therapist speaking to the subject and giving feedback about performance. Visual cues are given by encouraging the subject to look at the muscles as they function, and by using a mirror. Kinaesthetic cueing is accomplished by encouraging the subject to 'feel' the particular action, for example, to 'feel the stomach being pulled in'. Tactile cues are provided by the therapist touching the subject's abdomen as muscle contraction begins.

The action is held for two seconds initially, building to five, ten and eventually thirty seconds, breathing normally. Although initially the action may demand high levels of muscle work to facilitate learning, the eventual aim is to use minimal muscle activity. A useful teaching point is to contract the abdominal muscles as hard as possible and then to relax by half (50 per cent MVC) and then half again (25 per cent MVC). The therapist should monitor the ribcage to ensure that it does not move substantially, and the feeling should be one of the umbilicus drawing inwards and slightly upwards rather than of bulging (doming) or spinal flexion.

Once this has been achieved, the holding capacity of these muscles is built up until the patient can maintain the contraction for ten repetitions, each held for ten seconds (Richardson 1992). Several other starting positions may be used (see Treatment Note 8.1) and the most suitable position is chosen for the particular patient being treated.

Several errors can occur when a patient practises abdominal hollowing. Essentially, the ribcage, shoulders and pelvis should remain still throughout the action. The contour of the abdomen will flatten if a deep breath is taken and held, but the therapist should see the chest expansion involved. Where this occurs, the patient is instructed to exhale and hold this chest position as the exercise is performed. Placing a belt around the lower chest is useful to give feedback about chest movement.

Another substitution action is to use the external oblique to brace the abdomen. However, these muscles will pull on the lower ribs and depress them at the same time, slightly flexing the thoracic spine. A horizontal skin crease is often visible across the upper abdomen. Where this occurs, the patient is encouraged to perform pelvic floor contraction at the same time as abdominal hollowing. Simultaneous contraction of the gluteus maximus must be avoided with this action, as this will teach an inappropriate motor pattern for trunk stability during dynamic sports activity.

Key point
When performing the abdominal hollowing action, monitor the patient's lower ribs. As the action is performed, the ribs should stay still and neither raise nor lower.

Use of pressure biofeedback
Restoration of the abdominal hollowing mechanism can also be enhanced by the use of pressure biofeedback. The biofeedback unit consists of a rubber bladder and pressure gauge similar to a sphygmomanometer.

Treatment note 8.3 *continued*

Prone lying

In prone lying, the pressure biofeedback unit is placed beneath the abdomen, with the lower edge of the bladder level with the anterior superior iliac spine, and the centre of the bladder over the umbilicus . The unit is inflated to 70 mmHg and abdominal hollowing is performed. The aim is to reduce the pressure reading on the biofeedback unit by 6–10 mmHg, and to be able to maintain this contraction to repetition (10 repetitions of 10-second hold) to ensure that endurance of the target muscles is adequate.

Crook lying

As a further test, a crook lying position is used. The bladder of the unit is placed beneath the subject's lumbar spine and inflated to show a constant figure of 40 mmHg. The subject is instructed to contract the abdominal muscles without performing a posterior pelvic tilt. If the lordosis is unchanged, a constant pressure is shown on the pressure unit. Increasing pressure shows flattening of the lordosis (lumbar flexion), while reducing pressure shows increased lordosis (lumbar extension). Excessive motion in either direction represents loss of lumbar stability. Alteration of starting position and the addition of simultaneous limb movement encourages body awareness and movement control.

Heel slide

The ability of the deep abdominals to maintain spinal stability may be accurately assessed using the heel slide manoeuvre. The subject starts in crook lying, with the spine in a neutral position and the pressure biofeedback unit positioned beneath the lower spine. One leg is then gradually straightened, sliding the heel along the ground to take the weight of the leg. During this action, the hip flexors are working eccentrically and pulling on the pelvis and lumbar spine. If the strong pull of these muscles is sufficient to displace the pelvis, the pelvic tilt is noticeable by palpation of the anterior superior iliac spine (ASIS) and by an alteration of the pressure biofeedback unit. The action must be completed without using the substitution actions described above.

Multifidus muscle retraining

Traditionally, measurement and enhancement of multifidus function is begun in prone lying. The fibres of multifidus are palpated medial to the longissimus at L4 and L5 levels. The spinous processes are identified, and the fingers then slide laterally into the hollow between the spinous process and the longissimus bulk. The difference in muscle consistency is assessed, and then the patient's ability to isometrically contract the multifidus in a 'setting' action is determined. The patient is encouraged to use multifidus setting in a sitting position with a neutral lumbar spine. Palpation is with the therapist's thumb and knuckle of the first finger placed on either side of the lumbar spinous process at any one level. The instruction to the patient is to 'feel the muscle swelling' without actively flexing the lumbar spine. The patient's own thumbs may be used to give feedback for home practice.

Although some patients will benefit from direct intervention targeted at the multifidus, changes in this muscle associated with CLBP have been shown to remain after symptom resolution (MacDonald et al. 2009). In addition, EMG studies of even elite athletes show lumbar muscle asymmetry (Roy et al. 1990), so its relevance to symptoms may be questioned. Further, general exercise on a labile base (stability ball) has been shown to effectively recruit lumbar multifidus, demonstrating that muscle isolation is not the only way to train this muscle (Scott, Vaughan and Hall 2015).

Key point

Exercising on a Swiss ball can enhance multifidus muscle action.

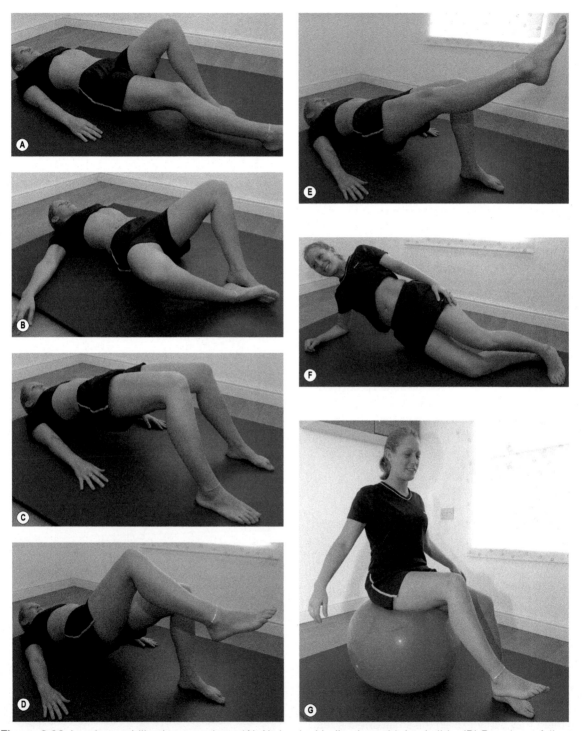

Figure 8.36 Lumbar stabilization exercises. (A) Abdominal hollowing with heel slide. (B) Bent knee fallout. (C) Bridging. (D) Single-leg bridge. (E) Single-leg bridge with leg straightening. (F) Side support. (G) Gym ball.

Phase III

When symptoms are subsiding and back fitness is enhanced, the subject is required to maintain or adopt the stable position only when it is required, relaxing at times when the spine is not under stress. For this to occur, muscle reaction time must be reduced through proprioceptive training in functional positions. The aim here is to move the spine out of alignment and impose stress upon it so that the stabilizing muscles react quickly to realign the spine and protect it from excessive stress, in a similar approach to that used for the ankle and knee.

More complex activities can now be used which draw the subject's attention away from the spine and into the environment. The aim now is to use proprioception to monitor the position and stability of the spine so that stability becomes more automatic and less attention-demanding.

More complex resistance training appropriate to individual sporting requirements may also be used (Fig. 8.37). The correct relationship between lumbar alignment and pelvic alignment is no longer rigorously maintained. A convex contour of the abdominal wall (doming or bow-stringing) suggests that the deep abdominals are failing to balance the action of rectus abdominis.

The speed and complexity of movements is increased and the subject is required to adopt lumbar positions which do not cause symptoms. The athlete's attention is fully taken up by focusing on the complexity of the exercise task (see information-processing bottleneck).

Cognitive functional therapy

Cognitive functional therapy (CFT) aims to apply a biopsychosocial model to the rehabilitation of lower back pain. Back pain is a multifactorial condition encompassing physical, lifestyle and psychological elements and limiting treatment to any one single element may partly explain the small effect sizes often seen in studies investigating back-pain interventions (Vibe Fersum et al. 2013).

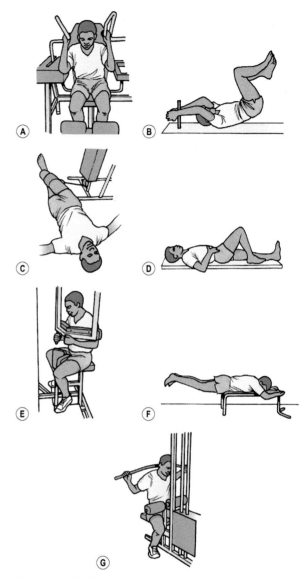

Figure 8.37 Examples of resistance exercises. Stage II (A) sitting abdominal curl, (B) reverse crunch, (C) lying cable trunk rotation, (D) heel slide, (E) sitting trunk rotation, (F) prone leg extension, (G) lateral pull-down. From Norris, C.M. (2008) *Back Stability*. Human Kinetics, Champaign, Illinois. With permission.

Pain and disability are often related to behaviours which are modifiable, and have been described in six domains, shown in Table 8.11 (O'Keeffe et al. 2015, O'Sullivan 2017).

Table 8.11 Interacting factors in CLBP

Physical	Cognitive	Psychological	Lifestyle	Social	Co-morbidities
Maladaptive posture & movement patterns	Beliefs	Fear	Inactivity	Socioeconomic status	Obesity
Pain behaviour	Catastrophizing	Anxiety	Sleep disturbance	Family	Chronic fatigue
Deconditioning	Hypervigilance,	Depression	Life stress	Work	Irritable bowel syndrome
	Self-efficiency			Culture	Inflammatory disorders
	Coping strategies				Peripheral sensitization

Data from O'Keefe et al 2015, O'Sullivan 2017

In addition, targeting therapy to a subject's individual needs would appear more appropriate than applying a blanket treatment approach, using standard exercises, for example, and several classification systems are available to do this. In the case of CFS, the classification system is multidimensional and uses patient examination (subjective and objective) within the four components of treatment used in the approach, shown in Figure 8.38.

Greater emphasis is placed on the cognitive component of CFT, where yellow flags (psychosocial factors) have been identified in subjects during subjective examination. Neuroscience education (Treatment Note 8.4) is used to explain negative beliefs such as fear of movement, mood state and protective behaviours. Functional movement exercises can be used to develop alternative strategies to normalize posture based on movement classification, which encompasses impairment of *movement* or impairment of *control* around the lumbo-pelvic and/or thoraco-lumbar regions (O'Sullivan 2005). Movement impairment focuses on peripheral pain sensitization, where pain is of rapid onset and increased by a movement in a defined direction (flexion, extension, rotation or lateral shift) or central pain sensitization, where fear avoidance or hypervigilance limits motion. Control impairment is again assessed in relation to both peripheral and central pain sensitization, and each is direction-specific, as before. Pain will be of gradual onset now, with a lack of awareness of pain triggers (peripheral), or limited by beliefs or behaviours (central). In each case, a graded exposure model is used, making the subject aware of negative

Cognitive functional therapy (CFT)

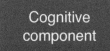

Figure 8.38 Components of cognitive functional therapy programme (Data from Vibe Fersum et al. 2013).

strategies such as muscle guarding or breath holding.

Movements from Stage 2 are integrated into functions applicable to the subject's daily living to increase body awareness, reduce avoidance and lessen fear of movement. In Stage 4, general exercise such as walking is used to increase the level of exercise tolerance. This may be augmented by actions from Stage 2 relevant to the subject's daily living – for example, bending, lifting, twisting.

Identifying modifiable influences

During subject assessment, modifiable influences on persistent back pain may be identified in six interrelating domains (Table 8.11). Within the *physical* domain are items such as alteration to movement patterns, maladaptive postures and general deconditioning. *Cognitive* factors include beliefs which the subject has about their condition, which have led to catastrophizing, hypervigilance

Treatment note 8.4 Neuroscience education in lower back rehabilitation

Patient education aims to improve treatment outcomes by encouraging a more active partnership between therapist and patient in the management of a health condition. In the management of lower back pain, educational approaches in three main categories have been used (McAuley 2015).

(i) Biomedical education focuses on biomechanical factors such as ergonomics and postural advice, which were typical of back school approaches in the 1970s.

(ii) Biopsychosocial (BPS) approaches focus on the interaction of biological, psychological and social factors. Biological factors include nociceptive activation and tissues changes, while psychological factors relate to beliefs/knowledge and psychological states and traits (anxiety, depression, stress). Social factors encompass subject interactions with others, both as individuals and within society as a whole (friends and family, work colleagues, cultural influences).

(iii) Neurophysiological approaches aim to reconceptualize a patient's understanding of pain by focusing on several key concepts, outlined below.

An explanation that pain is a normal sensation, and does not necessarily indicate harm within the body, can help. Rather than seeing pain as an indicator of tissue damage, with more pain implying greater damage, pain can be seen as the body's alarm system to threat or danger. Using examples from exercise may be helpful. When an individual lifts a weight in the gym, they may feel a burn in their muscles. This is interpreted as positive (I am working hard) rather than negative (I am injuring myself) because of the context. The same sensation (nociception) could be interpreted negatively in the presence of a worrying X-ray or scan, for example.

Because each person will have their own opinion of what is and is not a threat to them, past experiences can influence the perception of pain greatly. Where a person has had a history of back pain, any new pain may create images (often exaggerated) of their previous suffering. Realizing that the pain may be an entirely separate episode, and will usually clear up quickly within a normal timescale, can reduce the threat of the sensation and therefore the perception of pain. This resolution of symptoms is important, as back pain typically produces fragility, with subjects believing that their back is delicate and likely to

Table 8.12 Pain concepts

Concept	Description
Pain is normal	Pain is the body's warning system.
Pain is not directly related to tissue damage	Pain implies threat, not damage. Hurt does not mean harm.
Pain depends on perceived threat or danger	Past experience will colour how a threat is viewed.
Pain involves many brain areas at the same time	Several areas of the brain are involved (neuromatrix), including sensory, emotional and memory.
Pain relies on context	Pain can be influenced by things we hear, do and believe.
Pain is one of several protective outputs	Pain is often accompanied by immune system, autonomic, emotional and respiratory changes (fight or flight).
Body systems can change	All the body's protective systems can be increased or reduced and are trainable.
Active treatment strategies promote recovery	Pain can be controlled by seeking things which make you feel safe and avoiding things which make you feel threatened.

(Mosely and Butler 2017, Davies 2017)

Treatment note 8.4 *continued*

fail and so needs to be protected. One of the functions of neuroscience education is to dispel the myth of the spine being an 'at risk' body part and encourage subjects to view their spine as strong and resilient.

Pain is only one of several protective systems available to the body, and making subjects aware of different and equivalent mechanisms can be helpful. Noticing changes in breathing rate, heart rate, the immune system and emotional changes (anxiety and fear) associated with the fight or flight mechanism can help to put pain into perspective. Importantly, many of these changes are outside conscious control, providing the opportunity to teach subjects about conscious and unconscious mechanisms. Relaxing breathing and encouraging diaphragmatic breathing can reduce sympathetic drive, relax muscle and reduce pain. Linking conscious ('I can chose') to unconscious ('It controls me') thought can help to give subjects back control of their clinical condition.

Encouraging subjects to see pain as part of a physiological process within the body, and one which can change, is important. Change indicates the possibility of reducing pain and suffering

using a user-controlled form of training. Active strategies such as exercise, relaxation, pacing and seeking actions which reduce threat level can all be helpful and increase self-efficacy.

Systematic reviews of educational approaches have produced conflicting results, and in general shown only small effect sizes. However, neuroscience education has been found to decrease pain catastrophizing (*My pain has a serious cause*), fear-avoidance beliefs (*Rest when it hurts*), and self-efficacy beliefs (the confidence to perform a task) and these beliefs have in general been associated with poor outcomes in lower back treatment (McAuley 2015), so using an educational approach which aims to modify them would seem appropriate.

References

Moseley, G.L. and Butler, D.S. (2017) *Explain Pain Supercharged*. Noigroup Publications. Australia.

Davies, B. (2017) *Explain Pain*. Derby Royal Hospital. Noigroup. Lecture notes.

McAuley, J. (2015) Educational approaches to pain management. In Jull, G., Moore, A., Falla, D. et al. *Grieve's Modern Musculoskeletal Physiotherapy*. 4th edition. Elsevier.

and poor self-efficacy. Thoughts that pain relates to tissue condition (*hurt equals harm*), the back is naturally fragile, something has 'slipped out', that discs are 'worn', will all limit recovery and must be addressed. *Psychological* influences include *emotional* responses, such as fear, anxiety and depression, and these may drive associated *lifestyle* changes, such as sleep disorders and chronic stress responses. The *social* domain reflects influences from work and home/family especially, and this may be either positive (support) or negative (judgemental). Finally, *co-morbidities* may be important, with some (such as obesity) influencing back pain and being modifiable, and others (such as chronic fatigue, irritable bowel

syndrome) being related to back pain but less directly modifiable.

Functional training of the lower back

The term functional training (FT) is often used in both popular sports culture and rehabilitation. Functional training aims to use exercises which mimic as closely as possible day-to-day activities (Norris 2015), and in so doing often has similarities to the sensorimotor approach highlighted above, and may be used alongside neuroscience-based education (Treatment Note 8.4). FT usually contrasts sharply with traditional gym-based exercise, which frequently uses movements which exist in the gym alone. In general, functional movements are whole-body actions involving several joints and muscle groups at the same time. Because of this, the amount of coordination and skill required is much higher. If we take as an example a leg-extension movement, using a machine in the gym involves starting in a sitting position with the shin pressed against a pad. The action is to extend the knee to work the quadriceps muscles in isolation. For rehabilitation, this movement has value following injury, where the quadriceps muscles are working poorly and isolating them can help ensure recruitment. However, in a healthy uninjured individual, training on a leg-extension machine alone strengthens muscle without rehearsing normal movements. For this reason, we can categorize the leg extension machine as a *non-functional* action. In contrast, a step-up exercise involves movement at the ankle, knee, hip and lower spine. The quadriceps muscles are still used, as with the leg extension, but now the stepping action is one used daily when climbing the stairs. In addition, the quadriceps muscles are working in tandem with the hip extensors, calf muscles and upper body. Because this action mimics a day-to-day movement, the exercise can be categorized as a *functional* movement.

> **Key point**
> Functional training mimics day-to-day action, and typically involves whole-body movements.

Functional movements can be both open and closed kinetic chain (see Kinetic Chain Exercise, Chapter 1). In an *open-chain* action, the end of the limb moves freely in space, the proximal end of the limb is fixed, while the distal end moves. This type of action is used in rapid movement, such as throwing or the forward limb movement of running. A *closed-chain* action occurs when both ends of the limb are fixed, the proximal end by the body and the distal end by an object or surface, for example

a squat or step-up action. Open-chain actions are generally faster, involving ballistic actions, the joints of the moving limb are free to move, and mobility is emphasized. Closed-chain movements are slower and the joint surfaces are under compressive load, emphasizing stability.

The complexity of an exercise is important for coordination during functional actions. A simpler exercise should be used initially as it is easier to understand, control and correct. Gradually, as confidence is gained, more complex actions are used. Where a movement is complex, it can be divided into several component movements. Each individual movement can be practised and mastered and then the components put together. This type of training is called *part-task*, and is a useful method for rehabilitation where individuals may not be skilled in movement production. However, it has a disadvantage because sometimes putting the components together does not result in a smooth single action. Another method of learning a complex action is *whole-task* training. Here, the complex action is used and the subject and therapist accept that initially the performance of the action will be poor. Gradually, the action improves as parts which are incorrect are removed. The analogy here is of creating a statue. Part-task training would build it from blocks or bricks one at a time, while whole-task training would begin with a solid block of stone and chip away, as with a sculpture, to reveal the whole statue.

> **Definition**
> In functional training, *part-task* training divides a movement up into a number of components, while *whole-task* training performs the action as a single movement.

We have seen (in Chapter 2) that following overload a muscle will adapt over time. The adaptation caused closely mimics the overload which is used, a process represented by the SAID mnemonic (Specific Adaptation to Imposed Demand). The change within the body (adaptation) will closely match, or be specific to, the overload placed upon the body tissues (imposed demand). Functional training is designed to match the action required by an athlete in sports or a subject in daily living. In many ways, functional training is one of the oldest forms of training available and the one which was used widely prior to the development of more specialist exercise equipment. Many field athletic events, such as the javelin and discus, for example, have their roots in the use of weaponry, while others evolved from fighting and involved pulling, pushing, reaching and striking. Actions involving running and jumping are natural to our existence on the land and are simply extensions of fundamental gait patterns. Rather than using complex machines, we can achieve a good functional training workout using items which were commonplace in our pre-computer-age society and choosing whole-body actions. Examples of movement and equipment types are shown in Table 8.13.

Table 8.13 Functional training exercise

Exercise types	Example equipment
▶ Lift	▶ Dumb-bell & barbell
▶ Push & pull	▶ Kettlebell
▶ Reach	▶ Medicine ball/sand bag
▶ Squat & lunge	▶ Stability ball
▶ Moving & carrying	▶ Wobble or rocker board
▶ Twist	▶ Foam roller
▶ Strike	▶ Slide trainer
▶ Locomotion (walk/run/stairs)	▶ High bar/suspension frame
	▶ Agility ladder & hurdles
	▶ Rope/chain
	▶ Pulley
	▶ Resistance band
	▶ Weighted vest
	▶ Object (tyre/box)
	▶ Tools (hammer, shovel)
	▶ Trampette/vibration platform

(Data from Norris 2015)

Treatment note 8.5 Neuroscience approach to treating CLBP

We saw in Chapter 2 that pain has both peripheral (tissues) and central (brain) elements, and to be effective treatment must be targeted at both areas. The use of a neuroscience approach to the management of CLBP, which combined neuroscience education (see Treatment Note 8.4) with motor control training, has been described by Nijs et al. (2014). The initial management requires early neuroscience education/communication to explain any imaging findings and to confirm that these may not be related to symptoms. The process of hypervigilance is highlighted and the concept of pain reconceptualized. The inconsistent relationship between pain and tissue change is emphasized, with vocabulary such as 'hurt and harm' and 'sore but safe' being used.

▶ Exercise is given using a time-contingent rather than symptom-contingent approach. With a time-contingent approach the action is continued for a set time or number of repetitions, while a symptom-contingent approach is stopped when pain occurs. We have seen (Chapter 2) that pain can be viewed as a warning signal or alarm system. Hypervigilance is the process by which the brain overreacts to an action, providing a warning signal (pain) when it is not required (allodynia or hypersensitivity). Symptom-contingent approaches may facilitate hypervigilance, while time-contingent approaches deactivate top-down pain facilitation and reduce hyperexcitability.

▶ The second phase of the programme is to use sensorimotor/motor-control training which is progressive. Each exercise is again performed in a time-contingent fashion, and where fear-avoidance beliefs are encountered motor imagery may help. Time is taken to discuss the subject's beliefs about the outcome of an exercise prior to its practice. For example,

415

Treatment note 8.4 *continued*

does the subject believe that performing an exercise may make their condition worse, increase their pain, or damage their spine? These beliefs are challenged using pre-exercise communication.

▶ The third phase of the approach is to incorporate dynamic and functional exercises which mimic the functional requirement the subject has in daily living. The exercises are progressed and targeted at movements which the subject is fearful of, for example forward bending and lifting. Imagery may again be used prior to exercise practice to reduce the threat level of an action, and actions are regressed to ensure safety. For example, forward flexion to couch level, building to stool level, and finally floor level. Actions which the subject is fearful of may be identified during discussion and using photographic examples such as the PHODA (Photograph Series of Daily Activities) scale, which has been used successfully with CLBP patients exhibiting kinesiophobia (Trost, France and Thomas 2009). Table 8.14 summarizes the approach.

Table 8.14 Neuroscience-based rehabilitation for chronic lower back pain

▶ Neuroscience education and communication precede treatment and are used throughout
▶ Exercise performed in a time-contingent not symptom-contingent fashion
▶ Motor imagery used prior to exercise with subjects demonstrating fear avoidance
▶ Perception about an action (process) more important than consequences (outcome)
▶ Use action which subject is fearful of in a graded manor
▶ Used PHODA scale and/or discussion to identify threat level of a movement

(After Nils et al. 2014)

Table 8.15 Integrated back stability model

Phase	Content
Correction of movement dysfunction	▶ Posture evaluation ▶ Muscle balance tests ▶ Begin muscle balance corrective exercise ▶ Pain relieving physiotherapy modalities ▶ Back protection and unloading using taping/bracing ▶ Stability foundation movements
Development of back fitness	▶ Progress muscle balance corrective exercise ▶ Stability exercise using limb loading ▶ Begin functional starting positions ▶ General exercise to build CV fitness ▶ General strength exercise machine based ▶ Begin simple lifting and gross movement re-education
Functional restoration	▶ Functional exercise to match work/life requirements ▶ Multi-joint and whole-body resistance training ▶ Free weight training ▶ Build muscle strength/power and endurance ▶ Lifting re-education (combined movements) ▶ Increasingly complex actions to reduce fear of movement

References

Adams, M., Bogduk, N., Burton, K., Dolan, P., 2002. *The Biomechanics of Back Pain*. Churchill Livingstone, Edinburgh.

Adams, M.A., Hutton, W.C., 1983. The mechanical function of the lumbar apophyseal joints. *Spine* **8**, 327–330.

Adams, M.A., Hutton, W.C., Stott, J.R.R., 1980. The resistance to flexion of the lumbar intervertebral joint. *Spine* **5**, 245–253.

Airaksinen, O., Brox, J.I., Cedraschi, C., 2005. *European Guidelines for the Management of Chronic Non-specific Lower Back Pain*. European Commission Publications, Brussels.

Airaksinen, O., Brox, J.I., Cedraschi, C., Hildebrandt, J., Klaber-Moffett, J., Kovacs, F., Mannion, A.F., Reis, S., Staal, J.B., Ursin, H., Zanoli, G., 2006. COST B13 Working Group on Guidelines for Chronic Low Back Pain. Chapter 4. European guidelines for the management of chronic nonspecific low back pain. *European Spine Journal Mar*, **15** (2): S192–300.

Albert, H.B., Kjaer, P., Jensen, T.S. et al., 2008. Modic changes, possible causes and relation to lower back pain. *Medical Hypotheses* **70**, 361–368.

Alexander, L.A., Hancock, E., Agouris, I. et al., 2007. The response of the nucleus pulposus of the lumbar intervertebral discs to functionally loaded positions. *Spine* **32** (14), 1508–1512.

Bardin, L.D., King, P., Maher, C.G., 2017. Diagnostic triage for lower back pain: a practical approach for primary care. *Medical Journal of Australia* **206** (6), 268–273.

Beattie, P.F., Arnot, C.F., Donley, J.W. et al., 2010. The immediate reduction in lower back pain intensity following lumbar joint mobilization and prone press-ups is associated with increased diffusion of water in the L5-S1 intervertebral disc. *JOSPT*, **40**, 256–264.

Beattie, P.F., Brooks, W.M., Rothstein, J.M., 1994. Effect of lordosis on the position of the nucleus pulposus in supine subjects: a study using MRI. *Spine* **19** (18), 2096–2102.

Becker, C., 2006. Lumbar spondylolysis. *Sportex Medicine* **Jan**, 6–9.

Bergmark, A., 1989. Stability of the lumbar spine. *Acta Orthopaedica Scandinavica Supplementum* **230** (60), 3–54.

Bogduk, N., Engel, R., 1984. The menisci of the lumbar zygapophyseal joints: a review of their anatomy and clinical significance. *Spine* **9**, 454–460.

Bogduk, N., Jull, G., 1985. The theoretical pathology of acute locked back: a basis for manipulative therapy. *Manual Medicine* **1**, 78–82.

Bogduk, N., Twomey, L.T., 1987. *Clinical Anatomy of the Lumbar Spine*. Churchill Livingstone, Edinburgh.

Bogduk, N., Twomey, L.T., 1991. *Clinical Anatomy of the Lumbar Spine*, 2nd ed. Churchill Livingstone, Edinburgh.

Cappozzo, A., Felici, F., Figura, F., Gazzani, F., 1985. Lumbar spine loading during half-squat exercises. *Medicine and Science in Sports and Exercise* **17** (5), 613–620.

Cheung et al., 2009. Prevalence and pattern of lumbar magnetic resonance imaging changes in a population study of one thousand forty-three individuals. *Spine* **34** (9), 934–940.

Chiu, C., Chuang, T., Chang, K. et al., 2014. The probability of spontaneous regression of lumbar herniated disc: a systematic review, *Clinical Rehabilitation* **29**, 2.

Cramer, G.D., Tuck, N., Knudsen, J. et al. 2000. Effects of side posture positioning and side posture adjusting on the lumbar zygapophyseal joints as evaluated by magnetic resonance imaging. *Journal of Manipulative and Physiological Therapeutics* **23**, 380–394.

CSP (2016) Mythbuster campaign. http://www.csp.org.uk/your-health/healthy-living/public-information-leaflets/back-pain-myth-busters. Accessed 04/04/2017.

Cusi, M., Saunders, J., Hungerford, B. et al. 2010. The use of prolotherapy in the sacro-iliac joint. *British Journal of Sports Medicine* **44** (2), 100–104.

Cyriax, J., 1982. *Textbook of Orthopaedic Medicine*, **Vol. 1**, 8th ed. Baillière Tindall, London.

Darlow, B. and O'Sullivan, P.B., 2016. Why are back pain guidelines left on the sidelines? Three myths appear to be guiding management of back pain in sport. *Br J Sports Med* **50** (21), 1294–1295.

Deville, W.L., van der Windt, D.A., Dzaferagic, A. et al. 2000. The test of Lasegue: systematic review of the accuracy in diagnosing herniated discs. *Spine* **25** (9), 1140–1147.

Don Tigny, R.L., 1985. Function and pathomechanics of the sacroiliac joint. *Physical Therapy* **65**, 35–44.

Dreyfuss, P., Dreyer, S., Griffin, J., Hoffman, J., Walsh, N., 1992. Positive sacroiliac screening tests in asymptomatic adults. *Proceedings of the First Interdisciplinary World Congress on Lower back Pain and its Relation to the Sacroiliac Joint.* San Diego, CA.

Edmondston, S.J., Song, S., Bricknell, R.V., 2000. MRI evaluation of lumbar spine flexion and extension in asymptomatic individuals. *Manual Therapy* **5** (3), 158–164.

Evans, D.W., 2002. Mechanisms and effects of spinal high velocity low amplitude thrust manipulation: previous theories. *Journal of Manipulative and Physiological Therapeutics* **25**, 251–262.

Evans, D.W., Breen, A.C., 2006. A biomechanical model for mechanically efficient cavitation production during spinal manipulation: pre-thrust position and the neutral zone. *Journal of Manipulative and Physiological Therapeutics* **29** (1), 72–82.

Farfan, H.F., Cossette, J.W., Robertson, G.H., Wells, R.V., Kraus, H., 1970. The effects of torsion on the lumbar intervertebral joints: the role of torsion in the production of disc degeneration. *Journal of Bone and Joint Surgery* **52A**, 468.

Farfan, H.F., Osteria, V., Lamy, C., 1976. The mechanical etiology of spondylolysis and spondylolisthesis. *Clinical Orthopaedics and Related Research* **117**, 40–55.

Fennell, A.J., Jones, A.P., Hukins, D.W.L., 1996. Migration of the nucleus pulposus within the intervertebral disc during flexion and extension of the spine. *Spine* **21** (23), 2753–2757.

Frigerio, N.A., Stowe, R.R., Howe, J.W., 1974. Movement of the sacro-iliac joint. *Clinical Orthopaedic and Related Research* **100**, 370.

Gal, J.M., Herzog, W., Kawchuk, G.N., et al. 1997. Movements of vertebrae during manipulative thrusts to un-embalmed human cadavers. *Journal of Manipulative and Physiological Therapeutics* **20**, 30–40.

Giles, L., Taylor, J., 1987. Human zygapophyseal joint capsule and synovial fold innervation. *British Journal of Rheumatology* **26**, 93–98.

Gomes-Neto, M., Lopesa, J.M. Conceiçãoa, C.S. et al. (2017) Stabilization exercise compared to general exercises or manual therapy for the management of lower back pain: a systematic review and meta-analysis. *Physical Therapy in Sport* **23**, 136–142.

Gregory, P., Batt, M., Wallace, W., 2002. Comparing injuries of spin bowling with fast bowling in young cricketers. *Clinical Journal of Sports Medicine* **12** (2), 107–112.

Grieve, G.P., 1970. Sciatica and the straight leg raising test in manipulative treatment. *Physiotherapy* **56**, 337.

Gutke, A., Hansson, E.R., Zetherström, G. et al. (2009) Posterior pelvic pain provocation test is negative in patients with lumbar herniated discs. *Eur Spine J.* **18** (7), 1008–1012.

Harreby, M., Hesseloe, G., Kier, J., Neergaard, K., 1997. Lower back pain and physical exercise in leisure time in 38-year-old men and women. *European Spinal Journal* **6**, 181–186.

Herzog, W., Scheele, D., Conway, P., 1999. Electromyographic responses of back and limb muscles associated with spinal manipulative therapy. *Spine* **24**, 146–153.

Herzog, W., Symons, B., 2001. The biomechanics of spinal manipulation. *Critical Reviews in Physical and Rehabilitation Medicine* **13**, 191–216.

Hill, J.C., Dunn, K.M., Lewis, M., Mullis, R., Main, C.J., Foster, N.E. et al., 2008. A primary care back pain screening tool: identifying patient subgroups for initial treatment. *Arthritis Rheum* **59** (5), 632–641.

Hirsch, C., Nachemson, A., 1954. New observations on mechanical behaviour of lumbar discs. *Acta Orthopaedica Scandinavica* **22**, 184–189.

Hodges, P. (2015) The role of motor control training. In: Jull, G., Moore, A., Falla, D. et al., (eds) *Grieve's Modern Musculoskeletal Physiotherapy*. Chapter 45.5. pp. 482–487.

Hodges, P., Falla, D., 2015. Interaction between pain and sensorimotor control. In: Jull, G., Moore, A., Falla, D et al. (eds) *Grieve's Modern Musculoskeletal Physiotherapy*. Chapter 6. pp. 53–67.

Holm, S., Maroudas, A., Urban, J.P.G., Selstam, G., Nachemson, A., 1981. Nutrition of the intervertebral disc: solute transport and metabolism. *Connective Tissue Research* **8**, 101–119.

Hoshina, H., 1980. Spondylolysis in young athletes. *Physician and Sports Medicine* **8**, 75–79.

Hukins, D.W.L., 1987. Properties of spinal materials. In: Jayson, M.I.V. (ed.), *The Lumbar Spine and Back Pain*. Churchill Livingstone, London.

Janda, V., Schmid, H.J.A., 1980. Muscles as a pathogenic factor in back pain. *Proceedings of the International Federation of Orthopaedic Manipulative Therapists, 4th Conference*, 17–18, New Zealand.

Klein, J.A., Hukins, D.W.L., 1981. Functional differentiation in the spinal column. *Engineering in Medicine* **12** (2), 83.

Klein, J.A., Hukins, D.W.L., 1983. Relocation of the bending axis during flexion–extension of the lumbar intervertebral discs and its implications for prolapse. *Spine* **8**, 659–664.

Koumantakis, G.A., Watson, P.J., Oldham, J.A., 2005. Supplementation of general endurance exercise with stabilization training, versus general exercise only. *Clinical Biomechanics* **20**, 474–482.

Kraemer, J., Kolditz, D., Gowin, R., 1985. Water and electrolyte content of human intervertebral discs under variable load. *Spine* **10**, 69–71.

Laslett, M., 1997. Pain provocation sacroiliac joint tests. In: Vleeming, A., Mooney, V., Dorman, T., Snijders, C., Stoeckart, R. (eds), *Movement Stability and Lower Back Pain*. Churchill Livingstone, Edinburgh.

Laslett, M., Williams, M., 1994. The reliability of selected pain provocation tests for sacroiliac pathology. *Spine* **19**, 1243–1249.

Leatt, P., Reilly, T., Troup, J.G.D., 1986. Spinal loading during circuit weight-training and running. *British Journal of Sports Medicine* **20** (3), 119–124.

Lee, D.G., 1994. Clinical manifestations of pelvic girdle dysfunction. In: Boyling, J.D., Palastanga, N. (eds), *Grieve's Modern Manual Therapy*, 2nd ed. Churchill Livingstone, Edinburgh.

Lewit, K., 1985. The muscular and articular factor in movement restriction. *Man Medicine* **1**, 83–85.

MacDonald, D., Moseley, G.L., Hodges, P.W. (2009) Why do some patients keep hurting their back? Evidence of ongoing back muscle dysfunction during remission from recurrent back pain. *Pain* **142** (3),183–188.

Maitland, G.D., 1986. *Vertebral Manipulation*, 5th ed. Butterworth, London.

Markolf, K.L., Morris, J.M., 1974. The structural components of the intervertebral disc. *Journal of Bone and Joint Surgery* **56A**, 675.

Masci, L., Pike, J., Malara, F., Phillips, B., et al. 2006. Use of the one-legged hyperextension test and magnetic resonance imaging in the diagnosis of active spondylolysis. *British Journal of Sports Medicine* **40**, 940–946.

McKenzie, R., May, S., 2003. *The Lumbar Spine: Mechanical Diagnosis and Therapy*. Spinal Publications New Zealand, Waikanae.

McKenzie, R.A., 1981. *The Lumbar Spine: Mechanical Diagnosis and Therapy*. Spinal Publications New Zealand, Waikanae.

Mens, J.M.A., Vleeming, A., Snijders, C.J., Stam, H.J., 1997. Active straight leg raising test: a clinical approach to the load transfer function of the pelvic girdle. In: Vleeming, A., Mooney, V., Dorman, T. (eds), *Movement Stability and Lower Back Pain*. Churchill Livingstone, Edinburgh.

Mercer, C., Jackson, A., Hettinga, D., Barlos, P., 2006. *Clinical Guidelines for the Physiotherapy Management of Persistent Lower Back Pain Part 1: Exercise*. Chartered Society of Physiotherapy, London.

Miller, M.I., Madeiros, J.M., 1987. Recruitment of internal oblique and transversus abdominis

419

muscles during the eccentric phase of the curl-up exercise. *Physical Therapy* **67**, 1213–1217.

Mooney, V., Robertson, J., 1976. The facet syndrome. *Clinical Orthopaedics* **115**, 149–156.

Mulligan, B.R., 1989. *Manual Therapy – Nags, Snags, and PRPs etc.* Plane View Services Wellington, New Zealand.

Nachemson, A., 1987. Lumbar intradiscal pressure. In: Jayson, M.I.V. (ed.), *The Lumbar Spine and Back Pain*. Churchill Livingstone, London.

Nachemson, A., Evans, J., 1968. Some mechanical properties of the third lumbar inter-laminar ligament (ligamentum flavum). *Journal of Biomechanics* **1**, 211.

Nelson, M.A., Allen, P., Clamp, S.E., De Dombal, F.T., 1979. Reliability and reproducibility of clinical findings in lower back pain. *Spine* **4**, 97–101.

NICE (2016) Lower back pain and sciatica in over 16s: assessment and management. National Institute for Health and Care Excellence. NICE Guidance NG59. Accessed 03/04/2017.

Nijs, J., Meeus, M., Cagnie, B. et al., 2014. A modern neuroscience approach to chronic spinal pain: combining pain neuroscience education with cognition-targeted motor control training. *Phys Ther* **94** (5), 730–738.

Norris, C.M., 1995. Spinal stabilisation 2. Limiting factors to end-range motion in the lumbar spine. *Physiotherapy* **81** (2), 4–12.

Norris, C.M., 2000. *Back Stability*. Human Kinetics, Champaign, Illinois, USA.

Norris, C.M., 2008. *Back Stability* (2nd edition). Human Kinetics, Champaign, Illinois.

Norris, C.M. (2015) *The Complete Guide to Back Rehabilitation*. Bloomsbury.

Norris, C.M., Matthews, M., 2008. The role of an integrated back stability program in patients with chronic lower back pain. *Complementary Therapies in Clinical Practice* **14**, 255–263.

O'Keeffe, M., Purtill H, Kennedy N, et al. (2015) Individualised cognitive functional therapy compared with a combined exercise and pain education class for patients with non-specific chronic lower back pain: study protocol for a multicentre randomised controlled trial. *BMJ Open* **5**, e007156.

O'Sullivan, P.B., 2000. Lumbar segmental instability. *Manual Therapy* **5**, (1) 2–12.

O'Sullivan, P., 2005. Diagnosis and classification of chronic lower back pain disorders: maladaptive movement and motor control impairments as underlying mechanism. *Manual Therapy* **10** (4), 242–255.

O'Sullivan, P., 2017. Making sense of back pain: a cognitive functional approach. Course notes. Royal Free Hospital, London.

O'Sullivan, P.B., Twomey, L.T., Allison, G.T., 1997. Evaluation of specific stabilizing exercise in the treatment of chronic lower back pain with radiologic diagnosis of spondylolysis or spondylolisthesis. *Spine* **22**, 2959–2967.

Oliver, J., Middleditch, A., 1991. *Functional Anatomy of the Spine*. Butterworth-Heinemann, Oxford.

Ostgaard, H.C., Zetherström, G. and Roos-Hansson, E., 1994. The posterior pelvic pain provocation test in pregnant women. *Eur Spine J* **3** (5), 258–260.

Panjabi, M.M., 1992. The stabilizing system of the spine. Part 1. Function, dysfunction, adaptation, and enhancement. *Journal of Spinal Disorders* **5** (4), 383–389.

Panjabi, M.M., Hult, J.E., White, A.A., 1987. Biomechanical studies in cadaveric spines. In: Jayson, M.I.V. (ed.), *The Lumbar Spine and Back Pain*. Churchill Livingstone, London.

Panjabi, M.M., Jorneus, L., Greenstein, G., 1984. *Lumbar Spine Ligaments: An In Vitro Biomechanical Study*, ORS Transactions.

Potter, N.A., Rothstein, J.M., 1985. Intertester reliability for selected clinical tests of the sacroiliac joint. *Physical Therapy* **65**, 1671–1675.

Ranson C, Burnett A, and Kerslake R., 2010. Injuries to the lower back in elite fast bowlers. *J Bone Joint Surg Br* **92**, 1664–1668.

Richardson, C.A., 1992. Muscle imbalance: principles of treatment and assessment. *Proceedings of the New Zealand Society of Physiotherapists Challenges Conference*, Christchurch, New Zealand.

Roy, S.H., Deluca, C.J., Snyder-Mackler, L. et al., 1990. Fatigue, recovery and lower back pain in varsity rowers. *Medicine and Science in Sport and Exercise*, **22** (4), 463–469.

Sahrmann S.A., 2002. *Diagnosis and Treatment of Movement Impairment Syndromes*. Mosby, St. Louis.

Saragiotto, BT., Maher, CG., Yamato, Tiê P et al., 2016. Motor control exercise for nonspecific lower back pain: a Cochrane review. *Spine* **41** (16), 1284–1295.

Scott, I.R., Vaughan, A., Hall, J., 2015. Swiss ball enhances lumbar multifidus activity in chronic lower back pain. *Physical Therapy in Sport* **16** (3), 40–44.

Smith, B.E., Littlewood, C., May, S., 2014. An update of stabilisation exercises for lower back pain: a systematic review with meta-analysis. *BMC Musculoskeletal Disorders* **15**, 416.

Spitzer, W.O., LeBlanc, F.E., Dupuis, M., 1987. Scientific approach to the assessment and management of activity related spinal disorders: a monograph for clinicians. Report of the Quebec Task Force on Spinal Disorders. *Spine* **12**, 7s.

Sturesson, B., 2007. Movement of the sacroiliac joint with special reference to the effect of load. In: Vleeming, A., Mooney, V., Stoeckar, R. (eds), *Movement, Stability and Lumbopelvic Pain*. Churchill Livingstone, Oxford.

Sturesson, B., Selvik, G., Uden, A., 1989. Movements of the sacroiliac joints. A Roentgen stereophotogrammetric analysis. *Spine* **14**, 162–165.

Taylor, J.R., Twomey, L.T., 1986. Age changes in lumbar zygapophyseal joints. *Spine* **11**, 739–745.

Teraguchi et al., 2014. Prevalence and distribution of intervertebral disc degeneration over the entire spine in a population-based cohort: the Wakayama Spine Study. *Osteoarthritis Cartilage* **22** (1), 104–110.

Thompson, B., 2002. How should athletes with chronic lower back pain be managed in primary care? In: MacAuley, D., Best, T. (eds), *Evidence Based Sports Medicine*. BMJ Books, London.

Tkaczuk, H., 1968. Tensile properties of human lumbar longitudinal ligaments. *Acta Orthopaedica Scandinavica* **115** (Suppl.).

Trost, Z., France, C.R., Thomas, J.S., 2009. Examination of the photograph series of daily activities (PHODA) scale in chronic lower back pain patients with high and low kinesiophobia. *Pain* **141** (3), 276–282.

Turner, H., 2002. *The Sacro Iliac Joint*. Course notes, Manchester, UK.

Unsworth, A., Dowson, D., Wright, V., 1971. A bioengineering study of cavitation in the metacarpophalangeal joint. *Annals of the Rheumatic Diseases* **30**, 348–358.

Urban, L.M., 1986. The straight-leg raising test: a review. In: Grieve, G.P. (ed.), *Modern Manual Therapy of the Vertebral Column*. Churchill Livingstone, London.

Van Duersen, L.L., Patijn, J., Ockhuysen, A.L., Vortman, B.J., 1990. The value of some clinical tests of the sacroiliac joint. *Manual Medicine* **5**, 96–99.

Vernon, H.T., 2000. Qualitative review of studies of manipulation induced hypoalgesia. *Journal of Manipulative and Physiological Therapeutics* **23**, 134–138.

Vibe Fersum, K., O'Sullivan, P., Skouen, J.S., Smith, A., Kvåle, A., 2013. Efficacy of classification-based cognitive functional therapy in patients with non-specific chronic lower back pain: a randomized controlled trial. *Eur J Pain* **17** (6), 916–928.

Vicenzino, B., Hing, W., Rivett, D., Hall, T., 2011. *Mobilisation with Movement – the Art and the Science*. Churchill Livingstone

Vleeming, A., Mooney, V., Dorman, T., Snijders, C., 1997. *Movement Stability and Lower Back Pain*. Churchill Livingstone, Edinburgh.

Waddell, G., Feder, G., Lewis, M., 1997. Systematic reviews of bed rest and advice to stay active for acute lower back pain. *British Journal of General Practice* **47**, 647–652.

Wang, X.Q., Zheng, J.J., Yu, Z.W. et al., 2012. A meta-analysis of core stability exercise versus general exercise for chronic lower back pain. *PLOS ONE* **7** (12), e52082.

Weber, M.D., Woodall, W.R., 1991. Spondylogenic disorders in gymnasts. *Journal of Orthopaedic and Sports Physical Therapy* **14**, (1) 6–13.

Webster et al., 2010. Relationship of early magnetic resonance imaging for work-related acute lower back pain with disability and medical utilization outcomes. *Journal of Occupational and Environmental Medicine* **52** (9), 900–907.

Wynne-Jones, G. et al. 2014. Absence from work and return to work in people with back pain: a systematic review and meta-analysis. *Occupational and Environmental Medicine* **71** (6), 448–456.

Yang, K.H., King, A.I., 1984. Mechanism of facet load transmission as a hypothesis for low-back pain. *Spine* **9**, 557–565.

CHAPTER 9

The thorax and thoracic spine

Thoracic spine

The unique feature of the vertebrae in the thoracic region is the presence of facets, both on the sides of the vertebral bodies and the transverse processes. These are for articulation with the ribs, forming the costovertebral (CV) and costotransverse (CT) joints (Fig. 9.1). Most of the ribs articulate with two adjacent vertebral bodies and one transverse process. The facets on the head of the ribs articulate in turn with demi-facets on the upper and lower borders of the vertebrae, and the crest on the rib head butts onto the intervertebral disc. The joint capsule is loose and strengthened anteriorly to form the three portions of the radiate ligament. The costovertebral joint cavity is divided into two by the intra-articular ligament, except for ribs one, ten, eleven and twelve, which articulate with a single vertebra and have a single joint cavity.

The costotransverse joints are formed only with the upper ten ribs. The joint is made between the articular facet of the transverse process and the oval facet on the rib tubercle. The thin joint capsule is strengthened by the costotransverse ligaments.

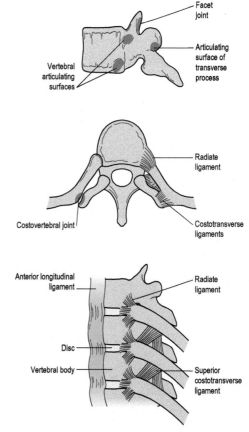

Figure 9.1 Joints between the ribs and thoracic spine.

Definition

The costovertebral (CV) joint is formed between the rib and the vertebral body; the costotransverse (CT) joint is formed between the rib and the transverse process of the vertebra.

Sternal articulations

The sternocostal joints are formed between the medial end of the costal cartilages of ribs one to seven. The joint between the first rib and the sternum is cartilaginous, but all the others are synovial. Each is surrounded by a capsule and supported by radiate ligaments. The fibres of these ligaments fan out and intertwine with those of the ligaments above and below, and also with those of the opposite sternocostal joints. In addition, the radiate ligament fibres fuse with the tendinous fibres of the pectoralis major. The eighth, ninth and tenth ribs form interchondral joints between their costal cartilages.

The costochondral joints are formed between the end of the rib and the lateral edge of the costal cartilage. The joint formed is cartilaginous, its perichondrium being continuous with the periosteum of the rib itself. Only slight bending and twisting actions are possible at this joint. The manubriosternal articulation is that between the upper part of the sternum and the manubrium. The joint is cartilaginous, with a hollow disc in its centre, and is strengthened by the sternocostal ligaments and longitudinal fibrous bands. About 7 degrees of movement occurs at the joint in association with breathing.

Rib movements

Movement of the diaphragm, ribs and sternum increases the volume within the thorax with inspiration. Each rib acts as a lever, with one axis travelling through the costovertebral and sternocostal joints, and another through the costovertebral and costotransverse joints. The two axes permit two types of motion, known as 'pump-handle' and 'bucket-handle'. In the pump-handle action the upper ribs and sternum are raised, increasing the anteroposterior diameter of the thorax. With bucket-handle motion the lower ribs move both up and out, widening the infrasternal angle and increasing the transverse diameter of the thorax. In the lower ribs (eight to twelve) a third motion called 'caliper action' may also occur, where the lateral diameter of the chest is increased without significant joint motion.

The variation in movement between the upper and lower ribs is due, in part, to the differing structure of their respective costotransverse joints. The upper joints are cup-shaped, permitting mainly rotation (pump-handle), while those lower down are flat, permitting both rotation and gliding movements (bucket-handle).

Key point

The ribs can move forwards and upwards, increasing the anteroposterior diameter of the thorax (pump-handle), and outwards, increasing the lateral diameter of the thorax (bucket-handle).

In addition to respiratory motion, the ribs also move in association with the thoracic spine. With flexion of the spine the ribs move closer together and with extension they are pulled further apart, flattening the ribcage. This latter action in the upper ribs is important for the correct movement of the scapulothoracic joint. Lateral flexion causes the ribs on the concave side to move together and those on the convex side to move apart. Rotation gives horizontal gliding of one rib relative to another.

Ribcage shape at rest

The general shape of the ribcage will change as a result of thoracic mobility, with an increased thoracic kyphosis causing a general flattening of the ribcage. In addition, congenital abnormalities occur, including pigeon chest, funnel chest and barrel chest.

424

- *Pigeon chest* is seen when the sternum is orientated *downwards* and the ribcage becomes pointed because the anteroposterior (AP) diameter is increased.
- *Funnel chest* occurs when the sternum is pushed *backwards* in relation to the ribcage, often due to an overgrowth of the ribs. On inspiration, the depression of the sternum may become more noticeable.
- *Barrel chest* deformity occurs when the sternum is orientated *forwards and upwards*, increasing the AP diameter. This deformity is seen in some pathological lung conditions.

The ribcage will also alter shape in cases of scoliosis. The vertebral bodies rotate towards the convexity of the curve, dragging the ribs with them. The ribs on the convex side of the curve are pushed backwards, creating a 'hump', and those on the concave side of the curve move anteriorly, causing a 'hollow' (Fig. 9.2). Rotation of the vertebral body causes the spinous processes to move away from the mid-line, in the opposite direction to the scoliosis. Right rotation of the vertebra therefore sees the spinous process deviating to the left.

> **Definition**
>
> Scoliosis is a deformity of the spine where a single or multiple lateral curvature is seen. The scoliosis is named according to the convexity (sharp point) of the curve.

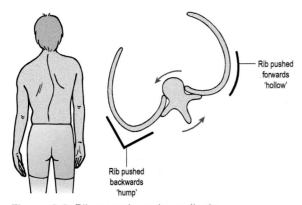

Rib pushed forwards 'hollow'

Rib pushed backwards 'hump'

Figure 9.2 Ribcage shape in scoliosis.

Movement of the thoracic spine

The relative thinness of the discs in the thoracic region, coupled with the presence of the ribs, makes movement here more limited than in other spinal areas. Extension is limited to about 30 degrees, with slightly more flexion being possible – roughly 40 degrees. Flexion is freer in the lower thoracic region but still restricted by the ribs. Extension is limited by approximation of the facets and spinous processes, as well as tissue tension, and causes the thoracic cage to become flatter. Lateral flexion is limited to roughly 25 degrees to each side, a greater range being available in the lower region. Lateral flexion is accompanied by the same amount of rotation, which occurs contralaterally. For example, right lateral flexion is accompanied by right axial rotation, causing the tip of the spinous process to rest to the left of the mid-line. Rib movements accompany lateral flexion, with the ribs on the concave side compressing and those on the side of the convexity being pulled apart.

The range of rotation is larger than other movements, with 35 degrees being possible to either side. However, when the spine is extended, both lateral flexion and rotation are dramatically reduced. As rotation occurs, the inferior facets of the upper vertebra slide laterally with respect to the lower vertebra, towards the direction of the rotation. Movement of the vertebra is accompanied by distortion of the ribs. The ribcage becomes more rounded on the side to which the rotation is occurring, and flattens on the opposite side.

Rotation of the thoracic spine is an important constituent of locomotion. In walking, when the right leg swings forward, the lower trunk and the pelvis rotate to the left about the fixed left leg. To keep the head facing forwards, the upper spine must rotate to the right, pulling the shoulders back into a forward-facing direction. As the upper and lower parts of the spine are rotating in opposite directions, there is a point at which the two movements cancel each other out. This point is the intervertebral disc between T7 and T8, which is not subjected to any rotation, while those vertebrae immediately above and below rotate maximally, but in opposite directions.

> **Key point**
>
> During walking and running, the pelvis rotates to one direction and the shoulders and trunk to the other. The two movements cancel each other out at the T7/8 spinal disc, where no rotation occurs at all.

Examination

Subjective assessment is used to highlight potential red flags (Table 9.1), always remembering that pain in the thoracic region can be referred from the viscera. Potential visceral referral areas are shown in Fig. 9.3. The screening examination is essentially similar to that of the lumbar spine, except that rotation is the movement most likely to be revealing as this normally has the greatest range. Rotation is performed in a sitting position, with overpressure being given through the shoulders. Resisted flexion and extension may be performed in a lying or a sitting position. Resisted lateral flexion is tested in a standing position with

Table 9.1 Red flags in the examination of the thoracic spine

Signs and symptoms	Investigate for
History of risk factors for CHD Angina pain Persistent nausea	Cardiac ischaemia
Severe unrelenting chest pain into upper back Pain not lessened when supine	Thoracic aneurysm
Epigastric pain travelling to thoracic region Symptoms altered at mealtimes Nausea or vomiting	Peptic ulcer
Right upper quadrant pain Fever, nausea and vomiting after eating fatty foods	Cholecystitis
Flank pain travelling to thoracic region Fever, nausea and vomiting	Kidney symptoms
Direct thoracic trauma History of severe coughing in >60	Fracture
History of cancer Unexplained weight loss Constant and/or night pain	Neoplasm
Limited chest movement Morning stiffness HLA-B27 test positive	Inflammatory disorder

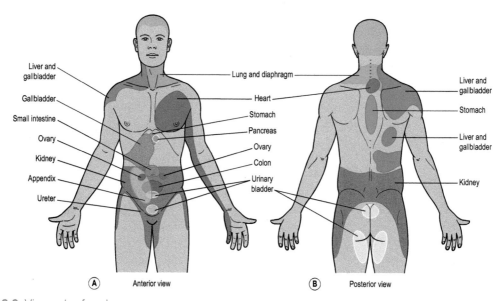

Liver and gallbladder
Gallbladder
Small intestine
Ovary
Kidney
Appendix
Ureter

Lung and diaphragm
Heart
Stomach
Pancreas
Ovary
Colon
Urinary bladder

Liver and gallbladder
Stomach
Liver and gallbladder
Kidney

(A) Anterior view

(B) Posterior view

Figure 9.3 Visceral referral areas.

the therapist initially at the patient's side. The patient's near wrist of the straight arm is gripped, as is the far shoulder. Stability is improved if the therapist widens his or her base of support by placing the near foot between those of the patient.

As rotation and lateral flexion accompany each other in the thoracic spine, it is often revealing to combine these movements at examination. Thoracic rotation is performed, and is followed by lateral flexion, first in one direction and then the other.

Palpation takes in the vertebrae, rib joints and ribs themselves, and is carried out with the patient in a prone position, with the arms over the couch side to move the scapulae apart. Alternatively, posteroanterior (PA) pressures may be used, with the thoracic spine extended using the elbow support prone-lying starting position. In a prone-lying position, the spinous processes of the thoracic vertebrae are angled downwards like the scales of a fish. The thoracic vertebrae may be considered in threes, with the transverse processes being found relative to the spinous processes, as shown in Table 9.2.

As an approximate guide to levels, the AC joint is normally aligned with the C7–T1 interspace, the spine of the scapula at T3 and the inferior scapular angle at T7.

The rib angles gradually spread out from the spine, with the eighth rib being furthest (about 6 cm) from the mid-line. The rib angles can be palpated at the same levels as the transverse processes down to the T8/T9, by pushing the soft tissue to one side. The facet joints lie in the paravertebral sulci, and the transverse processes, which overlie the

Table 9.2 Palpation of the thoracic vertebrae

T1, 2, 3	At the same level as spinous process
T4, 5, 6	Between two successive levels
T7, 8, 9	Level with spinous process of vertebra below
T10	Level with vertebra below
T11	Between two successive levels
T12	At same level

Table 9.3 Rib palpation

Rib structure	Region of palpation
1st rib	Above clavicle, within supraclavicular fossa
2nd	End level with manubriosternal joint (angle of Louis)
4th	Lies on nipple line
7th	End level with xiphisternal joint
11th	Tip lies in mid-axillary line
12th	Tip level with L1
Rib angle	3–4 cm lateral to end of transverse process
Costochondral (CC) joint	3 cm lateral to parasternal line at 2nd rib, 12 cm lateral at 7th rib, 18 cm lateral at 10th rib
Costotransverse (CT) joint	Depression between transverse process and rib

costotransverse joints, are found 3–4 cm from the mid-line. Guidelines for rib palpation are shown in Table 9.3.

Modifications to the slump test for the thoracic spine

A variation of this test for the cervical and thoracic spine is to perform it in the long sitting position (Fig. 9.4A). From this position, thoracic and lumbar flexion are added, followed by cervical flexion (Fig. 9.4B). Altering the order of movement will change the neurodynamic demands, enabling the practitioner to refine the test. For example, performing cervical flexion before lumbar and thoracic flexion will challenge the cervical neural tissues more. The test can be further refined to place emphasis on the sympathetic trunk. This is especially relevant in the presence of sympathetic signs in conditions such as T4 syndrome, thoracic outlet syndrome and Raynaud's syndrome, and in cases where cervicothoracic conditions mimic cardiac disease. Sympathetic testing is achieved by adding components of lateral flexion and rotation of the thoracic spine and lateral flexion of the cervical spine. Additional stress may be imposed by adding a minimal straight leg raise (SLR).

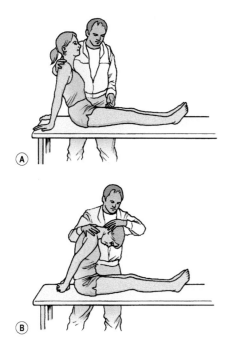

Figure 9.4 The slump test (long sitting). (A) Start. (B) Finish. From Butler (1991) with permission.

> **Key point**
> Where sympathetic signs (skin changes, sweating, swelling) are present in conditions such as thoracic outlet syndrome (TOS) and Raynaud's syndrome, modify the slump test to emphasize the sympathetic trunk. Add thoracic lateral flexion and rotation, and cervical lateral flexion, to the standard slump test.

Injury to the ribcage

Direct trauma to the ribcage can result in damage to the ribs, intercostal muscles or, indirectly, to the rib joints. Deep breathing will usually reproduce the pain of rib or intercostal injury, and palpation can be used to reveal the exact site of injury as these structures are superficial. Trunk extension will open the ribcage and cause pain, and intercostal muscle tearing will generally give pain to resisted trunk flexion. Rib springing at a distance from the point of injury usually produces pain from a rib fracture.

Rib fracture

With rib fracture it is the tearing of the intercostal muscles which can give the pain rather than the fracture itself. The acute pain may be relieved by local strapping. Pre-stretched elastic adhesive strapping is applied across the area to restrict ribcage expansion and give the athlete a feeling of support. In the subacute phase, active mobilization is required. If scar tissue formation is excessive and the source of pain, transverse frictions to the intercostal muscles along the line of the ribs can be helpful to modulate pain. In addition, holding the rib down with the fingertips and practising deep inspiration will help to stretch the injured area. Exercises to expand the ribcage, such as deep inspiration and overhead reaching, or trunk lateral flexion to the contralateral side, with or without rotation, is also helpful to stretch the area.

> **Key point**
> Following rib injury, intercostal muscle stretching is useful. Deep breathing exercises, coupled with manual therapy to isolate the movement to a single pair of ribs, may also be used.

Where rib trauma is severe, there is a danger of *pneumothorax*. Here, air enters the pleural cavity, changing the pressure within the thorax. The mediastinum is pressed away from the injured lung (mediastinal shift), with the potential to compress vital structures.

> **Definition**
> The mediastinum is the central compartment of the thoracic cavity, lying between the lungs. It contains the heart, major blood vessels, trachea, oesophagus, thymus and lymph nodes of the chest.

The subject experiences severe chest or back pain and becomes breathless. They may begin to cyanose (lips going blue) and panic. First-aid treatment is to cover the injured chest region with an airtight seal, such as a sterile plastic film or watertight dressing. Examination with a stethoscope (auscultation) can reveal an absence of lung sounds on the injured side, indicating that air is not entering the lungs. Hospitalization is required, where a chest X-ray may reveal a deep sulcus sign, showing that the costophrenic angle (junction of diaphragm and ribs) is abnormally deep. Treatment is by inserting a chest drain into the area outside the affected lung. The drain tube has a one-way valve, allowing excess air to escape and the lung to re-expand.

Rib joints

The sternocostal joints may be sprained, giving local swelling and tenderness, as may the costochondral joints (Tietze's syndrome). True Tietze's syndrome is a swelling of the costrochondral joints, which contrasts to costrochondritis, which is inflammation alone. Clinically, however, the two names are interchangeable.

Pressure on the sternum, or applied to the lateral aspect of the thorax, reproduces the pain, and palpation localizes the lesion. The injury can occur when performing exercises which force the arms into extension and abduction. Weight-training movements such as bench pressing and gymnastic exercises such as dips on parallel bars may both cause problems. Both the costovertebral and costotransverse joints may be subject to sprain, with pain occurring to rib movements and local palpation.

Costochondral pain must be differentiated from pain referral into the area from myocardial infarction, and from pathologies such as psoriatic arthritis or ankylosing spondylitis. In chest pain from myocardial infarction there is no history of sports trauma, and pain is vice-like and often described as a 'clenched fist' feeling, which may refer up into the jaw. Pain of rib origin will be affected by rib movement and posture, and is generally well localized. Medical pathologies affecting the ribs will generally have been present for some time and are differentiated by blood tests. Tests include the HLA-B27 genetic marker and erythrocyte sedimentation rate (ESR), which tests for non-specific inflammation throughout the body.

> **Key point**
> Ribcage pain must be differentiated from medical conditions affecting the ribs, and referred pain of visceral (internal organ) origin.

First rib injury

The first is the shortest and roundest of the ribs. It slopes downwards and forwards from its attachment to the first thoracic vertebra. It forms attachment for the scalene muscles, serratus anterior, and subclavius. Its superior surface bears a deep groove for the subclavian artery (posterior) and the subclavian vein (anterior). The arterial groove is the weakest part of the rib.

Fractures of the first rib may either be traumatic or the result of overuse. Overuse injuries have been reported as a result of repeated arm movements, such as heavy lifting and repetitive throwing. Symptoms are of pain associated with deep breathing, tenderness in the root of the neck, posterior aspect of the shoulder or axilla. Often the patient hears or feels a snap in the shoulder, as when performing a sudden violent movement. Range of shoulder movement will usually be full but painful, especially to extension. Accurate diagnosis by radiographs in traumatic lesions is essential because of the proximity of the major vessels, nerves and lung.

> **Key point**
> First rib injury gives pain on deep breathing. Tenderness is common at the root of the neck, posterior aspect of the shoulder or axilla. Shoulder extension may also cause pain.

429

Management is by rest from the causal action, with shoulder support in a sling if pain is limiting. Gentle isometric shoulder exercises are used, and the condition usually resolves within four to six weeks. Examination of breathing mechanics may be required, and ribcage expansion exercises given in less active individuals.

Rib displacement

Respiratory movements of the ribs may be used to assess anteroposterior position, by comparing one side of the body to the other. If a rib on one side stops moving before the rib on the other side during inhalation, the rib is said to be *depressed*. Inhalation involves an upward movement of the rib, so if the rib stops moving, it has been held down. Similarly, if the rib stops moving during exhalation

(downward movement) it is said to be *elevated*, because it is being held in an upward position.

Movement may also be forward or backward. An *anterior displacement* may occur, with a subluxation of the costovertebral joint, and the rib is sheared forwards. The rib will appear more prominent than its neighbour. This can occur in sport due to a blow to the back, typically when a knee hits the player on the back of the chest in rugby. A *posterior displacement* is more common and presents as a prominence of the rib angle. This is normally due to a blow to the chest, again from a tackle or through seatbelt or steering-wheel trauma in a road traffic accident (RTA). Management of rib displacement is by the use of muscle energy techniques (MET) and rib joint mobilization (see Treatment Note 9.1).

Treatment note 9.1   Manual therapy techniques for rib displacement

Manual therapy techniques encourage correct rib movement during respiration. Essentially, they force the rib into the opposite direction to the one in which they are being held. The rib may be bound down by scar tissue, requiring continuous stretching, or through muscle tightness/shortness, requiring PNF stretching. The intercostal muscles (forced expiration), oblique abdominals (trunk rotation), serratus anterior (scapular protraction), latissimus dorsi (arm adduction), scalenes (first rib, neck-side flexion) and quadratus lumborum (twelfth rib, trunk-side flexion) should all be considered.

Elevation

An elevated rib does not move down far enough during expiration. The aim is to encourage this movement and draw the rib down as the patient breathes out. For the first rib, pressure is placed over the rib with the knuckle (key grip) (Fig. 9.5). The head is side flexed to relax the anterior

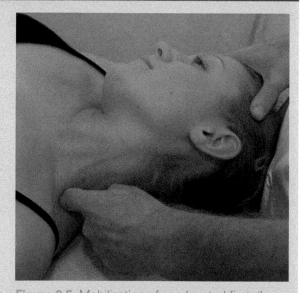

Figure 9.5 Mobilization of an elevated first rib.

scalene and the rib is pressed downwards with expiration. The second rib is gripped within the axilla and pulled downwards as the patient exhales powerfully (Fig. 9.6). The remaining ribs

Treatment note 9.1 *continued*

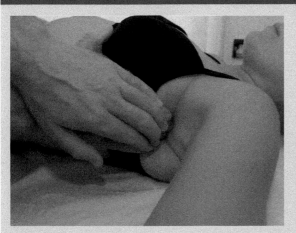

Figure 9.6 Mobilization of an elevated second rib.

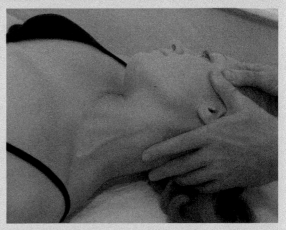

Figure 9.8 Treatment for a depressed first rib using anterior scalene stretch.

may be gripped with the fingertips or pushed downwards using the knife edge of the hand (Fig. 9.7).

Depression

The depressed rib is bound down and stops moving upwards during inspiration. The aim is therefore to encourage further upward movement as the patient breathes in. For the first rib, stretch of the anterior scalenes

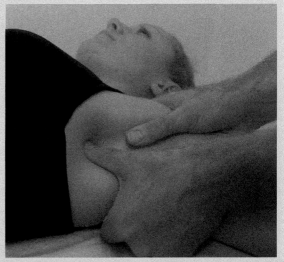

Figure 9.9 Treatment of a depressed second rib using thumb pressure.

is used (side flex the neck to the opposite side) to pull the rib upwards (Fig. 9.8). For the second rib, the finger or thumb pads press on the rib within the axilla (Fig. 9.9), and for the remaining ribs the thumb pad or pisiform presses on the rib undersurface within the intercostal space (Fig. 9.10).

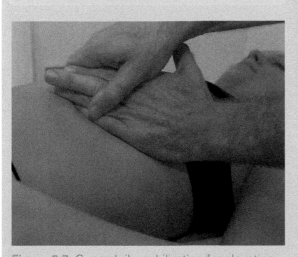

Figure 9.7 General rib mobilization for elevation.

Treatment note 9.1 *continued*

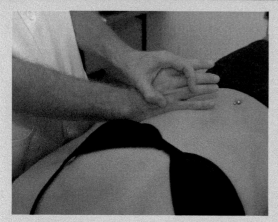

Figure 9.10 Treatment for general rib depression using pisiform grip.

open the ribcage and pull the rib backwards. For an anterior rib on the right, the patient sits at the end of the couch with the therapist to the left. The patient folds the arms across the chest. The therapist hooks his or her fingers over the anterior rib and side-bends the patient to the left to open the ribcage, and rotates to the right to encourage the rib to move back (Fig. 9.11).

Posterior displacement

For a posterior rib, the contact area is with the heel of the hand over the rib angle. For a right posterior displacement, the action is to side-bend to the left to open the ribcage and rotate to the left to draw the rib forwards (Fig. 9.12). An alternative

Anterior displacement

Where the rib lies further forward than the rib on the other side of the body, the aim is to

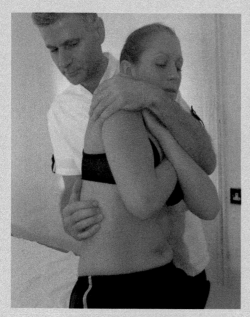

Figure 9.11 Treatment of anterior rib displacement using side-bending.

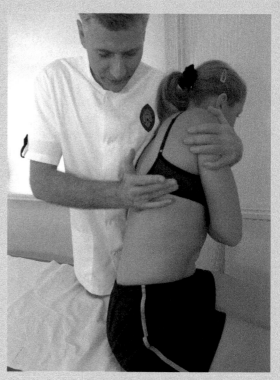

Figure 9.12 Treatment of posterior rib displacement using side flexion.

Treatment note 9.1 *continued*

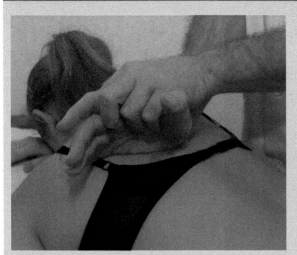

approach is to perform a posteroanterior mobilization on the rib angle while the patient is prone. The pisiform of one hand performs the action while the pisiform of the other presses over the transverse process of the vertebra on the opposite side to prevent the vertebra from rotating as the rib is mobilized (Fig. 9.13).

Figure 9.13 Treatment of a posterior rib in prone lying.

Manual therapy

Joint mobilization

A variety of procedures may be used for the thoracic spine (Fig. 9.14).

- ▶ *Posteroanterior central vertebral pressure* (PAVP) is often the technique used first, in the presence of both unilateral and bilateral symptoms. In the thoracic spine the spinous processes are larger than those of the cervical spine, and so the therapist may use the thumbs either side by side or one in front of the other. For the upper thoracic spine, the therapist stands at the patient's head, and for the lower regions at the patient's side. An oscillatory motion is given, with the range of movement being particularly great in the middle and lower thoracic areas, but somewhat limited between T1 and T2.
- ▶ The *costovertebral* and *costotransverse* joints are mobilized by springing the rib. The therapist places his or her thumbs, or the ulnar border of the hand and little finger, along the line of the rib to be mobilized to give a broad (and more

comfortable) area of contact. The mobilization must take the patient's respiratory movements into account, pressure for higher-grade movements coinciding with expiration.

- ▶ *Anteroposterior movements* (AP) may be performed on any of the costal joints (costochondral, interchondral, sternocostal). The therapist's thumbs are placed over the joint to be mobilized, with the fingers fanning out over the patient's chest. The movement may be directed towards the patient's head or feet to reproduce the symptoms, and then continued in this direction at a lesser grade.
- ▶ *Intervertebral rotations* may be applied both locally and generally. Local rotation may be carried out using pressure over the transverse processes. The thenar eminence of one hand is placed on the transverse process of one vertebra with the fingers pointing towards the patient's head. The hypothenar eminence of the other hand is placed on the transverse process on the opposing side of the spine either of the same vertebra or that of the vertebra below, with the fingers towards the patient's feet. A

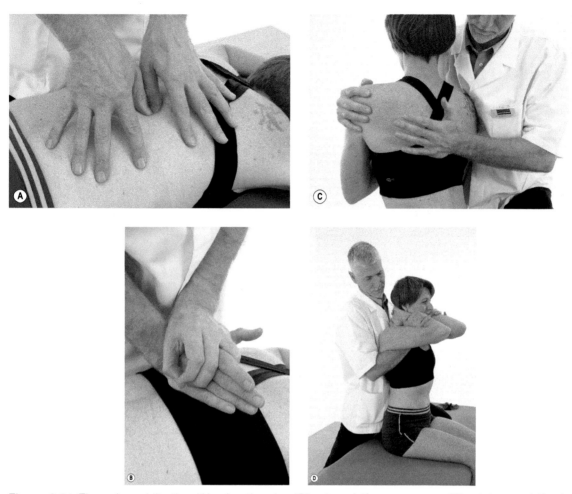

Figure 9.14 Thoracic mobilization (A) using thumbs, (B) using pisiform pressure, (C) rotatory mobilization using heel of hand, (D) extension using leverage.

number of techniques are used. Rotation may be applied by using alternating pressure from one hand and then the other with the hands over the same spinal level, or occasionally a high-velocity, low-amplitude thrust may be applied as the patient breathes out, with the hands over the transverse processes of two levels.

▶ *General rotation* may be performed with the patient seated over the couch end, with the arms folded and the hands gripping the shoulders. The therapist stands to the side of the patient. The patient rotates as far as is possible away from the therapist, who reaches across the patient's chest and grasps the patient's far shoulder. Overpressure is applied as the therapist pulls the far shoulder towards him- or herself and presses the far scapula away with the flat of the hand. Slight traction may be applied by gripping the far elbow rather than the shoulder. The therapist bends his or her knees before applying the grip and then straightens them as he or she pulls up and round. This technique may be used for mobilization or contract–relax stretching.

▶ *Longitudinal mobilization* or traction may be applied to the thoracic spine with the patient sitting and the therapist standing behind them.

434

The patient interlocks their fingers and places their hands behind their neck, elbows pointing forwards rather than outwards. The patient's neck should be comfortably flexed, with the ligamentum nuchae not fully stretched. The therapist winds their arms through the triangular space created by the patient's arms and draws the patient against their chest, adducting their arms to grip the patient's chest slightly. The therapist flexes their knees and rocks the patient forwards and backwards gently. As the patient is drawn backwards, they contact the therapist's chest and are pressed into thoracic extension. The traction force is generated by the therapist straightening their legs. No distraction force should be created by the therapist's arms – an attempt should not be made to lift the patient.

As a general note, the close proximity of structures in the thoracic region makes it difficult to assess precisely whether a patient's symptoms are coming from the intervertebral joint, the costotransverse joint, the costovertebral joints or a combination of all three. For this reason, many of the mobilizations affect all of these joints.

Key point

Mobilization techniques for the thoracic spine affect several joints simultaneously.

Trunk muscles

The trunk muscles are open to injury in the same way as any other muscle in the body, but muscle conditions are often overlooked in the search for signs of more complex injuries involving the intervertebral joints. Injury to the intercostal muscles has already been mentioned, but the abdominal muscles and erector spinae may also give pain from injury or muscle soreness.

Injury to the rectus abdominis has been described in tennis players especially. During the cocking phase of serving, the arm is reached overhead and the spine hyperextended, stretching the rectus and imposing high leverage forces upon the muscle. This action requires highly coordinated sequential muscle activity, which may break down in the presence of fatigue. Injury to the internal oblique can occur as part of a *side strain syndrome* during activities such as cricket, hurdling and javelin throwing, for example. Injury to the lateral abdominals is shown as a positive-resisted side flexion test. MRI scan has shown separate involvement of the internal oblique, external oblique and transversus abdominis (Humphries and Jamison 2004), and in each case the non-dominant side was affected. Isolated injury to the internal oblique has also been described in tennis (Maquirriain and Ghisi 2006), although it is less common. Differential diagnosis must be made from rib fracture and iliac crest avulsion injury, both of which are revealed radiographically.

Key point

In side-strain syndrome the side (lateral) flexor muscles are affected. The condition must be differentiated from rib fracture and iliac crest avulsion injury.

The abdominal muscles are tested isometrically to eliminate involvement of the spine. A crook-lying position may be used to relax the hips and aid comfort. Straight-trunk flexion taxes the rectus abdominis, while flexion–rotation works the oblique abdominals more. Pure rotation is tested in a sitting position, while lateral flexion is tested either in a sitting or standing position.

The upper (supra-umbilical) portion of the *rectus abdominis* is emphasized from a sit-up position, while the lower (infra-umbilical) portion is assessed by lowering the straight or bent legs from 90 degrees hip flexion to work the muscle in a reverse origin to insertion fashion. Comparison is made between the right and left sides of the rectus by palpation and watching the displacement of the umbilicus, which will be pulled to the side of the stronger muscle.

Key point

During abdominal muscle contraction, movement of the umbilicus may be used to identify muscle contraction asymmetry. The umbilicus will deviate towards a stronger muscle, rather than moving inwards (abdominal hollowing), or straight upwards (upper rectus) or downwards (lower rectus).

The *oblique abdominals* are worked by performing rotation and lateral flexion. Rotation may be gauged using a twisting trunk curl action, for example reaching the right arm towards the left knee, or isometric trunk rotation in sitting. Rotation to the left works the right external oblique and left internal oblique, and vice versa. Resisted side flexion is performed grasping the patient's hand and asking them to reach the other hand down to the side of their knee. The *transversus abdominis*

acts to support the viscera and is active in forced expiration. It may be tested with the patient in a prone-kneeling position. From this position, the subject breathes out against a resistance (balloon or spirometer) and pulls the abdominal wall in.

The *erector spinae* are tested in a prone-lying position, the subject being asked to extend the trunk and lift the chest from the couch. Isometric contraction is assessed by having the patient (in a prone-lying position) maintain a horizontal position of the trunk, with only the legs supported. Alternatively, the patient should rest the chest over the couch end and attempt to straighten the legs to a horizontal position. The *quadratus lumborum* is tested with the subject prone, leg extended and slightly abducted, to elevate the pelvis laterally. Traction is placed through the elevated leg to oppose the pull of the quadratus lumborum.

Treatment Note 9.2   Changes to breathing mechanics

We have seen that movement of the ribs and thoracic spine is intimately linked to the mechanics of breathing. Bucket-handle movement occurs when the ribs flare outwards, while pump-handle movement occurs as the sternum is lifted (Fig. 9.15). These two actions expand the ribcage, reducing intrathoracic pressure to allow air to rush into the lungs. This mechanism is further enhanced as the diaphragm descends and the abdominal wall relaxes.

Injury to the ribs, rib joints or thoracic spine can affect the mechanics of breathing, causing a breathing pattern disorder (BPD), sometimes called dysfunctional breathing.

The act of breathing is intimately linked to psychological state and trait, with fear and anxiety tending to speed up both respiration and heart rate. In addition, anxiety states can cause shallow breathing and breath restricted to the upper regions of the chest.

Assessment of breathing can therefore be useful following injury to the thorax, and in persistent pain states.

Dysfunctional breathing may be assessed using the Manual Assessment of Respiratory Motion (MARM). This is a manual technique designed to differentiate between upward movement of the sternum (length breathing) and sideways expansion of the ribcage (width breathing). In addition, any asymmetry existing between the two sides of the ribcage is noted. The MARM has been compared with respiratory inductance plethysmography (RIP), and to be reliable for assessing breathing pattern in a small study (twelve subjects, two examiners). High levels of agreement were found between examiners comparing MARM to RIP when measuring upper ribcage relative to lower ribcage/abdomen motion, but not for measures of volume.

Treatment note 9.2 *continued*

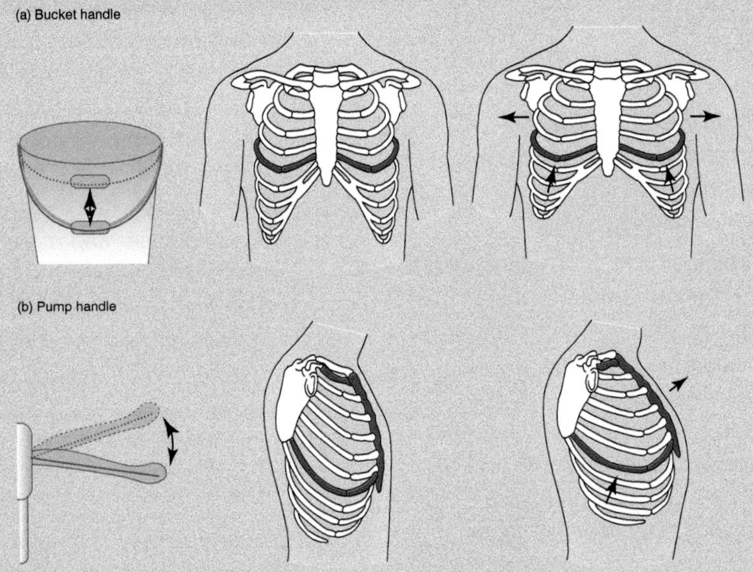

Figure 9.15 Ribcage movement during breathing.

Definition

Respiratory inductance plethysmography (RIP) is a method of evaluating chest motion during breathing (ventilation). It measures movement of the chest and abdominal wall, using elastic transducer bands placed around the chest (mid-axillary level) and abdomen (umbilical level).

Dysfunctional breathing is said to occur when a subject presents with breathlessness (dyspnoea) in the absence of respiratory disease. Five main classifications have been described (Boulding et al. 2016), as shown in Table 9.4.

Management of the condition includes assessing and treating any ribcage or thoracic spine movement restrictions, and changing the breathing pattern using respiratory exercises such as selective rib area expansion, diaphragmatic breathing, breath retention and breath timing. A respiratory-muscle training device may also be useful. These can provide loading to inspiration or expiration to develop muscle strength and/or endurance.

Table 9.4 Classification of dysfunctional breathing

Classification	Symptoms
Hyperventilation syndrome	Associated with symptoms that are related to respiratory alkalosis (such as dizziness, numbness in the hands and feet, and discomfort in the chest) but independent of hypocapnia (reduced CO_2 in the blood).
Periodic deep sighing	Frequent sighing with an irregular breathing pattern.
Thoracic dominant breathing	High (apical) thoracic wall movement with little evidence of lateral expansion.
Forced abdominal expiration	Subject utilizes inappropriate and excessive abdominal muscle contraction to aid expiration.
Thoraco-abdominal asynchrony	Delay between ribcage and abdominal contraction resulting in ineffective breathing mechanics.

CO_2 – carbon dioxide.
(Data from Boulding et al. 2016)

Hernia

A hernia is a protrusion of the contents of a cavity through the cavity wall. Most usually an organ or peritoneum is forced through the muscular layer of the abdominal wall at sites of natural weakness where nerves and blood vessels leave the abdomen. The most common types are femoral, inguinal and incisional. Less common types include umbilical, epigastric and hiatus herniae.

▶ *Inguinal herniae* occur as a result of damage or malformation of the structures forming the inguinal canal (see below). The herniated tissue passes through the *myopectineal orifice* (MPO). This area is bordered by the internal oblique and transversus above, rectus abdominis medially, iliopsoas laterally, and the pectineal ligament below. The hernia may be either *direct* or *indirect*, and is far more common in men than women. As the testis descends during foetal life, it drags with it a tube-like covering of peritoneum, the processus vaginalis, which is usually obliterated. If this tube remains, it constitutes a weakness which may lead to an indirect inguinal hernia. This usually occurs in males and on the right side of the body. Direct inguinal herniae are more common in older men, and rupture through the weak abdominal wall. They are precipitated by obesity, persistent coughing, and straining. Symptoms of an inguinal hernia are of a dragging sensation in the groin, especially when straining. A swelling may be noticeable over the external ring of the inguinal canal above and medial to the pubic tubercle, the point of attachment of adductor longus. In the case of an indirect hernia, the bulge may be in the upper scrotum. A bulge may be palpated over the hernia when the patient coughs. It is possible in principle to pass the little finger through the skin of the upper scrotum to the external ring of the inguinal canal, following the line of the spermatic cord, although this procedure in practice is painful. The patient is supine, and the examining finger is directed upwards, backwards and laterally. Again,

coughing will produce a bulge when hernia is present.

▶ *Femoral hernia* is a protrusion of abdominal contents through the femoral ring, which is the point below the inguinal ligament where the blood vessels enter the leg. The condition is more common in women than men. The features are essentially similar to those of the inguinal hernia, except that the femoral hernia is generally smaller and more difficult to detect.

▶ *Epigastric hernia* travels through the linea alba. A small bulge (usually of fat) is found between the two recti above the umbilicus.

▶ *Umbilical hernia* is due to failure of the umbilical ring to close completely. Later in life this may dilate as a result of a rapid increase in intra-abdominal pressure. These hernias may be very large.

▶ *Hiatus hernia* is a rupture of a portion of the stomach through the oesophageal hiatus in the diaphragm. This type of hernia generally gives no symptoms in itself, but may, in turn, cause reflux and oesophagitis, giving heartburn. In addition, reflux of bitter irritating fluid into the pharynx and mouth may occur. Antacids are used to neutralize gastric contents, and weight loss and dietary modification (small frequent meals, avoidance of foods inducing symptoms) are used initially.

▶ *Incisional hernias* occur after abdominal surgery through the weak area created by the incision.

Initial management of hernias is conservative, and involves instruction on actions to avoid increasing intra-abdominal pressure. When symptoms persist, surgery may be required.

Key point
Inguinal hernia is more common in men, femoral hernia more common in women.

Surgical management and rehabilitation

Open repair is performed under a full anaesthetic and usually results in an 8 cm incision. The hernial sac is either pushed back inside the body or removed, and a plastic mesh placed over the back of the weakened area to create a tension-free repair. The skin covering the mesh is closed using dissolving sutures. Using keyhole surgery, three cuts (0.5–1.5 cm) are made into the lower abdomen. Again, a plastic mesh is secured over the hernia area and the skin is repaired using dissolving sutures. As the keyholes are much smaller than the incision of an open repair, skin healing is faster.

Following surgery, it is essential that abdominal muscle contraction is redeveloped, as pain inhibition will often prevent spontaneous recovery. During the *immediate post-operative period* there are two main concerns: the effect of the anaesthetic and the activities of daily living. Fluid intake should be increased to avoid dehydration, which will result in a dry stool. Advise the subject to support their scar with the flat of their hand or a large soft pillow. Standard checking of the dressing should be made to ensure no leakage is occurring. Scar-site infection should be suspected where body temperature rises, requiring urgent medical referral. Deep breathing exercises are used to avoid air stagnation within the lungs.

By two to five days post-surgery, walking should be normal, with the patient encouraged not to stoop to try to protect the repair area. Ice or cold may be used over the scar area to ease swelling but temperature should be monitored closely as local skin sensation will be impaired. Pelvic floor exercise and abdominal hollowing should be begun as pain allows. Muscle retraining should use tactile cueing (touch and skin brushing), visualization and visual cueing, and repeated contractions. For this latter technique, the deep abdominal muscles are tightened (hollowing), relaxed partially and then tightened again, this time to a greater intensity. From seven to ten days, exercise intensity and functionality should be increased progressively.

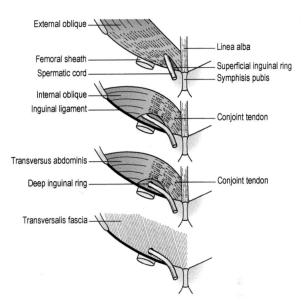

Figure 9.16 Formation of the inguinal canal. From Palastanga, Field and Soames (1994), with permission.

Sportsman's hernia

Sportsman's hernia, or groin disruption, is a condition which may mimic inguinal hernia in many ways. To understand the condition, we need to look at the structure of the region.

The inguinal canal (Fig. 9.16) is approximately 4 cm long, and transports the spermatic cord in the male, the round ligament in the female, and in both sexes the ilioinguinal nerve. Its anterior wall is formed from the aponeurosis (tendon sheet) of the external oblique, supported by the internal oblique muscle at its lateral third. The posterior wall is from the transversalis fascia, reinforced by the conjoint tendon at its medial third. The roof of the canal is formed by the internal oblique and transversus abdominis as they merge to form the conjoint tendon running from the pubic crest to the pectineal line of the pelvis. The deep inguinal ring is about 1.5 cm above the mid-point of the inguinal ligament and is an opening in the transversalis fascia. The superficial inguinal ring is a hole in the external oblique aponeurosis and lies at the medial end of the tendon above the pubic tubercle.

Table 9.5 Sportsman's hernia: tissue pathology and history

Tissues affected	Typical signs and symptoms	Differential diagnosis
Transversalis fascia	Deep pain to groin/lower abdomen	Hip structures
Posterior inguinal wall	Pain exacerbated by sport-specific activities	Bone injury
Insertion of distal rectus abdominis		Neurological involvement
Conjoined tendon at its attachment to the anterosuperior pubis	Palpable tenderness over rectus insertion	Inguinal hernia
External oblique aponeurosis	Pain with resisted hip abduction	Osteitis pubis
	Pain with resisted trunk curl	Adductor strain
		Iliopsoas teninosis
		Rectus abdominis strain

Unverzagt, Schuemann and Mathisen (2008); Kachingwe and Grech (2008).

Definition

The transversalis fascia is part of a membranous bag lining the abdomen; (i) it lies on the deep surface of the transversus abdominis muscle, (ii) its thick lower portion is attached to the inguinal ligament, (iii) the femoral vessels drag the fascia with them as they travel into the leg, forming the femoral sheath.

Sportsman's hernia (athletic pubalgia) has been described as injury of the muscular and fascial attachments to the anterior pubis (Kachingwe and Grech 2008). Several structures may be involved (Table 9.5), with up to 85 per cent of injuries involving the posterior wall of the inguinal canal (Sheen et al. 2014). The condition can include a tearing of the external oblique aponeurosis and the conjoint tendon, causing the superficial inguinal ring to dilate (Fig. 9.17). There may be a dehiscence (separation) between the conjoint tendon and the inguinal ligament but no hernial sac (Gilmore 1995). As the condition is not a true herniation, the term inguinal disruption (ID) is to be preferred (Sheen et al. 2014). The transversalis fascia may weaken and separate from the conjoint tendon and the external oblique has been said to tear at

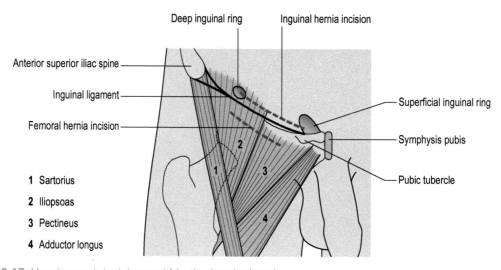

Figure 9.17 Hernia repair incisions within the inguinal region.

the site of emergence of the anterior ramus of the iliohypogastric nerve (Williams and Foster 1995).

The condition was originally described in soccer players but may occur in other sports. As many as 28 per cent of soccer players may experience the condition (Kemp and Batt 1998), and 50 per cent of male athletes presenting with groin pain lasting longer than eight weeks have been found during surgery to have sports herniae (Lovell 1995).

There is a gradual onset of pain, with a third of patients reporting a specific injury which may have resulted in tearing. Pain (in the inguinal, adductor or perineal region close to the pubic tubercle) is exacerbated by sports-specific kicking actions and sudden changes in movement direction.

> **Key point**
>
> Inguinal disruption gives pain (insidious or acute onset) in the groin area near the pubic tubercle.

The superficial inguinal ring is often dilated to palpation. Tenderness to palpation over the conjoint tendon and inguinal canal is increased by a resisted sit-up action. It is usual for several pathologies to coexist, with sportsman's hernia occurring alongside adductor tendinitis. In a study of athletes with groin pain for more than three months, 19 out of 21 were found to have two or more separate pathologies (Ekberg, Persson and Abrahamson 1988), and in general 25–30 per cent of athletes with this condition can be expected to have a secondary diagnosis (Lovell 1995).

> **Key point**
>
> A sportsman's hernia is a separation of the external oblique aponeurosis from the inguinal ligament. It is a muscle attachment injury rather than a true hernia, and no protrusion (hernial sac) is present.

Imaging may not identify the tissue affected, but is important to rule out alternative diagnoses (Sheen et al. 2014). Endoscopic examination may be used, and followed by immediate repair where a defect is found. Ultrasonography may be used to identify the tissue changes at the exact point of tenderness. Coupled with a Valsalva manoeuvre, ultrasound can differentiate true herniation from simple tissue overstretch. The use of colour Doppler permits the visualization of the epigastric vessels, and can assist in the differentiation of sports hernia from inguinal hernia. Direct inguinal hernia is said to lie medial to the inferior epigastric vessels, while indirect hernia lies laterally to this vessel (Hagan et al. 2007).

Treatment

The British Hernia Society's 2014 position statement on Sportsman's groin (Sheen et al. 2014) stated that a 'full physiotherapy rehabilitation regime (should be) undertaken prior to any surgery being contemplated'. Surgical (open or laparoscopic) treatment aims to release abnormal tension in the inguinal canal and to reconstruct the posterior wall weakness. Repair is often performed using polypropylene mesh, with the external oblique repaired and the inguinal ring reconstituted. Surgical success rates have been reported between 63 and 93 per cent (Kemp and Batt 1998), possibly reflecting the presence of additional pathologies.

Both prevention (Gilmore 1995, Norris 1995) and successful rehabilitation of this condition rely heavily on correct abdominal training. One of the factors in the development of this condition may be a muscle imbalance which favours tightness in the hip flexors, combined with preferential recruitment of the rectus abdominis and poor recruitment of the deep abdominals. Such imbalance may leave the lower abdominal area open to injury. Increasing the training emphasis on abdominal hollowing actions and reducing the emphasis on lumbar flexion actions may be a key factor which should be combined with stretching where hip flexor tightness is apparent.

In addition, dominance of the adductor muscles in certain sports such as soccer should be considered.

Table 9.6 Muscle balance exercises for sports hernia

Hip adductor stretch – straighten and slightly hollow the back by tilting the pelvis forwards. Press the knees downwards and hold the position for 30 s. Repeat 5 times.	
Hip flexor stretch – tighten abdominal muscles to stabilize pelvis and avoid low back extension. Lunge forwards forcing the hip into extension. Hold for 30 s and repeat 5 times.	
Hip abductor inner range work – lift bent knee upwards and outwards (abduction and lateral rotation) avoiding movement of the pelvis or spine. Hold the outer position for 10 s and repeat 10 times.	
Hip extensor (gluteal) inner range work – tighten abdominal muscles to prevent pelvic tilt, and lift bent leg. Maintain position for 10 s and then release.	
Isolation and re-education of the deep abdominals (core stabilizers) – maintain the neutral position of the spine. Draw the abdominal wall inwards in a hollowing action, hold for 10 s (breathing normally). Repeat 10 times.	
Building endurance of the core stabilizers – perform an abdominal hollowing action and maintain the neutral position of the spine. Allow one leg to slide out straight, avoiding pelvic tilt. Perform 5 times on each leg.	

Stretching the tight adductors and working the abductors proportionally should be considered. It has been suggested that repeated adductor actions create a shearing force across the pubic symphysis that places stress on the posterior inguinal wall (Simonet, Saylor and Sim 1995). In support of this hypothesis, it is common clinically to find athletes who have coexisting osteitis pubis and/or adductor tendinitis. Muscle balance exercises relevant to the prevention and rehabilitation of this condition are shown in Table 9.6.

Key point

Muscle balance assessment is essential in the management of sports hernia. Tight hip flexors and hip adductors, together with dominance of the superficial abdominals over the core stabilizers, is often found.

Table 9.7 presents an example rehabilitation programme for inguinal disruption with and without operative repair.

Thoracic outlet syndrome

Thoracic outlet syndrome (TOS) affects the *superior thoracic aperture*, a region bordered by the T1 vertebra posteriorly, the medial edge of the first rib and the manubrium of the sternum. TOS is a compression of the neurovascular structures travelling to the axilla from the cervical region and typically involves the brachial plexus rather than the nerve roots (Fig. 9.18). Symptoms appear in the arm rather than the neck, with the lower cervical and upper thoracic area (C7/T1) most commonly affected. Bilateral tingling appears over the median or ulnar nerve distributions into the forearm and hand. The anatomy of the region favours compression. The nervous structures travel through the costoclavicular space, formed by the inner clavicle, first rib and insertions of the scalene muscles. The lower trunk of the brachial plexus and the subclavian artery travel through the outlet formed between the scalenus anterior and scalenus medius to rest on the first rib. Symptoms

Table 9.7 Example rehabilitation programme of inguinal disruption (ID)

	Timescale	Activity
Non-operative	▶ Range of motion tests of spine, hip, and muscle length	▶ Strengthening/lengthening with or without soft-tissue work
	▶ Strength tests of gluteals, and deep abdominals	▶ Re-education of deep muscle control
	▶ Spine and hip muscle assessment	▶ Re-strengthening where weakness/asymmetry found
Post-operative	Week 1	▶ Isometric deep abdominals and pelvic floor (no breath hold)
		▶ Isometric hip musculature (no breath hold)
		▶ Re-education of diaphragmatic breathing
		▶ Spinal (ROM exercise)
		▶ Early walking programme
	Week 2	▶ Increase walking distance/time
		▶ Static cycle as tolerated
		▶ Continue isometrics and active spinal ROM
	Week 3	▶ Begin functional work emphasis
		▶ Swiss ball activities
		▶ Active mobility
		▶ Swimming where wound healed
		▶ Begin running programme (run/walk initially)
	Week 4	▶ Active assisted work to re-educate concentric/eccentric patterns
		▶ Multidirectional running
		▶ Begin and progress sports specific rehab
	Week 5	▶ Continue and progress concentric/eccentric patterns
		▶ Begin and progress light weight training
		▶ Introduce early jumping/landing/pushing/pulling actions

ROM – range of motion
(Data modified from Sheen et al. 2014)

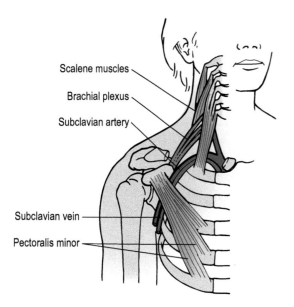

Scalene muscles

Brachial plexus

Subclavian artery

Subclavian vein

Pectoralis minor

Figure 9.18 Thoracic outlet syndrome.

from vascular compression are less common than those from neurological involvement, but alteration in blood flow may be used as a test for the condition (see below).

Predisposing factors

The more oblique slope of the first rib in the female changes the costoscalene angle, and may account for the increased incidence of the condition in females. Lower down, the neurovascular structures pass into the axilla beneath the coracoid process and the tendon of pectoralis minor.

Table 9.8 Postural presentation in thoracic outlet syndrome

Descended scapulae, compressing the subclavian artery and lower trunk of the brachial plexus over the first rib
Possible complication of cervical rib seen on X-ray
Soft tissue contracture limiting range of motion at shoulder joint and girdle
Reduced movement in upper/mid-thoracic region (dowager's hump)
Tenderness to palpation of upper/mid-thoracic segments and costal joints
Head protraction

Adapted from Grieve (1986).

In the non-athlete, middle-aged women are most commonly affected, with the typical clinical picture consisting of a round shouldered posture displaying a 'dowager's hump' between C7 and T1. The thoracic kyphosis is usually stiff, showing tight pectoral tissues and limited shoulder movements. The thoracic segments and rib angles are often exquisitely tender. The pectoral girdle muscles may have weakened through prolonged disuse, and a 'poking chin' head position is common. This postural complex is summarized in Table 9.8.

In the athletic population, postural changes due to the nature of a sport will make the condition more likely, especially in overhead sporting actions. Excessive shoulder depression or overdevelopment of the trapezius and neck musculature in sports such as American football, rugby and throwing sports will put the athlete at risk. Tightness in the pectoralis minor may occur in swimmers. In tennis players, asymmetrical development with excessive scapular depression has been described (Zachazewski, Magee and Quillen 1996). Subjects complain of pain and difficulty in gripping.

Carrying heavy objects or wearing a heavy coat exacerbates the problem, and simply allowing the arm to hang freely by the side can cause aching. The condition is seen commonly as an occupational injury, with the subject often noticing increased pain when reaching overhead. Typically, this pattern also occurs when a middle-aged woman takes up exercise in a keep-fit class. When severe, vascular signs such as coldness, blueing or whiteness of the skin may occur if the subclavian artery is affected. Equally, the patient may be woken at night with pain, or can experience numbness first thing in the morning.

Provocative tests for TOS

Various provocative tests are available which aim to reproduce the patient's symptoms. Sustained scapular elevation, or simply holding the arms overhead, may increase the signs. The *Adson test* examines the radial pulse while the patient breathes in deeply and holds the breath, at the same time extending the neck and rotating it either towards

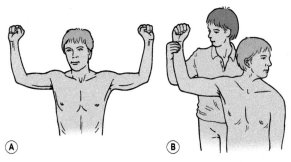

Figure 9.19 Provocative tests for thoracic outlet syndrome. (A) EAST test. (B) Modified Adson's test.

or away from the affected side. Abduction of the shoulder to 90 degrees with full external rotation, combined with vigorous hand movements, may give rise to symptoms if compression is significant. This is sometimes called the elevated arm stress test (*EAST*) or abduction–external rotation (AER) position test (Fig. 9.19). In addition, exaggerating the military posture and at the same time placing longitudinal traction through the arms may limit the costoclavicular space and reproduce symptoms.

Examination of the thoracic spine should also be made to differentiate the condition from T4 syndrome (see below), and the long-sitting slump test and upper limb tension tests should be performed.

Treatment

Conservative management is to elevate the scapulae in the first instance. Simply strengthening the trapezius may have little effect, first because the trapezius, as an anti-gravity muscle, is usually very strong, and second because the stronger muscle may still not be used correctly. Postural re-education may be more successful, teaching a less depressed shoulder girdle resting position. Enhancement of scapular stability with scapular repositioning exercises, and modification of sport technique, will also be required.

Tightness of the scalenes and pectoral muscles can respond to gentle PNF stretching techniques, and trigger-point deactivation. Mobilization procedures

of the thoracic spine are also helpful. Where neural tension tests are positive, mobilization of the neural tissues is required.

Vascular involvement

Vascular conditions which affect the upper limb in sport and daily living, although rare, are important, and are described in this chapter rather than Chapter 13. If missed, these conditions can lead to vascular insufficiency, with serious long-term effects. Early retirement from sport may be one result, but the worst-case scenario is death as a result of a thromboembolus (Taylor and Kerry 2003). Five more common vascular conditions are described below.

▶ **Occlusion of the subclavian artery** may be either external or internal. External occlusion within the thoracic outlet may be due to muscle imbalance, typically with overactivity of the anterior scalene, pectoralis minor or subclavius muscles. Bone changes within the area include those of the cervical rib or altered shape of the first rib. Internal occlusion occurs as a result of underlying atherosclerotic disease.

▶ **Subclavian-axillary artery aneurysm** carries the risk of exacerbation into thrombosis or embolism into the hand. The aneurysm may present as a pulsating mass within the supraclavicular or infraclavicular regions. Typically, repetitive trauma damages the vessel and the thrombosis forms as part of the repair process, involving fibrin and platelets to block up the damaged region. If part of the clot breaks loose, it will migrate into the vessels of the hand.

▶ **Posterior circumflex humeral artery** injury occurs through external compression of the distal portion of the axillary artery. The condition most usually occurs in conjunction with humeral head damage or subluxation. Symptoms are exacerbated during motions which combine abduction with external rotation of the upper arm.

▶ **Vascular trauma to the hand** may occur through repeated striking or catching actions which gives a localized compression of the vessels with signs of ischaemia (whitening of the skin and cold fingers) in the hand.

▶ **Deep vein thrombosis** (DVT) may occur within an upper limb vein (Paget-Schroetter syndrome), and is thought to account for 3 to 7 per cent of all DVTs (Taylor and Kerry 2003). A combination of hypercoagulability, blood flow (haemodynamic) changes and vessel wall (endothelial) damage must have occurred to form a thrombosis, a principle known as *Virchow's triad*. Changes in blood coagulation may occur through drug usage, in pregnancy, following trauma and with heavy smoking. Interruption in blood flow includes turbulence and stasis, while damage to the vessel wall lining (endothelium) may occur with hypertension or trauma. Upper limb DVT is more common in sports such as bodybuilding where marked muscle hypertrophy occurs.

Definition

A thrombosis is a blood clot which forms within a blood vessel, occluding its flow. An embolism occurs when part of the thrombosis clot breaks loose and blocks a vessel further down.

Assessment of vascular involvement

The presentation of vascular injury can closely mimic other musculoskeletal conditions, but closer observation of the patient is often revealing. *Skin changes*, including temperature and colour alterations, may be noticed, with distal symptoms increasing on exertion. Symptoms will most commonly be provoked by placing the athlete's limb into positions with a history of pain and increasing effort. Examination of the *nail bed* will often show capillary refill time to be prolonged. Here, the athlete's nail is compressed until it goes white and then is released. Normal pink skin colour should return immediately on pressure release; failure to do so suggests vascular insufficiency.

Key point

Capillary refill time is assessed by compressing the nail beds on the affected limb and comparing to the unaffected side. The nail goes white on compression and should return to normal skin colour upon release. Slowing of colour restoration indicates vascular involvement.

Distal pulses should be examined during positional changes and after exertion. Pulses on both sides of the body should be taken and compared. Following exertion, the pulse strength should increase. Where vascular insufficiency results from compression by muscle, pulse strength can reduce in the distal limb following exertion. Assessment of the pulse is refined by using *Doppler ultrasound*. This measures the velocity of blood flowing towards and away from the machine probe to give an audible signal. The *Allen test* is also commonly used for upper limb vascular conditions. The test measures the collateral circulation in the hand, which is supplied by the radial and ulnar arteries. To perform the test the athlete lifts their hand overhead and opens and closes their fist for 30 seconds. The therapist applies pressure over both the radial and ulnar arteries to cut off the blood flow to the hand. Keeping the hand elevated, the hand is opened, and it appears whitened. Pressure is released from the ulnar artery and colour should return in seven to ten seconds, showing that the artery is normal. The test is repeated releasing the radial artery. The *arm to arm blood pressure index* (AABI) may also be used, which measures the systolic pressure of the symptomatic arm and compares this to the unaffected arm, both before and after effort. A difference greater than 30–50 mmHg in systolic pressure is said to indicate reduced subclavian blood flow (Alan and Kerry 2003).

T4 syndrome

The T4 syndrome produces vague widespread symptoms of pain and paraesthesia in the upper limbs and head, possibly with autonomic involvement. Any region between T2 and T7 may be affected, but the focus is normally around T4. The distribution of symptoms in the hand is glove-like, in contrast to that of thoracic outlet syndrome, but many subjects have sensations extending from the wrist and forearm. Head symptoms appear in a 'skull cap' distribution, and the patient is commonly woken with pain. Onset may be due to unaccustomed activities or trauma (road traffic accident), but in many cases there is no specific history of injury. As with thoracic outlet syndrome, a predisposing factor is postural. Head protraction, shoulder girdle protraction and accentuated thoracic kyphosis are common, and place a stretch on the thoracic tissues.

Key point

Thoracic outlet syndrome gives bilateral tingling over the median or ulnar nerve distributions into the forearm and hand, but generally no head symptoms. T4 syndrome gives glove-like symptoms affecting the whole hand, and altered sensation in a skull-cap distribution over the head.

On examination, movements can be localized by performing rotations and flexion/extension from a slumped sitting starting position. Palpation is carried out with the patient prone, head in mid-position, with the therapist standing at the patient's head. The patient's forearms hang over the couch side and the upper arms are abducted to 90 degrees to widen the interscapular space. Signs of joint localization include pain, resistance to passive movement and guarding muscle spasm. Common findings include alteration of the alignment of one spinous process in comparison with its neighbours, with local pain to palpation. Examination must take in the cervical spine and first rib. The first rib is palpated above the centre of the clavicle, with the direction of pressure aimed towards the patient's lower scapula.

Mobilization is used for any joints which exhibited signs at examination, and may be carried out with the subject in prone or supine (Fig. 9.20). In prone, the therapist places their hands either side of T4 using a pisiform contact. The hands aim to contact the transverse processes (TP), with the fingers of one hand pointing outwards (laterally) and those of the opposite hand towards the head (cephalad). The hands move in opposition to produce the joint mobilization. In a supine position, the subject's arms are folded across the chest and hands placed over the anterior aspect of the shoulders. The

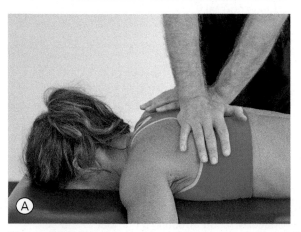
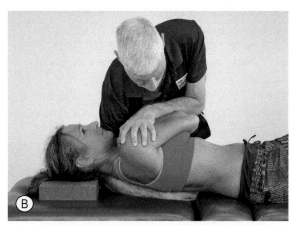

Figure 9.20 Thoracic spine mobilization techniques (A) PA rotary mobilization in prone, (B) PA mobilization in supine.

therapist places one hand beneath the patient's thoracic spine, with the side of the hand in contact with the area to be mobilized. Alternatively, a mobilization wedge may be used. Downward pressure is exerted through the patient's arms onto the therapist's hand. Postural correction may be carried out as with thoracic outlet syndrome.

Posteroanterior (PA) rotary joint mobilization (Grade III) to the T4 vertebra has been shown to produce sympathoexcitatory effects in the hand in a small (n=36) double blind, placebo-controlled trial. Skin conductance was measured continuously, and results demonstrated a significant difference between groups (Jowsey and Perry 2010). A meta-analysis of eleven papers assessing manual therapy to the cervical and thoracic spines has shown statistically significant changes in skin conductance, skin temperature, pain and range of motion (ROM) during upper-limb neurodynamic testing (Chu et al. 2014). These finding suggest that manual therapy may be useful for modifying symptoms in T4 syndrome.

Scheuermann's disease

Scheuermann's disease (juvenile osteochondrosis of the spine) is a condition predominantly affecting the thoracic spine around T9, although the lumbar levels may be involved. The condition is more common in males, and occurs in about 6 per cent of the adolescent population in the 12–18 age group. There is a disturbance of the normal ossification of the vertebrae. The vertebrae ossify from three centres, one at the centre of the vertebral body and two secondary centres (the ring epiphyses) in the cartilage end plates. In Scheuermann's disease there is an alteration of the normal development of the ring epiphyses, but avascular necrosis does not occur, in contrast to true osteochondrosis. Penetration of discal material is often seen through the cartilage end plate of the disc and into the vertebral body (Schmorl's nodes). The changes are largely developmental, but trauma may play a part in exacerbating the condition. In contrast, when the central bony nucleus is affected, Calve's vertebral osteochondritis is present, a much less common condition affecting a single vertebra. To make the radiographic diagnosis of Scheuermann's disease, three consecutive vertebral bodies must be wedged to at least 5 degrees.

Definition

Scheuermann's disease affects several vertebrae, Calve's affects a single vertebra.

The changes in Scheuermann's disease are primarily to the anterior margins of the thoracic vertebrae as these bear greater weight. The disc narrows anteriorly, and deficient growth of the vertebral body occurs as a result of epiphyseal malformation. The vertebra gradually takes on a wedged formation. Normally, several vertebrae are affected in the thoracic spine. The athlete is usually a skeletally immature adolescent, with a 'rounded back' posture. In the active stage of the condition there may be localized pain, often provoked by repeated thoracic flexion as occurs in certain swimming strokes (butterflier's back) and aerobic dance classes. Deep notches are visible over the anterior corners of the vertebrae on X-ray, and these appear sclerotic rather than rarefied (Fig. 9.21). The ring epiphyses are irregular, but the erythrocyte sedimentation rate (ESR) is normal.

Key point

In Scheuermann's disease, several thoracic vertebrae take on a wedged formation, giving a rounded back posture. Pain is exacerbated by repeated thoracic flexion.

The condition is self-limiting, with pain generally ceasing at the end of skeletal growth. In the active stage rest is required, and thoracic taping may reduce pain through deload. In more severe cases, especially those affecting a number of thoracic segments where kyphosis exceeds 30 degrees, a spinal brace (Milwaukee brace) may be required to

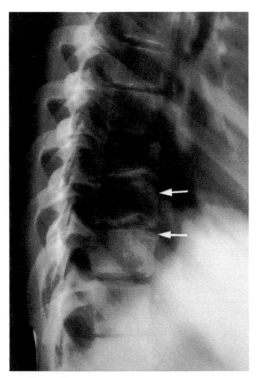

Figure 9.21 Radiographic appearance of Scheuermann's disease. From Read (2000), with permission.

prevent gross deformity. An exercise programme to prevent further deformity is important. This normally involves strengthening in extension and patient education to avoid repeated flexion during activities and prolonged flexion in sitting and lying. Assessment should also be made of soft tissue length and strength and rehabilitation planned accordingly.

A four- to six-week rehabilitation programme consisting of postural re-education, physiotherapy pain modalities (including acupuncture) and psychological support has been shown to reduce pain by 16–32 per cent in a study of 351 patients with Scheuermann's disease (Weiss, Dieckmann and Gerner 2002). The maximum kyphotic angle was reduced from an average of 60.7 degrees prior to treatment to 54.9 degrees following physiotherapy treatment (Weiss, Dieckmann and Gerner 2003).

Exercise therapy for the thoracic spine

As well as restoring fitness components to this body area (such as mobility and strength) following injury, posture can be a prime consideration. One of the common postural faults in this region is an increase in kyphosis. The increased thoracic curve often begins with scapular abduction, which moves the centre of gravity of the upper body forwards. In time, the thoracic spine flexes further as a result of the change in equilibrium. The increased curvature has a direct effect on scapulohumeral rhythm by limiting scapulothoracic motion and preventing the final degrees of abduction and extension of the glenohumeral joint (see Chapter 12). Reversing this trend requires a reduction in thoracic curvature to move the centre of gravity posteriorly, shortening of the shoulder retractors, and often restoration of correct shoulder depressor action. In the following section, examples are given of exercises to correct thoracic curvature by increasing extension. General examples of mobility exercises are also given for use in the restoration phase of injury.

Thoracic extension can be performed in a lying or kneeling position. The pelvis is posteriorly tilted to flatten and block the lumbar spine, and the arms are lifted to the side and eventually overhead (Fig. 9.22A). Lifting the sternum to extend the thoracic spine without expanding the ribcage (Fig. 9.22B) is also a useful exercise and may be practised in a sitting, high kneeling or standing position. In high kneeling (Fig. 9.22C), thoracic extension is performed by pressing (thrusting) the chest forwards and up, while at the same time drawing the scapulae downwards (depression). Passive extension may be performed by lying over a rolled towel, with the towel positioned at the apex of the thoracic curve. If the head does not rest on the mat, a thin pillow is used to prevent a protracted head position.

Thoracic mobility to rotation and lateral flexion may be localized to various segmental levels (Fig. 9.23). Mobility to rotation is performed in a sitting position, and may be localized by changing the position of the arms. Leaving the arms at the sides

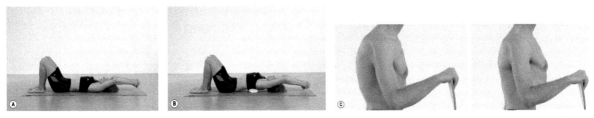

Figure 9.22 Exercise therapy for thoracic extension. (A) Thoracic extension, (B) Thoracic extension using towel as pivot, (C) Sternal lift.

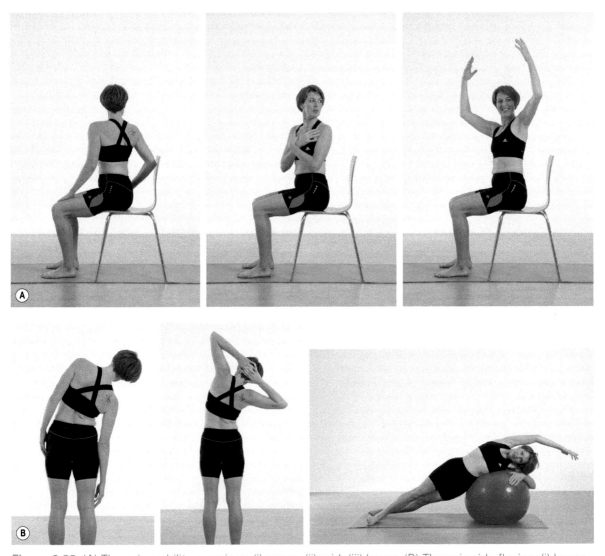

Figure 9.23 (A) Thoracic mobility exercises: (i) upper, (ii) mid, (iii) lower. (B) Thoracic side flexion: (i) lower region, (ii) upper region, (iii) side flexor stretch.

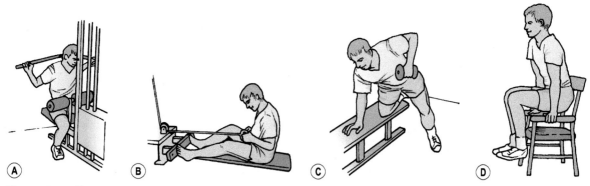

Figure 9.24 Resistance exercises for the thorax. (A) Lateral pull down. (B) Seated rowing. (C) One arm dumb-bell row. (D) Modified dip.

and leading the movement with the head (looking around to the direction of movement) will focus movement to the upper thoracic spine. Holding the elbows horizontally stresses the mid-thoracic spine, while when reaching overhead the pull is through the thoracolumbar fascia to stress the lower thoracic spine. Side (lateral) flexion may be mobilized by side-bending against a wall to prevent flexion/extension. With the hands by the sides (reach for the side of the knee), the lower thoracic region is stressed. Placing the hands behind the head and reaching up with the elbow transfers the centre of rotation higher up. Side-lying over a cushion or gym ball with the upper arm reaching overhead will stretch the muscles of side flexion as well as mobilizing the thoracic spine.

Examples of strength exercises for the thoracic spine musculature include single- or double-handed rowing actions, pull-downs and modified dips (Fig. 9.24).

References

Alan, P., Kerry, R., 2003. Vascular issues in sports. Part 1: the lower limb. *Sportex Medicine* **14**, 32–37.

Boulding, R., Stacey, R., Niven, R., et al., 2016. Dysfunctional breathing: a review of the literature and proposal for classification. *Eur Respir Rev* **25**, 287–294.

Chu, J., Allen, D.D., Pawlowsky, S., et al., 2014. Peripheral response to cervical or thoracic spinal manual therapy: an evidence-based review with meta analysis. *J Man Manip Ther* **22** (4), 220–229.

Courtney, R., Cohen, J., Reece, M., 2009. Comparison of the Manual Assessment of Respiratory Motion (MARM) and the Hi Lo breathing. *Int J Osteopath Med* 1–6.

Courtney, R., van Dixhoorn, J., Cohen, M., 2008. Evaluation of breathing pattern: comparison of a Manual Assessment of Respiratory Motion (MARM) and respiratory induction plethysmography. *Appl Psychophysiol Biofeedback.* **33** (2), 91–100.

Ekberg, O., Persson, N.H., Abrahamson, P., 1988. Longstanding groin pain in athletes: a multidisciplinary approach. *Sports Medicine* **6** (1), 56–61.

Gilmore, O.J.A., 1995. Personal communication.

Grieve, G.P., 1986. *Modern Manual Therapy of the Vertebral Column.* Churchill Livingstone, London.

Hagan, I., Burney, K., Williams, M., Bradley, M., 2007. Sonography reveals causes of acute or chronic groin pain. *Diagnostic Imaging* **29**, 33–40.

Humphries, D., Jamison, M., 2004. Clinical and magnetic resonance imaging features of cricket bowler's side strain. *British Journal of Sports Medicine* **38**, e21.

Jowsey, P., Perry, J. (2010) Sympathetic nervous system effects in the hands following a grade III poster-anterior rotatory mobilisation technique to

T4: a randomised control trial. *Manual Therapy* **15**, 248–253.

Kachingwe, A., Grech, S., 2008. Proposed algorithm for the management of athletes with athletic pubalgia (sports hernia): a case series. *Journal of Orthopaedic and Sports Physical Therapy* **38** (12), 768–781.

Kemp, S., Batt, M.E., 1998. The sports hernia: a common cause of groin pain. *Physician and Sportsmedicine* **26** (1), 1–6.

Lovell, G., 1995. The diagnosis of chronic groin pain in athletes. *Australian Journal of Science and Medicine in Sport* **27** (3), 76–79.

Maquirriain, J., Ghisi, J., 2006. Uncommon abdominal muscle injury in a tennis player: internal oblique strain. *British Journal of Sports Medicine* **40**, 462–463.

Norris, C.M., 1995. *Postural Considerations in Training, Presentation to the Football Association Medical Committee*. Lilleshall, England.

Sheen, A.J., Stephenson, B.M., Lloyd, D.M., et al., 2014. 'Treatment of the sportsman's groin': British Hernia Society's 2014 position statement based on the Manchester Consensus Conference. *British Journal of Sports Medicine* **48** (14), 1079–1087.

Simonet, W.T., Saylor, H.L., Sim, L., 1995. Abdominal wall muscle tears in hockey players. *International Journal of Sports Medicine* **16** (2), 126–128.

Taylor, A., Kerry, R., 2003. Vascular issues in sports. Part 2: the upper limb. *Sportex Medicine* **15**, 9–13.

Unverzagt, C., Schuemann, T., Mathisen, J., 2008. Differential diagnosis of a sports hernia in a high school athlete. *Journal of Orthopaedic and Sports Physical Therapy* **38**, 63–70.

Weiss, H.R., Dieckmann, J., Gerner, H.J., 2002. Effect of intensive rehabilitation on pain in patients with Scheuermann's disease. *Studies in Health Technology and Informatics* **88**, 254–257.

Weiss, H.R., Dieckmann, J., Gerner, H.J., 2003. The practical use of surface topography: following up patients with Scheuermann's disease. *Pediatric Rehabilitation* **6** (1), 39–45.

Williams, P., Foster, M.E., 1995. Gilmores groin— or is it? *British Journal of Sports Medicine* **29** (3), 206–208.

Zachazewski, J.E., Magee, D.J., Quillen, W.S., 1996. *Athletic Injuries and Rehabilitation*. Saunders, Philadelphia.

CHAPTER 10

The cervical spine

The cervical spine consists of eight mobile segments generally categorized into two functional units. The first comprises the occiput, C1 and C2 (the suboccipital region) and the second the segments from C2 to T1 (the lower cervical region) (see Fig. 10.1).

Within the suboccipital region, an important distinction is made between the atlanto-occipital (A/O) and atlantoaxial (A/A) joints. The atlanto-occipital joint, formed between the occipital condyle and lateral masses of C1, allows no rotation but free flexion/extension and some lateral flexion. There are three atlantoaxial joints. The median joint is formed between the odontoid peg of the axis and the anterior arch and transverse ligament of the atlas. The lateral two joints are between the lateral articular processes of the atlas and axis. The atlantoaxial joint allows free rotation to about 35 degrees, and only minimal flexion/extension. As rotation occurs, the head is depressed vertically by about 1 mm, causing ligamentous slackening and increasing the available range of motion.

> **Key point**
>
> The atlanto-occipital joint (C0–C1) allows no rotation, but free flexion/extension. The atlantoaxial joint (C1–C2) allows free rotation but only limited flexion/extension.

The discs of the lower cervical region are fairly thick, allowing free movement in all planes. Flexion and extension combined has a range of about 110 degrees, with only 25 degrees being flexion, and the least movement occurring between C7 and T1. With flexion, the upper vertebra of a pair slides anteriorly, pulling its inferior facet up and forwards, thus widening the facet joint space posteriorly. With extension the situation is reversed, the upper vertebra tilting and sliding posteriorly, gapping the facet joint anteriorly but narrowing

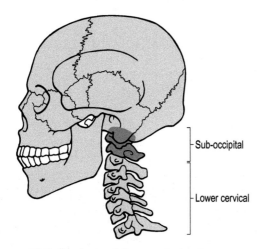

Figure 10.1 Regions of the cervical spine.

- Sub-occipital

- Lower cervical

the intervertebral foramen. Lateral flexion has a range of about 40 degrees to each side. This is not a pure movement, but is combined with rotation and slight extension. Rotation occurs in the lower cervical region in either direction to about 50 degrees, and is limited by grinding of the facets and torsion stress on the discs and facet capsules. The function size of the intervertebral foramen is increased on the opposite side to the rotation, but reduced on the same side. Thus, manual therapy to the cervical spine for unilateral pain often involves contralateral rotation to relieve root pressure.

The lateral edge of each vertebra in the cervical region is lipped to form an uncovertebral joint, lying anteriorly to the intervertebral foramen. Each joint is surrounded by a capsule which blends medially with the disc. The joints help to stabilize the neck and control its movements.

Within the total range of any cervical movement some regions move more than others. The upper cervical segments allow more rotation than the lower, but less lateral flexion. With head retraction

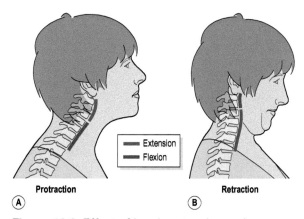

Figure 10.2 Effect of head protraction and retraction on cervical spine alignment.

the upper segments flex while the lower ones extend (Fig. 10.2). In fact, with this movement a greater range of upper cervical flexion is obtained than with neck flexion itself. As flexion occurs, the spinal canal lengthens, stretching the cord and nerve roots. Extension reverses this effect, relaxing the spinal structures.

Treatment Note 10.1 Surface marking of the cervicothoracic region

Cervical vertebrae

Most of the spinous processes of the vertebrae may be readily palpated (Fig. 10.3). Palpation is facilitated by having the patient draw their chin in and look down slightly (upper cervical flexion). The prominent point on the back of the skull is the external occipital protuberance (EOP), and below this the external occipital crest.

Moving the finger sideways, the mastoid process may be palpated behind the ear.

Travelling downwards (caudally) the prominent dip is the rudimentary spinous process of C1 (atlas) approximately 3 cm below the EOP. The palpable lump below this is the spinous process of C2 (axis), being the most prominent structure in the midline inferior to the skull. C3–5 are tightly pressed together due to the cervical lordosis and move apart with upper cervical flexion.

C7 forms the cervical prominens and can be differentiated from C6 by placing a finger on both spinous processes and asking the patient to extend their neck. The spinous process of C6 will disappear as it moves anteriorly. The transverse process of C1 may be palpated midway between the angle of the jaw (mandible) and the mastoid process.

Thoracic vertebrae

The spinous process of T3 lies approximately level with the root of the scapular spine, the inferior angle of the scapula is roughly level with T7, and T12 lies level with the midpoint of a line joining the inferior angle of the scapula and the iliac crest in the normal patient. The transverse processes lie some 3 cm lateral to the midpoint of the spine.

Treatment note 10.1 *continued*

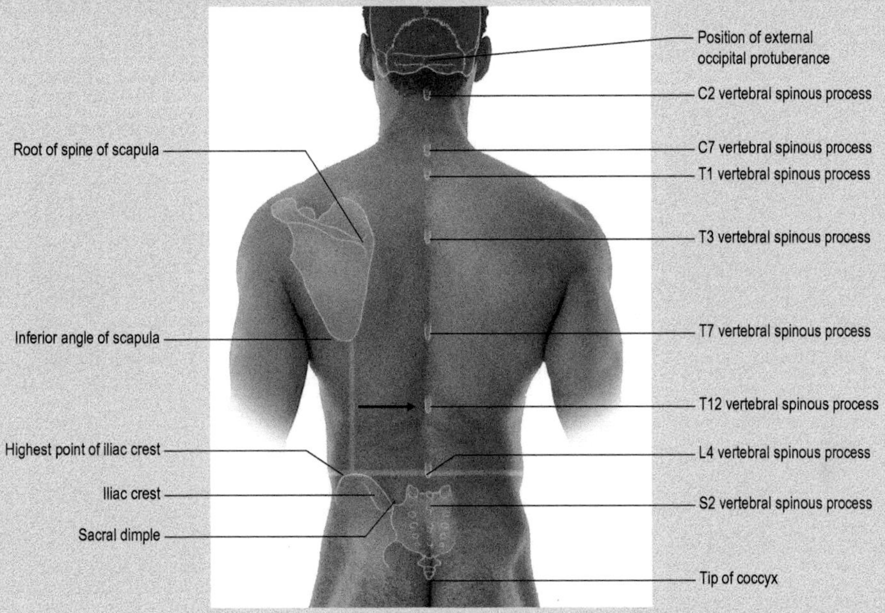

Figure 10.3 Surface marking of the spine. From Lumley (2008).

Ribs

The angle of the rib lies 3–4 cm lateral to the transverse process (86–87 cm from midline). The first rib lies deep to the clavicle and may be palpated within the supraclavicular fossa close to the midline of the clavicle, an area of particular tenderness as it lies close to the brachial plexus trunks and the subclavian artery. Palpating below the clavicle, the junction of the first rib and sternum may be found close to (1 cm) the medial end of the clavicle.

Anteriorly, the costal cartilages of the eighth, ninth and tenth ribs merge to join the sternum at the xiphoid process; the ends of the eleventh and twelfth ribs are free, hence the name 'floating ribs'. The sternum itself is easily palpated on the anterior chest wall. Superiorly, the suprasternal notch is found. Further, down the manubrium (upper portion of the sternum) joins the main body of the sternum at the sternal angle. The sternal angle is slightly flexible, exhibiting five to seven degrees of motion between full inspiration and full expiration (Field and Hutchison 2006). The second rib attaches to the sternum at this level, and the seventh rib is level with the xiphoid process.

References

Field, D., Hutchison, J.O., 2006. *Field's Anatomy, Palpation and Surface Marking*, 4th ed. Elsevier.

Lumley, J., 2008. *Surface Anatomy*, 4th ed. Churchill Livingstone, Edinburgh.

Vertebral arteries

One important difference between the cervical and other spinal areas is the presence of the vertebral arteries. These branch from the subclavian artery (Fig. 10.4A (i)) and pass through the foramina transversaria of each cervical vertebra from C6 and above (Fig. 10.4A (ii)). When the artery reaches the atlas, it runs almost horizontally (Fig. 10.4A (iii)) and

455

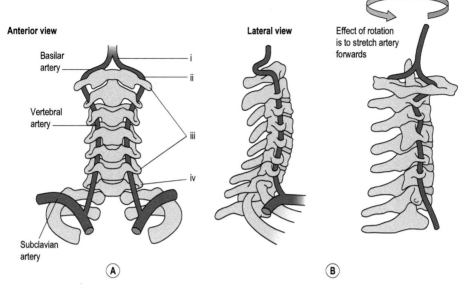

Figure 10.4 Structure of the vertebral artery. (A) Anterior and lateral view. (i) Branch from subclavian artery to C6. (ii) Vertical track through foramen transversaria. (iii) Horizontal section from C1. (iv) Entry to foramen magnum to join neighbour. (B) Effect of rotation is to stretch artery forwards. After Grant (1994a), with permission.

then enters the foramen magnum to join with its neighbour and form the basilar artery (Fig. 10.4A (iv)). The vertebral arteries supply about 11 per cent of the cerebral blood flow, the carotid system supplying 89 per cent (Grant 1994a).

Variations in the diameter of the vertebral arteries are common, and in some cases the basilar artery is supplied almost entirely by one dominant vertebral artery. During its course, the artery is in close relation to a number of structures, including the scalenus anterior and longus colli muscles, the uncinate processes, the superior surface of the facet joint, and of course the transverse process itself.

Cervical artery dysfunction (CAD) may occur with occlusion or dissection of either the vertebral artery itself, or the internal carotid artery.

Definition

Arterial *dissection* is the production of a flap-like tear in the inner lining of the artery, arterial *occlusion* is a blockage to the artery which may occur through external pressure or internal atherosclerosis.

The vertebral artery supplies the posterior part of the brain, while the internal carotid artery supplies the ventral part. Signs of dysfunction therefore vary, with the internal carotid presenting most commonly as neck pain, headache, Horner's syndrome, and retinal or cerebral ischaemia. Vertebral artery dissection frequently presents as cervical-occipital pain followed by vertigo, dysarthria, visual deficits, ataxia and diplopia (Kranenburga et al. 2017).

Definition

Horner's syndrome is damage to the sympathetic trunk. The condition may produce signs and symptoms such as constricted pupil (miosis), drooping eyelid (ptosis) and changes to the skin or eyeball position.

Table 10.1 Symptoms of vertebrobasilar insufficiency (VBI)

Dizziness (in over 60% of cases)
Visual disturbances
—spots before the eyes
—blurred vision
—hallucination
—field defects
Diplopia
Ataxia
Drop attacks
Visceral/vasomotor disturbances
—nausea
—faintness
—light-headedness
Tingling around lips (perioral dysaesthesia)
Nystagmus
Hemi-anaesthesia
Hemiplegia

From Grant (1994b), with permission.

One of the predominant symptoms of CAD is dizziness, although other symptoms occur as detailed in Table 10.1. Occlusion may be either intrinsic or extrinsic. Intrinsic causes include atherosclerosis blocking the artery, causing either focal narrowing or more extensive constriction over the whole length of the artery. Extrinsic causes of occlusion occur by compression to the vessel wall. This is most commonly caused during rotation of the neck if an anomaly of the artery exists. Three such anomalies have been described in the lower part of the artery (Bogduk 1986). First, an irregularity in the origin of the artery from the subclavian; second, bands of deep cervical fascia crossing the artery which tighten on rotation; and third, squeezing of the artery within the fascicles of either longus colli or scalenus anterior.

The major vertical portion of the artery (Fig. 10.4A) is most commonly affected by osteophytes and adhesive scar tissue, with neck rotation compromising the ipsilateral vessel. In the upper region (Fig. 10.4B), the artery may be occluded should the atlas move on the axis, through trauma, rheumatoid arthritis or abnormalities of the odontoid. Passive rotation of the neck can shut the contralateral artery by stretching it. Extension reduces cerebral blood flow less than rotation, but combined rotation–extension in the presence of traction increases the rate of occlusion significantly.

> **Key point**
>
> Abnormalities of the vertebral artery are common, with some patients having only one fully functioning artery.

Cervical artery dysfunction is a potential danger of any manual therapy procedure to the neck, particularly rotation manipulation. Trauma following manipulation occurs predominantly in the atlantoaxial component of the artery, which is stretched forwards during rotation. The more mobile neck of a younger adult will allow a greater range of rotatory motion and therefore greater stretch. Mechanical stress to the vertebral artery may lead to spasm (transient or persistent), subintimal tearing, perivascular haemorrhage or embolus formation leading to brainstem ischaemia. Repeated rotatory manipulation is especially dangerous as it builds on trauma which may already have occurred. In the UK between 1995 and 2003, 300 patients had adverse effects from cervical manual therapy, with the most frequent incident being stroke (Ernst 2004). Injury occurs typically through dissection of the internal carotid artery (ICA) or vertebral artery (VA) and may include cerebral ischaemia, stroke or death (Kerry et al. 2008). Dissection of the internal carotid artery begins as a tear of the inner lining of the artery wall (tunica intima). Blood under pressure is squeezed through the tear creating a haematoma. As a result the artery may narrow (stenosis) or dilate through aneurysm (ballooning). Arterial dissection is the most common cause of stroke and may be spontaneous or traumatic.

Cervical spine examination prior to manual treatment

Prior to mobilization, manipulation or exercise intervention on the cervical spine, a detailed

Table 10.2 Differential diagnosis in cervical spine examination

	Internal carotid artery disease	Vertebrobasilar artery disease	Upper cervical instability
Early presentation	▶ Mid-upper cervical pain. Pain around ear or jaw. ▶ Frontal/temporal head pain ▶ Ptosis ▶ Sudden onset unfamiliar pain	▶ Mid-upper cervical pain ▶ Occipital headache ▶ Sudden onset unfamiliar pain	▶ Neck & head pain ▶ Feeling of instability requiring constant support ▶ Cervical muscle hyperactivity
Late presentation	▶ Transient retinal dysfunction ▶ TIA ▶ CVA	▶ Changes to 5 'D's ▶ Vomiting, vagueness, clumsiness ▶ Cranial nerve dysfunction	▶ Altered sensation (dysthaesia) in hands & feet ▶ Feeling of lump in throat ▶ Arm & leg weakness

TIA - transient ischaemic attack, CVA - cerebrovasular accident,
5 'D's – Dizziness, Diplopia, Dysarthria, Dysphagia, Drop attacks.
(Data modified from Rushton et al. 2014).

examination is required. No single test is available to predict the presence or risk of cervical arterial dysfunction (Rushton et al. 2014) so a clinically reasoning approach must be taken involving the subject's presentation, patient preferences, and a risk-benefit analysis of the technique to be applied. Applying the simple 'Five D' method in subjective examination reminds the therapist of potential red flags. The 'D's stand for Dizziness, Diplopia (double vision), Dysarthria (difficulty speaking), Dysphagia (difficulty swallowing), and Drop attacks (sudden falling). Table 10.2 highlights more extensive information on differential diagnosis to screen out potentially more serious pathologies which may be disguised as musculoskeletal dysfunctions.

Nature of cervical injury in sport

One of the most common mechanisms of severe cervical injury is axial loading. This may be caused as a player hits another by using his or her head as a battering ram (spearing), or if the athlete falls onto his or her head or runs into an object head first. In this situation, the neck is slightly flexed, flattening the cervical lordosis. Now, the cervical spine absorbs considerably less energy than it would in its normal state as a flexible column. Initially, maximal discal compression occurs, and then the spine rapidly buckles and fails in flexion, resulting in fracture, subluxation or dislocation.

The contact area of the axial load on the skull can determine the nature and extent of cervical injury (Winkelstein and Myers 1997). Where the contact area is on the skull vertex, compression and cervical crush injury is likely to occur, even at slow velocities. The trunk continues to move while the head motion is abruptly stopped through ground contact. Where the ground contact area is at a distance from the skull vertex, the head will be forced into flexion or extension – the so-called escape direction. In this case direct compression along the length of the neck is reduced through cervical flexibility. Posterior element fracture more commonly occurs where force is directed *behind* the vertebral body, while direct compression forces acting *through* the vertebral body give rise to compression fracture. Anterior burst or wedge compression fractures occur where the cervical spine is forced into extension (Fig. 10.5).

An illustration of the importance of this mechanism and its preventive possibilities is found in American football. The incidence of cervical quadriplegia in this sport dropped dramatically, from a peak of 34 cases per year to 5, since head-first tackling and blocking were forbidden with the aim of reducing axial load injury (Torg et al. 1985).

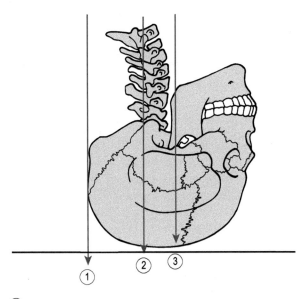

(1) Posterior element fracture

(2) Compression fracture

(3) Wedge fracture

Figure 10.5 Force line in relation to cervical injury during axial loading.

A similar mechanism has been described in rugby football. Cord injuries have occurred in scrum, ruck and maul situations when a player was attempting to pick the ball up from the ground, and as two forwards engage. The vertex of the head is restrained, either against another player or the ground, and the trunk continues to move forwards, forcing the cervical spine into flexion and dislocation. In ice hockey, axial loading again occurs, when a player hits the boards or an opponent with his helmeted head while the neck is slightly flexed. Where significant axial loading has occurred, permanent abnormalities exist within the cervical spine (Torg et al. 1993). These may include interspace narrowing at C5–C6 with deformity of the C5 end plate due to Schmorl's node formation. In addition, reversal of the cervical spine lordosis with fixation from C2 to C6 may be seen. Where these changes are present, they should preclude an athlete from participation in sports involving collision activities.

Definition

A Schmorl's node is a herniation of the nucleus pulposus of the spinal disc through the disc end plate and into the vertebral body.

In all full-body contact sports such as rugby, American football and ice hockey it is essential that players are taught that the initial point of contact in a tackle or block should be the shoulders or chest and not the head. In addition, strengthening the neck musculature may reduce the intensity of injury (Torg 1982).

Less severe trauma may occur to the neck with indirect impact or a sudden mistimed movement. A type of whiplash injury (see below) may occur in a rear impact where one player runs into another. Hyperextension of the neck can result, with varying degrees of tissue damage.

Diving into a shallow swimming pool or lake is also a common cause of injury, with fracture dislocation occurring as the neck is forced into flexion (or extension in some cases) when the head strikes the pool bottom. The condition may occur if a swimming pool is too shallow, especially if left unsupervised or without depth markings. In addition, this tragic injury is common in lakes and rivers with youngsters under the influence of alcohol or drugs.

In gymnastics the most usual mechanism of injury is flexion of the cervical spine, with injury occurring most commonly at C4 and C7 levels (Silver, Silver and Godfrey 1986). Again, there is an axial loading, with the gymnast landing on his or her head. Of note is the potential for abuse of the trampette by young athletes. This piece of equipment enables the young athlete to gain both height and speed in an inverted body position – a potentially lethal combination.

Whiplash

Pathology

Whiplash associated disorders (WAD) are normally associated with a road traffic accident (motor vehicle injury). However, rear-impact injury may also occur in sport. In a rear-impact vehicle accident of 7 mph, the head can be subjected to forces as high as 12–14 times that of gravity (12–14 g-force). This force occurs within milliseconds, which is outside the control of muscle reaction (Worsfold 2013). It is the acceleration of the head rather than the speed of the accident per se which is important. Rapid forces of this nature obviously occur in motorsports, cycling and skiing, but may also be seen when one player runs into another or a rugby scrum collapses, for example. Facet joint impaction may occur, giving both compression and shear forces, which will be worse where the head is rotated or side flexed at the time of the incident. Local bleeding, tissue rupture, synovial fold pinching, microfracture, muscle injury, vertebral artery strain, and nerve root sensitization have all been reported (Siegmund et al. 2009). Facet capsule strain can occur in up to 40 per cent of whiplash patients (compared to a 5 per cent occurrence in normal movements), with afferent nerve fibres within the capsule activated, leading to persistent sensitization. Collagen reorganization of capsule fibres has been observed even where ligament failure has not occurred. Both mechanoreceptors and nociceptive fibres are present in cervical ligaments, leading to whiplash symptoms. The dorsal root ganglia can become sensitized and inflamed (neuro-inflammatory cascade), leading to continued after-discharge from afferent nerve fibres even when joint loading has ceased. Altered blood flow rates through the vertebral arteries have been seen post whiplash, leading to symptoms of headache, blurred vision, dizziness and tinnitus/vertigo. During whiplash injury, vertebral artery elongation of 17.4 mm (side impact) and 30.5 mm (head rotated) have been reported, leading to a significant vessel diameter reduction (Siegmund et al. 2009). Direct damage to the dorsal root ganglia and nerve roots may occur due to transient pressure drops, with leakage of plasma membrane and interstitial haemorrhage seen, indicative of direct nerve cell damage. Muscle damage indicated by elevated serum creatine kinase levels have been shown, and alteration of neuromuscular control as a result of pain, tissue damage, and behaviour change is a common observation during physiotherapy examination.

Assessment and treatment

Poor recovery is more likely where pain levels are high, and where pain is neuropathic in nature. Increased sensitivity to stimuli (mechanical or thermal) is also a risk factor for poorer outcome, as is an unresolved post-traumatic stress reaction (Worsfold 2013). Psychological impact of whiplash may be determined using questionnaires as part of the subjective examination. Disability related to the neck may be assessed using the *Neck Disability Index* (Vernon and Mior 1991), while the *Impact of Event scale* (Horowitz et al. 1979) can be used to determine the presence of a post-traumatic stress reaction. Both questionnaires are widely available on the internet.

Treatment of WAD should take a biopsychosocial approach. Use of exercise, manual therapy and education is effective, but not more cost effective than simple advice from a physiotherapist (Lamb et al. 2013). Identification of sensorimotor changes in neck pain is a common finding, but these changes vary between individuals, making detailed assessment critical. A systematic review and best evidence synthesis of treatment of WAD concluded that mobilization, manipulation and clinical massage are effective interventions for the management of the condition, but passive physical modalities and acupuncture are not (Wong et al. 2016).

Cervical spine screening examination

The subjective assessment will give the practitioner an indication of the depth of examination required objectively. A great number of tests and procedures exist, but not all will be used with every patient. Following the subjective assessment, a screening examination is used to indicate where further tests, including palpation, should concentrate.

Initial objective examination includes posture and head position in both sitting and standing.

Muscle tension and both active and passive motions are examined. Flexion/extension, rotation and lateral flexion are examined for range and end-feel. Movements are isolated by eliminating unwanted shoulder elevation or trunk rotation. Resisted movements may be similarly tested, and the shoulder range to abduction and flexion/abduction assessed to determine if there is an associated shoulder or arm pathology. Pain referral and any sensation loss is mapped, and upper limb muscle power and reflexes assessed if the history suggests neurological involvement.

Two further movements and their adaptations are important with reference to mechanical therapy especially; these are head protrusion (protraction) and retraction. Flexion and extension of the cervical spine may be differentiated into suboccipital and lower cervical regions. Tucking the chin in (retraction) flexes the upper cervical spine, while drawing the chin to the chest flexes the lower cervical spine. Jutting the chin forwards (protraction) extends the upper cervical spine, while taking the head backwards (looking at the ceiling) while maintaining chin tuck (retraction) places greater extension stress on the lower cervical spine. Lateral flexion of the lower cervical spine draws the ear to the shoulder, while that of the upper cervical spine tips the head sideways around the nose as a pivot.

As with other tests, the location and intensity of symptoms is established prior to testing. Head protrusion is performed in a sitting position, with the patient instructed to slide the head forwards horizontally as far as possible by 'poking the chin out'. This is performed singly and to repetition. Head retraction is the opposite action, sliding the head back and 'pulling the chin in'. Again, overpressure may be used to assess end-feel and symptoms. Where postural pain is suspected, the movements are performed statically and maintained to load the structures and cause tissue deformation. The capsular pattern of the cervical spine is an equal limitation of all movements except flexion, which is usually of greater range.

Special tests

Further detail in cervical examination is gained by palpation to test accessory movements, and special tests such as the quadrant position and neurodynamic testing such as the upper limb tension test (ULTT). These two latter procedures are useful where the clinical picture is not clear, and to confirm or refute involvement of the cervical spine.

Quadrant test

The quadrant test combines extension, lateral flexion and rotation to the same side. For the *lower cervical spine*, the neck is taken back into extension and lateral flexion towards the painful side, and then rotated, again towards the pain. Testing the *upper cervical spine* is performed by extension with pressure to localize the movement to the upper cervical segments. When full extension has been gained, rotation is added towards the pain, and then followed by lateral flexion. Various sequences of combined movements may produce the patient's symptoms, and it is important that the same sequence of movements be used when making comparisons between both sides, or assessing prior to and following treatment (Fig. 10.6).

Adding compression to these test positions (*foraminal compression test*) can also be clinically revealing in cases where patients have intermittent

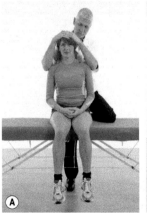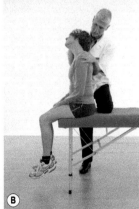

Figure 10.6 Cervical examination tests. (A) compression, (B) combined movement with overpressure.

symptoms not present at the time of examination. Initially, the head and neck are compressed (using a straight vertical force) with the head in neutral. If this fails to reproduce the patient's symptoms, compression is used in extension and finally in extension/rotation. In the latter case, the movement is to the unaffected side first; if symptoms are not reproduced, the affected side is then used. Where symptoms are present at the time of examination, a distraction test may be used in the neutral position with the aim of alleviating symptoms (*foraminal distraction test*).

Upper limb tension test

The upper limb tension test (ULTT) or brachial plexus provocation test (BPPT) (Elvey's test) is a neurodynamic test which may be thought of as the 'straight leg raise of the upper limb'. It develops tension in the cervical nerve roots and their sheaths and dura, and places greatest stress on the C5 and C6 structures. Four variations are used to place greater or lesser stress on particular nerves (ULTT 1, ULTT 2a, ULTT 2b, ULTT 3).

For ULTT 1 (Fig. 10.7) the patient is supine with the therapist facing the patient and standing at his or her side. The patient's shoulder girdle is depressed by caudal pressure from the therapist's hand. The forearm is supinated and the wrist and fingers extended, and then the shoulder is laterally rotated and the elbow extended. Finally, cervical lateral flexion (but not rotation) is added away from the tested arm. The instruction to 'keep looking at the ceiling but take your ear away' is helpful.

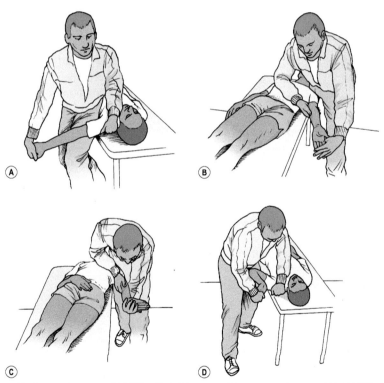

Figure 10.7 The upper limb tension test (ULTT). Finishing positions are shown. (A) ULTT 1: Median nerve. Shoulder abduction. (B) ULTT 2a: Median nerve. Shoulder girdle depression and external rotation of shoulder. (C) ULTT 2b: Radial nerve. Shoulder girdle depression and internal rotation of shoulder. (D) ULTT 3: Ulnar nerve. Shoulder abduction and elbow flexion. From Butler (1991), with permission.

Pain from two-joint muscle stretch over the shoulder is eliminated by altering the head or finger position (which will not affect the shoulder muscles but will alter the nerve tension) to establish if this affects the pain. In normal subjects an ache is usually felt in the cubital fossa, and some sensation on the radial side of the forearm and hand is common. The test is only positive if symptoms other than these, and similar to the patient's complaint, are produced.

ULTT 2a is used to place bias on the median nerve. The test is performed by depressing the patient's shoulder girdle and extending the elbow. The shoulder is laterally rotated and the wrist, fingers and thumb are then extended. Slight abduction of the shoulder may be added to sensitize the test. ULTT 2b places bias on the radial nerve. From the previous position, the shoulder is medially rotated and the forearm pronated. The wrist is then flexed, and ulnar deviation of the wrist further sensitizes the nerve.

ULTT 3 is used to test the ulnar nerve. The patient's wrist is extended and forearm supinated, and then the elbow is flexed. The shoulder girdle is depressed, and the glenohumeral joint abducted as though trying to place the patient's hand over his or her ear.

The ULTT is useful in patients with shoulder girdle or upper-limb involvement where the origin of the symptoms is unclear, or where other tests do not reproduce the symptoms. For a test to be positive, it must reproduce the patient's symptoms and be different from the uninjured side of the body. Furthermore, the test responses should be altered by movement of the distal body parts (forearm, wrist and fingers).

Examination test cluster

Patients presenting with cervical spine, shoulder and/or arm pain require an accurate diagnosis of mechanical pain which rules out serious pathology. Pain through nerve damage or inflammation (radiculopathy) may be examined using a variety of physiotherapy tests, but the reliability and accuracy of these tests is uncertain.

Table 10.3 Clinical test cluster for determination of cervical radiculopathy

Test	Performance
Spurling test	Passive side flexion of patient's neck towards symptomatic side. Patient's symptoms increase.
Neck distraction	Neck flexed for comfort and a distraction force of approximately 14 kg is applied. Patient's symptoms reduce or resolve.
ULTT 1	Test applied as detailed above. Symptoms production/elbow extension limited by >10° compared to uninjured side/symptom change with cervical side flexion.
Cervical ROM	Active cervical rotation in sitting. Range <60° on painful side.

ROM – range of motion; ULTT – upper limb tension test.
After Wainner et al. (2003), Cleland et al. (2005).

Key point

Radiculopathy is damage to or inflammation of a peripheral nerve and/or its root which gives rise to pain, weakness and/or numbness within the tissues supplied by the nerve.

In a study of 34 physiotherapy tests using 82 patients Wainner et al. (2003) determined that the ULTT 1 (median nerve bias) was the most useful test to determine radiculopathy. A test cluster of four examination items was identified and recommended for clinical usage, as detailed in Table 10.3.

Brachial plexus injury in sport

In sport, traction injury of the brachial plexus can occur, in a position similar to that of the ULTT. With blocking or tackling in rugby or American football, the shoulder may be forcibly depressed while the cervical spine is simultaneously laterally flexed to the contralateral side, imparting a traction force to the brachial structures. The upper trunk of the brachial plexus may suffer a neurapraxia as a result. Nerve function is temporarily disturbed and a burning sensation is felt in the upper limb.

The condition is often referred to as a 'stinger' or 'burner' by players, and recovery is usually full in a matter of minutes.

The stinger may also be associated with extension compression, and during this mechanism the athlete with cervical spine stenosis is more at risk. The presence of such stenosis also makes the likelihood of developing a stinger three times greater (Meyer et al. 1994). Decreased canal diameter is associated with a narrow intervertebral foramen, and it is this structure which is likely to cause compression of the nerve root. The ratio of the spinal canal diameter to the length of the vertebral body has been used as an important risk factor for the development of nerve pathology during collision sports. Spinal stenosis is defined as *a sagittal diameter of the spinal canal less than 14 mm from C4–C6* (Torg 2002). Variation in radiographic accuracy of this measurement has led to the development of the ratio method, where a ratio of 0.8 (spinal canal to vertebral body) is indicative of cervical spine stenosis.

Where a subject returns to sport too early following a stinger injury, further damage to the neural system may occur. Further investigation is required where neurological symptoms persist for 36 hours or more. Absolute contraindications to return have been given as: ligamentous instability of the cervical spine, MRI evidence of cord defect or swelling, neurological signs and symptoms for 36 hours or more, and more than one episode of neural injury (Torg 2002).

Key point

Following a stinger injury, a player should not return to collision sport if there are signs of cervical ligamentous instability, MRI evidence of cord defect or swelling, or where neurological signs and symptoms still exist.

Motion tests for the cervical spine

Following a traumatic injury such as occurs in sport or a road traffic accident (RTA), ligamentous tearing within the upper cervical spine (craniovertebral ligaments) can create structural instability. Testing the motion of the atlanto-occipital (C0–C1) and atlantoaxial (C1–C2) joints can therefore be revealing. The aim of the tests is to assess not specifically range of motion, but the reproduction of cord signs as the test is performed. Several tests are available (Pettman 1994), with movement of the skull on C1, or the skull and C1 on C2, forming the basis of each.

In the first test, the patient lies supine and the therapist sits at the patient's head. The transverse processes of C1 are palpated with the index fingers and the other fingers curl around the occiput. The action is for C2 to remain relatively fixed through body weight and for the therapist to lift the skull and C1 vertically away from the couch (Fig. 10.8A). Normally this movement is restricted by the *transverse ligament*, but if it is ruptured excessive motion will occur, giving symptoms.

The second test begins in the same starting position but this time the therapist palpates the spinous process of C2. The action now is to compress the top of the head (vertex) to lock the atlanto-occipital joint and then to side-bend the neck (Fig. 10.8B). As this occurs, the spinous process of C2 should move in the opposite direction (right side-bending giving left rotation) due to tightness in the *alar ligament*. If this ligament is ruptured, severe muscle spasm will be seen with cord signs.

For the third test, minimal distraction is used to test the *tectorial membrane*. The patient is sitting and the therapist stands behind. The side of the head is gripped and a distraction force imparted firstly in neutral and then in cervical flexion (Fig. 10.8C). Cord signs indicate a positive test.

Definition

The transverse ligament runs between the tubercles of the atlas (C1), the alar ligament runs from the sides of the odontoid peg of the axis (C2) to the base of the skull (occiput). The tectorial membrane is an extension of the posterior longitudinal ligament. It attaches

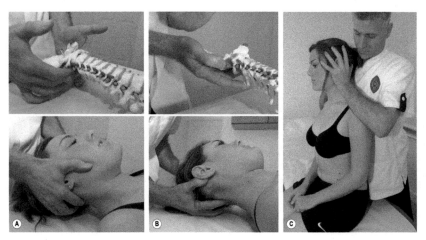

Figure 10.8 Craniovertebral ligament tests. (A) Transverse ligament. (B) Alar ligament test. (C) Tectorial membrane test.

to the vertebral body of atlas and onto the occiput (Fig. 10.9).

Manual therapy for the cervical spine

Manual therapy for the cervical spine broadly falls into three categories. Repeated passive movements (mobilization), mobilization combined with movement or exercise (MWM), and high-velocity low-amplitude thrust techniques (manipulation). The manual therapy techniques are normally designed to target stiffness / lack of movement or pain, either separately or in combination. Results from 27 randomized controlled trials (RCT) on mobilization or manipulation have been shown to be similar between techniques (Gross et al. 2010). An RCT considered 182 patients suffering non-specific neck pain of less than three months in duration who were assessed and judged suitable for manipulation. Even when patients were pre-selected for manipulation but received mobilization, no difference was found between the groups. The authors concluded that the use of neck manipulation could not be justified on the basis of superior effectiveness (Leaver et al. 2010).

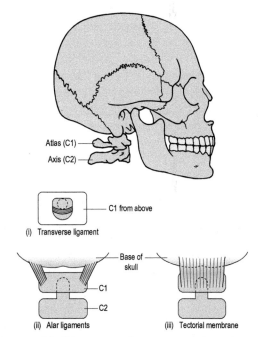

Figure 10.9 Diagrammatic representation of craniovertebral ligaments.

Physiological joint movements

One of the more useful lower-grade mobilization techniques for the cervical spine in the presence of unilateral symptoms is rotation, usually performed in a direction away from the patient's pain. The patient lies supine on the treatment couch with the

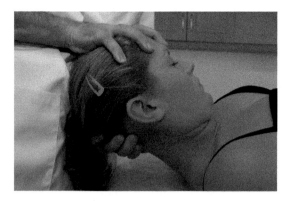

Figure 10.10 Physiological joint mobilization.

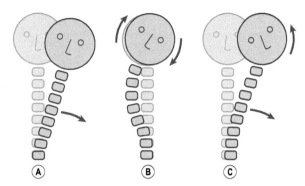

Figure 10.11 Lateral flexion of the cervical spine. (A) Lower cervical spine (C4–C7). (B) Upper cervical spine (C2–C4). (C) Atlanto-occipital joint (C0–C1).

head extending over the couch end. The therapist grasps the patient's occiput and chin (or side of the head), and rotates the head away from the painful side. The upper cervical (suboccipital) spine is better mobilized with the head and neck in line. With the lower cervical area, the neck is flexed further the lower down the spine the lesion is. The movement can be refined to rotate the atlantoaxial joint by flexing the cervical spine maximally and adding slight compression through the vertex (Fig. 10.10).

> ### Key point
>
> The upper cervical spine is mobilized with the head and neck in line (neutral). For the lower cervical area, the neck is flexed further the lower down the spine the lesion is.

Where pain is intense, or if the patient is particularly nervous, longitudinal oscillations are useful. The same grip may be used as with rotation movements, and the longitudinal motion is imparted by the therapist pulling through his or her arms. Stronger manual traction may also be of use to modulate pain. This may be applied with the patient's shoulders stabilized by body weight or using an assistant where larger forces are required. Traction is applied through straight arms by the therapist leaning back. The use of a belt or harness can reduce the strain on the therapist considerably (see Treatment Note 10.2).

Rotation mobilizations and manipulations have also been described with traction. Some authors have claimed that this procedure makes cervical manipulation safer by ensuring that any displaced fragment will move centrally (Cyriax and Cyriax 1983). Others dispute this claim, arguing that the mechanics of the vertebral arteries makes injury more likely with this technique (Grieve 1986, Grant 1994a). Certainly this procedure should not be applied unless other milder forms of manual therapy have been tried first, and even then a risk-benefit analysis would have to reveal that no other workable options were available.

Lateral flexion movements are useful for muscle stretching (especially the upper trapezius) as well as joint mobilization. For the lower cervical spine the whole head moves, the nose tracing the path of an arc. For the mid-cervical spine the head tips, the nose remaining still and representing the pivot point. For the suboccipital region (in particular C0–C1), the head and neck are side glided and lateral flexion is then imposed. Side gliding to the right is performed with lateral flexion (tipping) to the left (Fig. 10.11).

Accessory movements

Accessory intervertebral movements are traditionally performed with the patient in a prone lying position with the hands beneath the forehead. The chin is tucked in slightly to reduce the cervical lordosis. The tips or pads of the therapist's thumbs are used to impart the mobilization. Power for the movement comes from the shoulders and is transmitted through the arms and hands, so that the thumbs deliver rather than create the force.

▶ *Posteroanterior central vertebral* pressures are performed with the therapist's thumbs in contact with the patient's spinous process. More pressure is required to feel movement in the mid-cervical region than in the suboccipital or lower cervical areas. The atlas has no spinous process, but rather a posterior tubercle, and pressure here is through the overlying muscles and ligaments. The spinous process of C2 overhangs that of C3, so palpation is aided in this region by asking the patient to tuck the chin in further and so increase cervical flexion. The oscillation is repeated two or three times each second, and the direction of travel may be angled towards the patient's head or feet depending on comfort. Posteroanterior central pressures are very useful where symptoms are central, or evenly distributed to either side (Fig. 10.12).

▶ *Posteroanterior unilateral pressures* are similarly performed, but this time the therapist's thumbs are in contact with the patient's articular processes and angled towards the mid-line. The technique is used for unilateral symptoms over the painful side. Transverse vertebral pressures are given against the side of a single spinous process, with one thumb reinforcing the other. This technique is used mostly where there are unilateral symptoms which are well localized to the vertebrae. The movement is usually performed from the painless side pressing towards the pain.

▶ *Cervical lateral glides* may be performed by cradling the patient's head and performing a lateral translation away from the side of symptoms (see Fig. 10.18). Traditionally this is performed targeting a single spinal segment; however, studies have shown that mobilization

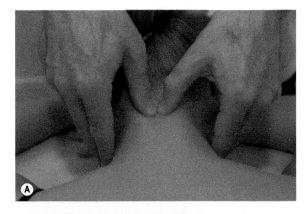
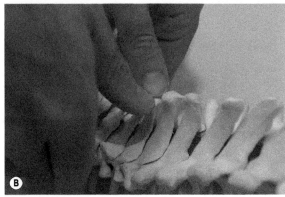

Figure 10.12 Accessory joint mobilization. (A) Surface palpation. (B) Position on skeleton.

procedures of this type are not specific to a single segment but mobilize all segments from C2 to C7 (Cleland et al. 2005). Lateral glide may also be performed with the patient's arm in the position of ULTT 1 and supported on a low table.

Mechanical therapy

Mechanical therapy was used for the lumbar spine in Chapter 8, and the same basic principles apply when using this technique for the cervical spine. Postural syndrome (pain eased by changing the subject's posture) is managed largely by modifying sitting posture with the slouch overcorrect exercise. This time, however, the elimination of head protrusion is thought to be an important aim. Standing with the back against a wall, the action is to use a head retraction (chin tuck) action, with

Treatment Note 10.2 Seatbelt techniques for cervical traction

Cervical traction is a technique which has traditionally been used in the treatment of cervical conditions, with recommended poundages being quite high in some cases (Cyriax 1982). Although mechanical traction may be used, it does not give the precision or variability that manual techniques can produce. However, to provide strong manual traction or repeated longitudinal mobilizations can be stressful to the practitioner's hands. The use of a seatbelt provides the advantages of manual techniques while reducing practitioner stress.

Starting position and grip

Counter-traction is provided by the patient's body weight and so they may be treated either with the couch flat, or in inclined sitting. Traction may be localized further down the cervical spine by adding flexion. The head may either be gripped with one hand cupped beneath the chin (ensure that the fingers are away from the trachea) and the other cradling the occiput (Fig. 10.14), or by both hands over the side of the head with the thumbs along the angle of the jaw (Fig. 10.13). The latter position is not as strong, but has the advantage that the patient can speak throughout the treatment.

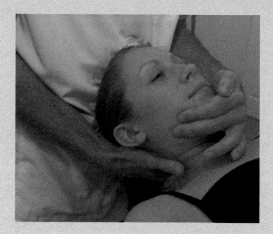

Figure 10.14 Hand grip using chin and occiput.

A stride standing position is taken up so that the therapist can transfer body weight from the front foot to the back foot to provide the force for the action. Make sure that a balanced gait is maintained throughout the action so that the therapist does not risk slipping.

Belt position

The belt is fastened and measured from the therapist's shoulder to his or her outstretched hand (Fig. 10.15). The belt then passes around the hips, on the outside of the forearms and the backs of the hands. The elbows are held out slightly to hold the belt away from the side of the head (Fig. 10.16). Once the belt is positioned, a powerful grip is not required from the therapist. As a measure, the therapist should be able to comfortably move the fingers while traction is on.

Variations

Several mobilization techniques may be given while traction is maintained. A gross AP glide may be given by bending and straightening the knees (Fig. 10.17) and a lateral glide may be

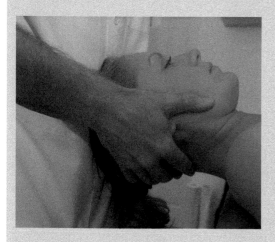

Figure 10.13 Hand grip on side of head.

Treatment note 10.2 *continued*

performed by tucking the elbows into the sides of the body and shifting the pelvis from side to side (Fig. 10.18).

Key point

For the suboccipital region, asking the patient to tuck the chin in (upper cervical flexion) flattens the cervical curve and aids PA mobilizations.

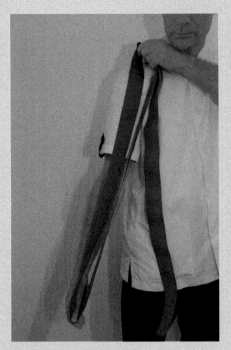

Figure 10.15 Measuring the belt.

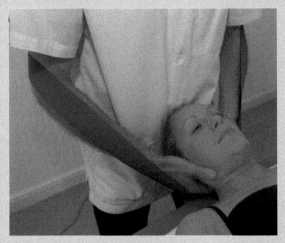

Figure 10.17 Anteroposterior (AP) glide using belt.

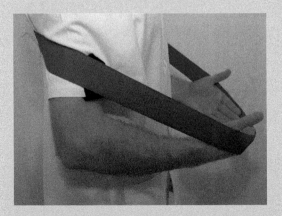

Figure 10.16 Belt position.

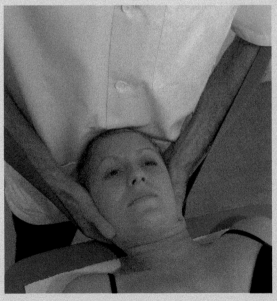

Figure 10.18 Lateral glide using belt.

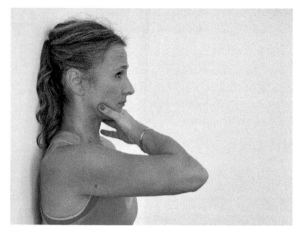

Figure 10.19 Chin tuck exercise using overpressure.

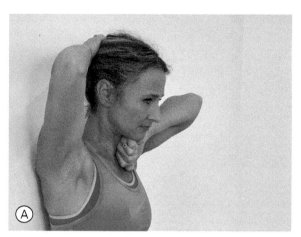

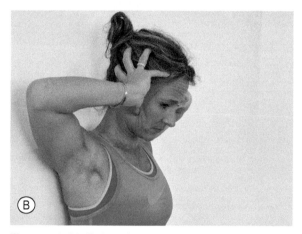

Figure 10.20 Enhancing sub-occipital flexion. (A) Fist traction. (B) Self-applied assisted skull rock.

or without overpressure. The action is for the subject to press onto their chin and jaw using the webspace of one hand (Fig. 10.19). The chin tuck action may be repeated as a rhythmic mobilization to centralize and/or reduce pain, or used as a sustained stretch (static stretch) to target tight soft tissue.

The chin tuck action moves the sub-occipital region from extension into flexion, but where posterior tissue is overly tight, further flexion may be added using two techniques. The first is fist traction. Here the subject places the fist of one hand (side on) between their chin/lower jaw and the top of their sternum. With the other hand active assisted cervical flexion is used, with the hand drawing the skull slightly upward (traction) and forward (flexion) over the pivot formed by the fist (Fig. 10.20A). A second action is the assisted skull rock. Now the subject uses the fingertips of their open hands on either side of the head with the centre of the hand over the ear. The action is to flex and apply traction (longitudinal force) by drawing the chin in and down towards the jugular notch of the sternum while at the same time drawing the occiput upwards (Fig. 10.20B).

Where asymmetry and tightness was apparent over the upper trapezius or sternocleidomastoid (SCM) muscles at assessment, stretching to rotation or lateral flexion may be used.

The action is more focused if the shoulder is stabilized by performing active depression before the neck is moved, and if the angle of rotation/lateral flexion is varied to feel the maximum benefit.

NAGs and SNAGs

The concept of NAGs, SNAGs and MWM was covered in Chapter 1. NAGs (natural apophyseal glides) are mid-range oscillatory mobilizations applied in the cervical region to the facet joints between C2 and C7, with a reverse NAG being applied for the upper thoracic spine. The procedures are used with the patient

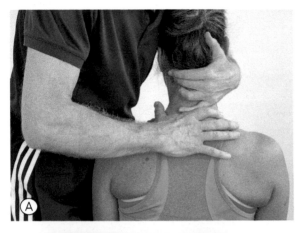

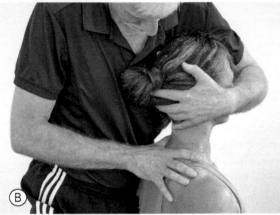

Figure 10.21 NAGs in treatment of the cervical region. (A) Cervical NAG. (B) Reverse NAG for upper Thoracic spine.

seated, placing the cervical spine in a functional weightbearing position.

Assuming the therapist is using the right hand, he or she stands to the right of the patient, blocking any unwanted shoulder movement with his or her own lower trunk. The patient's head is held in the therapist's cupped right hand, with the little finger hooked below the spinous process at the level to be treated. The therapist's left thenar eminence reinforces the pressure of the right little finger. The mobilization is applied through the hand and little finger at an angle of 45 degrees to the cervical spine (towards the eyes), and repeated six to ten times using an oscillation speed two to three per second (Fig. 10.21A).

Varying degrees of flexion, and traction, may be applied until a movement is found which reduces the patient's symptoms. The cradled head position is particularly useful in that it gives confidence to the especially nervous patient. For the reverse NAG, again the therapist reaches around the subject's head, but uses the thumb pad and distal interphalangeal joint to form a 'V' shaped contact area onto the articular pillar of the upper thoracic level selected (Fig. 10.21B).

SNAGs (sustained natural apophyseal glides) are sustained motions applied at end range. The therapist places the side of his or her thumb over the level to be treated, and presses upwards along the plane of the facet joint as the patient rotates or laterally flexes the head. The thumb follows the motion as the neck moves. Similar SNAGs may be used where flexion or extension is limited, and to C2 in the case of headaches. In this case the direction of movement is horizontal, again in line with the facet joint plane (Fig. 10.22A/B). To facilitate sub-occipital flexion following a SNAG procedure, the subject may be instructed to perform a SNAG using a towel at home. The edge of the towel is placed over the C2 spinous process and the towel is drawn upwards towards eye level. An active retraction action (chin tuck) is performed as gliding force from the towel is maintained (Fig. 10.22C).

Soft tissue techniques

Several muscles in the area can develop painful trigger points and shorten, requiring release. Direct pressure (ischaemic pressure), massage and muscle stripping, and dry needling are all useful. On the posterior aspect, many of the muscles run to the base of the skull (Fig. 10.23) and so massage must be extended right up onto the occipital rim. The suboccipital muscles may be massaged and stretched in the supine-lying position, and several trigger points may be identified. The therapist places his or her supinated forearms beneath the patient's head and grips the suboccipital structures with the pads of the flexed fingers. Gently gripping

471

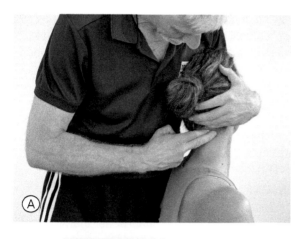

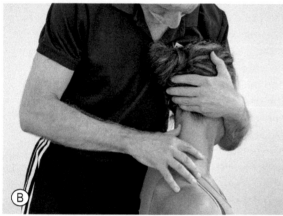

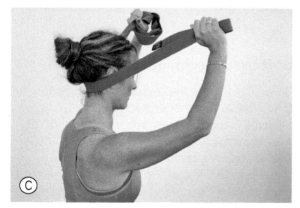

Figure 10.22 SNAGs in treatment of the cervical region. (A) Rotation. (B) Flexion. (C) Self-applied SNAG using webbing belt / towel.

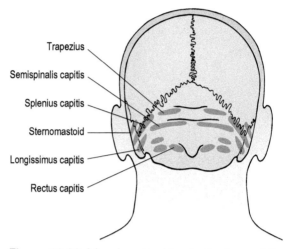

Figure 10.23 Muscles attaching to the base of the skull.

and relaxing the fingers imparts the massage. The muscles are stretched by retracting and flexing the neck, and then applying gentle overpressure. Transverse frictions may be given in prone lying or lean support sitting, using the thumb and forefinger, or forefinger supported by the middle finger to modulate pain (Fig. 10.24).

Four muscle layers are present (Table 10.4) and palpation will often identify trigger points at the muscle attachments or within their bellies. One of the main muscles to consider on the posterior aspect is the trapezius. Laterally, the sternomastoid may give pain as well as the scalenes. Trigger points (TrPs) for the sternomastoid may be found within the muscle belly or at the muscle attachment to the mastoid process. The clavicular portion of the muscle may give a TrP close to the clavicular attachment on the superior surface of the medial third of the clavicle. The scalenes may present TrPs close to the transverse processes of the cervical vertebrae. These are best located by drawing the sternomastoid muscle forwards and palpating behind it. The muscles may be stretched by combining neck and shoulder movements. The sternomastoid by depressing the shoulder then laterally flexing away from the tight side and rotating towards it, and the scalenes by stabilizing the first rib then rotating away from the tight side and flexing towards it. Where cervical pain is linked to shoulder changes, the pectoralis (major and minor) should also be considered (see Chapter 12).

Therapeutic exercise for the cervical spine

Restoration of cervical function using exercise therapy is an essential part of the treatment process, as automatic reversal of motor changes may not occur upon alleviation of a patient's symptoms (Jull et al. 2008). Cervical rehabilitation addresses the craniocervical, cervical and axioscapular muscles, and this later category is covered in Chapter 12. The topic of stabilization was covered for the lumbar spine in Chapter 8, and the principles are broadly similar for the cervical spine. The stabilizers of the cervical spine are the deep neck flexors (craniocervical flexors), longus coli, rectus capitis and longus capitis. These have a tendency to be poorly recruited following injury, while the superficial neck flexors (sternomastoid and scalenes) may be overactive, leading to substitution strategies. Retraining cervical stabilization depends on increasing the work of the deep neck flexors while reducing that of the superficial muscles, to focus on precision/control of movement.

Imbalance of the cervical region is usefully assessed by a screening test in a supine lying position. The patient is instructed to flex the neck ('look at your toes'). If the deep neck flexors are overpowered by the superficial neck flexors, rather than isolated craniocervical flexion, the chin juts forwards at the beginning of the movement (Fig. 10.25). This leads to hyperextension of the cervical spine in the suboccipital region, and the head then follows an arc-like movement as flexion continues in the lower cervical region only. This is more apparent when slight resistance is given against the forehead, and sternomastoid is seen to

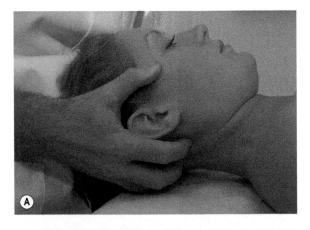

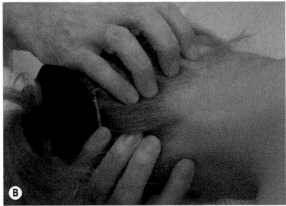

Figure 10.24 Soft tissue treatment of the suboccipital structure. (A) Whole hand position. (B) Detail of finger position.

Table 10.4 Posterior muscle layers of the neck

Layer	Category	Muscles
First	Superficial extrinsic	Trapezius, latissimus dorsi, levator scapulae, rhomboids
Second	Superficial intrinsic	Splenius capitis, splenius cervicis
Third	Erector spinae group	Longissimus capitis, longissimus cervicis (both part of erector spinae)
Fourth	Deep intrinsic	Semispinalis capitis, multifidus, rotatores

After Gunn (1996).

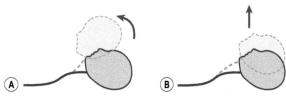

Figure 10.25 Neck flexion test. (A) Normal: cervical lordosis reverses and neck flexes. (B) Abnormal: cervical lordosis increases as chin juts forwards. Upper cervical spine hyperextends.

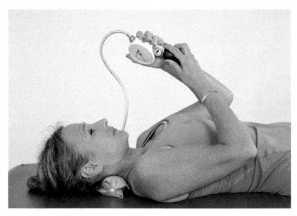

Figure 10.26 Use of pressure biofeedback unit (PBU) for deep neck flexor re-education.

stand out prominently as soon as the movement begins. Although this type of test is traditionally focused on muscle change, movement quality alteration does not depend on muscle alone. Where a subject has rehearsed a movement (through pain, habit or training) the familiarity of the action may dictate the preferential movement. Retraining the movement, rather than simply targeting the muscle, is clearly important.

> **Key point**
>
> Muscle imbalance of the cervical region may exist when the deep neck flexors are poorly recruited and the superficial flexors are overactive. Retraining movement, rather than muscle, is a key principle.

Craniocervical flexion

Re-education of deep neck flexor activity using craniocervical flexion begins in a supine-lying starting position. The head rests on the couch or small pad so that its weight does not act as a resistance to the movement. To reduce tension on mechanosensitive neural structures the patient may flex their knees and hips (crook lying) and place their arms across their abdomen to reduce neural tension. A pressure biofeedback unit (PBU) may be used to monitor head/neck movement, once the initial action has been learnt. The cuff of the unit is folded and placed behind the upper cervical spine (Fig. 10.26). The aim is to achieve suboccipital rather than lower cervical flexion. The action is a minimal flexion or 'nodding' action of the head alone

(dropping the chin to the throat), avoiding forceful actions or lifting the head from the couch. This action is popularly called a *skull rock* exercise. The cuff of the PBU is inflated sufficiently to fill the space between the cervical spine and couch, which is usually about 20 mmHg. The action is to slowly draw the chin inwards and downwards to increase the pressure by 6–10 mmHg. If the pressure reduces, the head is often being lifted by the sternomastoid and scalenes as a substitution strategy, so the exercise is restarted. The holding time of the movement is built up until the patient can maintain ten repetitions each of ten seconds duration. Several faults may be encountered during the execution of this movement, as detailed in Table 10.5.

Cervical flexion may be progressed in terms of loading by positioning the patient in crook lying with the head supported on a small foam block. The action is to curl the neck by performing upper and lower cervical flexion. The aim is to prevent any chin jutting (head protraction) movement and avoid upper cervical extension. A verbal cue of 'curling the neck vertebra by vertebra' from the head down is often useful.

Neck extensors

Neck extensor exercises begin in the four-point kneeling starting position (Fig. 10.27A). Where patients find this uncomfortable on their wrists,

Table 10.5 Correction of movement faults during craniocervical flexion

Fault	Teaching technique
▶ Cervical retraction (chin tuck) rather than craniocervical flexion (skull rock)	▶ (i) Use the tactile cue of drawing a number 1 on the couch with the back of the head. Occiput moves vertically. (ii) Encourage movement initiation with the eyes.
▶ Substitution strategy using excessive superficial cervical muscle activity.	▶ (i) Teach self-palpation of the sternocleidomastoid & anterior scalene muscles. (ii) Limit motion range and intensity to that which occurs prior to substitution strategy.
▶ Upper costal breathing action	▶ (i) Encourage muscle contraction during expiration. (ii) Teach abdominal/diaphragmatic breathing.
▶ Jaw clenching	▶ Perform action with lips together but teeth apart, tongue resting on roof of mouth
▶ Inability to reproduce required motion range accurately	▶ Teach knowledge of neural position and use reproduction of passive and then active movement.

(Data from Jull et al. 2008).

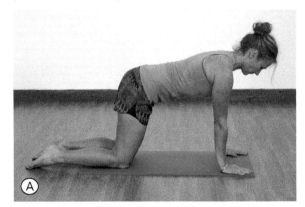

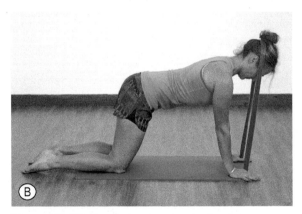

Figure 10.27 Cervical extension in 4 point kneeling. (A) Maintaining sub-occipital neural. (B) Using resistance band.

they may begin in prone lying, supporting the upper body on their arms (Sphinx position) instead. Upper cervical flexion for the rectus capitis muscles is practised using a small vertical nodding action (ask the patient to say 'yes' with their head). The obliquus capitus muscles are worked using a horizontal limited rotation movement (ask the patient to say 'no' with their head). Both of these muscle groups have important proprioceptive roles in the support and control of the upper cervical spine joints, and their role can be impaired following a whiplash injury.

Lower cervical extension is performed while the upper cervical spine is maintained in its neutral position. The distance between the base of the skull and C2 vertebra should remain unchanged to confirm that upper cervical (craniocervical) extension has not occurred. A key teaching point is to emphasize curling the neck and to limit movement of the chin. The chin should only move with the neck and not relative to it. Begin with the neck (lower cervical spine) in flexion and move just to the neutral position, keeping the eyes looking downwards rather than forwards. Once this action has been perfected, again begin with the neck in flexion, and instruct the patient to move through the neutral position into lower cervical extension, maintaining upper cervical neutral position. Greater resistance may be offered using a resistance band placed over the back of the head in the four-point kneeling (Fig. 10.27B) position initially, progressing to band usage in sitting and standing positions.

Sensorimotor and oculomotor training

Postural control involves both kinaesthesia and proprioception (Chapter 2), and from the perspective of the cervical spine three factors are key – muscle spindles within the sub-occipital muscles, the visual system (eyes) and the vestibular system (inner ear). Following injury, these systems may be disrupted, leading to loss of sensorimotor control. Symptoms include dizziness, nausea and light-headedness (cervical vertigo). Reproduction of active and passive positioning can be used to regain accurate proprioceptive control (see Chapter 2). Feedback is important to proprioceptive training, and using an inexpensive laser pointer placed on the patient's head and fixed using a headband can be effective. With a laser pointer attached to the subject's head, the action begins by establishing a starting point on the wall in front of the subject. The head is turned (rotation) or the subject looks up and down (flexion/extension) and tries to move back to the starting point. Passive movement with the therapist moving the subject's head (reproduction of passive positioning – RPP) and active movement with the subject performing the movement themselves (reproduction of active positioning – RAP) can both be performed with the eyes open and then closed. Training can be given by asking the subject to follow patterns on the wall using the laser dot.

Three types of exercise can be used for oculomotor training. First, the head is held still and the therapist moves an object horizontally and then vertically in front of the patient's face. The aim is for the patient to keep the head stable while fixing the gaze on the moving object (Fig. 10.28A). Once achieved accurately, this exercise is progressed so that the head moves with the eyes as the object is followed (Fig. 10.28B). This type of gaze fixation exercise may also be practised with simple upper-body movements, such as walking while the patient holds their finger or a pen up in front of their face. Finally, eye movements can be used to precede head movements in the same direction and then in opposite directions. All of these movements

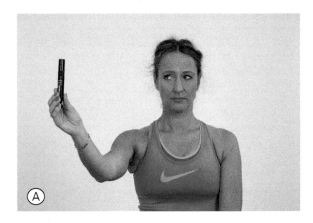

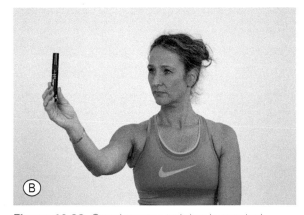

Figure 10.28 Occulomotor training in cervical rehabilitation. (A) Gaze fixation with head immobile. (B) Gaze fixation with head movement.

should be performed without an exacerbation of the patient's dizziness symptoms.

Cervical strengthening in sport

Following the restoration of appropriate stabilization and segmental control, many sports require general cervical muscle strengthening. This may be achieved by resisted movements (partner or resistance band) through range and static muscle work in bridging. Several exercise examples are given in Fig. 10.29. In each case it is essential to maintain cervical alignment. Once good alignment is lost the exercise should be stopped.

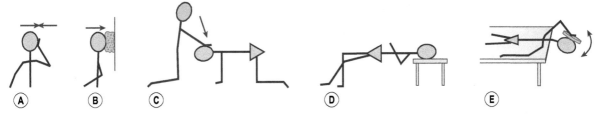

Figure 10.29 Examples of neck strengthening exercises. (A) Isometric resistance against the hand. (B) Pressing a sponge against a wall. (C) Resistance provided by a partner. (D) Neck bridge on a bench. (E) Resistance provided by a weight disc.

References

Bogduk, N., 1986. Cervical causes of headache and dizziness. In: Grieve, G.P. (ed.), *Modern Manual Therapy of the Vertebral Column*. Churchill Livingstone, Edinburgh.

Cleland, J.A., Whitman, J.M., Fritz, J.M., Palmer, J.A., 2005. Manual physical therapy, cervical traction, and strengthening exercises in patients with cervical radiculopathy: A case series. *Journal of Orthopaedic and Sports Physical Therapy* **35** (2), 802–808.

Cyriax, J., 1982. *Textbook of Orthopaedic Medicine*, 8th ed. Baillière Tindall, London.

Cyriax, J.H., Cyriax, P.J., 1983. *Illustrated Manual of Orthopaedic Medicine*. Butterworth, London.

Ernst, E., 2004. Cerebrovascular complications associated with spinal manipulation. *Physical Therapy Reviews* **9**, 5–15.

Grant, R., 1994a. Vertebral artery concerns: pre-manipulative testing of the cervical spine. In: Grant, R. (ed.), *Physical Therapy of the Cervical and Thoracic Spine*, 2nd ed. Churchill Livingstone, Edinburgh.

Grant, R., 1994b. Vertebral artery insufficiency: a clinical protocol for pre-manipulative testing of the cervical spine. In: Boyling, J.D., Palastanga, N. (eds), *Grieve's Modern Manual Therapy*, 2nd ed. Churchill Livingstone, Edinburgh.

Grieve, G.P., 1986. *Modern Manual Therapy of the Vertebral Column*. Churchill Livingstone, Edinburgh.

Gross, A., Miller, J., D'Sylva, J. et al., 2010. Manipulation or mobilisation for neck pain: a Cochrane review. *Manual Therapy* **15** (4), 315–333.

Gunn, C.C., 1996. *Treatment of Chronic Pain*, 2nd ed. Churchill Livingstone, Edinburgh.

Horowitz, M., Wilner, N., and Alvarez, W., 1979. Impact of event scale. *Psychosomatic Medicine* **41**, 209–218

Jull, G., Sterling, M., Falla D., Treleaven, J., 2008. *Whiplash, Headache and Neck Pain: Research Based Directions for Physical Therapies*. Churchill Livingston. Edinburgh.

Kerry, R., Taylor, A., Mitchell, J., McCarthy, C., 2008. Cervical arterial dysfunction and manual therapy: a critical literature review to inform professional practice. *Manual Therapy* **13**, 278–288.

Kranenburga, H.A., Schmitt, M.A., Puentedurac, E.J. et al., 2017. Adverse events associated with the use of cervical spine manipulation or mobilization and patient characteristics: a systematic review. *Musculoskeletal Science and Practice* **28**, 32–38.

Lamb, S.E., Gates, S., Williams, M.A., et al., 2013. Managing Injuries of the Neck Trial (MINT) Study Team. Emergency department treatments and physiotherapy for acute whiplash: a pragmatic, two-step, randomised controlled trial. *Lancet* **381** (9866), 546–556.

Leaver, A.M., Maher, C.G., Herbert, R.D. et al., 2010. A randomized controlled trial comparing manipulation with mobilization for recent onset neck pain. *Arch P.*

Meyer, S.A., Schulte, K.R., Callaghan, J.J., Albright, J.P., 1994. Cervical spinal stenosis and stingers in collegiate football players. *American Journal of Sports Medicine* **22**, 158–166.

Pettman, E., 1994. Stress tests of the craniovertebral joints. In: Boyling, J.D., Palastanga, N. (eds),

Grieve's Modern Manual Therapy, 2nd ed. Churchill Livingstone, Edinburgh.

Rushton, A., Rivett, D., Carlesso, L. et al., 2014. International framework for examination of the cervical region for potential cervical arterial dysfunction prior to orthopaedic manual therapy intervention. *Manual Therapy* **19**, 222–228.

Siegmund, G.P., Winkelstein, B.A., Ivanic, P., Svensson, M., Vasavada, A., 2009. The anatomy and biomechanics of acute and chronic whiplash injury. *Traffic Injury Prevention* **10**, 101–112.

Silver, J.R., Silver, D.D., Godfrey, J.J., 1986. Injuries of the spine sustained during gymnastic activities. *British Medical Journal* **293**, 861–863.

Torg, J.S., 1982. *Athletic Injuries to the Head, Neck and Face*. Lea and Febiger, Philadelphia.

Torg, J.S., 2002. Cervical spinal stenosis with core neurapraxia: evaluations and decisions regarding participation in athletics. *Current Sports Medicine Reports* **1** (1), 43–46.

Torg, J.S., Sennett, B., Pavlov, H., Leventhal, M.R., Glasgow, S.G., 1993. Spear tackler's spine: an entity precluding participation in tackle football and collision activities that expose the cervical spine to axial energy inputs. *American Journal of Sports Medicine* **21**, 640–649.

Torg, J.S., Vegso, J.J., Sennett, B., Das, M., 1985. The national football head and neck injury registry: 14-year report on cervical quadriplegia, 1971 through 1984. *Journal of the American Medical Association* **254**, 3439–3443.

Vernon, H., Mior, S., 1991. The neck disability index: a study of reliability and validity. *Journal of Manipulative and Physiological Therapeutics* **14**, 409.

Wainner, R.S., Fritz, J.M., Irrgang, J.J., et al., 2003. Reliability and diagnostic accuracy of the clinical examination and patient self report measures for cervical radiculopathy. *Spine* **28** (1), 52–62.

Winkelstein, B., Myers, B., 1997. The biomechanics of cervical spine injury and implications for injury prevention. *Medicine and Science in Sport and Exercise* **29** (2), 246–255.

Wong, J.J., Shearer, H.M., Mior, S., et al., 2016. Are manual therapies, passive physical modalities, or acupuncture effective for the management of patients with whiplash-associated disorders or neck pain and associated disorders? An update of the Bone and Joint Decade Task Force on Neck Pain and Its Associated Disorders by the OPTIMa collaboration. *Spine J* **16** (12),1598–1630.

Worsfold, C. (2013) Whiplash rehabilitation – an evidence-based approach. *In Touch. Journal for Physiotherapists in Private Practice* **144**, 14–21.

CHAPTER 11

The face and head

Ocular injury

Surface anatomy and basic muscle examination of the eye are shown in Treatment Note 11.1.

Eye injuries may arise from collisions in which a finger or elbow goes into the eye. Small balls in sport (squash balls, shuttlecocks) may cause ocular damage, while larger balls (cricket or hockey) are more likely to cause orbital fractures. Mud, grit or stone chips can enter the eye and cause both irritation and damage. It is interesting to note the speed at which a ball may move. In squash, the ball can travel at 140 mph, in cricket at 110 mph and in football at 35–75 mph. A small object travelling at these speeds obviously creates considerable force and potential for damage. This is borne out by the sad fact that over 10 per cent of eye injuries in sport result in blindness in that eye.

Where a foreign body is in the eye, quantities of water should be used to irrigate the eye and wash the object out (a squeeze bottle is particularly useful). Sit the subject down and get him or her to look up, right, left and then down as sterile/clean water is poured into the inner corner of the eye. No attempt should be made to probe the eye as this may cause the object to scratch the cornea.

> **Key point**
>
> An eyewash bottle (sterile water) is an essential item for first aid in sport. With the athlete sitting, pour water into the inner corner of the eye while they look up, right, left, and then down.

In some instances, particularly if the foreign body is an eyelash, the eyelid may be rolled back on itself. This procedure is carried out by first asking the athlete to look down. The therapist then grasps the lashes of the upper lid, pulling them gently down and out, away from the eye. A cotton swab is placed on the outside of the lid level with the lid crease. The lashes are then folded upwards over the swab to reveal the inside of the eyelid, and the foreign body is washed away. The eyelid goes back to its normal position when the athlete looks up and blinks.

A foreign body is one of the most common eye problems on the sports field, and is often seen in manual occupations. The reaction is usually pain and tear production. If the object is not removed, blinking may cause corneal abrasion and extreme pain for about 48 hours.

Treatment note 11.1   Surface examination of the eye

Lacrimal sac

Lacrimal gland

Flow of tears

Inferior canaliculus

Nasolacrimal duct

Upper eyelid   Pupil   Iris

Lacrimal lake   Lower eyelid   Sclera

(A)   (B)

Figure 11.1 Eye and lacrimal apparatus, indicating flow of tears. From Drake et al. (2010).

The sclera of the eye is the white portion at the side of the iris. It continues as the cornea, which is the clear central region of the eye through which the iris (eye colour) and pupil (black centre) may be seen. At the medial corner of the eye is the lacrimal lake, in which the tears collect. Tears originate in the lacrimal gland on the upper outer aspect of the orbit and flow downwards and inwards across the eye to hydrate the cornea. Once collected in the lacrimal lake, the tears drain into the nasal cavity. The eye and lacrimal apparatus is shown in Fig. 11.1.

Movement of the eye is controlled by the extrinsic or extraocular muscles, and each muscle may be tested by asking the patient to look in a particular direction (Fig. 11.2). This is most commonly carried out by having the patient follow the therapist's finger while keeping his/her head in a fixed position. The examination highlights abnormality of the third (oculomotor), fourth (trochlear) and sixth (abducent) cranial nerves, which supply the muscles.

Table 11.1 lists signs and symptoms which are indications for immediate ophthalmology referral.

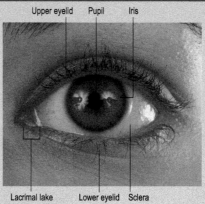

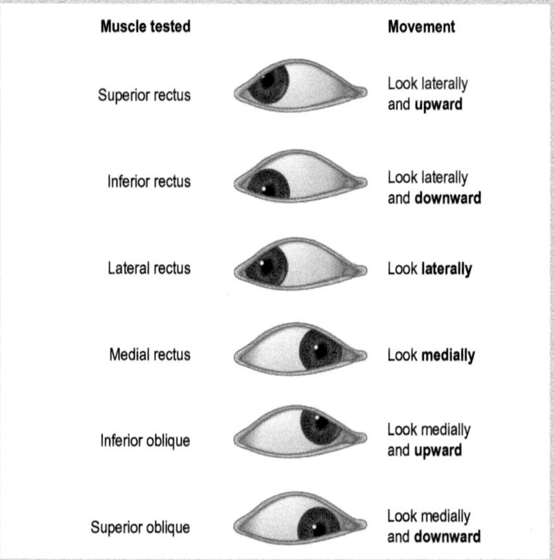

Muscle tested		Movement
Superior rectus		Look laterally and **upward**
Inferior rectus		Look laterally and **downward**
Lateral rectus		Look **laterally**
Medial rectus		Look **medially**
Inferior oblique		Look medially and **upward**
Superior oblique		Look medially and **downward**

Figure 11.2 Functional muscle testing of the extraocular muscles. From Drake et al. (2010).

Table 11.1 Indications for ophthalmic referral following eye injury

Severe eye pain
Peristant double vision (diplopia)
Persistent blurred vision or light sensitivity (photophobia)
Blood within the anterior chamber of the eye (hyphemia)
Penetrating injury (corneal laceration, misshaped pupil)
Embedded foreign object
Loss of part of visual field

(Data modified from French et al. 2017).

Definition

Corneal abrasion is a scratch on the clear region at the front of the eye.

Key point

Contact lenses should not be re-inserted until the eye has healed and been completely symptom free for 24 hours following injury.

It is important not to allow the subject to touch the foreign body as this will simply increase the area of abrasion. If the object cannot be washed out easily, cover the eye with a sterile dressing and take the subject to hospital. Encourage the subject to keep the eyes still as movement of the uninjured eye will also move the injured one, increasing tissue damage.

Contact lenses can cause problems. Hard lenses may break or become scratched or roughened, causing corneal damage. Soft lenses are easily torn. When the eye has been injured or infected, a contact lens should never be re-inserted until the eye has healed completely for at least 24 hours.

When contact lenses become dislodged, the wearer, with the aid of a mirror, is often the person most capable of removing them. Hard lenses may be removed with a small suction cup, available from an optician, and persistent soft lenses may be dislodged by water from a squeeze bottle, or by gently wiping with a cotton swab.

Following injury, basic vision assessment should be carried out and if any abnormalities are detected the subject should be referred to an ophthalmologist. A distance chart (placed six metres from the subject) and a near-vision chart (35 cm from the eyes) should be used. Failure to read the 20/40 line on either chart is

Table 11.2 Common eye symptoms encountered in sport

Symptoms	Possible cause
Eye itself	
Itching	Dry eyes, fatigue, allergies
Tears	Hypersecretion of tears, blocked drainage, emotional state
Dry eyes	Decreased secretion through ageing, certain medications
Sandy/gritty eyes	Conjunctivitis
Twitching	Fibrillation of orbicularis oculi muscle
Eyelid heaviness	Lid oedema, fatigue
Blinking	Local irritation, facial tic
Eyelids sticking together	Inflammatory conditions of lid or conjunctiva
Sensation of 'something in the eye'	Corneal abrasion, foreign body
Burning	Conjunctivitis
Throbbing/aching	Sinusitis, iritis
Vision	
Spots in front of eyes	Usually no pathology, but if persists consider possible retinal detachment
Flashes	Migraine, retinal detachment
Glare/photophobia	Iritis, consider meningitis
Sudden vision distortion	Macular oedema, retinal detachment
Presence of shadows or dark areas	Retinal haemorrhage, retinal detachment

Adapted from Magee (2002).

a reason for referral. Visual fields are tested in all four quadrants. One eye is covered, and the subject should look into the examiner's eyes. The examiner moves a finger to the edge of the visual field in both horizontal and vertical directions until the subject loses sight of it. Decreased visual acuity or loss of the visual field in one area warrants referral.

Pupil reaction may be tested with a small pen torch. Pupil size, shape and speed of reaction are noted. Pupil dilation in reaction to illumination requires immediate referral, as does any irregularity in pupil shape and an inability to clear blurring of vision by blinking. A number of common eye symptoms and possible causes are listed in Table 11.2.

Eye protection

Sports trauma accounts for 25 per cent of all serious ocular injuries (Jones 1989), and many could be prevented by wearing eye protection. Prevention of ocular trauma comes from two sources: sports practice and eye protection.

Changes in sports practice include rule modification and increasing player awareness. For example, rule changes in Canadian ice hockey to prevent high sticking have greatly reduced eye injury. Injury in badminton is more frequent at the net, so teaching young players to cover their face with the racquet when receiving a smash at the net would seem sensible.

Key point

Most sports injuries to the eye could be prevented if athletes wore eye protection.

Individual athletes should also protect themselves. The eye protectors worn must be capable of dissipating force, but should not restrict the field of vision or the player's comfort. In addition, if they are to be acceptable to a player they must be cosmetically attractive and inexpensive.

Each sport will have its own specific requirements. Where the blow is of great intensity, the eye protector must be incorporated into a helmet, and if there is a danger of irritation (chlorine in a swimming pool) the material used must be chemically resistant. Goggles for skiing must filter out ultraviolet light, while those for shooting may have to be suitable for low-light conditions or capable of screening out glare.

For general protection in racquet sports, polycarbonate lenses mounted in plastic rather than wire frames are the choice. The nasal bridge and sides of such a protector should be broad and strong to deflect or absorb force.

Dental injury

The simplest form of tooth injury is a concussion in which the anterior teeth are knocked against something. This may occur from a head butt, a punch, or someone running into a piece of apparatus. There is only minor soft tissue damage and the teeth and mouth are sore. The front teeth may be painful on eating, so the subject should avoid eating hard foods until the pain subsides.

Tooth subluxation occurs when a tooth becomes mobile after a direct injury, but is not displaced. On examination, the tooth may be loose and tender, and there may be some gum damage. It is usual for the teeth to tighten up and heal within a week, but the subject should see his or her dentist. A subluxed tooth may have damaged its dental artery or vein. When this happens, the venous blood can stagnate in the tooth and the haemoglobin seeps into the dentine, turning the tooth dull yellow and eventually grey.

Displacement of a tooth is more common when a gum shield is not worn. The displaced tooth should be washed briefly in sterile water or saline, taking care to put the tooth back the right way round. The subject may hold the tooth in place by biting on a cloth or handkerchief until specialist advice can be sought. In children, a displaced tooth may be soaked in whole milk until help is available.

The tooth should be handled by the crown to avoid further damage to the cells at its root. Good results may be expected if re-implantation is carried out within 30 minutes of trauma, but after 2 hours the prognosis is poor.

Examination of the tooth after an impact injury is initially by a pressure test. The biting edge of the tooth is gently pressed inwards towards the tongue and then outwards towards the lips. If the tooth is painless (but not numb) and moves only as much as its neighbours, injury is normally restricted to the gums alone. If the tooth is numb, painful, mobile, or depressed below the level of the other teeth, the subject requires dental referral.

> ### Key point
> After an impact injury affecting the teeth, tooth numbness, excessive mobility or depression below the level of the other teeth indicate the need for dental referral.

A number of tooth fractures may occur (Fig. 11.3). A small corner of the tooth may be chipped off, leaving a sharp edge which may cut into the tongue. Larger chips can expose the tooth dentine, causing pain when the subject sucks air into the mouth, or the tooth pulp, which can be seen by looking up into the mouth. This latter injury is a dental emergency, as are complete tooth fractures of the root apex or at gum level.

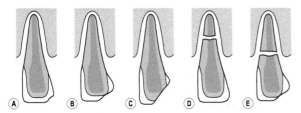

Figure 11.3 Tooth fractures. (A) Small corner fracture involving enamel only. (B) Larger corner fracture with dentine exposure. (C) Nerve root pulp exposed. (D) Fracture close to root apex. (E) Fracture at gum level. From Reid (1992), with permission.

Mouthguards

Custom-made mouthguards (gum shields) have been shown to reduce the incidence of dental injuries by as much as 90 per cent (Jennings 1990). In addition, they stop the teeth from cutting into the lips and cheeks. When the jaw is hit from below, the bottom teeth will impact into the guard, absorbing some of the impact force. A mouthguard will also modify the transmission of force through the temporomandibular joints. The combination of altered force transmission and shock absorption can reduce the likelihood of concussion and mandibular fracture. Any guard must cover the surfaces of the upper teeth, be comfortable to wear, and allow unhindered breathing and speech. Furthermore, it must show good properties of retention in the mouth, and give proper inter-maxillary positioning.

Mouthguards were originally worn in boxing, when they were simply curved pieces of rubber gripped between the teeth. Progress has been made in their design, and nowadays three types are available: custom-made, mouth-formed and ready moulded. Most protection is given to the upper front teeth, these being the ones most susceptible to injury.

For custom-made gum shields the first step is to take an impression of the upper teeth using a material such as alginate. Dental stone is poured into the impression to create a positive model of the teeth. Polyvinyl acetate-polyethelene (PVAc-PE) is vacuum formed over the model, and the mouthguard is trimmed and smoothed off.

Self-moulded guards come in two types. The first is soaked in hot water to soften it and moulded over the upper teeth ('boil and bite'). The second type consists of a preformed outer shell into which a plasticized acrylic gel or silicone rubber is added. The outer shell and fluid gel are placed over the teeth and pressed into position until the gel sets.

The dentally fitted type of mouth protector is better in terms of both safety and effectiveness. The model made from the impression of the subject's mouth can be reused to form a number of mouth shields.

The ready moulded kind are available off the shelf in many sports shops. They do not fit well, and have to be held in place by gritting the teeth. They should not be recommended to subjects as they are easily dislodged and may block the airway.

> **Key point**
> Ready moulded mouthguards (gum shields) which are held in place by gritting the teeth are dangerous. They are easily dislodged and may block the airway. Use a self-fitted (boil and bite) or dentally fitted unit instead.

Auricular injury

Cauliflower ear

Auricular haematoma ('cauliflower ear') is normally caused by a direct blow to the ear, in sports such as boxing and rugby. Blood and serum accumulate between the perichondrium and external ear cartilage, and secondary infection may arise. First aid treatment involves the use of ice and compression. As soon as possible the haematoma should be aspirated or drained through an incision, and the ear compressed to prevent further fluid accumulation. The injury occurs particularly in contact sports such as wrestling, boxing and rugby, and is very common. Schuller et al. (1989) found 39 per cent of high school and collegiate wrestlers from a group of 537 had one or both of the auricles permanently deformed by injury. Some degree of prevention may be achieved by wearing protective headgear.

Underwater diving injury

Air either side of the tympanic membrane should be at equal pressure. Externally, the air is at atmospheric pressure, and internally the Eustachian tube leads to the nasopharynx. Pressure changes such as those that occur in an aeroplane are equalized by swallowing or yawning, through the Eustachian tube mechanism. If the free exchange

of air is impaired, barotrauma may occur. If the outside air pressure rises, such as may occur in diving, and the Eustachian tube mechanism is unable to equalize pressure, pain will result, a condition referred to as 'the squeeze'. Small haemorrhages may occur in the middle ear and the tympanic membrane may burst in depths below three metres. With a severe cold, the Eustachian tube may be blocked, so a subject should not dive (or fly if the condition is severe).

Barotrauma to the inner ear secondary to decompression is less common, but considerably more serious. This type of trauma usually occurs at depths below 35 m. Symptoms may be caused by the formation of gas bubbles in the blood vessels supplying the inner ear (Renon et al. 1986).

The reduction in air volume at increasing depths is responsible for another danger with diving and underwater swimming, the phenomenon of 'mask squeeze'. A relative vacuum is created in a diving mask or swimming goggles as the diver descends. With a mask, this is equalized by breathing out through the nose into the mask, but with swimming goggles this is not possible. A swimming pool may be as deep as three or four metres. Children who dive down for objects at this depth face the very real danger of conjunctival haemorrhage and oedema. As the air space within the goggles is not connected to a body cavity, the air pressure will not be equalized. The pressure within the goggles will drop lower than that inside the body causing the ocular vascular system to over-distend and fluid to accumulate in the tissues covered by the goggles.

> **Key point**
> Conjunctival haemorrhage or oedema (bleeding or swelling of the eye membrane) may occur in children who wear swimming goggles and dive for objects in a deep pool.

Diving with ear plugs in or with an upper respiratory tract infection should also be avoided because of danger to the eardrum (tympanic membrane). Water pressure will press an ear plug further in, compressing the air between the plug and eardrum. This can cause severe pain and may even rupture the drum. During any change in air pressure, the pressure inside the eardrum is equalized through the Eustachian tube mechanism when swallowing or yawning. With upper respiratory tract infections, this tube can become blocked, giving severe pain (middle-ear squeeze) as the eardrum is stretched inwards.

Swimming pool ear

Swimming pool ear (otitis externa) is an irritable condition of the outer ear which can occur in subjects who swim regularly. The symptoms are mainly itching, bordering on pain, but in extreme cases discharge may occur and even partial hearing loss. The ear canal produces its own protective layer of cerumen (wax). With prolonged exposure to chlorinated water especially, the wax may degenerate and the skin of the inner ear can become macerated. This leaves the ear open to bacterial or fungal infection, especially as the skin is damaged by vigorous drying (corner of a towel or cotton swabs) or scratching (fingernail).

Prevention is the key to this condition. Ear wax should not be removed, and nothing should be inserted into the ear. To limit water contact, rather than using ear plugs a close-fitting swimming cap

can be used. Where itching is present, anti-bacterial eardrops should be used and the subject should avoid water contact until the symptoms settle.

Maxillofacial injuries

Sport accounts for about 12 per cent of maxillofacial injuries (Handler 1991), with fractures of the maxilla and zygomatic bones being more common in contact sports (Fig. 11.4). If the upper jaw has been subjected to a blow, injury should be suspected if the teeth are out of alignment or one half of the cheek feels numb. Direct palpation of these fractures is painful, and pain may be elicited as far back as the temporomandibular joint if the subject is asked to bite on a folded cloth or tongue depressor. Chewing will be painful and local swelling may be apparent.

> **Key point**
> To assess fractures of the maxilla or zygomatic bones, ask the subject to bite on a folded cloth or tongue depressor and palpate for pain.

Bony deformities are assessed as follows:

▶ The *zygoma* is often better assessed by looking at both cheekbones from the top of the patient's head (Fig. 11.5A). Gently palpate the

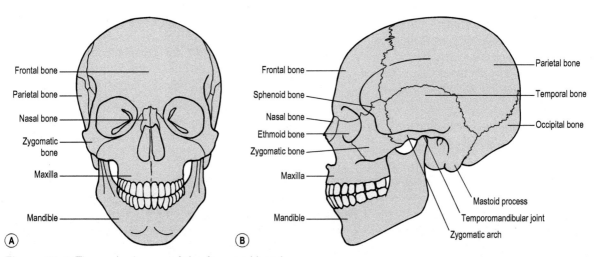

Figure 11.4 The major bones of the face and head.

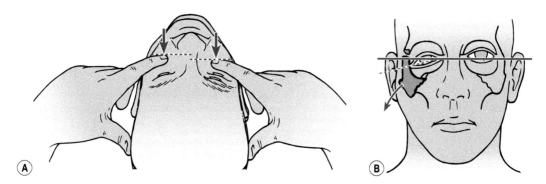

Figure 11.5 Assessing zygomatic fractures. (A) Checking for bone deformity. (B) Depression of the lateral canthus. After Magee (2002), with permission.

zygoma with the flat of the finger and compare finger levels. In addition, with fractures of the zygoma, as the bone drops inferiorly it will pull the lateral canthus down with it (Fig. 11.5B).

▶ The *maxilla* may be assessed by stabilizing the head with one hand and reaching up inside the mouth to grip the bone above the upper teeth. Assess for pain and anterior bony displacement.

▶ *Mandibular* fracture may occur with a direct blow to the chin, with pain being experienced as the mouth is opened or closed, in an area in front of the ear. There is malocclusion and abnormal mobility of the mandible.

Most of these fractures extend through the intraoral mucosa and so bleeding is often noticed from the mouth. The primary aim is to ensure a clear airway. Blood, bone and tooth fragments and saliva must be cleared from the mouth. The mobile jaw fragment may be temporarily secured with a bandage around the head and chin.

The local application of ice will ease pain, and direct pressure by the subject supports the area until hospitalization is achieved.

A severe blow such as occurs in contact sports (boxing and martial arts especially) may cause a *blowout fracture*. Here the floor or occasionally the medial wall of the orbit is fractured. If not identified, vision may be permanently impaired or lost through damage to the ocular nerves or development

of an abscess (Karsteter and Yunker 2006). The mechanism of injury is a severe blow directed to the ocular region.

> **Definition**
>
> A blowout fracture may occur in contact sports. The floor of the orbit is usually fractured, and the eyeball pushed backwards.

The force of the blow is conducted from the thicker orbital rim to the orbital floor, which, as the weaker segment, then gives way. In addition, the increased pressure within the eyeball (intraorbital hydraulic pressure) is transmitted to the wall of the orbit, causing the bone to give way. Following blunt trauma to the ocular region, suspicion of blowout fracture is raised in the presence of immediate eye swelling with a feeling of fullness in the eye, pain around the orbital rim, recession of the eyeball (enophthalmos), vision change and pain on eye movement, especially adduction and infraduction (look down and in). Confirmation is by X-ray or MRI.

> **Definition**
>
> Enophthalmos is sinking (recession) of the eyeball within the orbit. It is evaluated in comparison to the uninjured side and in relation to the orbital rim.

Temporomandibular joint pain

The temporomandibular joint (TMJ) can give rise to facial pain of various types, often resulting from alterations in the way the teeth come together (occlusion). This may be affected by mouthguards used in sports, as a reaction following dental work, or as a result of direct facial trauma.

Structure and function

The TMJ is a synovial condyloid joint found between the mandibular fossa of the temporal bone and the condyle of the mandible. The two bony surfaces are covered with fibrocartilage and separated by an articular disc. Movements of the jaw include protraction, retraction, elevation, depression and lateral gliding, all of which are used to some extent when chewing. The three main muscles contributing to TMJ motion are the temporalis, masseter and pterygoids, and deep tissue massage or acupuncture/dry needling may be used to treat trigger points within these (see Treatment Note 11.2). The temporalis fans out from the temporal fossa to insert into the coronoid process of the mandible. The masseter has both deep and superficial portions and attaches from the zygomatic arch and maxillary process to the angle of the mandible. The medial pterygoid is similar in position to the masseter, but the lateral pterygoid arises from the sphenoid bone and inserts into the mandibular condyle and articular disc, playing a large part in stabilization of the TMJ.

In the occluded position, the upper teeth are normally in front of the lower ones. As the mouth is opened, the lower incisors move downwards and forwards, a movement encompassing forward gliding and rotation at the TMJ. Depression of the mandible is controlled by eccentric action of the temporalis, but if resisted, the geniohyoid, mylohyoid and digastric muscles contract. The jaw is closed powerfully by masseter, temporalis and the medial pterygoid. The lateral pterygoid pulls the mandible forwards (protraction) while the temporalis is the main effector of retraction.

Pathology

Dysfunction of the TMJ may present as local muscle tenderness, limited motion and a general dull ache over the side of the face. Clicking may be present, and patients often protrude the mandible as the jaw is opened, or sublux the joint. When chronic, the condition may show reduced range of motion, with contracture of the masticatory muscles. Pain and muscle spasm are common, with the lateral pterygoids most usually affected. Emotional stress which presents as teeth clenching is a common factor, as is an alteration in bite pattern and chewing action.

Trauma to the area is common in contact sports, and soft tissue damage and subluxation/dislocation may occur. Whiplash injuries can also give rise to the condition. As the head tips back rapidly, the jaw flies open, stretching the masseter and joint structures. Immediately following this the jaw snaps shut, which may in turn compromise the articular meniscus.

Management

Joint mobilization

With the patient in a side-lying starting position (Fig. 11.6), the head of the mandible may be palpated just in front of the ear canal (external auditory meatus) and felt to move as the mouth is opened and closed. *Anteroposterior* and *posteroanterior* joint mobilization may be performed using one thumb pad as the other thumb monitors movement at the TMJ. By reaching inside the mouth (gloved hand) the thumb may be placed along the medial surface of the mandible (Fig. 11.6B) and can then be used to produce *lateral gliding*. By altering the thumb position slightly and gripping the mandible inside the mouth with the thumb and outside with the fingers, a *longitudinal* mobilization may be performed.

Home exercise/movement techniques

Normal functional opening of the mouth is between 25 and 35 mm depending on body size. This

487

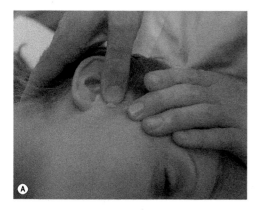

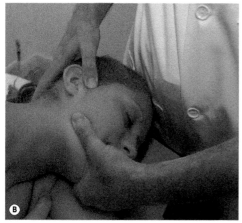

Figure 11.6 Mobilization techniques for the temporomandibular joint (TMJ). (A) Anteroposterior (AP) mobilization. (B) Lateral glide.

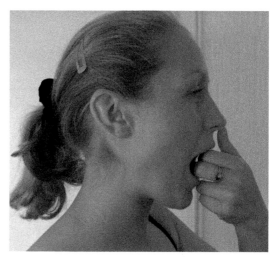

Figure 11.7 Self-stretching procedure for the temporomandibular joint (TMJ).

may be assessed by asking the patient to place two of their knuckles into their mouth (Fig. 11.7). Inability to do this indicates TMJ hypomobility. Self-stretching to increase maximal mouth opening (MMO) begins by asking the patient to simply open and close the mouth, gradually increasing the range until a yawning motion is used. Prolonged static stretch is used by placing a single knuckle and then two knuckles between the teeth. The stretched position is maintained for five to ten minutes until the muscles relax.

Translation movements occur when the mouth is opened further than about 1 cm. From this position the patient is instructed to protrude and retract the chin, and to use lateral gliding movements (Fig. 11.8).

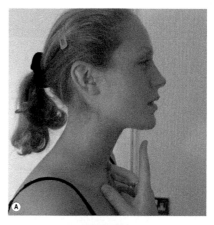

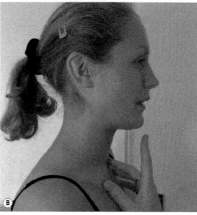

Figure 11.8 Temporomandibular joint (TMJ) home exercise. (A) Chin protraction. (B) Chin retraction.

Treatment note 11.2   Dry needling in the treatment of TMJ pain

The three muscles giving pain in TMJ conditions are the lateral pterigoid, masseter and the temporalis. All of these muscles may develop painful trigger points (TrP), which can be successfully treated using ischaemic pressure or dry needling. In addition, several traditional acupuncture points are found in this region which may be used in the treatment of TMJ pain and facial pain in general.

Trigger points

The lateral pterygoid muscle is claimed to be the main source of TrP pain to the TMJ (Simons, Travell and Simons 1999). It can only be effectively palpated through the masseter muscle, and then only with the mouth open by 2–3 cm. The muscle lies between the mandibular notch and the zygomatic arch.

TrPs for the temporalis muscle are found 1–2 finger breadths above the zygomatic arch and also towards the anterior aspect of the muscle at its attachment behind the supraorbital ridge. Interestingly, this is the precise location of a traditional acupuncture point (extra point) called Taiyang, meaning 'supreme yang' and regularly

used for the relief of frontal headaches. TrPs for the masseter are more easily found with the mouth open. Central TrPs are located on a diagonal bisecting the angle of the mandible, and attachment TrPs up towards the zygomatic process (Fig. 11.9).

Traditional acupuncture points

The stomach (ST), small intestine (SI) and gallbladder (GB) acupuncture meridians (channels) all travel on the side of the face and have important points which can be used in the treatment of TMJ pain. The point ST-6 lies within the belly of the masseter muscles and is often tender to palpation. The point GB-8 lies within the temporalis muscle and again may be painful. The point SI-19 lies directly behind the TMJ and the point ST-7 lies directly in front. Both may be used in TMJ treatment (Fig. 11.10).

Dry needling technique

The superficial nature of the structures in the face make precise needling essential. The point ST-6 should be needled no deeper than 0.5 cm, if needling perpendicularly, and deeper only if

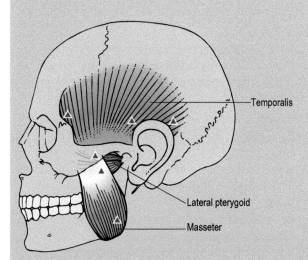

Figure 11.9 Trigger points in relation to the temporomandibular joint (TMJ).

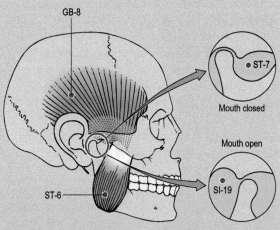

Figure 11.10 Traditional acupuncture points in relation to the temporomandibular joint (TMJ).

489

Treatment note 11.2 *continued*

a transverse insertion is used. For this type of insertion, a fold of skin is lifted and the needle placed into the skin only.

GB-8 lies 1.5 cm above the apex of the ear, and at this point there is a slight depression. Again needle insertion is superficial: 0.5–1.0 cm, angled transversely. Both SI-19 and ST-7 are located by first palpating the condyle of the mandible just in front of the ear. As the mouth is opened

the condyle slides down and forwards and SI-19 is located in the gap behind the condyle. The point is then needled with the mouth slightly open to a depth of no more than 1 cm. ST-7 is located in the hollow in front of the condyle when the mouth is closed and is then needled to a depth of 0.5–1.0 cm. Importantly, both points are not needled at the same time: palpation will reveal the more tender point, which is then chosen.

Nasal injury

Nasal injuries mainly require treatment for haemorrhage (nose bleed). Direct pressure should be applied to the distal part of the nose with the head held forward. The subject is able to breathe through the mouth. In cases where bleeding is severe, a cotton-wool ball or compress may be placed inside the nostril, providing the pad is large enough not to be inhaled. If bleeding continues, hospitalization may be required to cauterize the ruptured vessels or apply vessel-constricting agents.

Nasal fracture is one of the most common maxillofacial injuries in sport. Often the nasal bones are obviously deviated to one side or depressed. Gently running the finger down the edge or bridge of the nose may reveal a step deformity, but this can easily be disguised when oedema is excessive (frequently the case). Generally, reduction is only required where there is obstruction of the nasal passages, or to improve the cosmetic outcome. Reduction of a displaced fracture should be performed within seven days because, after this, fibrosis makes accurate realignment of the bony fragments difficult.

The nasal septum and orbit must be examined at the same time as the nose, as concurrent injuries here can often go unnoticed. Septal haematoma may expand to block the air passage. Treatment is usually by evacuation of the clot, followed by nasal packing using a nasal tampon or gauze.

Definition

A septal haematoma is bleeding and bruising (haematoma) between the two layers of mucosa covering the nasal septum.

Concussion

Unconsciousness is the result of an interruption of normal brain activity. In sport this may be a result of both *head injury* and *sport related concussion (SRC)*. The condition is more common in horse riding (equestrian) and striking sports such as boxing and freestyle martial arts, but is also seen in rugby and football with player collisions.

Sports-related concussion is a traumatic brain injury induced by biomechanical forces. Table 11.3 outlines common features of SRC.

Concussion occurs when the brain is rapidly 'shaken', and the condition can be present even though the patient is still conscious. Often, the period of unconsciousness is so brief that it may go unnoticed, and there is only transient memory loss. This is frequently the case with contact injuries, where an athlete collides with another and hits his or her head, or where the head is shaken violently. Clinically, concussion may occur from a direct blow to the head or from impulsive force which is transmitted to the head from other regions of the body. There is an impairment of neurological function, which is usually short lived and resolves

Table 11.3 Common features of sports-related concussion (SRC)

▶ SRC may be caused by a direct blow to the head, face, neck.
▶ A blow to the body may create an impulsive force transmitted to the head.
▶ Typically, a rapid onset and short-lived impairment of neurological function that resolves spontaneously.
▶ In some cases, signs and symptoms evolve over a number of minutes/hours.
▶ Signs and symptoms normally reflect a functional disturbance rather than a structural injury.
▶ No abnormality is generally seen on standard structural neuroimaging.
▶ Loss of consciousness may or may not occur.
▶ Resolution of clinical and cognitive features typically follows a sequential course.
▶ Signs and symptoms cannot be explained by drug, alcohol or medication use, or other injuries or co-morbidities.

(Data modified from McCrory et al. 2017)

spontaneously. In SRC there is a *functional disturbance* rather than structural damage, and as such neuroimaging is generally normal (McCrory et al. 2017).

> **Key point**
>
> In sport-related concussion the disturbance is functional not structural. Neuroimaging is therefore normal.

The Glasgow coma scale (see below) is traditionally used to assess head injury. However, due to the mild nature of sport concussion this type of scale is no longer considered, by itself, an appropriate evaluation measure for sport concussion. A sport concussion assessment tool (SCAT) was developed at the International Conference on Concussion in Sport, Prague 2004, and has been updated several times, culminating most recently, at the Berlin conference 2016, with the development of the SCAT5 for subjects over the age of 13, and the Child SCAT5 for children aged 5–12 years (McCrory

Table 11.4 Factors to be aware of following a concussion incident

Worsening headache	Persistent irritability
Drowsiness or inability to wake up	Seizures (arms and legs jerk uncontrollably)
Inability to recognize people or places	Weakness or numbness in the arms or legs
Repeated vomiting	Unsteadiness on feet
Unusual behaviour or confusion	Slurred speech

(Data modified from McCrory et al. 2017)

et al. 2017). Originally, a Pocket SCAT was developed for non-medical professionals, and this has been replaced with the concussion recognition tool (CRT5).

The SCAT5 takes a minimum of 10 minutes to complete, and consists of on-field and off-field tests. On-field testing identifies red flags, observable signs, memory assessment (Maddocks questions), examination (Glasgow coma scale) and cervical spine assessment. Off-field testing details athlete background, symptom evaluation, cognitive screening, neurological screening, delayed recall testing, and decision making. The SCAT5 is available for free download at http://bjsm.bmj.com/content/bjsports/early/2017/04/28/bjsports-2017-097506SCAT5.full.pdf.

The CRT5 is shown online here: http://bjsm.bmj.com/content/early/2017/04/26/bjsports-2017-097508CRT5. This looks at similar signs and symptoms to the SCAT5 but is targeted at non-medical personnel. The CRT5 looks at red flags, observation, symptoms and memory assessment, and advises on courses of action dependent on the outcome of findings. The aim of assessment is to quickly recognize the presence of SRC and remove a subject from the field of play.

> **Key point**
>
> Where concussion is suspected the athlete should be immediately removed from play and medical assessment made.

Table 11.5 The Glasgow coma scale

Function	Response	Score
Eye opening	Spontaneous eye opening	4
	Eyes open to command	3
	Eyes open to pain	2
	No eye opening	1
Verbal response	Coherent appropriate response	5
	Coherent but inappropriate response	4
	Incoherent speech	3
	Non-speech noises (moans and groans)	2
	No vocalization	1
Motor response	Obeys commands	6
	Localizing purposeful response to pain	5
	Non-localizing purposeful withdrawal from pain	4
	Reflex flexion to pain (arm, decorticate posturing)	3
	Reflex extension to pain (arm, decerebrate posturing)	2
	No motor response	1
Total score		**46**

The final section of the SCAT5 gives athlete information and draws attention to things to look for in the 24-48 hour period following the concussion incident, as detailed in Table 11.5.

As recovery occurs, return to play should be graded, with recommendations for a graded return to play included on the SCAT5. Initially the subject should rest until asymptomatic and return to limited activities, including only those which do not promote symptoms. Light aerobic activities (walking, static cycle) may be used to maintain cardiopulmonary fitness, and sport-specific non-contact skills may be gradually re-introduced. When full-contact practice is begun (following medical clearance) it is important to both assess functional skills and restore the subject's confidence.

Multiple concussion incidents

The cumulative effects of concussion can be important in sports such as boxing, steeplechase and football. EEG disturbances due to neuronal damage through repeated trauma may be seen, especially where a series of EEGs are performed.

In addition, neuropsychological performance can be impaired, often in the presence of a normal CT scan.

Failure to allow adequate recovery from a concussion incident may result in *second impact syndrome* (SIS), where a second blow to the head causes further swelling and bleeding. The second blow may be minor and may not appear sufficient to affect the brain. However, the two combined impacts cause rapid and profuse swelling. Athletes usually develop respiratory failure and collapse. The mortality rate for this condition is as high as 50 per cent (Cantu 1998).

Definition

Second-impact syndrome occurs when a second blow is received before the effects of the first concussion have worn off. Massive swelling develops in the brain, the athlete collapses and may go into respiratory failure. The syndrome is often fatal.

Because of the risk of persistent swelling or late bleeding, the return to sport should be delayed following multiple concussion. The SCAT5 highlights the importance of medical examination where red flags have been identified, but the existence of SIS as a distinct condition has been disputed (McCrory and Berkovic 1998).

Intracerebral lesions

The danger from any head injury is an expanding intracranial lesion resulting from a torn blood vessel, causing epidural (extradural) haemorrhage, subarachnoid haemorrhage or subdural haematoma (Fig. 11.11), so assessment is vital.

Definition

The brain has three covering membranes called (from inner to outer) the pia, arachnoid and dura mater. *Epidural haemorrhage* is bleeding between the skull and the dura mater. *Subdural haemorrhage* is bleeding between the arachnoid and dura mater. *Subarachnoid haemorrhage* is bleeding between the pia and arachnoid mater.

These conditions are indicated by an alteration in consciousness (lucid state). Normally, the intracranial pressure is 4–15 mmHg and an intracranial pressure of 40 mmHg will cause neurological impairment.

After such an incident, the CRT5 should be applied and a subject only be allowed to continue providing he or she does not present with red flags, including neck pain, double vision, weakness or tingling in the arms, severe headache, convulsions, disorientation, vomiting and increasingly agitated state. The Glasgow coma scale (which forms part of the SCAT5 for sport concussion) is typically used to assess head injury.

The Glasgow coma scale

The Glasgow coma scale (Teasdale and Jennett 1974) is a series of tests that are given a numerical value which can then be used to objectify an athlete's state of consciousness (Table 11.6). The first test relates to the eyes, and determines whether the athlete opens the eyes spontaneously or in response to sound (verbal command) or pain. Opening the eyes to verbal command merely means that the person has registered sound; it does not imply that they necessarily understand the command. The second test is of verbal response, and assesses the athlete's reaction to simple questions such as 'Where are you?' or 'What is your name?'. The test assesses whether the athlete is aware of him/herself and the environment. The third test is of motor response. The maximum score is 6 if the athlete is able to perform actions correctly to verbal commands such as 'Move your arm.' If the athlete fails to respond, a painful stimulus is applied by the practitioner pressing their knuckles into the athlete's sternum, or pressing the athlete's fingers together around a pen. Painful stimuli to the face or palm of the hands should be avoided as these can give reflex eye closing and hand closing respectively. Where reflex responses alone result, flexion of the arms and hands together with adduction of the upper limb and extension of the lower limb with plantarflexion of the feet (decorticate posturing) indicates a lesion above the red nucleus. Extension of the arms with pronation of the forearm (decerebrate posturing) indicates a lesion of the brainstem. The time of the test should be noted and the test repeated every 15–30 minutes to note any degeneration of results.

Where the score is between 3 and 8 on the coma scale, emergency care is required immediately as a severe head injury is present. Those with scores

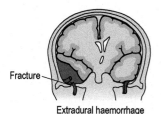
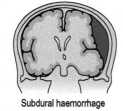

Fracture

Extradural haemorrhage   Subdural haemorrhage

Figure 11.11 Intracranial haematoma.

of 9–11 are considered to have a moderate head injury, and those with a score of 12 or higher are considered to have a mild head injury.

Caution must always be exercised with head injuries. Unfortunately, the practitioner or coach who has to decide whether to allow an athlete to continue playing has no way of knowing if secondary brain damage is going to develop. At the time of injury, bleeding may have occurred which could accumulate and give rise to a subdural haematoma.

On the sports field, an athlete who remains unconscious should be placed in the recovery position until an ambulance is available to take him or her to hospital. If there is bleeding or discharge from an ear, the athlete should be turned so that the affected ear is dependent. Nothing should be given by mouth, and the athlete should not be left unattended. Testing for responses should continue regularly (every 10 minutes or more frequently) and any changes in the athlete's condition should be recorded.

Headache

Headaches may be broadly classified as primary or secondary types. Primary headaches are the most common type seen (90 per cent), are generally benign and are not caused by an underlying disease or structural problem. This type includes migraine and tension-type headaches, but also medication-induced and exercise-related headache, as well as trigeminal headache (trigeminal neuralgia). Secondary headaches give symptoms in the head, but the cause is elsewhere, for example cervicogenic headache, where pain stems from the neck, and temporomandibular headache, coming from the TMJ. Although less common (10 per cent), secondary headaches also include more serious pathologies such as tumour, intracranial haemorrhage and meningitis.

Cervicogenic headache

A cervicogenic headache is one which stems from the upper neck. The sub-occipital nerve

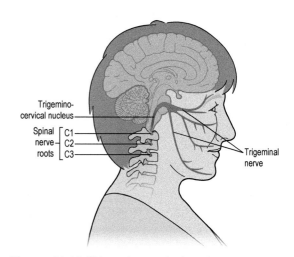

Figure 11.12 Trigeminocervical nucleus.

roots (C1–C3) converge into the same region of the brain as the trigeminal nerve, an area called the *trigeminocervical nucleus* (Fig. 11.12). Impulses from the upper neck can therefore be misinterpreted as head or face pain (Bogduk and Govind 2009).

> **Definition**
> The *trigeminal* is the fifth cranial nerve. It gives off three branches – the ophthalmic nerve, the maxillary nerve and the mandibular nerve.

Patient history and examination frequently highlights unilateral headache, often with a change in neck posture, with coexisting neck and/or shoulder symptoms. Pain is commonly changed by neck movement or sustained postures, and autonomic features such as dizziness and photophobia may also be present. Cervical range of motion is often reduced and asymmetrical. An overriding feature is that treatment targeted at the cervical spine is able to modify the subject's familiar symptoms.

The flexion rotation test is a useful examination tool in cases of cervicogenic headache (Fig. 11.13). Flexing the neck maximally from supine (bringing

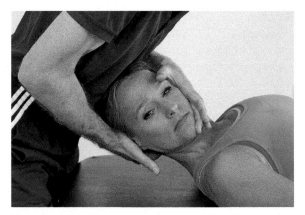

Figure 11.13 Flexion-rotation test.

the chin towards the sternum), the head is turned to each side (flexion-rotation) to assess for symmetry and symptom reproduction (Hall and Robinson 2004).

Typically, subjects with cervicogenic headache present with a forward head posture (sub-occipital extension) and may lack control of deep-neck flexor activity (see Chapter 10). Treatment may include cervical mobilization in sitting (NAGs and SNAGs), and self-mobilization procedures such as fist traction and chin-tuck actions using a towel or wall. See Chapter 10.

Migraine

Migraine is a headache which typically presents as a persistent throbbing (pulsating) sensation. It is more common in women, and often accompanied by light sensitivity (photophobia), dizziness and nausea. Migraine is sometimes preceded by an aura (warning sign) such as flashing lights or paraesthesia. Some subjects find their attack follows an alteration in homeostasis which acts as a trigger, such as menstruation, stress, prolonged tiredness or in some case certain types of foods. Migraine was previously thought to be a vascular disorder, but evidence is now emerging linking it to abnormal brain functioning (information processing) leading to the interpretation of sensory stimuli incorrectly. In this respect, migraine can be viewed as a type of central sensitization (Gantenbein and Sándor 2006).

Treatment for migraine typically includes rest/sleep in a dark room. Medication includes aspirin and antiemetics. Aerobic exercise (40 min, 3 times per week) has been shown to reduce migraine episodes equally to medication, so may be viewed as an option for prophylaxis (Varkey et al. 2011). A Cochrane review which included 22 trials involving 4,985 individuals concluded that acupuncture reduced the frequency of migraine headaches, and was similarly effective to treatment with prophylactic drugs (Linde et al. 2016).

References

Bogduk, N., Govind, J., 2009. Cervicogenic headache: an assessment of the evidence on clinical diagnosis, invasive tests, and treatment. *Lancet Neurol* **8** (10), 959–968.

Cantu, R.C., 1998. Second impact syndrome. *Clinics in Sports Medicine* **17**, 37–44.

French, R., St George, G., Needleman, I. et al., 2017. Face, eyes and teeth. In: Brukner, P., Clarsen, B., Cook, J. et al. (eds) *Clinical Sports Medicine*. 5th ed. McGraw Hill.

Gantenbein, A.R., Sándor, P.S., 2006. Physiological parameters as biomarkers of migraine. *Headache* **46** (7),1069–1074.

Hall, T., Robinson, K., 2004. The flexion-rotation test and active cervical mobility – a comparative measurement study in cervicogenic headache. *Manual Therapy* **9** (4),197–202.

Handler, S.D., 1991. Diagnosis and management of maxillofacial injuries. In: Torg, J.S. (ed.), *Athletic Injuries to the Head, Neck, and Face*, 2nd ed. Mosby Year Book, St Louis.

Jennings, D.C., 1990. Injuries sustained by users and non-users of gum shields in local rugby union. *British Journal of Sports Medicine* **24**, 3.

Jones, N.P., 1989. Eye injury in sport. *Sports Medicine*, **7**, 163–181.

Karsteter, P.A., Yunker, C., 2006. Recognition and management of an orbital blowout fracture in an amateur boxer. *Journal of Orthopaedic and Sports Physical Therapy* **36** (8), 611–618.

Linde, K., Allais, G., Brinkhaus, B., et al., 2016. Cochrane Database of Systematic Reviews 2016, Issue 6. Art. No.: CD001218.

Magee, D.J., 2002. *Orthopedic Physical Assessment*, 4th ed. Saunders, Philadelphia.

McCrory, P.R., Berkovic, S.F., 1998. Second impact syndrome. *Neurology* **50** (3), 677–683.

McCrory, P., Meeuwisse, W., Dvorak, J. et al., 2017. Consensus statement on concussion in sport – the 5th international conference on concussion in sport held in Berlin, October 2016 *British Journal of Sports Medicine* Published Online First: 26 April 2017. doi:10.1136/bjsports-2017-097699.

Renon, P., Lory, R., Belliato, R., Casanova, M., 1986. Inner ear trauma caused by decompression accidents following deep sea diving. *Annals of Otolaryngology (Paris)* **103**, 259–264.

Schuller, D.E., Dankle, S.K., Martin, M., Strauss, R.H., 1989. Auricular injury and the use of headgear in wrestlers. *Archives of Otolaryngology: Head and Neck Surgery* **115**, 714–717.

Simons, D.G., Travell, J.G., Simons, L.S., 1999. *Travell and Simons' Myofascial Pain and Dysfunction*, **vol. 1**, 2nd edn. Lippincott, Williams and Wilkins, Philadelphia.

Teasdale, G., Jennett, B., 1974. Assessment of coma and impaired consciousness. *Lancet* **ii**, 81–84.

Varkey, E., Cider, A., Carlsson, J., Linde, M. 2011. Exercise as migraine prophylaxis: a randomized study using relaxation and topiramate as controls. *Cephalalgia*. Oct; **31** (14): 1428–1438.

CHAPTER 12

The shoulder

Functional anatomy

The upper limb attaches to the trunk via the shoulder (pectoral) girdle. The shoulder complex in total consists of the scapula and clavicle, articulating with the ribcage and sternum to form four joints, all of which require attention in the management of shoulder pain. The clavicle forms a strut for the shoulder, holding the arm away from the side of the body and allowing a greater range of unencumbered movement. At one end, the clavicle joins the sternum through the sternoclavicular joint, while at the other it joins the scapula via the acromioclavicular joint.

Definition

The acromioclavicular (A/C) joint is formed between the acromion process of the scapula and the lateral (outer) end of the clavicle. The sternoclavicular (S/C) joint is formed between the top of the sternum and the medial (inner) end of the clavicle.

The scapula rests on the ribcage through muscle tissue alone, an essential point when dealing with stability of the shoulder complex. The glenohumeral joint is the articulation between the head of the humerus and the shallow glenoid fossa of the scapula.

The glenoid fossa is only one third the size of the humeral head, but the fossa is extended by the glenoid labrum attached to its periphery. This fibrocartilage rim is about 4 mm deep, with its inner surface lined by, and continuous with, the joint cartilage. The joint itself is surrounded by a loose capsule with a volume twice as large as the humeral head. The anterior capsule is strengthened by the three glenohumeral ligaments. The lower portion of the capsule is lax in the anatomical position and hangs down in folds. It has two openings, one for the passage of the long head of biceps and the other between the superior and middle glenohumeral ligaments, which communicates with the subscapular bursa (between subscapularis and the joint capsule). The capsule is further strengthened by the rotator-cuff muscles, which act as 'active ligaments' and blend with the lateral capsule. The 'roof' of the joint is formed by the bony coracoid and acromion processes and the coracoacromial ligament, which runs between them, the three structures together forming an arch. Surface marking of the shoulder is shown in Fig. 12.1.

Rotator-cuff action

Most joints have a high degree of passive stability provided by their capsules and ligaments. The

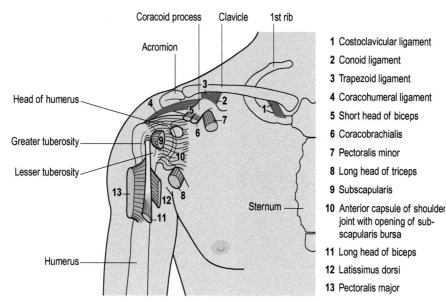

Coracoid process   Clavicle   1st rib

Acromion

Head of humerus

Greater tuberosity

Lesser tuberosity

Humerus

Sternum

1 Costoclavicular ligament
2 Conoid ligament
3 Trapezoid ligament
4 Coracohumeral ligament
5 Short head of biceps
6 Coracobrachialis
7 Pectoralis minor
8 Long head of triceps
9 Subscapularis
10 Anterior capsule of shoulder joint with opening of sub-scapularis bursa
11 Long head of biceps
12 Latissimus dorsi
13 Pectoralis major

Figure 12.1 Major palpable structures of the shoulder.

shoulder, however, depends more on the active stability provided by its muscles to maintain joint integrity. With the arm hanging by the side, the weight of the arm is largely supported passively by the coracohumeral ligament, superior portion of the glenohumeral ligament, and the superior capsule. When the arm moves away from the side of the body, tension in the superior capsule and superior portion of the glenohumeral ligament is lost, and inferior translation of the joint is restricted by the inferior glenohumeral ligament. The joint now comes to rely more on active stability provided by the rotator-cuff muscles.

The fibres of the joint capsule are angled forwards and slightly medially when the arm is hanging by the side of the body. As abduction progresses, tension within these fibres causes the shoulder to passively externally rotate. This movement prevents the humeral head from being pulled closer to the glenoid, and facilitates a greater range of movement. Importantly, the external rotation also allows the greater tuberosity to clear the acromion process (see below).

> **Key point**
>
> The fibres of the joint capsule, angled downwards and slightly medially, are under slight tension at rest. Recoil of these fibres produces a passive lateral rotation force during abduction.

Active abduction of the humerus is accomplished by the supraspinatus and deltoid, acting as the prime movers. With the arm dependent, contraction of the deltoid (particularly the middle fibres) merely approximates the joint (upward translation), because the medial muscle fibres run almost parallel with the humerus. Unopposed, this pull would force the head of the humerus into the coracoacromial arch, resulting in impingement. Contraction of the infraspinatus, subscapularis and teres minor (Fig. 12.2) causes compression and downward translation to offset the upward translation of deltoid (Culham and Peat 1993). In an overhead throwing or serving action (Fig. 12.3) the subscapularis moves superiorly, because the humerus has externally rotated and the muscle

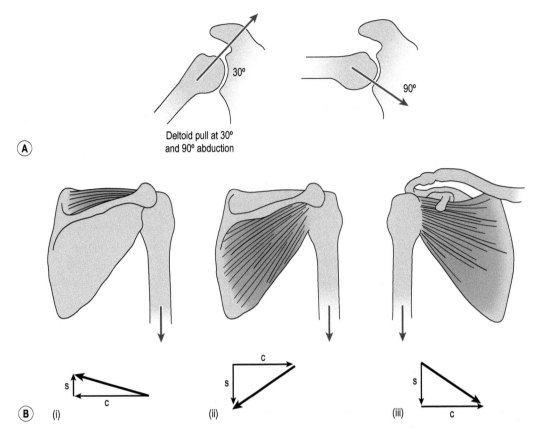

Figure 12.2 Rotator cuff muscle action. (A) Deltoid pull at 30° and 90° abduction. (B) Muscles counteracting pull of deltoid. (i) Supraspinatus, (ii) infraspinatus and teres minor, (iii) subscapularis. Resolution of muscle force: S, shear; C, compression.

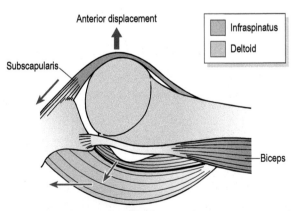

Figure 12.3 Muscular restraints to anterior displacement of the humeral head in an overhead throwing action. Adapted from Reid (1992), with permission.

can no longer effectively control the humeral head. The infraspinatus, and to a lesser extent the teres minor, stabilize the joint anteriorly in this position (Cain, Mutschler and Fu 1987). For this reason, sEMG can address this muscle in stabilization programmes targeted at throwing sports. By 90 degrees abduction, the pull of the deltoid no longer tends to cause impingement, as shear forces are exceeded by compression, and the humeral head is stabilized into the glenoid (Perry and Glousman 1995).

The supraspinatus is better placed to produce a rotatory action, and therefore initiates abduction for the first 20 degrees. The line of action of supraspinatus is such that less translation is caused, and its contribution to abduction is to reduce the reliance on deltoid and, as a consequence, reduce translation. After 30 degrees of abduction, the scapula starts to rotate to alter the glenoid position.

> **Key point**
>
> The rotator-cuff muscles downwardly translate the humeral head to guard against the risk of impingement caused by upward translation initiated by the deltoid.

Scapulohumeral rhythm

Motion of the shoulder girdle as a whole changes the position of the glenoid fossa, placing it in the most favourable location for the maximum range of humeral movement. When the glenoid cavity moves it does so in an arc, the diameter of which is the length of the clavicle. The medial border of the scapula moves in a similar but smaller arc, and as a consequence the positions of the shoulder girdle structures change in relation to each other.

As the scapula moves medially and laterally towards and away from the vertebral column, the curvature of the ribcage forces the scapula to change from a frontal to a more sagittal position. This, in turn, alters the direction in which the glenoid cavity faces. With elevation, the scapula is accompanied by some rotation, the glenoid cavity gradually pointing further upwards as the scapula gets higher.

With both shoulder abduction and flexion, the clavicle axially rotates. As the scapula twists, the coracoclavicular ligament 'winds up' and tightens, causing the clavicle itself to rotate. As the arm is abducted to 90 degrees (stage I and II, see below) the clavicle elevates by 15 degrees, but does not rotate. Above 90 degrees (stage III), further elevation of the clavicle occurs (up to 15 degrees) but marked posterior rotation now occurs to 30–50 degrees (Magee 2008). For this reason, a diminished range of movement at either SC or AC joints that reduces clavicular rotation will also impair scapular, and therefore glenohumeral, motion.

> **Key point**
>
> Clavicular rotation about the sternoclavicular and acromioclavicular joints is essential to full-range shoulder abduction. Stiffness in these joints will limit abduction range.

The abduction cycle

Movement of the arm into abduction may be divided into three overlapping stages (Table 12.1), and alterations to this cycle are associated with various pathologies as detailed below.

Table 12.1 Movement of the arm into abduction

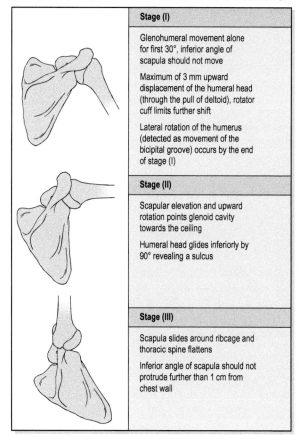

Stage (I)
Glenohumeral movement alone for first 30°, inferior angle of scapula should not move
Maximum of 3 mm upward displacement of the humeral head (through the pull of deltoid), rotator cuff limits further shift
Lateral rotation of the humerus (detected as movement of the bicipital groove) occurs by the end of stage (I)
Stage (II)
Scapular elevation and upward rotation points glenoid cavity towards the ceiling
Humeral head glides inferiorly by 90° revealing a sulcus
Stage (III)
Scapula slides around ribcage and thoracic spine flattens
Inferior angle of scapula should not protrude further than 1 cm from chest wall

Stage (I)

In stage (I), no significant movement of the scapula should occur. The scapular stabilizers (serratus anterior especially) should hold the scapula firmly on the ribcage, providing a stable base for the humerus to move upon. As the arm abducts, lateral rotation of the humerus may be detected by palpation of the bicipital groove (intertubercular sulcus). If the humerus is maintained in a neutral position, abduction in the frontal plane is limited to about 90 degrees. Laterally rotating the humerus increases this range to 120 degrees. When the arm is elevated in the sagittal plane, abduction is accompanied by medial rotation due to tightness in the coracohumeral ligament. No rotation is required for elevation in the scapular plane (30–45 degrees anterior to the frontal plane). In this position, the joint capsule does not undergo torsion and the deltoid and supraspinatus are optimally aligned.

At the beginning of abduction in the frontal plane, slight approximation of the humerus should occur (maximum 3 mm) to overcome the weight of the arm, as the fibres of the joint capsule are taken off stretch and no longer support the arm through elastic recoil. No noticeable elevation of the shoulder should occur, unless the upper fibres of trapezius dominate the movement. The instantaneous axis of rotation in stage (I) is near the root of the scapular spine, and moves superiorly and laterally as abduction progresses.

Key point

Stage (I) of the abduction cycle is the stage of scapular stability. The scapula should remain fixed to the ribcage, and no winging or marked elevation of the scapula should occur.

Stage (II)

By the beginning of stage (II), from 30 degrees of abduction, the scapula should be upwardly rotating to maintain clearance between the acromion and the approaching greater tuberosity of the humerus.

Scapular rotation in the beginning of stage (II) occurs as a result of elevation of the clavicle on the SC joint. Between 80 and 140 degrees, the instantaneous axis of rotation (IAR) migrates towards the AC joint along the upper central scapular area. Movement then occurs as elevation of the clavicle on the SC joint, and rotation of the scapula on the clavicle at the AC joint. More movement occurs at the glenohumeral joint than at the scapulothoracic joint. Ratios of 2:1 are thought to be optimal, giving 120 degrees of movement at the glenohumeral joint and 60 degrees at the scapulothoracic joint in a total abduction range of 180 degrees. However, changes to this ratio often occur in non-symptomatic subjects, so adaptation occurs to different movement ranges.

Scapular rotation occurs as a result of force-couples between the various muscles attached to the scapula (Fig. 12.4). Upward (lateral) rotation accompanying shoulder-joint abduction or flexion is brought about by contraction of the upper and lower fibres of trapezius and the lower portion of serratus anterior. Serratus anterior is probably the most important of the group. It has two sets of fibres. The fibres of the upper portion run horizontally and slightly upwards, while those of the lower portion are aligned downwards. Both sets pull powerfully on the scapula, anchoring it to the ribcage and causing scapular upward rotation as trapezius lifts the lateral end of the clavicle and acromion process. If serratus anterior and the lower fibres of trapezius are ineffective, the upper trapezius will dominate the movement. In this case, these fibres show increased tone and can be tight. As the abduction moves further into stage (II), the moment arm of lower trapezius is lengthened and this portion of the muscle becomes increasingly active in the movement.

Downward (medial) rotation frequently occurs as a result of eccentric action of the above muscles. However, in activities such as hanging and chinning a beam, active scapular rotation is accomplished by levator scapulae and the rhomboids pulling upwards on the medial side of the scapula together with pectoralis minor pulling the coracoid process

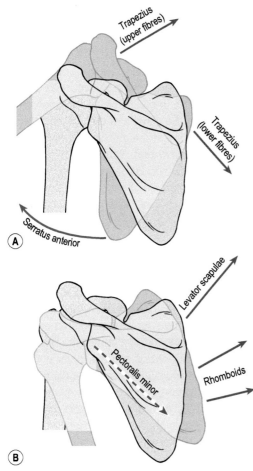

Figure 12.4 Muscle force couples which create scapular rotation. (A) Lateral rotation. (B) Medial rotation. From Palastanga, Field and Soames (2013), with permission.

down. In cases where these muscles are tight or overactive, upward rotation of the scapula will be limited during abduction.

As scapular rotation progresses, lateral rotation of the humerus should be apparent as the cubital fossa and thumb orientate towards the ceiling. Ineffective scapular upward rotators, especially lengthening of the lower fibres of trapezius, will prevent correct orientation of the glenoid and may increase the risk of impingement. Tightness in the medial rotators, especially the pectoralis major and subscapularis, combined with lengthening

and weakness of the lateral rotators, may lead to delayed lateral rotation at the glenohumeral joint. This type of motion change may be associated with impingement of the greater tuberosity against the inferior acromion.

During stage (II), as the humerus reaches 90 degrees abduction, its head slides beneath the acromion and a noticeable dip is formed in the skin. Failure of the shoulder musculature to pull the humerus into this position may result in the head slipping beneath the acromion with a sudden thud as the arm raises above 90 degrees, and similarly in this position during descent.

> **Key point**
> In the first half of stage (II) the scapula is seen to upwardly rotate. At the end of stage (II) the humeral head is pulled beneath the acromion forming a noticeable sulcus.

Stage (III)

During stage (III), as the arm approaches 120 degrees abduction, no further movement is available from the glenohumeral joint. Additional range to reach the arm overhead is achieved by sliding the scapula over the thorax into further upward rotation and abduction. To facilitate this movement, the thoracic spine must reverse its kyphosis and flatten. A kyphotic posture and inflexibility in the thoracic spine will therefore limit the final degrees of abduction. As a simple test for this, the patient is asked to stand with the back flat against a wall and the pelvis posteriorly tilted to avoid any possibility of hyperextension at the lumbar spine. Both arms are then abducted, keeping them in full contact with the wall. If thoracic extension is limited, the subject will be unable to perform pure abduction to full range. Instead, the arm moves through flexion-abduction to bring it in front of the forehead. In conditions where abduction is limited, therefore, greater range may often be gained by mobilizing the thoracic spine as well as working on the glenohumeral joint.

As the arm moves into its final overhead position and the scapula rotates maximally, the inferior angle of the scapula juts out through the outer edge of the thorax. However, no more than 1–2 cm of the inferior angle should ideally be visible at this point. During this final phase the IAR moves to the AC joint. Clavicular elevation is limited by tension in the costoclavicular ligament. As the coracoid process moves away from the clavicle, tension in this ligament causes dorsal rotation of the clavicle about its long axis.

> **Key point**
>
> To reach the arm overhead, the scapula must slide over the thorax. To facilitate this movement, the thoracic spine should reverse its kyphosis and flatten. An increased kyphotic curve and/or reduced flexibility of the thoracic spine may therefore limit the final degrees of abduction.

Scapular dyskinesis

Scapular dyskinesis is an alteration in position or movement of the scapula (Kibler et al. 2013). Observation of the medial and inferior borders of the scapular may reveal winging or prominence of the medial border. Disruption to the smooth movement of the scapula during arm lifting or lowering such as early scapular elevation (shrugging) or rapid downward rotation (twisting) are indications that dyskinesis may exist. This type of yes/no observational analysis has been shown to have high sensitivity (76 per cent) and positive predictive value (74 per cent) to show asymmetries in both symptomatic and non-symptomatic subjects (Uhl et al. 2009). Both static and dynamic changes may be seen, with static changes typically the result of alteration in tissue length, and dynamic changes due to muscle sequencing. Scapular tipping is characteristically associated with shortening of the pectoralis minor muscle (assessed by the prominence of the corocoid process and tissue tension comparing

the symptomatic and non-symptomatic side) and tightening of the posterior capsule (assessed by the cross-body and sleeper stretches, below). Alteration in upward rotation of the scapular during normal rhythm may be due to overactivity and/or tightening of the levator scapulae and rhomboid muscles (upward scapular rotators) and reduced or late action of the upper and lower trapezius and serratus anterior (downward scapular rotators).

Scapular dyskinesis has been shown to be associated with impingement pain and glenohumeral instability (Cools et al. 2014), but whether this is a consequence of pain or a causal factor of the conditions is not known. For this reason rehabilitation must be subject-specific and related to a patient's familiar symptoms (those that they are seeking treatment for).

> **Key point**
>
> Scapular dyskinesis (alteration in position or movement of the scapula) is associated with both subacromial impingement syndrome and glenohumeral instability. It may be either a result of the condition and/or a factor in its development.

An algorithm for rehabilitation of scapular dyskinesis has been proposed (Cools et al. 2014) which focuses intervention on lack of soft-tissue flexibility or lack of muscle performance. Flexibility intervention (manual therapy and exercise) targets both the scapular and glenohumeral structures, depending on assessment findings. Muscle performance addresses both control of force couples and muscle strength, again determined by clinical assessment.

Assessment of dyskinesis

Dyskinesis may be assessed by position changes of the scapula in different postures, and by the effect of scapular repositioning on symptoms. Scapular position change in varying postures is assessed using the lateral scapular slide test (LSST). The distance from the medial scapula

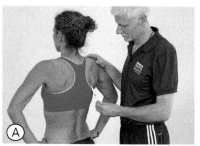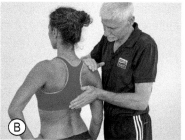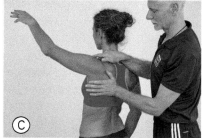

Figure 12.5 Tests of scapular dyskinesis. (A) Lateral scapular slide test (LSST). (B) Scapular retraction test (SRT). (C) Scapular assistance test (SAT).

to the spine is measured at the superior ankle, scapular spine (T3) and inferior angle (T7). These measurements are taken in sitting, standing with the hands on the hips (thumbs posterior), and in 90-degree abduction and internal rotation (scarecrow position). The test is positive if there is variance greater than 1.5 cm between positions (Fig. 12.5A). Although this test can be useful clinically if it highlights changes which may modify subject symptoms, it has been shown to be unreliable with poor sensitivity and specificity (Odom et al. 2001).

The scapular retraction test (SRT) assesses the ability of the serratus anterior and lower trapezius to posteriorly tilt the scapula and hold it against the chest wall (see above). The test is normally used with impingement pain to determine if scapular stability can modify the result of the empty-can test. The empty-can test is performed, and if positive (reproduction of the subject's familiar pain) the SRT test is used. The therapist draws the upper scapula backwards (grasping over the clavicle) and presses the lower scapula to the chest wall (inferior angle). These combined movements can be achieved by the therapist placing their cupped hand over the subject's shoulder and laying their forearm along the medial scapular border. If pain to the empty-can test is reduced, the test is positive (Fig. 12.5B).

The scapular-assistance test (SAT) is used to determine if optimizing scapular movement (abduction, retraction and lateral rotation) affects a subject's symptoms. The subject abducts the

arm and assesses their symptoms. The SAT is performed by stabilizing the upper scapula using the cupped hand as above, and pressing the inferior angle onto the chest wall (posterior tilt) and outwards (lateral rotation) as the arm is abducted. The test is positive if the subject's symptoms are modified (Fig. 12.5C). The SAT has been shown to be reliable in the clinical setting with percentage agreement of 77 per cent (testing in scapular plane) and 91 per cent (sagittal plane) between two testers assessing 46 subjects (Rabin et al. 2006).

The biomechanics of throwing

In sport, throwing is to the upper limb what gait is to the lower limb. It is an activity seen in many sports in some form, and there are similarities between all types of throw and with shots in racquet sports. In addition, rapid overhead actions can occur in daily living in manual occupations especially.

Throwing-type actions can be divided into five stages that form a single, continuous motion (Fig. 12.6). In the early stages, up to ball release, the body is accelerating the object. By the later stages, following release, the aim is to decelerate and reduce the effect of stress on the body. The phases are as follows:

▶ WIND-UP (phase i) – the subject positions him/herself in the best position for the throw. A right-handed thrower will plant the back foot on the ground and turn the body perpendicular

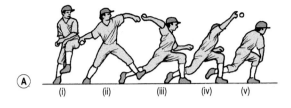

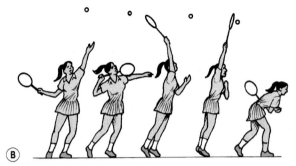

Figure 12.6 (A) Stages of throwing. (i) wind-up – athlete positions him- or herself for the throw; (ii) cocking – lead leg moves forwards, arm moves backwards, stretching body; (iii) acceleration – body drives forwards, leaving arm behind; (iv) deceleration – object released. Elbow continues to extend and shoulder to internally rotate; (v) follow through – trunk and lead leg show eccentric activity to dissipate energy. (B) Similarity to tennis serve. After Fleisig, Dillman and Andrews (1994), with permission.

to the direction of throw (left side of the body forward). The thrower then steps towards the target and begins to move the arms.

▶ COCKING (phase ii) – the front leg moves forwards and the throwing arm moves backwards, effectively stretching the body out and building elastic energy. The shoulder is abducted to 90 degrees and taken into extension and external rotation. The elbow is flexed to 45 degrees.

▶ ACCELERATION (phase iii) – the body moves forwards leaving the arm behind. The elbow begins to extend, and the shoulder internally rotates.

▶ DECELERATION (phase iv) – this sees the release of the object being thrown, and the

energy built up to throw the object must now be effectively dissipated to reduce stress on the body tissues. The arm continues to extend at the elbow and internally rotate at the shoulder, bringing the knuckles up. The rotator cuff (external rotators) decelerate the internal rotation motion, and limit distraction to the glenohumeral joint. The elbow flexors similarly decelerate extension and limit hyperextension of the elbow joint.

▶ FOLLOW-THROUGH (phase v) – the trunk is flexed eccentrically and the lead leg is extended, pushing into the ground eccentrically to absorb energy. The throwing arm continues to move, giving a longer period over which to dissipate energy, and the hand may end up near the knee of the lead leg. Angular displacement for the shoulder and elbow throughout the throwing action is shown.

Screening examination of the shoulder complex

Clinical assessment begins by taking a subjective history, being mindful of possible red flags which may imply referral where present in clusters. Common red flags for the upper quadrant are shown in Table 12.2.

A screening examination is performed to enable the examiner to focus more closely on the injured area. The history suggests tissue irritability where the subject is unable to sleep on the painful side, pain extends into the upper arm past the elbow, and/or pain occurs at rest. Pain control and tissue unloading or protection may then be a primary aim (McClure and Michener 2015).

The patient's posture and actions are noted while undressing, and the area is inspected for swelling, colour and deformity. A combination of active, resisted and passive movements are used to assess the shoulder complex. The patient is viewed from behind to note scapulohumeral motion. It is helpful to have the patient facing a full-length mirror, so the anterior aspect of the shoulder and the patient's facial expression may

Table 12.2 Red flags in shoulder assessment

Suspect condition	Findings on subjective or objective assessment
Tumour	History of cancer
	Unexplained weight loss or fatigue
	Pain not related to mechanical stress
	Mass or deformity
Infection	Red skin
	Fever or chills
	Systemically unwell
Fracture or dislocation	Significant trauma
	Seizure
	Acute disabling pain
	Acute loss of motion
	Deformity
Neurological lesion	Unexplained sensory or motor deficit
Visceral pathology	Pain unrelated to mechanical stress to the shoulder
	Pain with physical exertion or respiratory stress
	Pain associated with GI symptoms
	Scapular pain associated with eating
Haemodynamic consideration	Unexplained exercise-induced pain
	Unexplained numbness or tingling
	Non-dermatomal pain distribution
	Skin discoloration – blue or white
	Pulsatile or throbbing pain nature

GI – gastrointestinal
(Data from McClure and Michener 2015, Taylor and Kerry 2015)

also be assessed. Active abduction and flexion-abduction are performed with overpressure applied at end-range, to assess end-feel. Positional changes of the scapula, either at rest or during movement, may warrant closer inspection. Active GH rotation may be performed by asking the patient to place a hand behind the back (medial rotation) and then behind the head (lateral rotation). Passive lateral rotation is performed with the elbow flexed and upper arm held into the side. This is also the position for resisted lateral and medial rotations. Passive medial rotation is performed with the patient placing a hand into the small of the back. The examiner stabilizes the upper arm and keeps the patient's elbow tucked

into the side of the body. The examiner then gently pulls the patient's forearm away from the body, increasing medial rotation. Any limitation of movement is noted, and the percentages of limitation relative to each other reveal if a capsular pattern exists. The capsular pattern for the GH joint is gross limitation of abduction with some limitation of lateral rotation and little limitation of medial rotation.

> **Key point**
> The capsular pattern for the glenohumeral (shoulder) joint is gross limitation of abduction, with some limitation of lateral rotation and little limitation of medial rotation.

Resisted abduction and adduction are performed in mid-range, the examiner stabilizing the subject's pelvis to prevent any lateral trunk flexion occurring at the same time as the shoulder moves. Elbow flexion, extension and forearm rotation may be assessed at the same time with the elbow flexed and the upper arm held close to the body. The patient's forearm rests on the examiner's when testing the triceps, and resistance is given from above when testing the biceps. Resisted shoulder shrugging tests the trapezius. When a smaller therapist is examining a larger subject, it is particularly important that resistance is applied from a position which gives maximum mechanical advantage to the therapist.

Referred pain from the neck must always be considered in cases of shoulder pain, and the neck-screening examination is performed to establish whether movement is painful or reproduces the patient's shoulder symptoms. This simple but methodical examination should take no more than two to three minutes and tells the examiner whether the shoulder is the cause of pain, if a contractile or non-contractile structure is affected, and if a capsular pattern exists to suggest an intracapsular lesion.

Locking test and quadrant test

Should movement apparently be full and painless at the glenohumeral joint, two further procedures are sometimes useful to reproduce the patient's symptoms. These are the locking test and the quadrant position (Fig. 12.7). Both tests refer to the position of the greater tuberosity relevant to acromial arch and glenoid. Each should be assessed for pain and end-feel, and compared with the uninjured side.

Locking test

The locking position combines internal rotation, extension and abduction of the shoulder with the scapula fixed. In this position the subacromial space is compressed, and will give pain should an impingement syndrome be present. Cadaveric studies have shown that in the locking position the posterosuperior tip of the glenoid is in contact with the humeral head (Mullen, Slade and Briggs 1989).

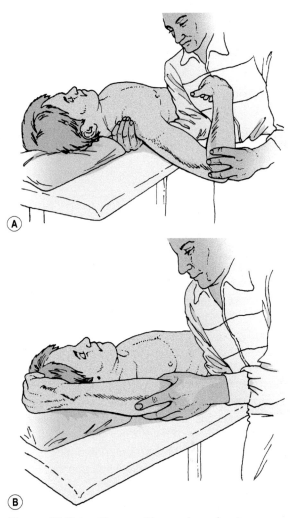

Figure 12.7 Locking position and quadrant position.

To perform the test, the patient is in a supine position and the practitioner stands by the patient's side towards the shoulders. The therapist places the palmar aspect of his or her forearm beneath the patient's shoulder and grips the trapezius muscle to stop the shoulder shrugging. The therapist holds the patient's elbow, slightly medially rotates the arm, and lifts it into abduction.

Quadrant test

The quadrant position stresses the anterior and inferior capsule, and combines external rotation, slight flexion and full abduction of the shoulder. The therapist's forearm grips the patient's shoulder to prevent shrugging. The action is to hold the elbow and move the patient's arm into abduction, allowing the humerus to move from medial rotation (palm to chest) to lateral rotation (palm to ceiling). The point at which the humerus begins to change from medial to lateral rotation marks the beginning of the quadrant (Petty and Moore 2001). From this point, horizontal extension is examined by pressing the elbow to the floor, releasing it, and then moving into further abduction before pressing again. Both

507

the quality and the range of motion are assessed, as well as the occurrence of muscle spasm. The affected shoulder is compared to the unaffected side.

> **Key point**
>
> The quadrant position stresses the joint capsule and indicates capsular tightening.

Sternoclavicular joint

The sternoclavicular (SC) joint provides, via the clavicle, the only structural attachment of the scapula to the rest of the body. The joint performs functionally as a ball and socket. The medial end of the clavicle articulates with the clavicular notch of the sternum, and the adjacent edge of the first costal cartilage. The congruity of the joint is enhanced by the presence of an interarticular fibrocartilage disc, which separates the joint cavity into two. In addition to improving the congruity of the joint, the disc also provides cushioning between the two bone ends. Furthermore, it holds the medial end of the clavicle against the sternum, preventing it moving upwards and medially when pushing actions are performed.

The joint is strengthened by a capsule attached to the articular margins and four ligaments (anterior SC, posterior SC, interclavicular and costoclavicular). Three degrees of movement are possible at the joint: elevation-depression, protraction-retraction and axial rotation. The axis of rotation for the first two movements (not rotation) is lateral to the joint itself, passing through the costoclavicular ligament. Consequently, when the lateral end of the clavicle moves in one direction, its medial end moves in the opposite direction, an important consideration with clavicular joint dislocation.

A total of about 60 degrees of elevation and depression is available, elevation being limited by tension in the costoclavicular ligament,

and depression by the interclavicular ligament and articular disc. When the lateral end of the clavicle is protracted, the medial end moves backwards, the opposite movement occurring with retraction. The total range of motion here is about 35 degrees. This fact may be used in the emergency situation where posterior SC dislocation is causing asphysia (blocked oxygen intake). A folded towel is placed on the ground between the subject's shoulders to act as a fulcrum, and the arm on the injured side is pushed firmly backwards to draw the medial aspect of the clavicle forwards and away from the trachea.

> **Key point**
>
> When the lateral (outer) end of the clavicle moves forwards in a protraction movement, the medial (inner) end moves back. In retraction, the movement is reversed.

Axial rotation is purely a passive action accompanying scapular movements. The range of rotation is small (20–40 degrees), but increases slightly as the lateral end of the clavicle is pulled back.

Injury

Injury to the SC joint is unusual, forming about 3 per cent of all shoulder-girdle trauma. Anterior dislocations occur more commonly than posterior dislocations, in a ratio of 20:1 (Zachazewski, Magee and Quillen 1996). Normally, the clavicle will fracture or the acromioclavicular joint will give way before the SC joint is seriously injured. However, when damage does occur, it is frequently the result of direct lateral compression of the shoulder, such as occurs when falling onto the side of the body. The injury is more common in horse-riding and cycling where sufficient force is produced, but is seen in rugby and wrestling. First- and second-degree injuries involve overstretch to the ligaments and capsule, while third-degree injuries represent subluxation or dislocation with ligamentous rupture.

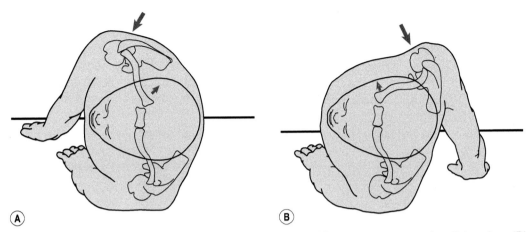

Figure 12.8 Sternoclavicular dislocation. (A) Anteriorly directed force causes posterior dislocation. (B) Posteriorly directed force causes anterior dislocation. From Garrick and Webb (1990), with permission.

The SC joint will dislocate in the opposite direction to the applied force, thus an anterior force (falling onto the back) will dislocate the joint backwards (Fig. 12.8). Several important structures lie in close proximity to the joint, including the oesophagus, trachea, lungs, pleurae, brachial plexus and major arteries and veins. Posterior dislocation, therefore, if it is severe, may be potentially life-threatening. In contrast, anterior dislocation can occur in the absence of trauma, and frequently results only in slight discomfort.

Key point

The SC joint can dislocate in a fall onto the side of the body. The joint will move in the opposite direction to the applied force, an anteriorly directed force causing the joint to move backwards. If severe, this may be potentially life-threatening as the trachea may be damaged.

Initial examination (of posterior dislocation) on the field must obviously be aimed at ruling out life-threatening injury. The presence of stridor, dyspnoea, cyanosis, difficulty with speech, pulsating vessels and neurological signs may all necessitate immediate hospitalization.

Definition

Stridor is a high-pitched breath sound caused by obstruction of the windpipe (larynx). Dyspnoea is difficult or laboured breathing, and cyanosis is a blue discoloration of the skin resulting from poor oxygenation of the blood.

If these are not present, joint examination may continue. Pain is generally well localized, and may become progressively more limiting over time. Anterior dislocation leaves a visible step deformity, and with posterior dislocation the usual prominence over the medial clavicle is lost. Local swelling is sometimes present, with crepitus and pain to motion, especially horizontal flexion. The shoulder is frequently held protracted.

Radiographic investigation will rule out clavicular fracture and may enable differentiation between fracture and epiphyseal injury in the younger subject (under 25). Closed reduction is often possible immediately after injury if pain is not too severe and muscle spasm has not yet set in. Anterior dislocation may be reduced using traction through the abducted arm and will sometimes spontaneously reduce with active shoulder retraction. The joint often reduces with an audible

509

thud. After reduction, the joint is immobilized (figure-of-eight bandage or sling depending on severity) and anti-inflammatory medication and the POLICE protocol applied.

Posterior dislocations, even where spontaneous reduction occurs, will still require hospital referral and observation. Posterior dislocations usually stay reduced, but anterior dislocations can recur. Reductions are generally stable, and results are comparable to surgical fixation with fewer complications.

Following immobilization, manual therapy and exercise is helpful. Anteroposterior gliding may be performed with the therapist placing his or her thumbs over the sternal end of the clavicle, and range-of-motion exercise is used progressively as strength is increased.

Acromioclavicular joint

This joint is formed between the oval facet on the lateral end of the clavicle and the similarly shaped area on the acromion process. The lateral end of the clavicle overrides the acromion slightly. The joint capsule is fairly loose, and strengthened above by fibres from trapezius and by capsular thickenings which make up the superior and inferior acromioclavicular (AC) ligaments. As with the SC joint there is an intra-articular disc, but this

time it does not divide the cavity in two. The joint is further stabilized by the coracoclavicular ligament, divided into its conoid and trapezoid parts. The conoid ligament is fan-shaped and resists forward movement of the scapula, while the stronger trapezoid ligament is flat and restricts backward movements. As with the SC joints, the AC joint moves only in association with the scapula. Three types of movement are again present: protraction–retraction, elevation–depression and axial rotation.

Examination

Following general shoulder examination, the AC joint may be specifically targeted using the 'cross-body' or 'scarf' test (Fig. 12.9A). Here, the patient's hand is taken across their chest (horizontal adduction) and placed on top of their other shoulder. Where the joint is especially painful, this is carried out as a passive movement with the therapist supporting the weight of the patient's arm. In cases of high irritability, minimal horizontal adduction is all that is required to provoke symptoms.

> **Key point**
>
> Where the AC joint is suspected to be the source of pain, horizontal adduction with overpressure ('cross-body' or 'scarf' test) can be used as a confirmatory test.

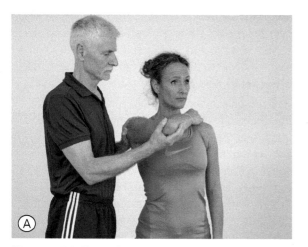
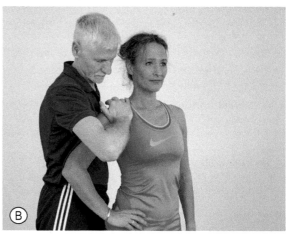

Figure 12.9 Tests for acromioclavicular (AC) joint dysfunction. (A) Cross-body test. (B) Shear test.

The cross-body test has been shown to gap the AC joint by an average of 6.4 mm, measured using ultrasonography, compared to a gap of 7.7 mm with passive end-range humeral external rotation. However, greater direct stress is placed on the AC joint using the cross-body manoeuvre than with humeral rotation (Park, Park and Bae 2009). The cross-body test has been shown to have a sensitivity of 77 per cent, compared to 41 per cent for the active compression test (Chronopoulos et al. 2004). This latter test was designed to assist the diagnosis of labral tears and to differentiate them from AC joint involvement, depending on the patient's description of their pain location as 'on top' or 'inside' the shoulder (O'Brian et al. 1998).

Definition

Sensitivity is a measure of how well a test identifies those who have a condition (positives), in contrast to specificity, which measures how well a test identifies those who do not have a condition (negatives). Combining sensitivity and specificity gives diagnostic accuracy.

Where the Scarf test is too painful, or shoulder-motion range is limited, the Shear test can be useful (Fig. 12.9B). The subject sits with their affected arm resting on their lap. The therapist clasps the subject's shoulder between their cupped hands and presses inwards, pushing the clavicle and scapula towards each other to impart a shearing stress to the AC joint. Pain localized to the joint, and reproduction of the subject's familiar symptoms, is positive.

Injury

The most common conditions affecting the AC joint are traumatic injury (sprains or dislocation) and non-traumatic degeneration. AC joint sprains vary in intensity between minor grade I injuries to grade III ruptures representing complete disruption of the joint (sprung shoulder). The injury is traditionally classified radiographically into six types (Table 12.3). Type I injury is a mild sprain, with type II giving acromioclavicular ligament rupture with no displacement. In a type III injury the joint is displaced, but the coracoclavicular distance is less than twice that of the uninjured side. In addition, the deltoid and/or trapezius muscles may become detached from the distal end of the clavicle.

Definition

The coracoclavicular distance (assessed on X-ray) is the space between the superior aspect of the coracoid process and the undersurface of the clavicle where the coracoclavicular ligaments attach.

Types IV, V and VI are variations of type III with greater amounts of displacement or changed displacement direction. They are often assessed using weight-lifting radiographs, where the anterior deltoid is contracted by having the subject hold a weight with the elbow flexed and arm next to the body. If the clavicular attachment of the deltoid is intact, the joint may reduce as weight is taken, and if the lateral end of the clavicle becomes more prominent, the clavicular attachment of the deltoid may be detached.

Injury is usually the result of a superiorly directed force, as occurs with a fall onto the point of the shoulder, being struck from above, or typically a mistimed rugby tackle. The force drives the scapula downwards, an action resisted by the coracoclavicular ligament.

Key point:

AC joint dislocation normally occurs with a downwardly directed force such as a fall, or blow, onto the point of the shoulder.

Examination reveals local tenderness over the AC joint, sometimes with a noticeable step deformity. The deformity may occur later, if initial muscle spasm reduces acromioclavicular separation.

Table 12.3 Classification of acromioclavicular injuries

Type	Radiographic appearance	Soft tissue injury
I	Clavicle not elevated with respect to the acromion	AC ligament mild sprain
		CC ligament intact
		Joint capsule & muscles intact
II	Clavicle elevated but not above superior border of the acromion	AC ligament ruptured
		CC ligament sprain
		Joint capsule ruptured
		Deltoid & trapezius minimally detached
III	Clavicle elevated above superior border of the acromion. Coracoclavicular distance is less than twice normal (<25 mm)	AC & CC ligaments ruptured
		Joint capsule ruptured
		Deltoid and trapezius detached
IV	Clavicle displaced posteriorly into trapezius	AC & CC ligaments ruptured
		Joint capsule ruptured
		Deltoid & trapezius detached
V	Clavicle markedly elevated. Coracoclavicular distance is more than double normal (>25 mm)	AC & CC ligaments ruptured
		Joint capsule ruptured
		Deltoid & trapezius detached
VI	Clavicle inferiorly displaced behind coracobrachialis and biceps tendons.	AC & CC ligaments ruptured
		Joint capsule ruptured
		Deltoid & trapezius detached

AC – acromioclavicular, CC – corococlavicular

Initial treatment aims to reduce the symptoms. Cold application, rest and a sling support is used to take the weight of the arm. The joint is immobilized in the sling initially, and then gradually mobilized within pain-free limits. With grade I and II injuries, some relief may be provided by taping.

Acromioclavicular taping

Stress may be taken off the AC joint by a simple taping, designed to press the clavicle down and take some of the weight of the arm away from the distal shoulder structures. The subject is positioned in sitting at the side of the couch with the elbow flexed to 90 degrees and the shoulder abducted to 30 degrees. The shoulder is slightly elevated and the arm rests on the couch. The shoulder and chest on the injured side of the body should be shaved of long hair, and spray adhesive may be applied if required. The nipple area is protected with a non-adhesive pad.

A felt pad is placed over the acromion to protect it from abrasion. Two anchors of 7.5 cm elastic adhesive tape are applied. The first runs horizontally from the sternum to the paravertebral area on the side of injury. The second is placed around the mid-humerus with light tension, ensuring that the limb is not excessively compressed (Fig. 12.10A). Two stirrups of 7.5 cm elastic adhesive tape are placed (pre-stretched) from the front to the back of the chest anchor, passing over the acromion (Fig. 12.10B). These are then reinforced by two strips of 5 cm zinc oxide taping. Two further strips of elastic adhesive tape are placed (pre-stretched) laterally from the arm anchor across the anterior aspect of the shoulder to join the chest stirrups over the acromion, and laterally from the anchor, passing posteriorly over the shoulder to the acromion (Fig. 12.10C). Again, these stirrups are reinforced by 5 cm zinc oxide taping. If the shoulder stirrups have been applied correctly, their tension will tend to lift the arm into abduction slightly. The chest and

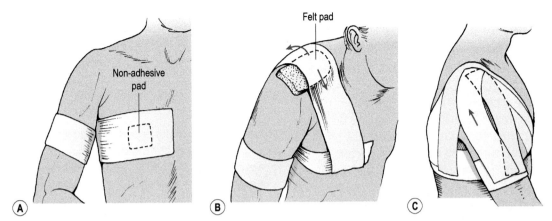

Figure 12.10 Acromioclavicular joint taping. (A) Anchors. (B) Stirrup applied under tension. (C) Arm stirrups.

arm stirrups are closed by reapplying the chest and arm anchors (7.5 cm elastic adhesive tape) to act as fixing strips. Sensation and pulse should be re-tested after tape application.

In the acute phase of injury, the forearm weight may also be taken by a collar and cuff sling. With time, when pain-free arm motion to 90 degrees is available, the humeral portion of the tape may be dispensed with.

Specific exercise therapy

As inflammation subsides, exercise therapy is commenced to restore function. This is used initially to maintain muscle tone in the absence of joint movement. Isometric contractions of the scapular and glenohumeral muscles are used, and the subject maintains general fitness and lower-body strength by exercising with the AC joint taped. When pain subsides and movement commences, gentle scapular actions are used such as shoulder shrugging and bracing, within the limits of pain. These may progress to a scapular-stabilization programme. Range-of-motion exercises for the glenohumeral joint are begun, ensuring that correct scapulohumeral rhythm is maintained.

When full pain-free motion is obtained, the subject may be seen to have a permanent step deformity, and some joint degeneration may occur in later years. The major problem resulting from this injury is lack of confidence when falling in contact sports. The effects of direct trauma may be limited by placing a felt doughnut pad over the joint. Confidence is built using progressive closed-chain exercises and rehearsal of falling actions. These may begin with forward rolls onto the outstretched arm on a mat, initially from a kneeling position, progressing to standing and finally a diving forward-roll over a bench. Pressure over the point of the shoulder begins with log-rolling on the floor, and builds up to shoulder blows onto a rolled mat or punch bag.

Surgical intervention

There is some controversy concerning the treatment of this condition. Both conservative and surgical approaches restore function to a similar degree (Bannister et al. 1989), and some surgical methods have been shown to give long-term functional detriment. Certainly, removal of the distal end of the clavicle will disrupt the acromioclavicular ligament, a main stabilizer of the joint (Fukuda et al. 1986). In the literature, the main argument for surgery has been the development of degenerative changes in the joint as a result of non-operative management. However, degeneration does not occur in all patients, and when it does occur, it is not necessarily a limitation (Dias et al. 1987). In

513

addition, surgery is often as effective if done in the acute or chronic condition, so there is normally no advantage to operating immediately.

In a literature review of 11 papers detailing the long-term results of both surgical and conservative management of this injury, Dias and Gregg (1991) found poor results to have occurred in 13 out of 247 patients treated conservatively (5.3 per cent), and 22 out of 233 managed surgically (9.4 per cent). These authors argued that, as comparable results were obtained regardless of the method used, conservative management was the treatment of choice for most AC injuries. Looking at strength-testing following grade III AC injuries treated conservatively (average 4.5-year follow-up), Tibone, Sellers and Tonino (1992) found no subjective complaints in patients, all of whom were able to participate in sport. Full motion occurred in all subjects, and no significant differences were found in muscle strength of injured and non-injured sides in rotation, abduction/adduction or flexion/extension. A meta-analysis of grade III injuries comparing operative versus non-operative management (Smith et al. 2011) showed better cosmetic outcome for operative treatment but no difference in strength, pain, throwing ability or development of osteoarthritis.

AC joint degeneration

Joint degeneration is common in later years following injury, regardless of the grade of damage that occurred, and particularly after repeated trauma. In addition, some sports, such as weightlifting, have a higher incidence of degenerative changes in the AC joint, even where no incidents of trauma may have occurred. Osteolysis of the distal clavicle may occur following repeated microtrauma in sports such as weightlifting. The condition presents as pain, usually dull and aching in nature, brought on by activities such as lifting and throwing. On examination there is point tenderness over the joint, with pain and crepitus to passive horizontal adduction (cross-body test).

> **Definition**
>
> Osteolysis is a pathological destruction of bone through active reabsorption of the bone matrix by osteoclast cells. It can be viewed as the reverse of ossification.

Where the diagnosis is uncertain, radiographs will frequently reveal degeneration, and injection of local anaesthetic into the joint is helpful to establish if the degeneration is the cause of the patient's symptoms.

Movements which stress the joint (for example, press-ups, weight training or throwing) should be limited. Initially, immobilization in a sling may be required in the acute/reactive stage of the condition. Later, joint mobilization can provide good results. Anteroposterior gliding may be performed with the patient in a sitting position. The therapist grasps the distal end of the clavicle with his or her thumb and forefingers of one hand, and the acromion process in a similar fashion with the other hand. The hands are worked against each other to glide the joint. Injection of corticosteroid may give many months of relief, a technique made easier if the shoulder is laterally rotated to distract the AC joint. Rehabilitation includes strength work in limited (pain-free) range, progressing range as symptoms allow.

Fractures of the clavicle

The most common mechanism of injury is a fall onto the outstretched arm, and occasionally direct trauma to the shoulder. Although common, these injuries should not be taken too lightly, as it must be remembered that the subclavian vessels and the medial cord of the brachial plexus lie in close proximity, as does the upper lobe of the lung (Fig. 12.11). Neurovascular and pulmonary examination may therefore be required.

There is usually a cracking sensation at the time of injury, with immediate pain over the fracture sight and rapid swelling. Signs of injury to vital structures are rare, but include dyspnoea and paraesthesia and obviously warrant immediate hospitalization. Laceration of the subclavian artery presents as a

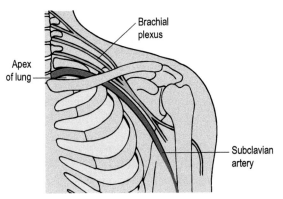

Figure 12.11 Structures close to the clavicle.

readily expanding pulsating haematoma. Deformity following clavicular fracture is common, as is crepitus.

> **Key point**
>
> Following suspected clavicular fracture, signs of altered sensation (paraesthesia) or breathlessness (dyspnoea) warrant immediate hospital referral.

Fractures of the proximal and middle thirds of the clavicle make up the largest proportion (80 per cent) of such injuries. If not displaced, these should be immobilized (bandage or sling depending on severity) generally for two to six weeks. Overlap of the bone fragments may shorten the clavicle (foreshortening), altering the biomechanics of the shoulder, and where this occurs a figure-of-eight bandage is often used to limit overlap. With young athletes, the risk of non-union may make it necessary to curtail activity for up to three months after injury. Traditional figure-of-eight bandages must not be applied so tightly as to constrict the blood or nerve supply to the arm. When little displacement is present, support in a sling is usually sufficient. Some step deformity usually occurs, as complete immobilization of athletes (other than in a cast) is difficult. This type of deformity is generally cosmetic rather than functional. Isometric exercise, and limited-range shoulder shrugs and shoulder flexion below 90 degrees may be allowed as healing progresses.

Distal fractures tend to be displaced by retraction immobilization, and are better wired. Internal fixation of the proximal clavicle carries with it similar complications to that of the sternoclavicular (SC) joint. Fractures to the extreme proximal end of the clavicle may be misdiagnosed as SC dislocations, and in the younger individual, epiphyseal injury should be considered in this region. It should be noted that the sternoclavicular epiphysis may remain open until the age of 25 (Zachazewski, Magee and Quillen 1996), so radiological examination must be accurate.

Winged scapula

During normal scapulohumeral rhythm, the scapula slides over the ribcage and is held in place by the serratus anterior. If weakness or paralysis of the serratus anterior occurs, the scapula will stand prominent from the ribcage when the arm is protracted against resistance. In addition to muscular weakness, there are a number of other causes, including damage to the long thoracic nerve, brachial plexus injury, conditions affecting the fifth, sixth and seventh cervical nerve roots, and certain types of muscular dystrophy (Apley and Solomon 1989).

Where weakness is due to nerve palsy, spontaneous recovery is to be expected. Re-education of scapulohumeral movement is required, as habitual alteration of scapulohumeral rhythm is often seen. Strengthening the shoulder musculature in general, and especially serratus anterior, is also useful.

Occasionally, a congenitally undescended scapula (Sprengel's shoulder) is seen, sometimes associated with marked thoracic kyphosis. Normally, the scapulae descend completely by the third month of fetal life. However, if undescended, the scapula appears slightly smaller, higher and more prominent. Scapulohumeral rhythm is affected and abduction is limited, as a consequence. Minor cases respond to rehabilitation, although marked deformity may require surgery.

Apparent winging may occur when the scapulae abduct through lengthening of the scapular retractors and tightening of the protractors. As the scapulae move away from the mid-line they roll around the ribcage, lifting their medial border. This is not true winging, however, because the condition is present at rest and during muscle contraction. Treatment note 12.1 shows exercise-therapy and manual-therapy techniques used in the restoration of scapulothoracic stability.

Taping may be used to give feedback about the position of the scapula and lengthened muscle. A positional box tape may be used to facilitate position of the scapula (Fig. 12.13). The tape has

---

Treatment Note 12.1　Restoration of scapulothoracic stability

Scapular stability is enhanced by restoring the functional capacity of the lower trapezius and serratus anterior, which, as stability muscles, often show reduced activity and lengthening. Surface electromyography (sEMG) may be used, with the active electrode placed over the lower trapezius or serratus anterior. The patient is placed in prone lying and the scapula is passively positioned into its neutral position by the therapist. This often requires retraction and depression to neutralize the protraction/elevation often found (Fig. 12.12). The patient is encouraged to hold this position through his or her own muscle activity, gaining feedback from the sEMG readout. Enough muscle activity should be used to keep the anterior aspect of the shoulder off the treatment couch, but not to retract the scapulae. Once this position can be maintained actively, the holding time is built up until the patient can perform ten repetitions, holding each for ten seconds.

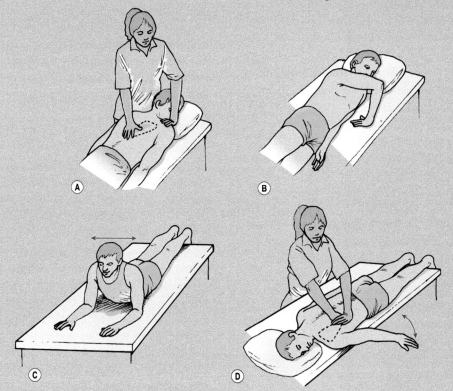

Figure 12.12 Enhancing scapulothoracic stability. (A) Scapular repositioning. (B) Rhythmic stabilization. (C) Trunk rocking. (D) Arm movement progressions.

Treatment note 12.1 *continued*

Key point

The main scapular stabilizers are serratus anterior and the lower trapezius. These muscles are worked using low-load scapular depression and retraction. The inner-range scapular position is held to build postural endurance.

two horizontal strips to draw the medial borders of the scapulae together, and two vertical strips to facilitate thoracic extension. Non-elastic taping is used to take up skin tension and act as a feedback system for the patient. Facilitatory taping may be used over the serratus anterior (Fig. 12.14A) or lower trapezius (Fig. 12.14B), or to increase patient awareness of body-segment position and facilitate underlying muscle action.

The scapular force couples may be maximally challenged using a side-lying, braced position (Wilk and Arrigo 1993). The patient begins in side lying with the arm flexed/abducted to 90 degrees and internally rotated. The hand is now flat on the couch with the fingers pointing towards the patient. Scapular fixation is maintained against the rhythmic stabilization provided by the therapist in all planes.

The next stage is to introduce a limited range of movements of the humerus onto the now-stable base of the scapular thoracic joint. Initially, the patient assumes elbow support prone-lying, to work the shoulder in closed kinetic chain format. He or she moves the body over the arm forward and backwards and side to side, to create closed-chain flexion/extension and abduction/adduction. At all times, the scapula must remain in contact with the thorax. The patient is now moved to the edge of the couch so the affected arm hangs over the couch side. Maintaining scapula thoracic stability, inner-range movements in all three planes are used, in an attempt to automatize stability.

The starting position is now changed to sitting or standing, and inner-range movements are used with sEMG monitoring of the lower trapezius. Home exercises may be used by asking the patient

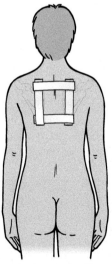

Figure 12.13 Box taping to facilitate correct scapular alignment.

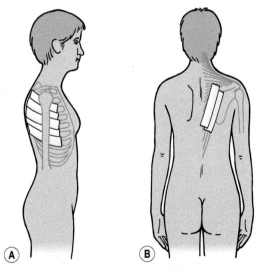

Figure 12.14 Faciliatory taping. (A) Serratus anterior. (B) Lower trapezius.

517

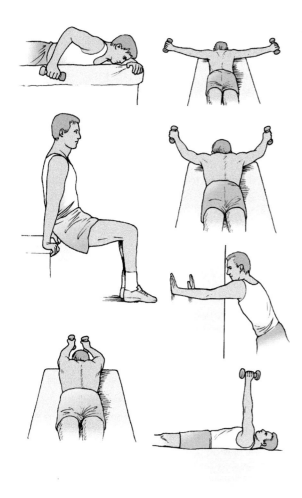

Figure 12.15 Exercises to selectively strengthen the scapulothoracic muscles. After Kamkar, Irrang and Whitney (1993).

to place the thumb of the opposite hand beneath the inferior scapular angle. The patient then gently keeps the inferior ankle pressed against the thumb (retraction and depression) while performing inner-range movements.

These initial actions, where stabilization ability is being re-educated, must keep the arm below 30 degrees abduction to prevent scapular movement. Later, greater glenohumeral range may be used as the patient can control scapulothoracic movement.

The scapulothoracic muscles may be selectively strengthened using the individual exercises shown in Figure 12.15.

Shoulder impingement

Prevalence of shoulder pain is high, with 30 per cent of individuals reporting pain in their lifetime, and over 50 per cent complaining that symptoms last beyond three years (Lewis 2009a). Up to 65 per cent of all shoulder pain can be attributed at least in part to impingement (Michener et al. 2003). The results of surgical treatment are comparable to those of conservative treatment, but in the long term up to one third of patients are left with persistent pain and disability (Seitz et al. 2011), making impingement one of the key challenges for therapists.

Biomechanics of impingement

We have seen that the shoulder joint has a larger ball (head of the humerus) than socket (glenoid fossa), with the glenoid fossa being one-third the size of the humeral head. The joint is surrounded by a loose capsule with a volume twice that of the humeral head. The roof of the joint (coracoacromial arch) is formed by the coracoacromial ligament together with the coracoid process and acromion process. The area below the coracoacromial arch is called the subacromial space, officially defined as having the humeral head as its base and the undersurface of the anterior acromion, coracoacromial ligament and the acromioclavicular joint as its roof. Within the subacromial space there are three structures, the supraspinatus tendon, subacromial bursa and long head of the biceps tendon.

> ### Key point
> The subacromial space is formed with the humeral head at its base, and the undersurface of the anterior acromion, coracoacromial ligament and the acromioclavicular joint as its roof. Within the space lies the supraspinatus tendon, subacromial bursa and long head of the biceps.

Subacromial impingement syndrome (SAIS) occurs when the tissues within the subacromial space generate pain or are compressed. Once general medical considerations have been eliminated,

Table 12.4 Factors associated with subacromial compression

Intrinsic	Extrinsic
▶ Tendon trauma (partial or full thickness tears)	▶ Referral from cervical spine
▶ Tendon degeneration	▶ Postural changes to thoracic spine
▶ Bursal swelling	▶ Altered scapular movement
	▶ Altered humeral movement
	▶ Tightness of posterior shoulder structures (rotator cuff/capsule)
	▶ Altered bony orientation (osteophytes)

mechanical compression may be considered either intrinsic, due to changes in the structures within the subacromial space, or extrinsic, resulting from external factors affecting the structures (Table 12.4).

The height of the subacromial space (acromiohumeral distance or AHD) is between 7 and 14 mm in healthy subjects (Seitz et al. 2011). A reduction in AHD may occur at rest, but only a measurement taken during active arm elevation is able to demonstrate functional narrowing. MRI studies of AHD have demonstrated smaller distances in the region of 3 mm during arm elevation in those with rotator-cuff tendinopathy due to SAIS (Graichen et al. 1999).

During the abduction cycle (above), decreased EMG activity in the infraspinatus and subscapularis together with the middle deltoid has been seen in subjects with SAIS from 30–60 degrees abduction (Reddy et al. 2000). The long head of the biceps has been shown to assist in stabilizing the head of the humerus in an anterior and superior direction and to decrease pressure within the subacromial space (Payne et al. 1997). Fluctuations of translation of the humeral head are relatively small in the healthy subject, with movement in the region of 1 mm being recorded. The humeral head should remain centred within the glenoid. Where the rotator-cuff muscles have reduced activity, or contract too late in the movement, upward displacement of the humerus occurs due to the unopposed pull of the deltoid. Anteroposterior movement of the humeral head varies, with values of 0.7–2.7 mm of anterior translation and 1.5–4.5 mm of posterior translation being recorded for different ranges of abduction (Ludewig and Cook 2002). Increased superior and/or anterior humeral head movement is associated with SAIS, with increased superior translation of 1.5 mm and increased anterior translation of 3 mm being quoted (Michener et al. 2003).

Tightness in the posterior capsule induced surgically in cadavers results in an increase in the superior and anterior humeral head translation (Harryman et al. 1990). This finding has been used to justify manual therapy aimed at the posterior capsule, and exercises such as the cross-body and sleeper stretch (see below). Although these techniques are often effective therapeutically in SAIS, they will probably affect both the posterior rotator cuff and capsule, as it is unlikely that the capsule can be selectively isolated non-operatively (Michener et al. 2003).

Anterior displacement of the head of the humerus relative to the glenoid may be compensated by posterior tightening of the posterior shoulder structures. This condition is especially common in those who use overhead movements, such as throwers, and the range of internal rotation and horizontal adduction at the glenohumeral joint is reduced as a result. Contraction of the posteroinferior capsule temporarily moves the head away from the painful anterosuperior region.

Definition

Obligate translation in the shoulder is tightening of the postero-inferior shoulder structures to unload the irritable antero-superior structures.

A reduction in internal rotation range occurs, the process being termed glenohumeral internal rotation deficit (GIRD). The motion change may be a result of humeral retroversion, posterior capsule thickening or increased muscle stiffness (Kibler et al. 2012). Although capsular tightening has been identified in elite baseball pitchers (Borso 2008), researchers have failed to identify this in the normal population (Gibson 2011). Increased muscle stiffness in the posterior rotator cuff and an alteration in synergistic movement patterns has been identified with the posterior deltoid, infraspinatus, and teres minor all affected (Hung et al. 2010).

GIRD is said to be present when there is a difference of 20–25 degrees in internal rotation range between the subject's two shoulders when rotation is measured at 90 degrees abduction. It has been suggested that overhead-throwing athletes such as baseball pitchers have a greater injury risk if they have this condition (Wilk et al. 2011). The loss of range of internal rotation (GIRD) is often associated with a glenohumeral external-rotation gain (GERG), and where the ratio between the two is greater than one, symptoms are said to be more likely (Magee 2008).

Key point

Glenohumeral internal rotation deficit (GIRD) and glenohumeral external rotation gain (GERG) may be associated with shoulder-impingement symptoms.

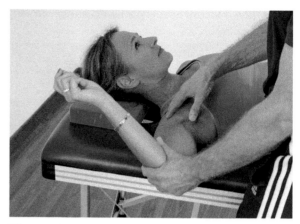

Figure 12.16 Assessment of GH internal rotation in supine.

Internal rotation range is measured, and a common field test is the scarecrow sign (Fig. 12.16), where the athlete stands with their back to the wall, elbows flexed to 90 degrees and upper arms abducted to the horizontal. Lowering the forearms maintaining 90 degrees elbow flexion provides visual information about the symmetry of internal rotation range, and any compensatory scapular elevation or tipping becomes apparent. In the clinic the test is performed with the subject supine, to provide some scapular fixation. Treatment of the condition can involve stretching out the reduced range of internal rotation, in parallel with re-strengthening of the rotator cuff and optimization of scapular alignment. Figure 12.17A & B shows

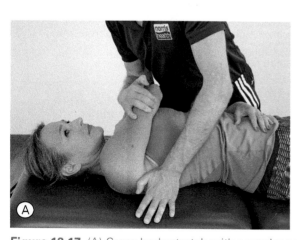

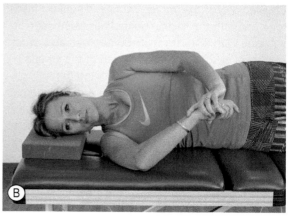

Figure 12.17 (A) Cross-body stretch with scapular counter pressure. (B) Sleeper stretches.

the cross-body stretch and the sleeper stretch. The cross-body stretch lengthens the posterior structures during horizontal adduction, while the sleeper stretch uses internal rotation and aids in passive scapular stabilization by taking the subject's bodyweight onto the scapula itself. Internal rotation range measured in the scarecrow position may also be used as an indicator of the effectiveness of other forms of therapy, such as cervical spine mobilizations and movement re-education, on the shoulder complex.

Decreased performance in the serratus anterior and lower trapezius has been identified in subjects suffering from rotator-cuff tendinopathy due to SAIS, with reduced total EMG activity and onset of activation (Seitz et al. 2011). This change has also been shown with overhead athletes demonstrating shoulder impingement (Cools et al. 2004).

Pathology

It is generally considered that compression of the soft tissues between the head of the humerus and the acromion during abduction and elevation causes pain, with the classic impingement test combining abduction and internal rotation (empty-can sign) to press the greater trochanter onto the undersurface of the acromion, sandwiching any impinging structure between the two.

The traditional view of the development of impingement syndrome is of mechanical compression through three progressive phases (Neer 1983). The condition has been said to begin (stage I) in the younger patient (under 25) with oedema and hemorrhage through persistent overhead activities, leading to deterioration of the tendon and bursa (stage II) in the 25–40-year-old, to final, full-thickness rupture and bone-spur formation in those over 40 years of age (stage III). However, this progressive pathology has been challenged (Lewis 2011). If compression of the supraspinatus tendon occurs beneath the subacromial arch, the direct mechanical strain should lead to abrasion to the tendon's upper surface. However, damage to the inferior (joint) side of the tendon has been found in over 90 per cent of cases in athletes

and over 80 per cent of cadavers, representing internal impingement (Edelson and Teitz 2000). The prevalence of partial thickness tears in cadavers has been shown to be roughly 30 per cent, with damage to the articular aspect of the tendon or intra-tendon substance (Loehr & Uhthoff 1987). The fibres on the lower (non-acromial) side of the tendon have a smaller cross-sectional area than those on the upper surface. The lower fibres are therefore more vulnerable to tensile loading, especially during elevation where tendon strain is increased. Movement of the upper tendon fibres upon the lower may result in intratendinous shearing, giving reaction through physiological failure of the lower tendon fibres rather than injury through external compression (Lewis 2011).

Where external compression is a cause of SAIS, the shape of the acromion becomes relevant. Three types of acromion have been described: flat (type I), curved (type II) and hooked (type III) (Ticker and Bigliani 1994). The suggestion is that rotator cuff tears as a result of SAIS are more common in those with a hooked acromion, justifying the need for surgical removal of the anterior/inferior aspect of the acromion (acromioplasty). However, many asymptomatic individuals have been found to have a curved or hooked acromion, and it has been suggested that the success of acromioplasty may be due to enforced rest following surgery rather than to the surgical procedure itself (Lewis 2011). The shape of the acromion itself may be a secondary rather than a primary effect. Bony-spur formation of the acromion seems to be at the insertion of the coracoacromial ligament. A repetitive upward translation force (due to impaired action of the rotator cuff) may create tension at the acromial insertion of the ligament which is smaller than the coracoid side. The ligament may be a source of pain as free nerve endings have been identified within it.

The subacromial bursa is innervated by the lateral pectoral nerve and subscapular nerve, and is capable of both nociception and proprioception. Removal of the bursa (bursectomy) alone gives the same degree of pain relief as bursectomy combined with acromioplasty, with no significant differences at two-and-a-half years' follow-up (Henkus et al. 2009).

Changes to the supraspinatus tendon seen in SAIS indicate that the condition is likely a tendinopathy rather than a tendinitis. No infiltration of cells associated with inflammation are seen within the tendon in specimens taken during surgery, but increased volume of the tendon seen experimentally may be the result of a reactive phase similar to Achilles or patellar tendinopathy. An increased vascular response (neovascularization) in degenerative areas of the supraspinatus has been noted with Doppler ultrasound (Levy et al. 2008), suggesting a healing response to microtrauma, as is seen in tendonitis in other body areas. The presence of tendinopathy and increased metabolic response during a reactive phase would suggest that relative rest and graduated loading should form part of the management of this condition.

> **Key point**
>
> Pathological changes in the supraspinatus tendon with impingement syndrome indicate a process of tendinopathy rather than tendinitis.

Patient assessment

Tests used to assess SAIS are effective at provoking the subject's pain, but may be less useful at identifying the pathological tissue responsible for the pain. Traditional passive tests aim to compress the structures within the subacromial space by combining some degree of abduction with internal rotation (Table 12.5).

With many conditions there can be a poor clinical correlation between pathology and pain, and the shoulder is no exception. Some subjects may have pain with few apparent indicators on imaging, while others are asymptomatic in the presence of marked bone or soft tissue changes. Systematic review, with meta-analysis of the Neer and

Table 12.5 Common clinical tests for SAIS

Test name	Action
Neer's sign	Also called the *forward flexion impingement test*. Stabilize the scapula and grip the arm below the elbow with the other hand. Passively elevate arm into full flexion. Positive if pain is produced at end of passive elevation.
Hawkins–Kennedy	Elbow flexed to 90°, shoulder passively forward flexed to 90°. Take shoulder into internal rotation.
Full/empty can	Also called *Jobe's test* and the *Scaption test*. Passively elevate arm to 90° in scapular plane. Turn hand down so thumb points towards floor for internal rotation (empty can) and apply resistance to abduction. Repeat with palm up for external rotation (full can).

Hawkins–Kennedy tests for impingement (and the Speed test for labral pathology), concluded that diagnostic accuracy is limited (Hegedus et al. 2008).

The use of clinical tests as symptom-provoking procedures to monitor treatment effect has been proposed for SAIS (Lewis 2009a) using the *shoulder symptom modification procedure*, which provides a logical synopsis of common tests and methods from several areas of physiotherapy, such as mobilization with movement (MWM), exercise therapy, manual therapy and taping. Techniques in four areas are used, as shown in Treatment Note 12.2. Patient-described outcome is normally that of pain measured on a numerical rating scale (NRS) or visual analogue scale (VAS), with a minimal clinical important difference (MCID) being set at a 30 per cent improvement from baseline to represent a meaningful change. Movement range may also be used to assess the effectiveness of subsequent treatment technique.

Rehabilitation

Rehabilitation aims to reduce the subject's symptoms during aggravating movements, and to improve movement quality. Loss of translational control of the humeral head within the glenoid is

Treatment Note 12.2 Shoulder symptom modification procedure.

The Shoulder symptom modification procedure (SSMP) consists of four components (Table 12.6)

Humeral head positioning

Pressure techniques are used on the humeral head which are similar to traditional mobilization with movement (MWM) procedures but used with manual pressure, belts or elastic tubing. Either anterior or posterior directed pressure is maintained during the subject's movement in an attempt to reduce symptoms.

Movements which caused pain during testing may be repeated using minimal humeral head pressure to modify symptoms. External rotation and humeral head depression are performed to restrict or modify internal rotation and elevation stresses which traditionally exacerbate SAIS. A posterior glide MWM applied manually has been shown to immediately reduce pain by 20.2 per cent and increase movement range by 15.3 per cent in a group of subjects with anterolateral shoulder pain which restricted shoulder elevation (Teys et al. 2006). In this study, the increase in motion range was not related to change in pain, leading the authors to suggest that joint or muscle mechanisms may be responsible for the movement change rather than pain.

Scapular positioning

Manual techniques and taping may be used to slightly modify scapular position, as altered scapular kinematics is often associated with impingement symptoms (Ludewig and Cook 2000). The same scapular modifications may then be used for re-education. Scapular position of elevation/depression, protraction/retraction, tipping (also called tilt, representing rotation about a mediolateral axis), and rotation (rotation about an anteroposterior axis) are all compared to the unaffected side and modified if required. Scapular winging may be modified by manual stabilization or taping, to assess the effect on the subject's symptoms.

Radiculopathy

If shoulder pain arises from the cervical spine, manual therapy to this region can affect pain and movement in the shoulder region. Both soft-tissue and joint-based techniques may be used. A study which used lateral mobilizations applied to the C5/C6/C7 spinous processes in sitting have been shown to both reduce pain (mean 1.3 cm measured in a VAS scale) and increase abduction motion range (mean 12.5 degrees measured using videoanalysis) in patients with shoulder pain of at least six weeks' duration (McClatchie et al. 2009). Cervical mobilization has been shown to increase lateral rotation motion range at the shoulder in subjects with restricted movement in the absence of shoulder treatment (Schneider 1989). Oscillatory mobilization was given to the C4/5 and C5/6 segments, with lateral rotation range at the shoulder increasing from 0–1/4 range to 1/2–3/4 range. It was suggested that pain referred from the cervical spine to the shoulder resulted in increased muscle tone to the shoulder musculature, restricting motion range at that joint. The restricted and/or painful shoulder movement should be performed, and cervical tissue treatment applied, to assess change in the shoulder symptoms.

Thoracic kyphosis

Changes to the thoracic kyphosis have been shown to alter scapular tipping and rotation, and to decrease the amount of elevation at the glenohumeral joint (Michener et al. 2003). Altering

Table 12.6 SSMP components

Body region	Mechanical technique
▶ Humeral head	▶ Application of mobilization with movement.
▶ Scapular position	▶ Passive stabilization or modification, with or without taping.
▶ Cervical spine	▶ Neuromodulation procedure to address pain and movement. quality
▶ Thoracic spine	▶ Reduction of increased kyphosis.

Data modified from Lewis (2009b).

Treatment note 12.2 *continued*

thoracic and scapular posture has been shown to significantly increase shoulder flexion and abduction range in the scapular plane, and to delay the point of onset of pain within the motion range in subjects with SAIS (Lewis et al. 2005). Manual techniques using overpressure and/or taping may be used to reduce the subject's kyphosis, and movement quality is reassessed. Where thoracic stiffness is present, localized manual therapy may be applied, as this has been shown to change impingement signs (Neer, empty can, Hawkins–Kennedy, and active abduction) in subjects with impingement syndrome (Boyles et al. 2009).

strongly associated with impingement symptoms, and poor co-contraction of the rotator cuff muscles during the abduction cycle is often found in symptomatic subjects. Over time, compensatory muscle strategies are put in place to maintain adequate function, and as glenohumeral and scapulothoracic movements are optimized, compensatory actions which have become habitual must be identified and reduced. With chronic conditions especially, *central sensitization* and altered *neuroplastic changes* are seen. Central sensitization occurs (see Chapter 1) when altered processing is seen within the dorsal horn cells of the spinal cord, while neuroplastic changes may include altered representation of the body part within the somato-sensory cortex, increased strength of internal neural connections, and reorganization of neuronal territory (Littlewood et al. 2013). Motor skill training which is functionally relevant to the patient may help normalize the representation of the body part in the somato-sensory cortex and so be instrumental in managing a subject's pain (Gibson 2011).

Rehabilitation aims to (i) re-establish muscle co-contraction and translational control of the humeral head, (ii) enhance scapular stability and positioning during the abduction cycle, (iii) reduce habitual compensatory movements and (iv) optimize body segment and whole-body alignment, and appropriate movement strategies.

Early rehabilitation begins with the techniques described in the shoulder symptom modification procedure (SSMP), which aims to reduce symptoms in aggravating movements. Isolation movements may be used to re-educate scapular stability and rotator cuff co-contraction during abduction actions. Movements in the scapular plane (30–45 degrees anterior to the frontal plane) are used with ranges below the horizontal to reduce pressure within the subacromial space. Passive or active lateral rotation of the humerus is maintained to distance the greater tuberosity from the anterior aspect of the acromion process.

Hand grip, tactile feedback of the wrist and hand, and closed-chain upper-limb actions can all lead to co-contraction of the rotator cuff musculature to initiate the pre-setting phase of muscle activity in the shoulder. Sensorimotor input may be enhanced by working the scapulothoracic joint and glenohumeral joint in unison, in contrast to isolation movements often prescribed.

Key point

Grip and tactile feedback to the wrist can be used to initiate rotator cuff activity prior to the performance of rehabilitation exercises for SAIS.

Through linked kinetic chains, movement of the whole body contributes to upper limb function. Fault in one part of the kinetic chain may cause compensation elsewhere in the chain, a feature called link fallout, and rehabilitation should reflect this. Movement and/or stability of the proximal body component is begun prior to the distal, with an emphasis on functional rotation patterns. Throughout the rehab programme, the therapist should aim to minimize compensatory patterns in the client, which may be localized to the shoulder and upper limb or appear in other body areas. Within traditional therapy approaches there is often a focus on isolation actions at the shoulder. Although this approach has a place within the whole programme, if rehab is restricted to isolation actions alone, it may fail to restore full function. The use of exercise, focusing on a dynamic whole-body approach, using both rotator cuff action and scapular stability as part of a kinetic chain movement, is likely to produce a better functional outcome. The use of complex exercise has been shown to be superior to isolation exercise for the rotator cuff, using a six-week programme with subjects training three times per week (Giannakopoulos et al, 2004). These authors suggested that rehabilitation for the shoulder should begin with isolation actions to stimulate the weaker muscles, and progress to complex actions to give greater overload, an approach also used successfully during the rehabilitation of other body areas (Norris and Matthews 2008). Treatment Note 12.3 shows example exercises which may be used as part of a structured rehabilitation programme following full client assessment.

Treatment Note 12.3   Example rehabilitation exercises used when managing subacromial impingement syndrome (SAIS)

Sternal lift

The action (Fig. 12.18) is to lift the anterior chest forwards and up using thoracic extension (sternal lifting), rather than ribcage expansion (taking a deep breath). The therapist uses tactile cueing by placing their hands onto the client's sternum, or uses an object placed flat against the sternum to show that the sternal plate is angled downwards as the thoracic kyphosis increases and upwards as the kyphosis reduces. If the subject has difficulty isolating the sternal lift action from deep inhalation, ask them to inhale, and then lift the sternum as they exhale. Where they sway their body forwards or backwards, ask them to stand or sit with their back pressed up against a wall and perform the sternal lift action from this starting position. The action is to draw the scapulae down the wall as the sternum lifts upwards.

Overhead stretch on gym ball

This exercise combines thoracic extension with full range flexion/abduction at the shoulder (Fig 12.19). The subject lies over a large (65 cm) gym ball. Have them reach overhead with their elbows straight but not locked completely. At the same time, encourage their chest to open and thoracic spine to extend. To increase overload, a light dumb-bell may be held between the hands. Where shoulder flexibility is limited, practise the movement close to a wall so the hands rest on the wall rather than overhead.

Gym ball superman with star arms

Again, the subject uses a gym ball with their chest on the ball surface, feet apart and on the floor (Fig. 12.20). Their arms should be out to

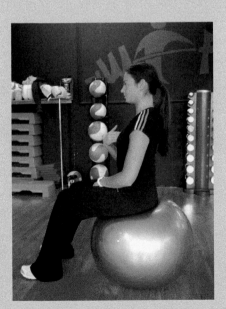

Figure 12.18 Sternal lift.

Treatment note 12.3 *continued*

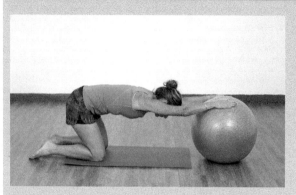

Figure 12.19 Overhead stretch on gym ball.

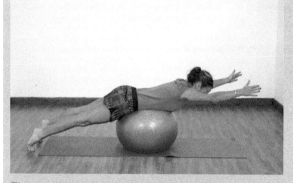

Figure 12.20 Gym ball superman with star arms.

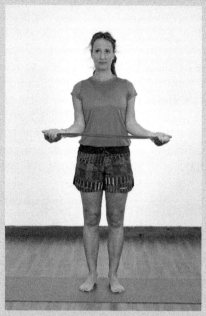

Figure 12.21 Pilates dumb waiter with band.

the side in a T-shape, hands resting on the floor. Raise the arms out to the sides (extension–abduction), turning them so the thumbs point to the ceiling (lateral rotation at the shoulder). At the same time, perform a thoracic extension movement by drawing the scapulae down and inwards and opening the chest. Raise the head slightly to look at the floor 1–2m in front of the ball. Hold the top position to 2–3 seconds, breathing normally (do not allow the subject to hold their breath), and then lower the arms and trunk under control.

Pilates dumb waiter with band

The subject stands with their feet hip-width apart, and elbows bent to 90 degrees, and tucked into the side of their trunk (Fig. 12.21). For the dumb waiter action, have the palms facing upwards and laterally rotate the shoulders to draw the forearms outwards in an arc away from the body. Pause at the outer-range position and then return to the starting position. To increase overload the subject should hold a resistance band between the hands and pull outwards against the resistance. Again, pause at the outer-range point and then move back to the starting position under control.

Abduction with lateral rotation using band

Begin by hooking a resistance band beneath a door using a door stop. This exercise has two parts (Fig. 12.22). For the first part, have the subject perform an isolation action with the shoulder, combining abduction and lateral rotation to draw their hand outwards and turn the palm forwards so their thumb moves towards the ceiling. When they have performed this action several times and are comfortable with it, they can move to part two of the action, which is a complex movement combining trunk rotation

Treatment note 12.3 *continued*

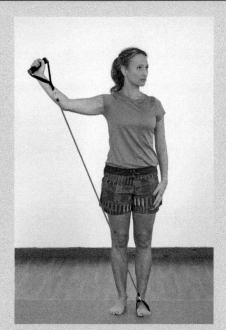

Figure 12.22 Abduction with lateral rotation using band.

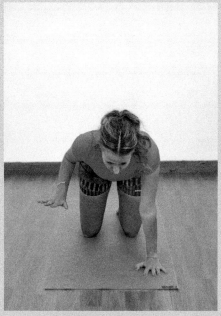

Figure 12.23 Pilates cat paws.

and arm movement. Now, they stand with their far foot turned outwards (lateral rotation at the hip) and reach downwards towards the door. They then turn their whole body outwards, away from the door, as they abduct their arm and turn it outwards. Their eyes should follow their hand throughout the action as the trunk turns inwards towards the door when the arm is lowered. The second action works the shoulder musculature with the core muscles at the same time. To increase overload on the core, perform the action in single-leg standing so that whole body balance is challenged.

Pilates cat paws

This exercise (Fig. 12.23) works the scapular stabilizers with the arm in flexion in closed-chain position (hand on the floor). The exercise begins in four-point kneeling (knee beneath the hip and hand beneath the shoulder). The subject stabilizes their scapula by drawing it down slightly and inwards. Verbal cues such as 'press your chest outwards'

or 'push your hand into the floor and make your arm longer' can be useful, and tactile cues have the therapist place a flat hand onto the scapula or using a book placed on the upper thorax are also suitable. The action is to shift the shoulders to the right to take the chest weight over the right hand and to lift the heel of the left hand, leaving the fingers just in contact with the mat. The right scapula must now work hard to remain fixed to the thorax and not wing outwards. Reverse the action taking the weight to the left. Once the action can be performed with good scapulothoracic alignment, have your client progress to lifting the hand by bending their elbow. Ensure that the shoulders remain level, and do not allow the shoulder on the lifted side to dip down.

Standing band pull

Begin with the subject standing, shoulders hip-width apart (Fig. 12.24). Have them hold the ends of a resistance band in each hand and loop the centre beneath their feet. Adjust the band so it is tight, and encourage them to draw their scapulae

Treatment note 12.3 *continued*

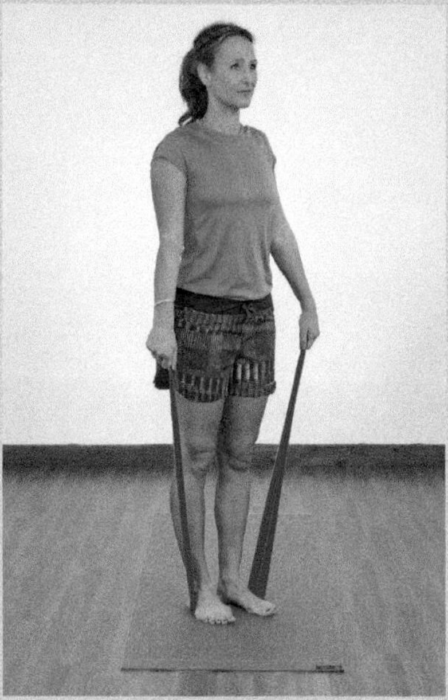

Figure 12.24 Standing band pull.

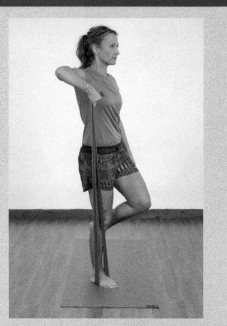

Figure 12.25 Single-arm row with single-leg stand.

down and inwards, at the same time lifting their sternum. Use verbal cues such as 'open your chest' and 'draw your shoulder blades down into the back pocket of your shorts'. Tactile cues can encourage both movements simultaneously by placing one finger between their scapulae and drawing the skin downwards and another finger on the sternum to draw the skin upwards. Ensure that they do not increase their lumbar lordosis as they lift their ribcage.

Single-arm row with single-leg stand

This action combines a shoulder movement with whole-body action to provide complex work of overall body balance and coordination (Fig. 12.25).

Begin with the subject facing a pulley machine or resistance tubing secured to a door frame. Have them take the slack up on the cable or tubing and stand on one leg, establishing their balance. They should maintain a good upright posture and draw the cable towards themselves, moving the shoulder blades downwards as they do so. The action is to stabilize the scapula as the arm moves, but not to overly brace the shoulders or thrust the chest forwards. The knee of the supporting leg should bend slightly (soften) and the hips are aligned horizontally. Do not allow the pelvis to dip towards the non-weightbearing side.

Manual Therapy

Manual therapy can be useful in the treatment of SAIS to modify symptoms identified at initial assessment. These may be directed at the shoulder, thoracic spine or cervical spine, as indicated by the SSMP. Initial management during the reactive phase of the condition may involve hands-on therapy, and as pain eases and function improves during the recovery phase, rehabilitation (hands-off techniques) becomes more important. Therapy aims to reduce the subject's symptoms during aggravating movements, and to improve movement quality as a lead-in to rehabilitation, which may begin either in parallel with manual therapy or subsequent to it. Tightness of the posterior shoulder tissues is often associated with anterior and superior translation of the humeral head, so soft tissue techniques aimed at the posterior tissues may be used in parallel with joint-based techniques. Lateral rotation is an important movement during rehabilitation, but this movement direction may be limited in subjects suffering from impingement.

Manual therapy aims to (i) reduce symptoms, (ii) mobilize the joint in an antero-posterior and inferior direction, (iii) release tight posterior structures and (iv) address the cervical and thoracic spine.

Cervical mobilization is traditionally carried out with the subject lying, with the head supported. However, where shoulder symptoms are referred from the cervical region they are usually experienced in the standing or sitting position. Choosing the sitting position for cervical mobilization has the advantage that the shoulder may be tested and re-tested for pain and movement after the cervical mobilization. Begin with the subject sitting in a hard-back chair, or support their back with your shin if they are sitting on a treatment couch (Fig. 12.26). Cradle the subject's head with your left arm (use a towel or paper sheet to protect their face), and use the thumb or flexed finger to apply a mobilization to the side of the spinous process. Target the levels from C4 to C7 as these refer to the shoulder region, and begin the mobilization pressing towards the non-painful arm (contralateral side). If symptoms remain unchanged, repeat the mobilization towards the side of pain (ipsilateral side). Small amounts of movement (small amplitude) are used at end range, traditionally called a Grade IV mobilization.

Where the thoracic kyphosis is accentuated and/or the thoracic spine is stiff to extension, mobilizing the thoracic vertebrae in a posteroanterior (PA) direction can be useful. The subject lies prone, with a folded towel or pillow for extra padding beneath the chest if preferred (Fig. 12.27). Using a pisiform bone contact, a localized force is applied to the spine, reinforcing one hand with the other. Target the spinous process or transverse process for localized central or unilateral PA mobilizations, or use one hand on each side of the spine for a more generalized extension force.

Whilst mobilization and exercise are able to produce fairly high forces applied over a relatively short period, the use of postural taping applies low-level force over an extended period for re-education. The time period is important as it gives the opportunity for the subject to adapt to the new posture and reinforces the new alignment to address symptoms. Begin with the subject either lying flat on their front (prone lying) with the couch end tilted upwards by 10–20 degrees or a folded

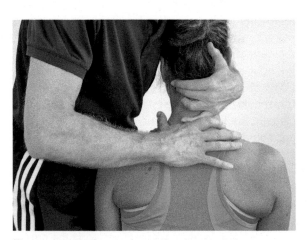

Figure 12.26 Cervical mobilization in sitting.

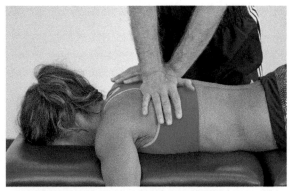

Figure 12.27 PA glide to thoracic spine using pisiform contact point.

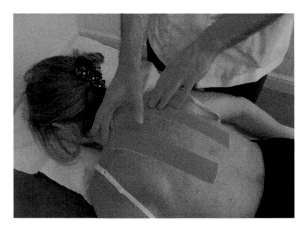

Figure 12.28 Thoracic taping applied in supine lying.

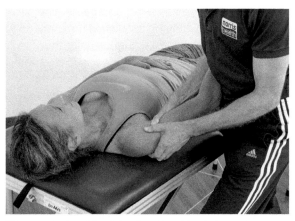

Figure 12.29 AP glide the shoulder joint using cupped-hand contact.

towel beneath their chest, in both cases to place the thoracic spine into extension. If the subject is able to perform and hold the sternal lift action (active thoracic extension), the taping may be applied in sitting or standing. The taping is placed on the skin with some tension to provide skin stimulation (Fig. 12.28). Where kinesiotape (K-tape) is used, it can be placed directly onto the skin, but where zinc oxide tape is used, an undermesh should be used to protect the skin. If using K-tape, the first part of the tape (2 cm) is placed on the skin under no tension to secure it firmly. The tape is then stretched to 25 per cent (some tension) or 50 per cent (greater tension) of its length and placed onto the skin. The end 2 cm of tape is again stuck to the skin under no tension to ensure a firm attachment. Where zinc oxide tape is used, the undermesh is placed onto the skin under no tension, and the zinc oxide, which is non-elastic, is attached to the mesh and pulled downwards to give tactile feedback for thoracic extension. Greater or lesser force may be used depending on the client's needs.

We have seen that one of the most common scenarios with shoulder impingement is that the humeral head moves forwards (anterior) and upwards (superior), increasing the likelihood of compression to the subacromial structures. Mobilization in the opposite direction (posterior

and inferior glides) can modify symptoms. AP gliding can be performed with the subject lying or sitting. The lying position supports the trunk and enables greater force to be applied, while the sitting position enables active shoulder movements to be performed more easily as a precursor to mobilization with movement (MWM) techniques. Use the heel of your hand as a contact area and cup the humeral head to make the technique more comfortable. The other hand may be placed over the clavicle to provide counter pressure and limit movement of the scapula and trunk (Fig. 12.29).

Inferior glides may be used at several GH joint angles, but as impingement pain typically occurs as the arm approaches the horizontal, progression to 90-degree abduction can be useful. Begin with the subject lying on their back (supine lying) on their affected shoulder close to the couch side. For right-shoulder symptoms, stand to their left side with your right hand cupped over the top of the shoulder (middle deltoid) and the left hand close to the top of their inner arm. Both hands are positioned close to the joint line, and the client's arm is abducted to 90 degrees, or the greatest range possible for them up to 90 degrees. The action is to move the arm straight downwards (inferiorly) by pressing with your right hand and guiding with your left. The action can combine both superior and inferior movement, drawing the arm

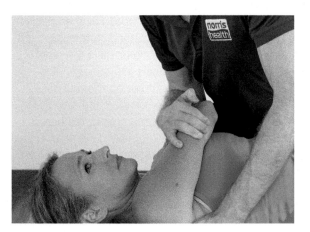

Figure 12.30 Soft tissue work in side lying for GIRD.

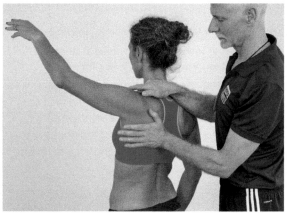

Figure 12.31 MWM for glenohumeral abduction.

superiorly slightly (10–20 per cent) providing there is no pain, and emphasizing the inferior direction (80–90 per cent). A rhythmic action is used within the free range of motion just moving to the point of restriction but not into it, traditionally called a Grade III mobilization.

Tightness of the posterior joint is associated with shoulder impingement and GIRD, as restriction posteriorly can press the humeral head anteriorly to reduce the subacromial space. Begin with the subject lying on their unaffected side. Fold their affected arm across their chest to place the posterior structures on stretch (Fig. 12.30). Target the structures in tissue layers from the superficial to the most deep, altering your massage depth accordingly. Work into the tissues gradually, beginning with the posterior deltoid, and then move more deeply to the teres major and minor. Deeper still are the supraspinatus and infraspinatus, and finally after working through the muscle tissue you will reach the posterior joint capsule. Use two or three fingers gripped together as your massage contact area to apply the required pressure, or choose a massage tool. Assess the effectiveness of the massage procedure by pain (assessed on a VAS scale from 1 to 10), joint stiffness (assessed by resistance to motion and joint end feel), and tissue tension (assessed by tissue resistance to palpation pressure). The

subject may use the crossbody position as a stretch for home use (see below). Ask them to take their affected arm across their body and apply overpressure with the non-affected arm. Hold the stretch for 20 to 30 seconds and perform three repetitions morning and evening.

Mobilization with movement (MWM) (see Chapter 1) combines passive movement of the joint with active movement to improve movement quality with the aim of reducing symptoms. In the case of shoulder impingement, the aim is to create a greater range of pain-free motion to flexion/abduction. Begin with the subject sitting or standing and stand behind them. Use the cupped hand over the top and front of their shoulder joint, approaching from the medial side (Fig. 12.31). Ask the subject to raise their arm forwards and outwards at an angle of 30 degrees to their body (scaption) with their thumb upwards (lateral rotation at the glenohumeral joint). As they do so, draw their shoulder joint towards you to impart a posterior glide. You may use the other hand to monitor their scapula, and if necessary gently press it against their ribcage to encourage stability or draw it downwards to discourage upward shifting (see scapular assistance test above). As an alternative to hand pressure, the therapist may use a webbing belt (yoga belt) looped over the client's shoulder.

Rotator cuff tendinopathy

As we have seen above, SAIS may affect the supraspinatus tendon, but tendinopathy of the rotator cuff muscles in general is also seen associated with the condition and separate from it. The pathology and rehabilitation principles underlying tendinopathy have been covered in Chapter 1, and in the sections of tendinopathy of the Achilles tendon (Chapter 6) and patella tendon (Chapter 4).

Supraspinatus

Pain on screening test may be elicited with resisted external rotation and initiation of abduction. The tendon is made up of six to nine independent fascicles (Fallon et al. 2002) containing proteoglycan lubricant, which facilitates independent sliding of each fascicle. During shoulder abduction the inner (joint-side) part of the tendon is subjected to traction, while the outer parts are compressed. The attachment of the tendon to bone is via a fibrocartilage enthesis, a tissue less capable of withstanding tension loading. The inner articular fibres have a smaller cross-sectional area compared to those on the superior (bursal) aspect. Stressing the two sets of fibres experimentally has shown the articular fibres to rupture with half the force of the bursal side fibres (Nakajima, Rokuuma and Hamada 1994). Intrinsic pathology of the rotator cuff tendons leads to decreased function and a lessened ability to control the humeral head position. This reduction in function may allow the humeral head to translate superiorly, increasing stress on any of the structures within the subacromial space. Changes to the bursa may therefore be secondary to the tendon itself (Lewis 2009a).

Palpation to the muscle insertion is performed with the injured arm medially rotated (hand behind the back) to bring the greater tuberosity forwards and make the tendon more superficial (Fig. 12.32A). This is also the most convenient position for transverse frictional massage, the

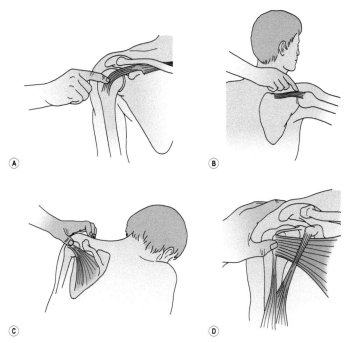

Figure 12.32 Palpation and treatment of rotator cuff tendon injury. (A) Supraspinatus: tendon. (B) Supraspinatus: musculotendinous junction. (C) Infraspinatus. (D) Subscapularis. After Cyriax and Cyriax (1983), with permission.

symptomatic area often being found by palpating about one finger's width below the anterior tip of the acromion. The musculotendinous junction is more conveniently palpated with the injured arm abducted to 90 degrees and supported (Cyriax and Cyriax 1983). The palpating finger is directed at the space between the posterior aspect of the lateral clavicle and the scapular spine. Again, this is the most convenient starting position for transverse frictional massage (Fig. 12.32B).

Calcification of the supraspinatus (or rarely the other rotator cuff tendons) may develop following chronic tendinopathy within the critical zone, an area claimed to be susceptible to injury due to reduced vascularity. This area, near the attachment of the supraspinatus (see Fig. 12.33), may be stressed when the arm is held in its resting position of adduction and neutral rotation. Compression of the tendon vessels and microtrauma may be associated with repetitive hypoxia. Fibrocytes within the tendon are transformed to chondrocytes, and collagen disintegration, coupled with the accumulation of mucopolysaccharides, begins. Hydroxyapatite mineral deposit deposition is then initiated (Lemak 1994).

During the reactive phase, the deposit is of toothpaste-like consistency, but may not be clinically relevant. Conservative management

(active rest followed by loading) is usually successful if the condition is caught early enough. Loading is performed in the pain-free range (Torstensen, Meen and Stiris 1994), avoiding both the resting position (adduction and neutral rotation) and internal rotation.

Remaining muscles

Pain on resisted lateral rotation but not abduction implicates the *infraspinatus*. Local pain may be found by palpation to the posterior aspect of the greater tuberosity with the patient's shoulder flexed, slightly adducted and laterally rotated. The most convenient position for this is elbow support in a prone-lying position, with the patient leaning forwards and outward over the injured shoulder.

If resisted medial rotation alone gives pain, the *subscapularis* is most likely affected, at its insertion into the lesser tuberosity. This structure may be palpated and treated along the inner edge of the intertubercular sulcus. The patient is in a long sitting position, and the therapist grasps the hand on the affected side. A transverse frictional mobilization is carried out by medial and lateral rotation of the patient's shoulder against the palpating finger of the therapist.

Pain in combination with resisted adduction implicates the muscles (pectoralis major, latissimus dorsi and teres major) attaching within the intertubercular sulcus. These muscles show tendinopathy less commonly than muscle tearing.

Treatment of rotator cuff tendinopathy consists of targeting both medial and lateral rotation of the glenohumeral joint in multiple arm positions. The focus is on progressive loading, and as with other forms of tendinopathy isometric contractions may be analgesic, and eccentric actions are often a way to impart high loads to the tendon which are well tolerated. Rotation actions may be performed using resistance tubing or pulley machines in varying starting positions (Fig. 12.34). As symptoms settle, abduction and lateral rotation may be performed within the scapular plane.

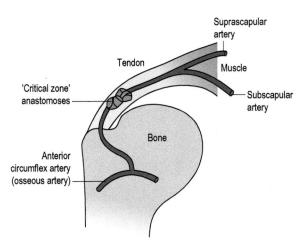

Figure 12.33 Vascularity of the critical zone. From Keirns (1994), with permission.

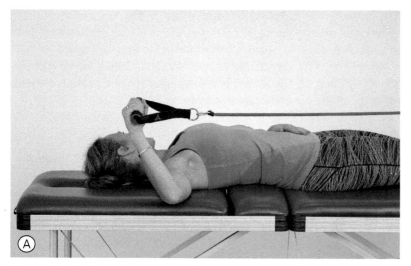
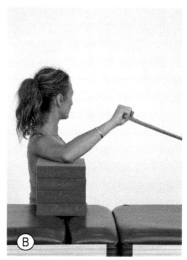

Figure 12.34 Resisted rotation training for rotator cuff tendinopathy. (A) Lying. (B) Table top.

Definition

The scapular plane is the normal resting position of the scapula on the ribcage. To perform exercise in the scapular plane, the arm is held 30–45 degrees to the midline (sagittal plane).

Biceps

The long head of the biceps originates at the supraglenoid tubercle and passes intracapsularly into the bicipital groove (intertubercular sulcus). The tendon is round at its origin, flattens as it passes over the shoulder joint, and narrows within the

Treatment Note 12.4   Rotator cuff trigger points

Trigger points (TrPs) within the rotator cuff muscles may occur in shoulder conditions, and some pain modulation may be produced by targeting them.

Supraspinatus

The supraspinatus may refer pain into the point of the shoulder and as far down the arm as the lateral epicondyle. TrPs may be found in the muscle bulk, which are usually very painful to palpation as the muscle is more superficial here (Fig. 12.35). As the muscle travels across the head of the humerus it is covered by the deltoid and so less painful to palpation, but at its insertion onto the superior aspect of the greater tuberosity again it may be tender. TrPs may be treated by ischaemic compression and

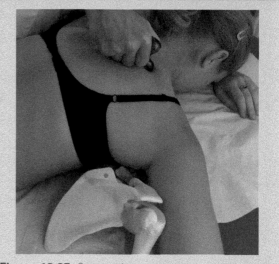

Figure 12.35 Supraspinatus.

Treatment note 12.4 *continued*

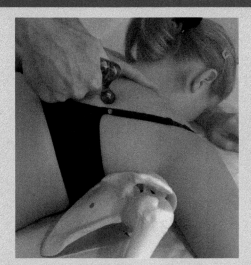

Figure 12.36 Infraspinatus.

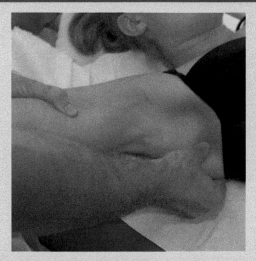

Figure 12.37 Subscapularis, anterior approach.

dry needling. When needling over the scapula, the possibility of incomplete ossification of the scapula surface must be considered and deep needling (greater than 1.0 cm) should be used with caution.

Infraspinatus

TrPs from the infraspinatus refer to the shoulder and arm in much the same way as the supraspinatus. Differentiation is through palpation and pain to abduction (supraspinatus). In addition, the larger origin of the infraspinatus can refer pain between the scapulae into the rhomboid region. TrPs may be in the belly of the muscle, normally located just below the medial third of the scapular spine, and occasionally right onto the medial border of the scapula (Fig. 12.36). To facilitate palpation, ask the patient to place the arm across the chest to grasp the opposite shoulder and place the muscle on slight stretch.

Teres minor

The teres minor has the same action as infraspinatus but a different innervation (teres minor the axillary nerve, infraspinatus the suprascapular nerve). TrPs are often secondary to those of infraspinatus and lie within the muscle belly. They are located at the lateral edge of the

scapula between the infraspinatus above and the teres major below.

Subscapularis

TrPs in this muscle have been described as 'the key to frozen shoulder' (Simons, Travell and Simons 1999) and this claim may coincide with pathological changes found within the rotator interval in frozen shoulder contraction syndrome (see Fig. 12.37). Referred pain is to the posterior aspect of the shoulder and can extend down the posterior aspect of the arm. TrPs are mostly beneath the scapula and only accessible by placing the patient supine with the arm abducted to 45 degrees. The therapist then places traction through the arm to draw the scapula laterally and locates the lateral edge of the scapula beneath the medial to the latissimus dorsi. A pincer grip is used between the thumb and forefinger.

East meets West

Many traditional acupuncture points correspond to TrPs. SI-12 (small intestine 12) lies directly within the belly of the supraspinatus, while SI-10 lies on the belly of infraspinatus, and SI-9 within teres minor. The small intestine acupuncture channel (meridian) is often used in cases of posterior shoulder pain (Fig. 12.38).

535

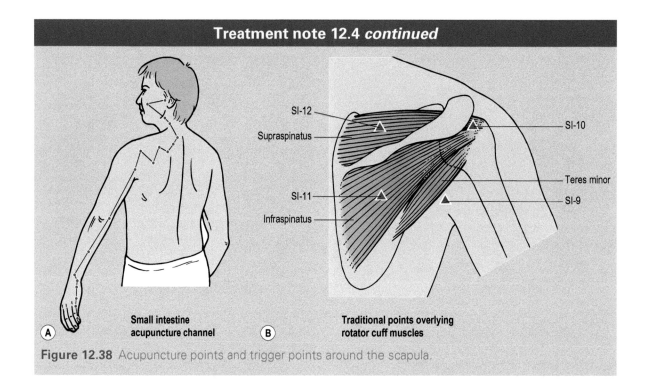

SI-12

Supraspinatus

SI-11

Infraspinatus

SI-10

Teres minor

SI-9

Small intestine acupuncture channel

(A)

(B)

Traditional points overlying rotator cuff muscles

Figure 12.38 Acupuncture points and trigger points around the scapula.

intertubercular sulcus. As the humerus moves, the tendon slides within its groove by as much as 3–4 cm. The tendon is held in the groove by the transverse ligament, which is a thickening of the capsule and bridges the gap between the greater and lesser tuberosities. The coracohumeral ligament travelling from the lateral edge of the coracoid to the lesser and greater tuberosities assists in retaining the long head. Anatomical dissection and MRI studies on this area have revealed that the transverse humeral ligament is not a true separate entity (Gleason et al. 2006) but rather a merger of fibres from the supraspinatus and subscapularis. These fibres fuse into a single unit, forming a tunnel over the long head of the biceps. In addition, the superior glenohumeral ligament folds into a U-shaped sling supporting the long head, and fibres of the supraspinatus tendon join the posterosuperior portion of this sling (Werner et al. 2000). The combination of several structures within this region allows load to be shared between the structural group rather than being taken in isolation by individual units.

Key point

In the region of the intertubercular sulcus, the long head of biceps has structural associations with the supraspinatus and subscapularis tendons, and with the superior glenohumeral ligament. These associations allow load sharing between the structures.

Cadaveric studies have shown that the biceps tendon will not displace when the transverse ligament is cut, if the coracohumeral ligament remains intact (Slatis and Alato 1979). The tendency for subluxation or dislocation of the tendon from the bicipital groove is dependent on a number of factors, including the depth of the groove, the angle of the medial wall of the groove, and the presence of a supratubercular ridge. Normally, the medial wall of the bicipital groove forms an angle of 60–70 degrees, and angles of less than 30 degrees, when combined with a shallow groove, have been shown to be associated

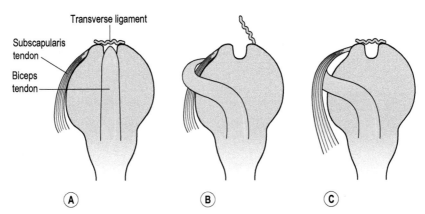

Figure 12.39 Biceps tendon subluxation. (A) Normal alignment. (B) Transverse ligament tears, biceps tendon rides over subscapularis. (C) Transverse ligament intact, biceps tendon slides beneath subscapularis. After Reid (1992), with permission.

with tendon subluxation (O'Donoghue 1973). A supratubercular ridge is present in 55 per cent of the population, and well developed in 18 per cent (Reid 1992). It is a proximal extension of the medial wall of the bicipital groove, and may force the biceps tendon against the transverse ligament, thus increasing tension. When the tendon subluxes, it does so in one of two ways, both normally associated with trauma to the humerus or rotator cuff. The tendon usually moves medially and will lie superficial to the subscapularis if the transverse ligament ruptures. If the subscapularis remains attached to the transverse ligament, the biceps tendon may end up deep to the subscapularis tendon itself (Fig. 12.39).

Biceps tendon dislocation typically occurs after a violent overhead action, with the subject feeling pain on the anterior aspect of the shoulder. The shoulder will feel weak or 'dead' and often the subject describes feeling 'something going out' or 'snapping'. On examination there is tenderness to palpation over the tendon, and medial and lateral rotation may elicit a palpable click. This may be further investigated using Yergason's sign or Speed's test. Yergason's sign may also be used to detect a labral tear.

▶ *Yergason's sign* – the patient attempts to supinate the flexed elbow while externally rotating the shoulder.

▶ *Speed's test* – shoulder flexion from a position of extension with the forearm supinated.

Management of biceps tendon dislocation is usually surgical followed by intensive rehabilitation to restore correct scapulothoracic and glenohumeral function.

> **Key point**
>
> Both Yergason's sign and Speed's test attempt to reproduce biceps tendon dislocation using resisted shoulder and elbow movements.

Tendinopathy of the long head of biceps presents as pain to resisted shoulder and elbow flexion and resisted forearm supination. Yergason's sign and Speed's test may again be used. The teno-osseous junction of the muscle at the supraglenoid tubercle and adjacent glenoid labrum is difficult to palpate directly, but the tendon itself within the intertubercular sulcus is easier. A painful arc is only present with these conditions if the inflamed area of tendon is within a pinchable position in mid-range abduction, in which case impingement tests will be positive.

Overuse is the predominant causal factor, with alteration in the biomechanics of overhead actions often being present. The synovial sheath of the

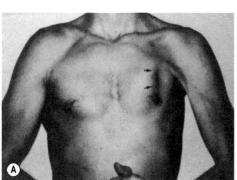
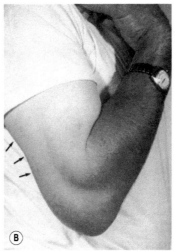
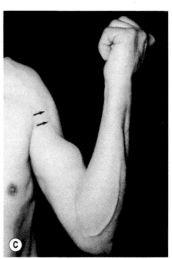

Figure 12.40 Ruptures to muscles in the shoulder region. (A) Pectoralis major. (B) Triceps. (C) Biceps. After Reid (1992), with permission.

tendon may become swollen and inflamed, with thickening and haemorrhaging frequently seen. Adhesions may be present. If the locking position and quadrant test reproduce pain, posteroanterior (PA) gliding should be assessed. If limited, PA pressures against the humeral head (see below) should be used.

Rupture of the biceps brachii occurs more commonly at the insertion of the long head into the supraglenoid tubercle, but tears to the short head, distal attachment or belly may occur (Fig. 12.40). The rupture more frequently follows SAIS and tendon degeneration. The mechanism of injury for proximal tendon injuries is normally a forced extension while the muscle is contracting. This can result from an arm tackle or block, where the arm is held abducted and then pushed back behind trunk level. Distal tendon injuries may occur as a result of heavy lifting with the elbow flexed to 90 degrees.

Key point

The bicep ruptures more commonly at its long head, attaching into the supraglenoid tubercle. The injury normally occurs with forced arm extension as the muscle is contracting.

On examination, pain is elicited to resisted elbow flexion and supination (which may be combined with shoulder flexion), and passive end-range extension. A visible defect may be noted in the muscle, with retraction of the tendon. In the case of the long head, the tendon may no longer be palpable in the intertubercular sulcus, and as the muscle is contracted the belly of the long head is seen to bunch up into a ball-shaped mass. Local swelling and bruising are noted, and lead to an increased arm girth measurement.

Both surgical and conservative management have been recommended, with surgical management normally favoured (in the young especially) because conservative treatment is often said to give a loss of supination power. However, the reason for this deficit may be the lack of adequate rehabilitation following conservative management (Bandy, Lovelace-Chandler and Holt 1991).

Conservative management consists of the POLICE protocol to minimize inflammation, with gentle mobility exercises to the elbow within the pain-free range. Exercise therapy is used to maintain shoulder function. Multi-angle isometric training begins as soon as possible to reduce muscle atrophy, the deciding factor for starting this being pain. As pain to resisted movement reduces, dynamic exercise is begun against manual, and later isokinetic, resistance. PNF techniques combining shoulder flexion/adduction/medial rotation with elbow flexion/supination are used, as well as static stretching to elbow and shoulder extension. The resistance-training programme is progressed with power actions, and functional sporting activities are introduced. The long-term prognosis is good in terms of restoration of function, but a palpable defect will usually remain in the muscle.

Surgery for distal tendon injuries includes re-inserting the tendon into the radial tuberosity, or the use of a fascia lata graft, where surgery has been delayed and the tendon has retracted. The long head may be re-inserted into the supraglenoid tubercle in the case of an avulsion or, in some instances, to the wall of the bicipital groove.

Pectoralis major

Rupture of the pectoralis major is unusual, but when it does occur, the muscle is usually already under tension when further force is imposed on it (Fig. 12.40A). The most common example of this scenario is the bench-press exercise in weight training. The injury normally occurs during the eccentric phase of the exercise as the bar is being lowered. During the last 30 degrees of humeral extension of this action, the inferior fibres of the muscle have been shown to lengthen disproportionately (Wolfe, Wickiewicz and Cavanaugh 1992). In addition, with fatigue, the athlete may move the whole body in an attempt to lift the weight, and so bring accessory muscle groups into action, enabling the athlete to exceed his or her safe limit. When lowering this excessive weight, the athlete loses control and the injury occurs.

Key point

The pectoralis major is most commonly ruptured while performing a bench-press action in weight training. The injury normally occurs during the last 30 degrees of the eccentric (lowering) phase of the movement.

A tearing sensation is felt, and a large haematoma is apparent over the anterior axilla. Weakness and pain to resisted adduction and medial rotation is noted to manual muscle testing. No defect may be seen at rest, but if the muscle is contracted isometrically by asking the athlete to press the hands together as if clapping, a defect may be apparent. Following injury, the muscle does not retract very far, perhaps due to its varied fibre direction and wide origin. The insertion into the humerus (just lateral to the intertubercular sulcus) of the non-dominant arm is more normally affected (Kretzler and Richardson 1989).

Non-surgical treatment can be successful for partial tears, and in the non-athletic individual. However, surgical management is more generally recommended (Reut, Bach and Johnson 1991). At operation, the deltoid is retracted and the tendon is reattached either via drill holes in the humerus or by suturing the tendon to the remnant of tissue insertion.

The arm is immobilized in a sling, and isometric contractions started as soon as the pain stabilizes. Assisted movements are begun one week after surgery, and thereafter the rehabilitation programme aims to restore strength, mobility and function. As strength training progresses, eccentric movements must be used to prepare the muscle for its action of decelerating the bar in the bench-press exercise. In addition, pectoral muscle stretches and retraction work must be used to avoid a protracted shoulder posture.

Triceps

In addition to the more common elbow site for triceps injury, occasionally the muscle may avulse from its glenoid attachment, especially in throwing athletes (Fig. 12.40B). Pain occurs to triceps stretching, often palpable at the inferior rim of the glenoid. With rest, a fibrous union will normally fix the fragment back in place, but surgery to remove the avulsed fragment and re-suture the tendon may be required where the injury recurs. When the muscle belly itself is injured, it is usually the medial head which is involved, and the treatment of choice is conservative (Kunichi and Torisu 1984).

It is important to note that the normal tendon is capable of sustaining considerable force before it will rupture, making avulsion fracture the more usual injury. Where tendon rupture occurs, an underlying pathology may be present. High-dosage oral steroids may weaken the tendons (Hunter, Shybut and Nuber 1986), a situation especially important with athletes using heavy-resistance exercise or power movements. Conditions such as rheumatoid arthritis, systemic lupus erythematosus and hormone disorders may also predispose to tendon rupture (Reid and Kushner 1989).

Shoulder instability

Classification

The stability of the glenohumeral joint lies very much on a continuum. At one end there is the stable, fully functional joint, and at the other the dislocated joint requiring surgery. In many cases, there is a progression which begins with a reduction of stability through alteration in static, dynamic or proprioceptive factors. Individual differences in bony or soft-tissue configuration can give some subjects a greater risk of instability, and training activities can alter the subtle muscle balance that exists around the joint. Trauma will cause both mechanical changes to stabilizing structures and alteration in proprioception and movement control. Any or all of these factors may coexist to push the subject from a position of stability to one of instability of some degree. The progression from minor instability to major instability may then occur with time, unless there is treatment intervention of some type.

Instability may be classified using the TUBS/AMBRI acronyms (Matsen, Harryman and Sidles, 1991). These acronyms represent two ends of the spectrum (Table 12.7), from instability through trauma to instability through congenital factors. The patient with a TUBS lesion will have suffered traumatic instability in one direction only (unidirectional). The glenoid labrum will have been detached from the anterior rim of the glenoid

Table 12.7 Classification of shoulder instability

TUBS	AMBRI
Born loose	Torn loose
T — Traumatic aetiology	A — Atraumatic aetiology
U — Unidirectional instability	M — Multidirectional instability
B — Bankart lesion	B — Bilateral condition
S — Surgical repair	R — Rehabilitation normally successful
	I — Inferior capsular shift if rehabilitation fails

(Bankart lesion) and surgery will probably be required, although rehabilitation should be tried first, as this can be successful with minor degrees of injury. The AMBRI patient has an atraumatic aetiology causing multidirectional instability in both shoulders (bilateral). Usually this patient responds well to intensive rehabilitation, but if surgery is required, an inferior capsular shift is normally the treatment of choice.

The TUBS/AMBRI classification does not take into account those patients who present with instability due to altered muscle balance or 'muscle patterning', so-called functional instability. An alternative classification is the Stanmore triangle (Lewis, Kitamura and Bayley 2004). Here, instability is classified as three polar types (Fig. 12.41). Polar type I covers the traditional TUBS lesion, where structural change has been induced through trauma. Polar type II is an instability through

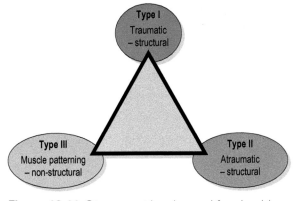

Figure 12.41 Stanmore triangle used for shoulder instability classification.

Table 12.8 Typical clinical finding of polar instability types

Polar I (Traumatic structural)	Polar II (Atraumatic structural)	Polar III (Muscle patterning)
▶ Positive apprehension (anterior) ▶ Rotator cuff weak especially subscapularis (belly press) ▶ Global posture & scapular alignment generally unchanged ▶ MRA may also show capsular detachment	▶ Positive apprehension (anterior) ▶ Capsular laxity – positive sulcus sign, excessive external rotation ▶ Test IR in 90° abduction (scarecrow position) and use DRST ▶ GIRD sometimes present – relevant if difference between sides > 25° (sleeper stretch) ▶ Anterior translation & posterior capsule tightness (obligate translation) ▶ Single-leg balance/squat (corkscrew test)	▶ Increase superficial (large) muscle activity and reduced deep (small) muscle activity ▶ Infraspinatus most often reduced, pec major/anterior deltoid/lat dorsi increased ▶ Often associated with swayback posture/increased thoracic kyphosis/scapular tipping ▶ Especially important for success of surgical repair ▶ Global posture work may help to initiate better shoulder patterning

(Data from Jaggi and Lambert 2010)
MRA – magnetic resonance arthrography, GIRD – glenohumeral internal rotation deficit,
DRST – dynamic rotatory stability test

atraumatic change which is still structural and equates to the AMBRI lesion mostly. Polar type III represents instability through alteration of muscle patterning. The sides of the triangle represent both rehabilitation and surgery, and the essential feature of this classification is that patients can change their position through degeneration or disuse on the one hand and rehabilitation on the other. This classification enables us to predict more accurately those who are likely to respond favourably to rehabilitation. This is important because on the one hand altered muscle patterning has been cited as an important factor in the failure of stabilization surgery (McAuliffe et al. 1988), while on the other hand inappropriate surgical stabilization has been associated with an increased incidence of glenohumeral degeneration (Malone 2004). Typical clinical findings for the three polar types are shown in Table 12.8.

Stability mechanisms

Shoulder stability is supplied by both static and dynamic factors. Static stability is provided by the glenoid labrum, joint capsule and ligaments, while dynamic stability comes from muscle action (Table 12.9). As the arm hangs by the side of the

Table 12.9 Stability of the glenohumeral joint

Dependent position	Coracohumeral ligament Superior glenohumeral ligament Supraspinatus muscle
Elevation	
Lower range (0–45°)	Anterior capsule Superior glenohumeral ligament Coracohumeral ligament Middle glenohumeral ligament Subscapularis, infraspinatus and teres minor muscles
Middle range (45–75°)	Middle glenohumeral ligament Subscapularis muscle (decreasing importance) Infraspinatus and teres minor muscles Inferior glenohumeral ligament (superior band)
Upper range (>75°)	Inferior glenohumeral ligament (axillary pouch)
Throughout elevation	Dynamic activity of rotator cuff

From Peat and Culham (1994), with permission.

body, the pull of gravity is resisted by the superior capsule and the coracohumeral ligament. If the arm is loaded – when carrying a bag, for example – the greater force is resisted by the supraspinatus which

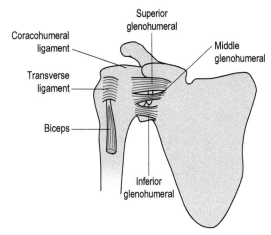

Figure 12.42 Anterior ligaments of the glenohumeral joint.

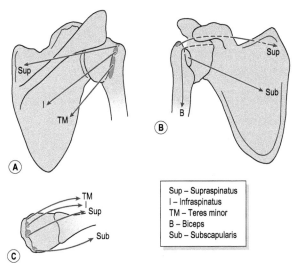

Figure 12.43 Active stabilizers of the glenohumeral joint. (A) Posterior. (B) Anterior. (C) Superior.

shares a common distal attachment with the two previous structures and has a line of action that is virtually identical to them.

The middle glenohumeral ligament lies directly under the tendon of subscapularis and is attached to it (Fig. 12.42). The ligament varies tremendously between subjects. In some it may be 2 cm wide, while in others it may be completely absent (Peat and Culham 1994). Both the subscapularis and middle glenohumeral ligament limit external rotation and are important anterior stabilizers in the lower and middle ranges of abduction.

The inferior glenohumeral ligament (the thickest position of the glenohumeral ligament in total) is the most important passive stabilizing structure in overhead actions. The ligament is divided into three bands, with the inferior portion forming the axillary pouch. The anterior band wraps around the humeral head at 90 degrees abduction with external rotation, and prevents anterior head migration (O'Brian et al. 1990). It is therefore the anterior band of the inferior glenohumeral ligament that is most significant in stabilizing the arm in overhead-throwing sports. As this ligament tightens, abduction is limited and the humerus must laterally rotate and move towards the scapular plane.

The glenohumeral and coracohumeral ligaments form a 'Z' shape on the anterior aspect of the

shoulder, with the middle glenohumeral ligament providing the crossbar of the Z. Above and below the crossbar are spaces that create areas of potential weakness. Superiorly (foramen of Weitbrecht) the opening allows the subscapularis bursa to communicate with the joint cavity. Inferiorly, a smaller bursa is sometimes present. In some subjects, if the Z crossbar (middle glenohumeral ligament) is missing, the anterior defect formed may contribute to anterior instability.

Active stability is provided by the rotator-cuff muscles (Fig. 12.43). As previously stated, the pull of the deltoid is almost vertical and it tends to cause upward translation of the humeral head. This is counteracted by the rotator-cuff muscles, which tend to downwardly translate the head. The combination of the two sets of muscle translation forces stabilizes the head of the humerus in the glenoid. These compressor forces are at their maximum between 60 and 80 degrees, and are minimal after 120 degrees (Comtet, Herberg and Naasan 1989). Where a massive tear of the rotator-cuff muscles occurs, stability of the joint can still be maintained by the middle deltoid alone compressing the humeral head into the glenoid (Gagey and Hue 2000).

Where instability exists through altered rotator-cuff or serratus anterior dysfunction, it is likely that compensatory muscle action will be seen. Anterior instability has been associated with change in pectoralis major activity and posterior instability with altered latissimus dorsi and anterior deltoid activity (Malone 2004). In addition, those with atraumatic instability show reduced proprioceptive ability of the upper limb (Barden et al. 2004).

Assessing instability of the shoulder

Passive stability

Passive (static) instability of the glenohumeral joint is traditionally assessed clinically by a number of drawer and apprehension tests. Anterior and posterior instability is initially tested with the subject in a sitting position. The therapist grasps the subject's upper arm over the humeral head, and applies forward and backward pressure while stabilizing the scapula (Fig. 12.44). The injured and uninjured sides are compared for range and end-feel. Excessive anterior glide leaves a posterior hollow, and the movement can be graded as mild (less than a third of the head coming off the

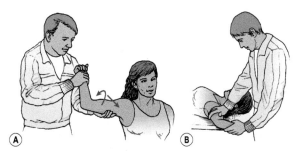

Figure 12.45 (A) Apprehension test – pain/apprehension increases as an anteriorly directed force is applied. (B) Modified apprehension test – pain reduces with posterior pressure.

glenoid), moderate (head riding on the edge of the glenoid, but spontaneously reduces when released), or severe (complete dislocation of the head). Posterior subluxation is considered abnormal when more than 50 per cent of the humeral head comes off the glenoid.

The apprehension test is again performed in a sitting position. The subject's arm is taken into 90 degrees abduction and externally rotated. At the same time, an anterior pressure is exerted on the proximal humerus (Fig. 12.45A). The test is positive in the presence of spasm or a feeling of impending (or actual) subluxation. A more rigorous procedure is to position the athlete in a supine-lying position, with the injured shoulder over the table edge. The arm is abducted to 90 degrees and externally rotated. From this position, the examiner applies an anteriorly directed pressure to increase pain and a posteriorly directed pressure to reduce pain (Fig. 12.45B).

Active stability

Muscle control of the glenohumeral joint may be assessed using the dynamic rotary stability test (DRST) described by Margarey and Jones (2003). The DRST assesses the ability of the rotator cuff to keep the humeral head centred in the glenoid. The subject sits on a couch (Fig. 12.46) with the therapist standing behind. The subject's arm is held in a scaption (flexion–abduction) position, with the elbow flexed to 90 degrees. The therapist monitors the position of the subject's humeral head whilst

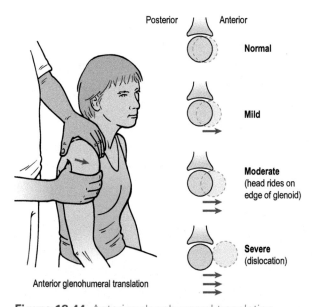

Posterior   Anterior

Normal

Mild

Moderate
(head rides on edge of glenoid)

Severe
(dislocation)

Anterior glenohumeral translation

Figure 12.44 Anterior glenohumeral translation.

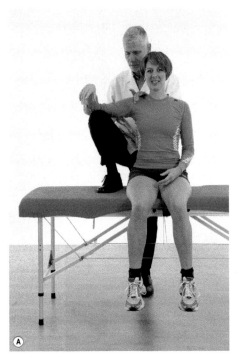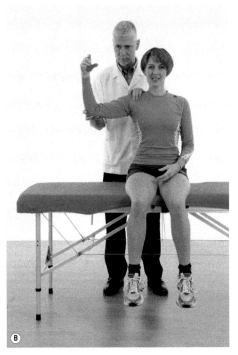

Figure 12.46 Assessing muscle control of the glenohumeral joint.

applying firstly resisted lateral rotation (subject twisting arm backwards) and then medial rotation (subject twisting arm forwards). The test is positive where anterior or posterior translation of the humeral head is detected and symptoms are provoked.

The DRST test may be extended to monitor which muscles are stabilizing the joint to differentiate between the local stabilizers (rotator cuff) and the global stabilizers (especially pectoralis major and latissimus dorsi). The subject and therapist take up the same starting position, but this time the subject's forearm is placed on a supporting surface. A small stool may be used, or the therapist's knee. Gentle longitudinal resistance is given to the subject's humerus (traction), with the instruction to 'stop me making your arm longer' or to 'suck your arm back into its socket'. The pectoralis and latissimus muscles are monitors for overactivity. The subject is then encouraged to 'suck the arm back into the socket' with minimal superficial muscle work, as part of a training programme to re-educate the local stabilizer muscles.

Scapular control

Assessment of the subject's ability to control the scapula throughout the three stages of abduction (scapular dyskinesis, above) can be important. Both static and dynamic scapular assessment can provide information which may be relevant to symptoms and/or rehabilitation planning. The abduction cycle (see Table 12.1) forms the baseline for comparison during movement. As the arm is abducted, the subject's posture is noted. Typically, instability at the shoulder will be compensated by postural change, with the subject weightbearing *away* from the painful side and shortening the trunk, indicating that the latissimus dorsi is overactive. Pectoralis major dominance often presents as a protracted and medially rotated shoulder position at rest.

The scapula should remain fixed to the ribcage through serratus anterior action. Where this muscle is underactive the scapula may appear to wing, and when the arm is placed under load

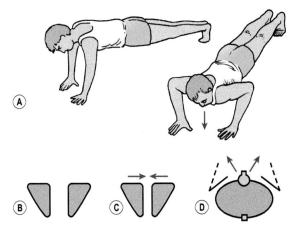

Figure 12.47 Eccentric push-up as a global assessment of scapulothoracic stability. (A) Athlete slowly lowers from a push-up position – note position of scapula. (B) Scapulae should remain apart and fixed to the ribcage as the body is lowered. (C) Scapulae fall together if rhomboids and levator scapulae are dominant. (D) True winging. The medial edges of the scapulae lift.

in a closed-chain position the rhomboid muscles may compensate by pulling the medial edges of the scapulae together (see eccentric push-up in Fig. 12.47). During open-chain actions the scapular position should be monitored as the glenohumeral joint is rotated. Where the latissimus is dominant, the subject will often fix the scapular by adducting the arm (elbow tight into side of the body). Where the pectoral muscle dominates, protraction and medial rotation often occurs, rounding the shoulder into a 'guarding' position. The ability to differentiate glenohumeral movement from scapulothoracic movement (segmental control) should be assessed in a number of functional positions such as sitting, standing and reaching. Importantly, changes to static position and dynamic control should be compared between the symptomatic and non-symptomatic sides. Alteration of alignment or movement may be either a cause or consequence of instability, or clinically irrelevant if symptoms are not affected. Restoration of scapular stability and control is shown in Treatment Note 12.1.

Enhancing glenohumeral stability

Initial management of glenohumeral (GH) instability addresses the reactive phase of injury and aims to protect soft tissues and facilitate healing. Traumatic injury (polar I) will usually require a greater focus on this component than non-traumatic (polar II and III) conditions where pain has progressed slowly. Active rest and restriction of exacerbating postures must protect the irritable joint, but at the same time avoid maladaptive behaviours and stiffness. Acute type I injury may require immobilization, while types II and III generally manage with protection in the form of taping or simply advice concerning activity modification. We have seen that the rotator-cuff muscles have lines of pull that tend to approximate the head of the humeral into the glenoid cavity to encourage joint stability (concavity compression), and work to adjust the head position to centre it. Working these muscles is therefore our starting point for rehabilitation.

> **Definition**
> Concavity compression is the process of centring and stabilizing the humeral head into the glenoid to resist the upward pull of the deltoid and downward pull of gravity.

Isometric actions may be used against passive resistance initially. The therapist grasps the subject's upper arm and applies a longitudinal force. The subject is encouraged to resist the force with imagery such as 'sucking the ball back into the socket', or 'don't let me lengthen your arm'. In addition, downward gliding forces may be encouraged by having the subject resist upward glide applied by the therapist, applying a force to draw the partially abducted arm outwards. The subject is encouraged to keep the pectoralis major and latissimus dorsi relaxed (Fig. 12.48A).

The belly-press action (resisted medial rotation) is useful to activate the subscapularis to provide anterior GH stability (Werner et al. 2007), but the therapist should monitor the anterior chest wall to ensure the pectoralis does not compensate. The

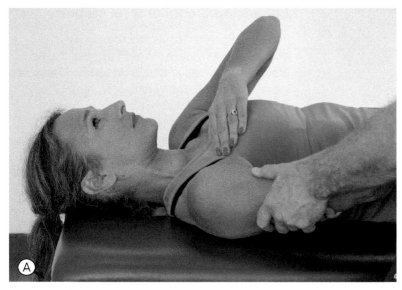
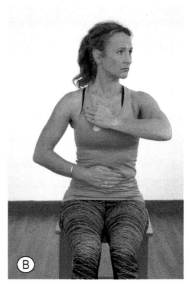

Figure 12.48 Resisted isometric exercise for glenohumeral stability. (A) Resistance against therapist longitudinal gliding force. (B) Belly press (subscapularis activation) self-monitoring pectoralis major.

subject is taught to self-monitor (Fig. 12.48B). This action uses a closed-chain format, which favours stability (see Chapter 2), and the holding time of the isometric action is progressed (5–10 seconds to 30–40 seconds) rather than the contraction force.

Although this action aims to recruit the local stabilizing muscles (see Chapter 2) such as subscapularis rather than the global muscles such as pectoralis or latissimus, polar III subjects often find this difficult. Activating postural tone using whole-body stability can be a useful technique in these cases (Jaggi and Lambert 2010). Practising rotator-cuff actions standing or sitting on an unstable surface (balance cushion, gym ball) or simply standing on one leg can help to de-activate the overactive global muscles. Where this fails, surface EMG biofeedback can be useful to discourage activity of the global muscles and/ or encourage activity of the local stabilizers. In addition, taping used for tactile feedback off scapular alignment (retraction and depression) may be used to optimize general shoulder alignment and discourage dyskinesia.

As we have seen above, stretching and manual therapy may be used to target GIRD to move the joint towards a more optimally aligned position and reduce symptoms. This approach also has its use where pain limits the progression of GH stability.

Progression is now towards GH stability through range, and the dynamic rotatory stability test described above can be used as a starting point for through-range motion. The scarecrow test position (above) may be used in lying with a small dumb-bell for through-range lateral rotation, monitoring the head of the humerus. In addition, this position may also be used for self-monitored MWM.

Bodyweight and partial bodyweight closed-chain actions can progress to Swiss-ball wall rolls (Fig. 12.49A) and kneeling hand walks (Fig. 12.49B). This begins the focus on more functional training, and progresses rehab towards early throwing actions, where rehabilitation is similar to that described for SAIS.

Proprioceptive training of the unstable shoulder

The principles behind proprioceptive training of the shoulder are similar to those described in Chapter 8 for the lumbar spine. The aim is to

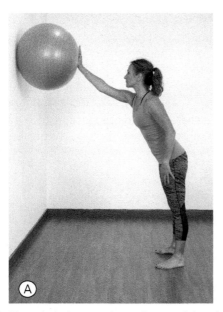 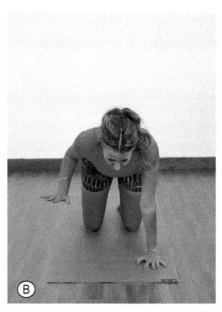

Figure 12.49 Closed chain exercise using partial and full bodyweight. (A) Swiss ball wall roll. (B) Kneeling hand walk.

re-educate local and global stabilizers of both the glenohumeral and scapulothoracic joints using multisensory cues. Proprioceptive training of the shoulder can involve four elements (Lephart and Henry 2000), shown in Table 12.10, which aim to re-educate neuromuscular control by stimulating actions at the level of spinal reflexes, brainstem and higher centres (see Chapter 2). Dynamic stabilization addresses both the glenohumeral and scapulothoracic joints. As we have seen above, co-activation of the local stabilizing muscles of the glenohumeral joint may be performed using pushing and pulling forces along the length of the humerus (long-axis resistance) encouraging the subject to 'suck the ball back into the socket'. Scapulothoracic stability is begun by maintaining the position of the scapula as the practitioner places it flat onto the thoracic wall in its optimally aligned position. Joint repositioning may be passive (therapist moves the limb) or active (subject moves the limb), beginning with the DRST test positions. Performing actions using a dynamometer for visual feedback, or a hand-held laser pointer, can also be helpful. Initially exercises are performed with the eyes open, and then closed. Reactive neuromuscular control

Table 12.10 Proprioceptive training of the shoulder

Element of retraining	Importance	Exercise type
Dynamic stabilization	Co-activation of muscle forces to (i) centre humeral head on glenoid and (ii) fix scapula to thoracic wall (local stabilizers)	Joint approximation, building isometric endurance
Joint position sensibility	Precision of hand placement	Reproduction of active and passive joint position
Reactive neuromuscular control	Maintenance of stability against external loading (global stabilizers)	Unstable base
Functional motor patterns	Specific to athlete's sport	Complex tasks

From Lephart and Henry (2000) and Gibson and Elphinston (2005).

is performed using unstable surfaces such as a Swiss ball or balance ball. Finally, functional motor patterns are used that may be open or closed-chain, involve resistance bands or pulleys in tri-plane motions, or complex whole-body actions.

Closed kinetic-chain activities

Essentially, closed kinetic-chain activity involves movement of the proximal body segment on a fixed distal segment (Chapter 2). This is common in the lower limb, during the stance phase of gait, for example. In the upper limb, the majority of daily actions occur in open-chain format, with the distal segment (arm) moving on a fixed proximal base (thorax). However, the upper limb must be able to work in a closed kinetic-chain pattern for 'fall' and 'push' actions. In many sports, for example, the subject is likely to fall onto the hand or elbow, and in some sports, such as gymnastics, complex closed kinetic-chain actions are involved (handstand/vault). During a closed-chain action, such as falling onto the outstretched arm, gravity assists in closing the chain of movement, approximating the joint surfaces. Following shoulder injury, subjects often have kinesiophobia (fear of movement) with respect to falling onto the hand, especially if this action caused the injury initially. As a consequence, they are often hypervigilant when walking over uneven surfaces or when in crowded areas. Targeting this fear can lead to a reduction in frailty.

> **Key point**
>
> Subjects with shoulder injuries often fear falling onto the outstretched arm. Targeting this fear in rehabilitation can reduce overall frailty.

The muscle action is primarily eccentric to control the deceleration of movement and provide a protective role. As concentric action begins to accelerate the body segment, the joint surfaces are still approximated (push-up), whereas during open-chain actions the joint surfaces are under traction (throwing).

Traditional closed-chain exercises include bodyweight (push-ups, dips) resistance and weights (bench and shoulder presses). Additional movements include the push-up with a press, and the sitting push-up. Hand-walking activities are useful and may be performed on a wall, floor, treadmill, stepper, static cycle or steps, either from a kneeling or prone falling position. Use of a rocker board for double-handed activities and a balance board for single-handed activities is also useful for closed kinetic-chain rehabilitation and is challenging to proprioception. The same would apply to activities on the Swiss ball and slide trainer (Fig. 12.50).

> **Key point**
>
> In closed kinetic-chain exercises the muscle action is mainly eccentric to control excessive movement and protect the joint.

Resistance training

A variety of weight-training exercises may be performed to re-strengthen the shoulder musculature. Fig. 12.51 illustrates four movements that work both the glenohumeral and scapulothoracic muscles in both open and closed chain. The movements minimize the risk of impingement by combining lateral rotation movements with abduction in the scapular plane.

In overhead motions, the cocking phase provides an eccentric pre-stretch to the muscles (adductors and internal rotators), closely followed by an explosive acceleration phase. Concentric–eccentric coupling of this type requires plyometric rehabilitation. As we have seen in Chapter 2, plyometrics involve a pre-stretch (eccentric) and short amortization phase where the movement direction is reversed, and finally a rapid facilitated concentric action. Activities include overhead soccer throws, basketball chest passes, single-arm tennis-ball throws, use of exercise tubing in PNF patterns and use of small medicine balls (Wilk and Arrigo 1993).

Use of surface EMG in throwing actions

In an overhead motion the arm externally rotates, causing the humeral head to move superiorly. In this position, the subscapularis is not able to control

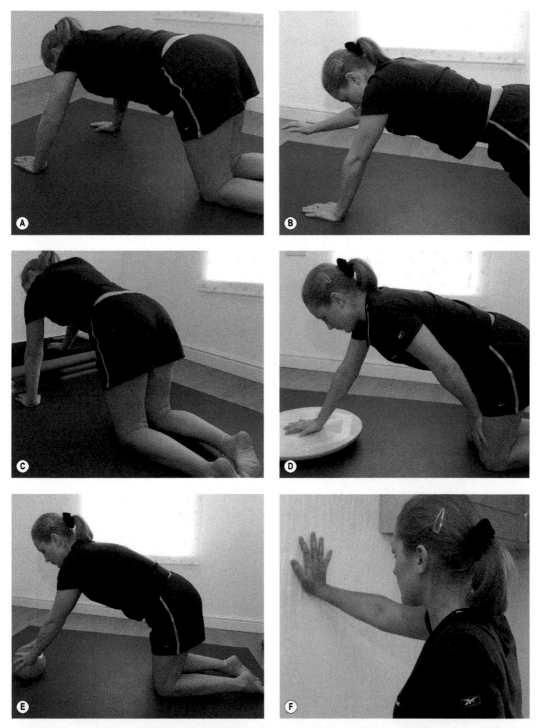

Figure 12.50 Closed-chain shoulder rehabilitation. (A) Knee push-up. (B) Hand walking flat. (C) Stool. (D) Wobble board. (E) Gym ball. (F) Single-arm wall lean. (G) Throw and catch on trampette. (H) Hand work on static cycle.

549

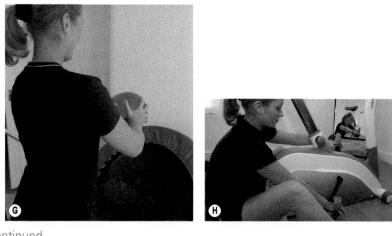

Figure 12.50 Continued.

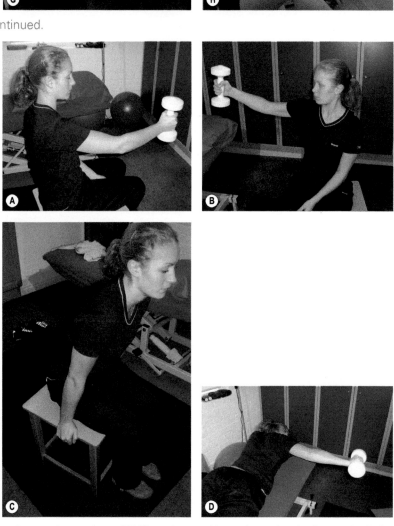

Figure 12.51 Glenohumeral exercises. (A) Elevation and lateral rotation in the sagittal plane. (B) Elevation and lateral rotation in the scapular plane. (C) Sitting press-up. (D) Horizontal abduction in lateral rotation.

the humeral head any longer and the tendency to anterior translation is therefore increased. The joint must depend on the inferior glenohumeral ligament for passive stability, the only effective active control coming from the infraspinatus. If the ligamentous control is failing, enhancement of infraspinatus action can effectively control the humeral head (Reid 1992).

> **Key point**
>
> When the arm is overhead and ligamentous stability of the humeral head is inadequate, the infraspinatus muscle can provide active stability.

The sEMG electrode is placed over the bulk of the infraspinatus below the scapular spine avoiding the posterior deltoid. The shoulder is flexed to activate the sEMG signal and the athlete is instructed to maintain the audible or visual signal from the machine by tightening the rotator-cuff muscles. Isometric rotator-cuff tightening is performed for multiple repetitions (10 sets of 10 repetitions), and then holding time is built (up to a 10-second hold) before active glenohumeral movements are commenced. Short-lever shoulder flexion (in neutral rotation) is performed between 70 and 90 degrees, as the subject tries to push the sEMG signal up as high as possible. If pain or apprehension occur, the exercise is regressed to isometric holding alone. As sEMG signals can be maintained with active shoulder flexion, further exercises are added in a progression (Table 12.11). When painless and confident full-range motion has been obtained, general shoulder rehabilitation is begun.

Taping and mobilization with movement

In shoulder conditions where the head of the humeral is pulled forwards (anterior) relative to the glenoid, (often with impingement or instability symptoms), mobilization with movement and taping may be of help. As we have seen (Chapter 1), mobilization with movement (MWM)

Table 12.11 Use of surface EMG in rehabilitation of anterior instability of the shoulder

1 Forward flexion with a straight elbow
2 Forward flexion with increasing external rotation
3 Abduction with flexion, progressing to elbow extension
4 Abduction with elbow extension with increasing external rotation
5 Abduction from flexion
6 Abduction from flexion with increasing external rotation
7 Reaching for objects behind the back or overhead

From Reid (1992), with permission.

is a technique where a sustained mobilization is applied to a joint, normally at 90 degrees to the plane of movement.

MWM was described above in the management of SAIS. Following therapist-applied MWM, both self-monitored MWM and taping can usefully maintain the tactile feedback provided. The taping consists of the strips of 5 cm zinc oxide taping placed over adhesive net tape (Fig. 12.52). The first strip passes from the anterior aspect of the shoulder

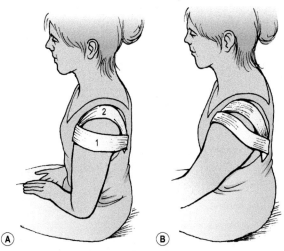

Figure 12.52 Proprioceptive taping of the shoulder. (A) Strip 1 passes from the anterior shoulder to the inferior angle of the scapula. Strip 2 passes over the middle trapezius. (B) Gap between the two strips corresponds to the humeral sulcus at 90-degree abduction.

around the lateral aspect of the joint and down to the inferior angle of the scapula. The second strip passes from the anterior aspect of the shoulder, over the middle fibres of trapezius and again down to the inferior angle of the scapula. The adhesive net tape is placed on the shoulder in a relaxed state, but the zinc oxide tape pulls the skin to give the subject the sensation of posterior gliding (strip one) and scapula depression (strip two). The gap between the two pieces of tape should correspond to the sulcus, which appears at the tip of the acromion at 90 degrees abduction. As with the MWM, the taping should modify symptoms to re-test.

Labral tears

The glenoid labrum (Fig. 12.53) is a 4 mm ring consisting of fibrocartilage which fastens to the rim of the glenoid fossa, and fibrous tissue which attaches to the joint capsule. The inner labral surface is lined with synovium, and the outer surface attaches to the joint capsule and merges with the periosteum of the humerus. The long head of biceps attaches to the supraglenoid tubercle and strengthens the labrum superiorly. This superior aspect of the labrum may not be attached to bone at all on its inner edge but can project into the joint forming a meniscus (Palastanga, Field and Soames 2006).

Tears of the labrum may be divided into Bankart tears affecting the anterior inferior portion of

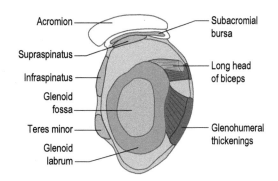

Figure 12.53 The glenoid labrum. From Palastanga, Field and Soames (2006).

the labrum and SLAP lesions affecting the superior portion, the pneumonic SLAP standing for Superior Labral tear travelling Anterior to Posterior. Bankart tears are usually associated with anterior shoulder dislocation, and a SLAP lesion with traction of the tendon of the long head of biceps.

SLAP lesions have been classified into several types (Table 12.12). The essential mechanism of injury involves force placed through the long head of biceps, either through trauma or repetitive loading, and the lesion extended from in front (anterior) of the biceps insertion to behind it (posterior). High eccentric loading occurs during overhead activities involving a combination of abduction and external rotation (cocking phase of throwing). This in combination with shoulder instability has been suggested as the most likely causal factor (Dodson and Altchek 2009).

Several tests exist to identify SLAP lesions clinically, with O'Brian's active compression test perhaps being the most common (O'Brian et al. 1990). Here, the shoulder is placed in 90 degrees forward elevation and 20 degrees horizontal abduction. The therapist places a downward force onto the subject's forearm with the arm firstly pronated (stretching biceps) and then supinated (relaxing biceps). The test is positive where pain is produced with the forearm in the pronated (biceps on stretch) position. This arm action is also a close-pack position for the acromioclavicular joint, so the AC joint must be discounted first. Research on the ability of clinical tests to evaluate the presence of a SLAP lesion suggests that a battery of several tests is required. A meta-analysis of 12 studies describing 14 tests concluded that the Yergason's test was the only test to have a significant ability to influence clinical decision-making (Walton and Sadi 2008). A systematic review of 17 papers concluded that no single test was sensitive or specific enough to determine the presence of a SLAP lesion, and suggested that a combination of two or more tests was required (Dessaur and Magarey 2008).

Table 12.12 SLAP lesion types

Type I	Fraying or degeneration to edge of superior labrum	
Type II	Detachment of biceps tendon and superior labrum from glenoid rim (most common type)	
Type III	Biceps tendon remains intact, superior labrum suffers bucket handle tear and displaces into joint	
Type IV	Bucket handle tear of superior labrum and part of biceps tendon, both of which displace into joint (least common type)	

Treatment of labral tears is conservative initially, with surgery only indicated for those who fail conservative management (Dodson and Altchek 2009). The aim is to restore normal shoulder motion (both glenohumeral and scapulothoracic) and stability. Where the causal action has involved repeated external rotation and abduction, there is likely to be a soft-tissue imbalance with a loss of glenohumeral internal (medial) rotation compared to external (lateral) rotation, a glenohumeral internal rotation deficit (GIRD, see above). In this case, stretching into GH internal rotation while stabilizing the scapula is required.

Surgical management is to re-attach the labrum using sutures and bone anchors. Following surgery, rehabilitation is vital. For the first three weeks post-surgery, subjects are normally protected in a sling for day-to-day usage. In this period, postural awareness, scapulothoracic stability and glenohumeral stability actions are taught. Stability exercise uses shoulder-joint control rather than motion range, with bracing actions, closed-chain positions and movement-awareness drills, as for instability. Abduction and external-rotation actions are generally avoided, with the arm kept predominantly in flexion and below shoulder height. Motion range progresses after three weeks, with extension and abduction re-introduced as tolerated. The aim is to progress to full active range by six to eight weeks post-surgery, and full daily-living or sport-specific function within three to four months, depending on subject/athlete preference. Tightness to the posterior joint in relation to GIRD, if found on assessment, is managed as above.

Glenohumeral dislocation

Dislocation (sometimes a progression from instability) is a commonly seen shoulder injury, with anterior displacement being encountered more often than posterior. Forced movements involving external rotation and abduction are common mechanisms, and a fall onto the outstretched arm is also a frequent aetiology.

At the time of injury, the glenoid labrum may become detached (together with the inferior glenohumeral ligament) giving a Bankart lesion, sometimes with a parallel fracture of the glenoid rim. Acute anterior dislocation gives considerable pain. The arm is usually held slightly abducted and externally rotated, and the normal rounded contour of the shoulder is lost. Close inspection shows the acromion process to be more prominent than usual, and a hollow is visible below it. The displaced humeral head can usually be felt on the anterior aspect of the shoulder.

Reduction

The question of whether to reduce an acute injury is one of debate. On the positive side, early reduction of an uncomplicated injury may be achieved without anaesthetic and with little discomfort. If left, muscle spasm sets in, making reduction under anaesthetic necessary. The main problem is the likelihood of further injury by reduction without X-ray by inexperienced staff. Fracture of the head or neck of the humerus may have occurred at the time of injury, and epiphyseal displacement is seen with adolescents. Displaced bone fragments may easily be pulled onto the circumflex or radial nerves, causing injury, and vascular damage may also occur.

Where an area of numbness is present over the deltoid, injury to the axillary nerve should be suspected, and swelling in the hand and fingers together with a loss of pulse suggests arterial damage as a result of humeral fracture (Reid 1992). For these reasons, an acute injury occurring for the first time should always be referred to an accident and emergency (casualty) department.

Recurrent anterior dislocation may be reduced more easily. The forces required to dislocate the shoulder in the first place are considerably less than with the acute injury, and so the chance of associated fracture is minimal. Spontaneous reduction may occur, and frequently the subject has learnt to reduce the dislocation themselves and the joint is fairly lax.

The simplest self-reduction procedure is for the subject to bend the ipsilateral leg and grasp the knee with both hands, keeping the arms locked straight. Slowly leaning back produces in-line traction, which usually allows the shoulder to reduce. It must be emphasized that these procedures should only be performed in the absence of pain and spasm. The traction is applied gently, brute force or 'yanking' the arm by another athlete being obviously contraindicated.

As an alternative, the subject may lie prone on a couch or gym bench with the arm hanging over the edge of the couch (hand off the floor). The weight of the arm will usually provide sufficient traction to initiate spontaneous reduction. Holding a weight in the hand (small dumb-bell) will assist the traction force. If the recurrently dislocated shoulder does not reduce readily, referral is still necessary.

Surgical repair

Surgical repair (Bankart repair) may be carried out to repair the torn glenoid labrum with sutures and reattach it to the glenoid, using anchors. In cases where there is capsular and/or ligamentous laxity,

the lax tissue may be tightened (capsular shrinkage) using either a radio-frequency heating probe or capsular plication (suturing).

Where bone damage has occurred to the glenoid, part of the coracoid process with its attached muscles may be surgically removed and transferred to fill the bone gap and reinforce the anterior joint. This is known as a Latarjet procedure. Bone damage may also occur to the posterior aspect of the humeral head (Hills-Sach lesion) at the time of injury if the head catches the front of the glenoid when dislocating.

Acute posterior dislocation is not as obvious as anterior. Pain is still intense, with the arm held adducted and internally rotated. Any attempt to move the arm is resisted by intense muscle spasm. In thin individuals the coracoid process is more visible than usual, and fullness is often apparent posteriorly. Heavy musculature in an athlete will, however, obscure these signs. Posterior dislocations require referral and reduction under sedation. Gentle in-line traction is applied to the adducted/internally rotated arm, with gentle pressure over the humeral head.

Rehabilitation following anterior dislocation

Following reduction, the POLICE protocol is applied to limit inflammation and facilitate healing. The arm is immobilized, and the initial period of immobilization is an important determinant of recurrence. Normally the recurrence rate for young (20–30 years) athletes may be as high as 85 per cent (Halbach and Tank 1990). However, this may be reduced considerably, with one study of 50 individuals showing a recurrence rate of 20 per cent after 6 weeks' immobilization (Reid 1992). Traditionally, immobilization is in a sling with the arm across the chest (adduction and internal rotation). However, immobilizing in abduction and external rotation has been claimed to reduce recurrence rate following primary anterior shoulder dislocation (Heidari et al. 2014). This claim has been challenged by other authors in two meta-analyses, one of five studies (Vavken et al. 2014), the other of six (Whelan et al. 2015).

Exercise therapy following immobilization is divided into four phases (Table 12.13).

▶ In phase one (0–3 weeks), isometric exercises are used. These are performed twice daily, with only minimal active abduction allowed to facilitate axillary hygiene. Limited flexion and extension are allowed, but external rotation is avoided. Scapular setting is used together with gentle, limited-range pendular swinging actions as tolerated. Whole-body stability exercise may be used to facilitate postural tone, as with instability rehab above.

▶ In phase two (3–6 weeks), active resisted internal rotation is used, and external rotation to neutral using elastic tubing. Abduction is usually limited to 45–90 degrees, and exercise for the rest of the body is progressed. Strengthening concentrates on medial rotation to strengthen the subscapularis and support the anterior joint, and limited-range adduction to work latissimus dorsi, teres major, the pectorals and coracobrachialis, to resist abduction forces.

▶ After 6–8 weeks (phase three), abduction increases to 90 degrees and limited external rotation is used to reduce stiffness. Only when strength has increased to 75 per cent of the uninjured shoulder should full-range motion be attempted. To reduce stiffness, self-stretches such as 'finger walking' along a table top or up a wall, and limited joint distractions are useful. Autotherapy distractions may be performed in a prone kneeling position, holding the couch end, and cane exercises may be useful.

Table 12.13 Guidelines for rehabilitation following anterior glenohumeral dislocation

Initial post-reduction period
Rest and ice
Immobilization
0–3 weeks
Isometrics twice daily
Minimal abduction for axillary hygiene only
Limited flexion and extension
Avoid external rotation
Gentle pendular swinging in transverse and sagittal planes
Scapular stability work
3–6 weeks
Resisted internal rotation
External rotation to neutral only
Abduction limited to 45°
Re-education of scapulohumeral rhythm
Extension/adduction/medial rotation pattern on pulley
Limited range resisted adduction
Pendular swinging giving way to automobilization techniques
Proprioceptive work including static joint repositioning
6–8 weeks
Abduction increased to 90°
External rotation gradually increased
Flexion/abduction/lateral rotation pattern on pulley
Full resistance training below shoulder height
Introduce fast throwing and catching below head height
Closed-chain work on balance board and trampette (two hands)
Final rehabilitation
Full range motion resisted
Ensure muscle balance (internal rotation: external rotation ratio)
Closed-chain work (single arm)
Push-up with clap
Fast reaction work — throwing/catching/blocking
Re-education of falling — forward roll/handstand/fall back

Frozen shoulder

Frozen shoulder (FS) or 'adhesive capsulitis' (also called frozen shoulder contraction syndrome) is an increasingly common pathology found in sport and exercise medicine. As the number of seniors involved in sport continues to rise, this condition is likely to be seen even more frequently. Exercise therapy is a key component to treatment of this condition, meaning that exercise professionals are very likely to see subjects who have suffered from this condition. In addition, the condition is often prolonged, impacting on general health and well-being.

Between 2 and 3 per cent of the adult population between the ages of 40 and 70 develop the problem, and the condition is more common in women. It presents as a gradual loss of shoulder movement, with or without pain. The initial loss of movement may go unnoticed until function is limited. Subjects complain that activities of everyday living become increasingly difficult. Combing the hair at the back of the head and fastening a bra strap are frequent sources of complaint. Active sports persons frequently notice the onset of the condition earlier than sedentary individuals, with end-range actions such as a golf swing or overhead badminton shot becoming limited and painful, for example.

The term 'frozen shoulder' (Codman 1934) is not an accurate diagnosis, but rather a description of the major symptom, which is lack of movement. 'Adhesive capsulitis' (Neviaser 1945) implies capsular thickening, contraction and adhesions. The condition may appear as a primary (insidious) or secondary (traumatic) adhesive capsulitis. Secondary types can be associated with a number of soft-tissue and medical pathologies, including rotator-cuff injuries, impingement syndrome, traumatic arthritis, osteoarthritis, shoulder-joint immobilization, autoimmune disease, diabetes and thyroid dysfunction. Up to 30 per cent of individuals develop the condition in the opposite shoulder (Sheridan and Hannafin 2006).

> **Key point**
> FS can be primary (idiopathic) or secondary. The condition may be secondary to shoulder injury or a number of medical pathologies, and has a tendency to recur in the opposite shoulder.

FS is normally categorized into three stages representing freezing (stage I), frozen (stage II) and thawing (stage III) (Table 12.14).

During stage I, pain is the predominant feature, with dull aching at rest. Movement range increases significantly when intra-articular injection or anaesthesia is given, showing that muscle spasm is a key feature. During stage II, there is an increase in synovitis and capsular tightening. No inflammatory infiltrates are present in this stage showing that the synovitis is burning out. The capsule can develop fibroplasia, with hypercellular collagenous tissue laid down, explaining the dense, rubbery end feel. Stage III is the thawing stage, showing an improvement in motion range, perhaps due to capsular remodelling.

On examination, movement is usually limited in a capsular pattern (subacute) or by muscle guarding (acute). Accessory movements are limited, particularly inferior and anterior gliding, and the quadrant position is limited and painful when compared to the uninvolved side. Clinically,

Table 12.14 Stages of frozen shoulder

Stage	Signs and symptoms	Pathology	Conservative intervention
Freezing (0–6 months)	Pain predominates. Movement limited by pain & muscle spasm	Hypervascular synovitis. Capsule normal	Pain relief. Joint mobilization. Pendular swinging exercise
Frozen (3–9 months)	Pain and stiffness equal. Leathery end-feel to passive motion	Diffuse pedunculated synovitis. Capsule develops fibroplasia	Joint mobilization. Extensive stretching exercise
Thawing (3–9 months)	Stiffness predominates with pain at end range only	Capsular remodelling. Chronic movement dysfunction	End range stretching. Re-education of shoulder function

After Sheridan and Hannafin (2006).

pain and stiffness are the two most common challenges. This two-stage classification has led some authors to propose two simple stages: pain greater than stiffness (stage I) and stiffness greater than pain (stage II) (Lewis 2015). A narrative review of 13 observational studies (Ryan et al. 2016) confirmed pathogenic findings in the anterior GH capsule, the coracohumeral ligament, axillary fold and rotator internal. The sub-coracoid fat triangle was obliterated, and immune, inflammatory and fibrotic changes were seen histologically.

Definition

The rotator interval is the space between the anterior border of the supraspinatus tendon and the superior border of the subscapularis tendon. The space is filled by the coracohumeral ligament. The sub-coracoid fat triangle lies between the coracohumeral ligament and the coracoid process.

Changes are summarized in Table 12.15.

Diagnosis must eliminate red flags, with those for general shoulder examination shown above

Table 12.15 Pathological and histological changes in Frozen shoulder

▶ Thickening/fibrosis of rotator interval
▶ Scarring within subscapular recess (area between biceps & subscapularis)
▶ Neovascularisaion
▶ ↑ cytokine concentration (cell signalling)
▶ Contraction of auxilary recess (anterior/inferior capsule)
▶ ↓ joint volume (15–35 cc downt to 5–6 cc)
▶ Fibrosis of corocohumeral ligament
▶ ↑ number fibroblasts
▶ Presence of contractile proteins resembling Dupuytren's
▶ Subcoracoid fat triangle (between CHL & coracoid process) obliterated.
▶ Immune, inflammatory and fibrotic changes seen histologically

↑ - increased, ↓ - decreased, CHL - coracohumeral ligament
(Data from Lewis 2015)

(Table 12.2). The specific diagnosis of FS normally involves clinical examination to show normal shoulder radiographs and an equal restriction of both active and passive GH external rotation (Zuckerman and Rokito 2011).

Management

Management of FS includes supervised neglect, physiotherapy, medication and surgery. A systematic review of conservative treatments (Barrett et al. 2016) that looked at 26 randomized controlled trials (RCTs) involving 1,488 subjects concluded that high (silver) level evidence was available to support the use of corticosteroid injection, therapeutic exercise, shoulder-joint mobilizations and acupuncture for improving pain, range of motion (ROM) and function in the short term with idiopathic FS of less than one year's duration. Capsular distension and shockwave therapy may be as effective as corticosteroids for short-term improvement.

Supervised neglect involves patient education (with neuroscience education) and allowing the condition to take its natural course. Physiotherapy tends to use joint mobilization (mid-range and end-range), acupuncture/dry needling and exercise. Surgical intervention is mainly by manipulation under anaesthesia (MUA), arthroscopic dissection, or hydro-distension (high-volume injection). Medication on the whole includes corticosteroid injection and the use of non-specific anti-inflammatory drugs (NSAIDs) or analgesics.

Corticosteroid injection (ultrasound guided) has been shown to be effective in the short term but to have little long-term (6–18 months) benefit (Van der Windt and Koes 2002). Effect is enhanced when combined with physiotherapy (Maund et al. 2012). Subjects treated with MUA have been shown to achieve a 50-point functional improvement score, while those treated with physiotherapy gained a 78 point score (Melzer et al. 1995). However, physiotherapy for adhesive capsulitis can be protracted, with studies reporting 12–29 treatment sessions on average (Cleland and Durall 2002). Following an active physiotherapy programme that includes home exercise, 90 per cent of subjects have reported a satisfactory result (Griggs, Ahn and Green 2000) and subjects rated their shoulder function improvement as excellent (57 per cent) or good (29 per cent) (Vermeulen et al. 2000). Although spontaneous recovery may occur, as many as 50 per cent of subjects can still have symptoms up to seven years later if not treated (Shaffer, Tibone and Kerlan 1992).

MUA has been criticized for the intra-articular lesions caused by this procedure. In an arthroscopic study of 30 subjects following MUA, Loew, Heichel and Lehner (2005) showed haemarthrosis in all subjects, local synovitis in the region of the rotator cuff, and capsular rupture. Acute intra-articular lesions were seen in 12 subjects, and these consisted of labral detachment, rupture of the glenohumeral ligament, tear of the subscapularis tendon and worsening of supraspinatus fraying. The trauma caused by MUA has made arthroscopic capsular release more popular. In this technique, the joint is evaluated arthroscopically making precise surgical release of the fibrosed capsular portion possible. In addition, hydro-distension (using sodium chloride) may be performed under local anaesthetic to mechanically distend the joint to stretch adhesions within the capsule. An increase in the intra-articular distance is visible on ultrasound scan following the technique. Manual therapy and exercise may be used following the procedure (Buchbinder et al. 2007).

> **Key point**
>
> Manipulation under anaesthesia (MUA) for frozen shoulder has been shown to cause considerable tissue damage, including labral detachment, glenohumeral ligament rupture and rotator-cuff injury.

Manual therapy

Pain may be modulated in stage I of FS by the use of joint-mobilization procedures. Antero-posterior (AP) glides may be used at multiple joint angles as tolerated. In addition, an AP glide may be applied with the arm held in external rotation (Lewis 2015). The scapula must be stabilized to focus the mobilization force on the GH joint (Fig. 12.54A).

Inferior glide mobilizations may be used again with the scapula stabilized. This may be coupled with internal rotation in the hand-behind-back position (Fig. 12.54B). As abduction range increases, inferior glide may be applied with the subject's shoulder flexed to 90 degrees (Fig. 12.54C). Lateral glides may be performed with the subject in supine or side-lying, using a padded seatbelt around the chest wall to stabilize the scapula (Fig. 12.54D)

In stage III stiffness, mobilization with movement (MWM) may be used to impart an AP glide while stretching into lateral rotation. The subject is positioned close to the couch edge with the affected shoulder free to move. The arm is taken into as much abduction and lateral rotation as can be comfortably tolerated. A padded seatbelt is wrapped around the upper arm in a large loop to form a stirrup, and the therapist's foot is placed into the stirrup to create the AP glide. Lateral rotation is encouraged, with the hands supporting upper arm and forearm while maintaining the AP glide (Fig. 12.54E). As lateral rotation range increases, the patient may perform active, assisted lateral rotation using a stick as an AP glide imparted by the therapist (Fig. 12.54F)

Exercise therapy

In stage I, the primary aim is to reduce pain and ensure that the joint is not irritated (Table 12.16). Pendular swinging actions may be used to allow the subject to self-manage the condition. The subject leans over a table with the unaffected hand supporting them. The affected arm is allowed to relax and 'go heavy', allowing arm weight to slightly traction the joint in its flexed-abducted position. The action is to sway the body and impart a gentle circling movement on the straight arm, which is transmitted to the glenohumeral joint (Fig. 12.55A). It must be emphasized that shoulder-muscle action should not create the movement, but rather body sway. The action should be performed in

Table 12.16 Movement therapy for adhesive capsulitis

Stage	Pathology and signs	Exercise therapy
(I) 'Freezing'	Scar tissue forming and maturing. External rotation of shoulder markedly reduced, abduction less limited. Spasm end-feel	Active range of motion exercise Joint mobilization for pain relief, not increased range Pendular swinging
(II) 'Frozen'	Scarring mature. Glenohumeral joint lost mobility. Patient unable to lie on affected side at night. Elastic end-feel	More aggressive joint mobilizations providing joint is not irritated Stretching Strengthening within pain-free ranges
(III) 'Thawing'	Arm pain dominates, shoulder painless intense. Gross reverse scapulohumeral rhythm. Hard leathery end-feel	Scapular stability Aggressive glenohumeral joint mobilization. End-range stretching Movement re-education

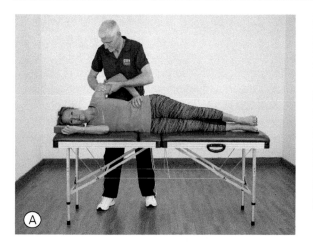
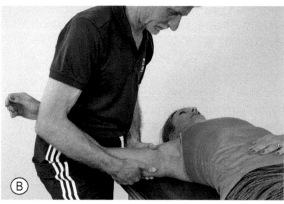
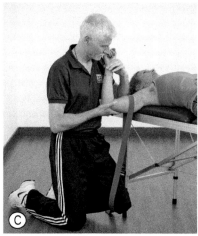
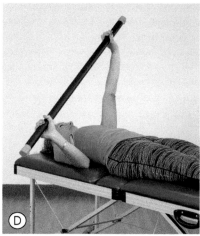

Figure 12.54 Mobilization techniques for frozen shoulder. (A) AP glide with arm in lateral rotation. (B) Inferior glide in abduction. (C) AP glide with lateral rotation MWM webbing belt. (D) AP glide with active lateral rotation using stick.

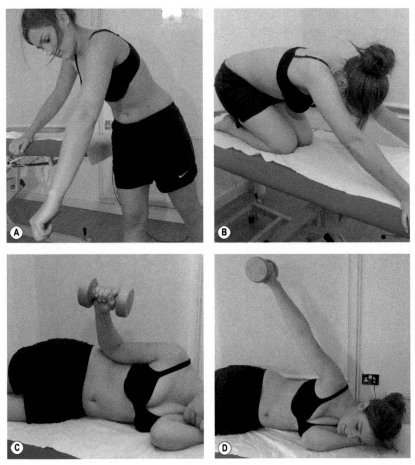

Figure 12.55 Exercise therapy for adhesive capsulitis. (A) Pendulum swinging. (B) Flexion–abduction with traction. (C) Resisted lateral rotation. (D) Initial range of abduction.

both clockwise and anticlockwise directions and repeated every two hours throughout the waking day. Isometric contractions have been shown to be anaesthetic in cases of shoulder tendinopathy (see above), and this can be tried. Results are very subject-specific, and should be used only where an anaesthetic effect is produced.

In stage II, pendular swinging may be continued for pain relief, but self-mobilization, stretching and strengthening should begin. Stretching focuses on the anterosuperior capsule and/or posterior capsule. Flexion-abduction with traction may be used in kneeling, holding onto an object, or simply gripping the floor with the fingertips and moving the bodyweight backwards to sit on the heels

(Fig. 12.55B). The aim is to encourage movement rather than force it. Resisted lateral rotation may be used in side-lying, with the weight of the arm initially and a light dumb-bell as pain allows (Fig. 12.55C). Abduction within the pain-free range should be used in side-lying (Fig. 12.55D) rather than standing at this stage. In standing, the increased leverage as the arm reaches the horizontal position encourages shoulder-shrugging and reverse scapulohumeral rhythm.

Scapular stability work should begin, and as abduction and lateral rotation-range increases, all three movements should be combined in sitting (Fig. 12.56). The subject begins the action by drawing the scapula down gently. While

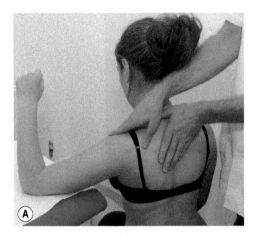

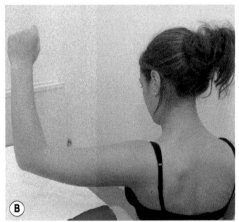

Figure 12.56 Combining shoulder lateral rotation and abduction with scapular stability. (A) Scapular repositioning. (B) Arm lifting.

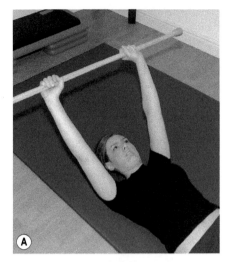

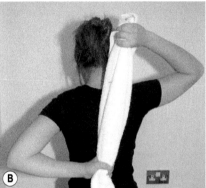

Figure 12.57 Full-range stretching exercises for the shoulder.

maintaining this position, the bent arm is laterally rotated and the elbow lifted from the couch. The distance between the ear and the shoulder should be maintained as shoulder-shrugging is avoided.

> **Definition**
> Normally in arm abduction there is more glenohumeral movement than scapulothoracic movement (ratio 2:1). With reverse scapulohumeral rhythm, glenohumeral movement is reduced and scapulothoracic movement increased to compensate.

In stage III, end-range stretching and further strengthening is used. The sit-to-heels exercise and sitting abduction-lateral rotation may be continued, with the aim of increasing range of motion in each. Passive abduction and lateral rotation using a stick or towel in lying (Fig. 12.57A) is useful, as the leverage involved assists in obtaining the final few degrees of movement. Both medial and lateral rotation may be gained using a hand-behind-neck (HBN) and hand-behind-back (HBB) action (Fig. 12.57B). The MWM actions used with shoulder impingement (above), both therapist and self-applied, can be useful to regain the final degrees of movement range. Muscle strength should also be a focus, as deconditioning produced by enforced

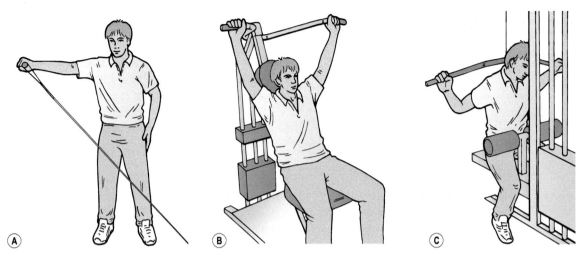

Figure 12.58 Weight-training actions for the shoulder. (A) Cable lateral raise. (B) Shoulder press. (C) Lateral pull-down. From Norris, C.M. (1996). Weight Training. CD-ROM Package. Exercise Association, London. With permission.

rest during stages I and II leads to muscle atrophy. Several weight-training exercises may be used both to regain shoulder strength and improve range of motion, including shoulder-presses, lateral pull-downs and pulley-abduction movements (Fig. 12.58).

Snapping scapulae

This unusual condition occurs especially in adolescent females just after skeletal maturity, and in both sexes following surgery. Subjects experience a snapping sensation, which is sometimes audible, near the vertebral border of the scapula. Pain is often localized to the rhomboids and levator scapulae over the medial scapular border, or the trapezius over the medial aspect of the scapular spine. One possibility is that tendinopathy occurs to the muscles, another that the bursa located beneath the medial border of the scapula becomes inflamed.

The condition occurs through microtrauma from excessive shearing forces beneath the scapula due to abnormal scapulothoracic rhythm. Management relies on the restoration of a more normal scapulothoracic rhythm.

Nerve-entrapment syndromes

Two relatively uncommon nerve-entrapments are seen around the shoulder – quadrilateral space syndrome and entrapment of the suprascapular nerve.

The quadrilateral (quadrangular) space lies between the teres minor and the subscapularis above, and the teres major below. The long head of triceps forms its medial wall and the surgical neck of the humerus lies laterally (Fig. 12.59A). Entrapment by tethering can occur to both the axillary nerve and circumflex humeral artery. The subject, frequently a throwing athlete, is usually young (22–35 years) and complains of shoulder pain of insidious onset. Muscle fatigue and loss of abduction power are apparent, and tenderness may be elicited to palpation over the involved quadrilateral space. Arteriograph frequently shows posterior circumflex artery occlusion. Most subjects respond to alteration of throwing technique, but some may go on to surgical decompression.

> **Definition**
>
> An arteriograph is an X-ray of an artery following injection of a radiopaque dye.

563

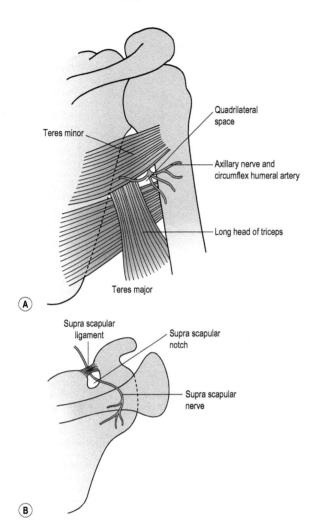

Teres minor

Quadrilateral space

Axillary nerve and circumflex humeral artery

Long head of triceps

Teres major

(A)

Supra scapular ligament

Supra scapular notch

Supra scapular nerve

(B)

Figure 12.59 Entrapment neuropathy in the shoulder. (A) Quadrilateral space. (B) Suprascapular notch.

The suprascapular nerve (Fig. 12.59B) is formed from the C5 and C6 nerve roots (superior trunk of the brachial plexus). It may be trapped as it passes through the suprascapular notch beneath the superior transverse scapular ligament (STSL), or as it winds around the lateral edge of the scapular spine (spinoglenoid notch). The roof of the suprascapular notch is formed by the STSL, which may thicken or ossify in later life causing nerve compression. Direct blows in contact sports can also cause the condition, as the nerve is superficial, and occult ganglions pressing on the shoulder

have been described (Gerscovich and Greenspan 1993). Entrapment can affect the motor response of both the supraspinatus and infraspinatus, either together or in isolation. The subject presents with visible muscular atrophy, and weakness is often noticed to backhand shots or in serving. Vague pain occurs deep in the posterior aspect of the shoulder. EMG is used to assess denervation of the involved muscles. Treatment involves physiotherapy to avoid positions that affect the nerve (scapular tipping and depression), and frequently taping is used to de-load the tissues. As nerve recovery occurs, the supraspinatus and infraspinatus are reactivated using rotator-cuff exercise. In non-responsive cases, decompression of the nerve at the suprascapular notch and scapular nerve block may be required.

References

Apley, A.G., Solomon, L., 1989. *Concise System of Orthopaedics and Fractures.* Butterworth, London.

Bandy, W.D., Lovelace-Chandler, V., Holt, A., 1991. Rehabilitation of the ruptured biceps brachii muscle of an athlete. *Journal of Orthopaedic and Sports Physical Therapy* **13** (4), 184–190.

Bannister, G.C., Wallace, W.A., Stableforth, P.G., Hutson, M.A., 1989. The management of acute acromioclavicular dislocation: a randomised prospective controlled trial. *Journal of Bone and Joint Surgery* **71B**, 848–850.

Barden, J.M., Balyk, R., Raso, V.J. et al. 2004. Dynamic upper limb proprioception in multidirectional shoulder instability. *Clinical Orthopaedics and Related Research* **420**, 181–189.

Barrett, E., de Burca, N., McCreesh, K. et al., 2016. The effectiveness of conservative treatments in the management of idiopathic frozen shoulder: a systematic review of randomised controlled trials. *Manual Therapy* **25**, e60–e61.

Borsa P.A., Laundner, K., Sauers, E., 2008. Mobility and stability adaptation s in the shoulder of the overhead athlete: a theoretical and evidence based perspective. *Sports Medicine* **38** (1): 17–36.

Boyles, R.E., Ritland, B.M., Miracle, B.M. et al., 2009. The short-term effects of thoracic spine thrust manipulation on patients with shoulder impingement syndrome. *Manual Therapy* **14**, 375–380.

Buchbinder, R., Youd, J., Green, J et al., 2007. Efficacy and cost-effectiveness of physiotherapy following glenohumeral joint distension for adhesive capsulitis: a randomized trial. *Arthritis & Rheum* **57**, 1027–1037.

Cain, P.R., Mutschler, T.A., Fu, F.H., 1987. Anterior stability of the glenohumeral joint: a dynamic model. *American Journal of Sports Medicine* **15**, 144.

Chronopoulos, E., Kin, T., Park, H., et al., 2004. Diagnostic value of physical tests for isolated chronic acromioclavicular lesions. *American Journal of Sports Medicine* **32** (3), 655–661.

Cleland, J., Durall, J.C., 2002. Physical therapy for adhesive capsulitis: systematic review. *Physiotherapy* **88** (8), 450–457.

Codman, E.A., 1934. *The Shoulder*, Thomas Todd, Boston.

Comtet, J.J., Herberg, G., Naasan, I.A., 1989. Biomechanical basis of transfers for shoulder paralysis. *Hand Clinics* **5**, 1.

Cools, A.M.J., Struyf, F., De Mey, K. et al., 2014. Rehabilitation of scapular dyskinesis: from the office worker to the elite overhead athlete. *British Journal of Sports Medicine* **48**, 692–697.

Cools, A.M., Witvrouw, E., Declercq, G., et al., 2004. Evaluation of isokinetic force production and associated muscle activity in the scapular rotators during a protraction-retraction movement in overhead athletes with impingement symptoms. *British Journal of Sports Medicine* **38**, 64–68.

Culham, E., Peat, M., 1993. Functional anatomy of the shoulder complex. *Journal of Orthopedic and Sports Physical Therapy* **18** (1), 342–350.

Cyriax, J.H., Cyriax, P.J., 1983. *Illustrated Manual of Orthopaedic Medicine*. Butterworth, London.

Dessaur, W.A., Magarey, M.E., 2008. Diagnostic accuracy of clinical tests for superior labral anterior posterior lesions: a systematic review. *Journal of Orthopaedic and Sports Physical Therapy* **38** (6), 341–352.

Dias, J.J., Gregg, P.J., 1991. Acromioclavicular joint injuries in sport. *Sports Medicine* **11**, 125–132.

Dias, J.J., Steingold, R.F., Richardson, R.A., Tesfayohannes, B., Gregg, P.J., 1987. The conservative treatment of acromioclavicular dislocation: review after five years. *Journal of Bone and Joint Surgery* **69B**, 719–722.

Dodson, C.C., Altchek, D.W., 2009. SLAP lesions: an update on recognition and treatment. *Journal of Orthopaedic and Sports Physical Therapy* **39** (2), 71–80.

Edelson, C., and Teitz, C., 2000. Internal impingement in the shoulder. *J Shoulder Elbow Surg* **9**, 308–315.

Fallon, J., Blevins, F.T., Vogel, K., Trotter, J., 2002. Functional morphology of the supraspinatus tendon. *Journal of Orthopaedic Research* **20** (5), 920–926.

Fukuda, K., Craig, E.V., An, K., Cofield, R.H., Chao, E.Y.S., 1986. Biomechanical study of the ligamentous system of the acromioclavicular joint. *Journal of Bone and Joint Surgery* **68A**, 434–439.

Gagey, O., Hue, E., 2000. Mechanics of the deltoid muscle. *Clinical Orthopedics*, **375**, 250–257.

Gerscovich, E.O., Greenspan, A., 1993. Magnetic resonance imaging in the diagnosis of suprascapular nerve syndrome. *Canadian Association of Radiologists Journal* **44**, 307–309.

Giannakopoulos, K., Beneka, A., and Malliou, P., 2004. Isolated vs complex exercise in strengthening the rotator cuff muscle group. *J Strength Cond Res* **18** (1), 144–148.

Gibson, J., 2011. The shoulder: evidence-based practice or reinventing the wheel? *In Touch Journal of for Physiotherapists in Private Practice*. **135** (June).

Gibson, J., Elphinston, J., 2005. Shoulder instability – treatment and rehabilitation of shoulder instability. *Sportex Medicine* 18–21.

Gleason, P.D., Beall, D., Sanders, T., et al., 2006. The transverse humeral ligament: a separate anatomical structure or a continuation of the osseous attachment of the rotator cuff? *American Journal of Sports Medicine* **34** (1), 72–77.

Graichen, H., Bonel, H., Stammberger, T., Haubner, M., Rohrer, H., Englmeier, K.H., 1999. Three-dimensional analysis of the width of the subacromial space in healthy subjects and patients with impingement syndrome. *Am J Roentgenol* **172** (4), 1081–1086.

Griggs, S.M., Ahn, A., Green, A., 2000. Idiopathic adhesive capsulitis: a prospective functional outcome of non-operative treatment. *Journal of Bone and Joint Surgery* **82**, 1398–1407.

Halbach, J.W., Tank, R.T., 1990. The shoulder. In: Gould, J.A. (ed.), 2nd edn *Orthopaedic and Sports Physical Therapy*. C.V. Mosby, St Louis.

Harryman, D.T., Sidles, J.A., Clark, J.M. et al., 1990. Translation of the humeral head on the glenoid with passive glenohumeral motion. *Journal of Bone and Joint Surgery [Am]* **72**, 1334–1343.

Hegedus, E.J., Goode, A., Campbell, S. et al., 2008. Physical examination tests of the shoulder: a systematic review with meta-analysis of individual tests. *British Journal of Sports Medicine* **42**, 80–92.

Heidari, K., Asadollahi, S., Vafaee, R et al., 2014. Immobilization in external rotation combined with abduction reduces the risk of recurrence after primary anterior shoulder dislocation. *Journal of Shoulder and Elbow Surgery* **23** (6), 759–766.

Henkus, H.E., de Witte, P.B., Nelissen, R.G. et al., 2009. Bursectomy compared with acromioplasty in the management of subacromial impingement syndrome: a prospective randomised study. *J Bone Joint Surgery [Br]* **91**, 504–510.

Hung, C., Hsieh, C., Yang, P., Lin, J., 2010. Relationship between posterior shoulder muscle stiffness and rotation in subjects with stiff shoulder. *Journal of Rehabilitation Medicine* **42** (3), 216–220.

Hunter, M.B., Shybut, G.T., Nuber, G., 1986. The effect of anabolic steroid hormones on the mechanical properties of tendons and ligaments. *Transactions of the Orthopaedic Research Society* **11**, 240.

Jaggi, A, and Lambert, S., 2010. Rehabilitation for shoulder instability. *British Journal of Sports Medicine* **44** (5), 333–340.

Kibler, W.B., Ludewig, P.M., McClure, P.W. et al., 2013. Clinical implications of scapular dyskinesis in shoulder injury: the 2013 consensus statement from the 'Scapular Summit'. *British Journal of Sports Medicine* **47** (14), 877–885.

Kibler, W.B., Sciascia, A., Thomas, S.J., 2012. Glenohumeral internal rotation deficit: pathogenesis and response to acute throwing. *Sports Med Arthrosc* **20** (1), 34–38.

Kretzler, H.H., Richardson, A.B., 1989. Rupture of the pectoralis major muscle. *American Journal of Sports Medicine* **17**, 453–458.

Kunichi, A., Torisu, T., 1984. Muscle belly tear of the triceps. *American Journal of Sports Medicine* **12** (6), 485.

Lemak, L.J., 1994. Calcifying tendonitis. In: Andrews, J.R., Wilk, K.E. (eds), *The Athlete's Shoulder*. Churchill Livingstone, Edinburgh.

Lephart, S.M., Henry, T.J., 2000. Restoration of proprioception and neuromuscular control of the unstable shoulder. In: Lephart, S.M., Fu, F.H. (eds), *Proprioception and Neuromuscular Control in Joint Stability*. Human Kinetics, Champaign, Illinois.

Levy, O., Relwani, J., Zaman, T. et al., 2008. Measurement of blood flow in the rotator cuff using laser Doppler flowmetry. *J Bone Joint Surg [Br]* **90**, 893–898.

Lewis, A., Kitamura, T., Bayley, J.L., 2004. The classification of shoulder instability. *Current Orthopaedics* **18**, 97–108.

Lewis, J.S., 2009a. Rotator cuff tendinopathy/subacromial impingement syndrome: is it time for a new method of assessment? *British Journal of Sports Medicine* **43**, 259–264.

Lewis, J.S., 2009b. Rotator cuff tendinopathy. *British Journal of Sports Medicine* **43**, 236–241.

Lewis, J.S., 2011. Subacromial impingement syndrome: a musculoskeletal condition or a clinical illusion? *Physical Therapy Reviews*.

Lewis J., 2015. Frozen shoulder contracture syndrome – Aetiology, diagnosis and management. *Manual Therapy* **20** (1), 2–9.

Lewis, J.S., Wright, C. and Green, A., 2005 Subacromial impingement syndrome: the effect of changing posture on shoulder range of movement. *JOSPT* **35** (2), 72–87.

Littlewood, C., Malliaras, P., Bateman, M. et al., 2013. The central nervous system – an additional consideration in rotator cuff tendinopathy and a potential basis for understanding response to loaded therapeutic exercise. *Manual Therapy* **18**, 468–472.

Loehr, J.F. and Uhthoff, H.K., 1987. The pathogenesis of degenerative rotator cuff tears. *Orthopedic Translation* **11**, 237.

Loew, M., Heichel, T., Lehner, B., 2005. Intraarticular lesions in primary frozen shoulder after manipulation under general anesthesia. *Journal of Shoulder and Elbow Surgery* **14**, 16–21.

Ludewig, P.M. and Cook, T.M., 2000. Alteration in shoulder kinematics and associated muscle activity in people with symptoms of shoulder impingement. *Phys Ther* **80** (3), 276–291.

Ludewig, P.M. and Cook, T.M., 2002. Translations of the humerus in persons with shoulder impingement symptoms. *J Orthop Sports Phys Ther* **32**, 248–259.

Magee, D.J., 2008. *Orthopaedic Physical Assessment*, 5th ed. Saunders, Elsevier. Philadelphia.

Malone, A.A., 2004. Muscle patterning instability – classification and prevalence in a tertiary referral shoulder service. *Proceedings of the International Congress of Shoulder Surgery*, Washington DC.

Margarey, M.E., Jones, M.A., 2003. Dynamic evaluation and early management of altered motor control around the shoulder complex. *Manual Therapy* **8** (4), 195–206.

Matsen, F.A., Harryman, D.T., Sidles, J.A., 1991. Mechanics of glenohumeral instability. *Clinical Sports Medicine* **10** (4), 783–788.

Maund, E., Craig, D., Suekarran, S., Neilson, A., Wright, K., Brealey, S., Dennis, L., Goodchild, L., Hanchard, N., Rangan, A., Richardson, G., Robertson, J., McDaid, C., 2012. Management of frozen shoulder: a systematic review and cost-effectiveness analysis. *Health Technology Assessment* **16** (11): 1–264.

McAuliffe, T.B., Pangayatselvan, T., Baylet, I., 1988. Failed surgery for recurrent anterior dislocation of the shoulder. Causes and management *Journal of Bone and Joint Surgery* **70B** (5), 798–801.

McClatchie, L., Laprade, J., Martin, S., Jaglal, S., Richardson, D., Agurd, A., 2009. Mobilizations of the asymptomatic cervical spine can reduce signs of shoulder dysfunction in adults. *Manual Therapy* **14** (4), 369–374.

McClure, P.W., Michener, L.A., 2015. Staged approach for rehabilitation classification: shoulder disorders (STAR-shoulder). *Phys Ther* **95** (5), 791–800.

Melzer, C., Wallny, T., Wirth, C.J., Hoffman, S., 1995. Frozen shoulder: treatment and results. *Archives of Orthopaedic Trauma Surgery* **114**, 87–91.

Michener, L.A., McClure, P.W., Karduna, A.R., 2003. Anatomical and biomechanical mechanisms of subacromial impingement syndrome. *Clinical Biomechanics* **18**, 369–379.

Mullen, F., Slade, S., Briggs, C., 1989. Bony and capsular determinants of glenohumeral locking and quadrant positions. *Australian Journal of Physiotherapy* **35**, 202–208.

Nakajima, T., Rokuuma, N., Hamada, K., 1994. Histological and biomechanical characteristics of the supraspinatus tendon. *Journal of Shoulder and Elbow Surgery* **3**, 79–87.

Neer, C.S., 1983. Impingement lesions. *Clinical Orthopedics* **173**, 70–77.

Neviaser, J.S., 1945. Adhesive capsulitis of the shoulder. *Journal of Bone and Joint Surgery* **27**, 211.

Norris, C.M. and Matthews, M., 2008. The role of an integrated back stability program in patients with chronic low back pain. *Complementary Therapies in Clinical Practice* **14**, 255–263.

O'Brian, S.J., Neves, M.C., Arnoczky, S.P. et al., 1990. The anatomy and histology of the inferior glenohumeral ligament complex of the shoulder. *American Journal of Sports Medicine* **18**, 451.

O'Brian, S.J., Pagnani, M.J., Fealy, S., et al., 1998. The active compression test: a new and effective test for diagnosing labral tears and acromioclavicular joint abnormality. *American Journal of Sports Medicine* **26**, 610–613.

O'Donoghue, D.H., 1973. Subluxing biceps tendon in the athlete. *Journal of Sports Medicine* **1**, 20.

Odom, C.J., Taylor, A.B., Hurd, C.E., Denegar, C.R., 2001. Measurement of scapular asymmetry and assessment of shoulder dysfunction using the lateral scapular slide test: a reliability and validity study. *Physical Therapy* **81** (2), 799–809.

Palastanga, N., Field, D., Soames, R., 2006. *Anatomy and Human Movement—Structure and Function* 5th ed. Butterworth-Heinemann, Edinburgh.

Park, G.Y., Park, J.H., Bae, J.H., 2009. Structural changes in the acromioclavicular joint measured by ultrasonography during provocative tests. *Clinical Anatomy* **22** (5), 580–585.

Payne, L.Z., Deng, X.H., Craig, E.V. et al., 1997. The combined dynamic and static contributions to subacromial impingement: a biomechanical analysis. *American Journal of Sports Medicine* **25**, 801–808.

Peat, M., Culham, E., 1994. Functional anatomy of the shoulder complex. In: Andrews, J.R., Wilk, K.E. (eds), *The Athlete's Shoulder*. Churchill Livingstone, Edinburgh.

Perry, J., Glousman, R.E., 1995. Biomechanics of throwing. In: Nicholas, J.A., Hershman, E.B. (eds), *The Upper Extremity in Sports Medicine*, 2nd edn. C.V. Mosby, St Louis.

Petty, N.J., Moore, A.P., 2001. *Neuromusculoskeletal Examination and Assessment*, 2nd edn. Churchill Livingstone, Edinburgh.

Rabin, A., Irrgang, J., Fitzgerald, K. et al., 2006. The intertester reliability of the scapular assistance test. *JOSPT* **36**, 653–660.

Reddy, A.S., Mohr, K.J., Pink, M.M., Jobe, F.W., 2000. Electromyographic analysis of the deltoid and rotator cuff muscles in persons with subacromial impingement. *J Shoulder Elbow Surg* **9**, 519–523.

Reid, D.C., 1992. *Sports Injury Assessment and Rehabilitation*. Churchill Livingstone, Edinburgh.

Reid, D.C., Kushner, S., 1989. The elbow region. In: Donatelli, R., Wooden, M.J. (eds), *Orthopaedic Physical Therapy*. Churchill Livingstone, Edinburgh.

Reut, R.C., Bach, B.R., Johnson, C., 1991. Pectoralis major rupture: diagnosing and treating a weight-training injury. *Physician and Sports Medicine* **19** (3), 89–96.

Ryan, V., Brown, H., Minns Lowe, C.J., Lewis, J. S., 2016. The pathophysiology associated with primary (idiopathic) frozen shoulder: a systematic review. *BMC Musculoskeletal Disorders* **17**, 340.

Schneider, G., 1989. Restricted shoulder movement: capsular contracture or cervical referral – a clinical study. *Australian J Physiotherapy* **35** (2), 97–100.

Seitz, A.L., McClure, P.W., Finucane, S. et al., 2011. Mechanisms of rotator cuff tendinopathy: Intrinsic, extrinsic, or both? *Clinical Biomechanics* **26**, 1–12.

Shaffer, B., Tibone, J.E., Kerlan, R.K., 1992. Frozen shoulder: a long-term follow-up. *Journal of Bone and Joint Surgery* **74**, 738–746.

Sheridan, M.A., Hannafin, J.A., 2006. Upper extremity: emphasis on frozen shoulder. *Orthopedic Clinics of North America* **37** (4), 531–539.

Simons, D.G., Travell, J.G., Simons, L.S., 1999. *Travell and Simons' Myofascial Pain and Dysfunction*, Vol. 1, 2nd edn. Lippincott, Williams and Wilkins, Philadelphia.

Slatis, P., Alato, K., 1979. Medial dislocation of the tendon of the long head of biceps brachii. *Acta Orthopaedica Scandinavica* **50**, 73.

Smith, T.O., Chester, R., Pearse, E.O. et al., 2011. Operative versus non-operative management following Rockwood grade III acromioclavicular separation: a meta-analysis of the current evidence base. *J Orthopaedics and Traumatology* **12**, 19.

Taylor, A., Kerry, R., 2015. Haemodynamics and clinical practice. In: Jull, G., Moore, A., Falla, D., et al. (eds) *Grieves Modern Musculoskeletal Physiotherapy*. Elsevier.

Teys, P., Bisset, L., Vicenzino, B., 2006. The initial effects of a Mulligan's mobilisation with movement technique on range of movement and pressure pain threshold in pain-limited shoulders. *Manual Therapy* **13**, 37–42.

Tibone, J., Sellers, R., Tonino, P., 1992. Strength testing after third-degree acromioclavicular dislocations. *American Journal of Sports Medicine* **20**, 328–331.

Ticker, J.B., Bigliani, L.U., 1994. Impingement pathology of the rotator cuff. In: Andrews, J.R. and Wilk, K.E. (eds) *The Athletes Shoulder*. Churchill Livingstone. Edinburgh.

Torstensen, T.A., Meen, H.D., Stiris, M., 1994. The effect of medical exercise therapy on a patient with chronic supraspinatus tendinitis. Diagnostic ultrasound-tissue regeneration: a case study. *Journal of Orthopaedic and Sports Physical Therapy* **20**, 319–327.

Uhl, T.L., Kibler, W.B., Gecewich, B. et al., 2009. Evaluation of clinical assessment methods for scapular dyskinesis. *Arthroscopy* **25** (11), 1240–1248.

Van der Windt, D., Koes, B., 2002. Are corticosteroid injections as effective as physiotherapy for the treatment of a painful shoulder? In: MacAuley, D., Best, T. (eds), *Evidence Based Sports Medicine*. BMJ Books, London.

Vavken, P., Sadoghi, P., Quidde, J., 2014. Immobilization in internal or external rotation does not change recurrence rates after traumatic anterior shoulder dislocation. *J Shoulder Elbow Surg* **23** (1),13–19.

Vermeulen, H.M., Obermann, W.M., Burger, B.J., Kok, G.J., 2000. End range mobilisation techniques in adhesive capsulitis of the shoulder joint. *Physical Therapy* **80**, 1204–1213.

Walton, D.M., Sadi, J., 2008. Identifying SLAP lesions: a meta-analysis of clinical tests and exercise in clinical reasoning. *Physical Therapy in Sport* **9** (4), 167–176.

Werner, C.M., Favre, P., Gerber, C., 2007. The role of the subscapularis in preventing anterior glenohumeral subluxation in the abducted, externally rotated position of the arm. *Clin Biomech* **22**, 495–501.

Werner, A., Mueller, T., Boehm, D., Gohlke, F., 2000. The stabilizing sling for the long head of the biceps tendon in the rotator cuff interval. A histoanatomic study. *American Journal of Sports Medicine* **28** (1), 28–31.

Whelan, D., Kletke, S., Schemitsch, G. et al., 2015. Immobilization in external rotation versus internal rotation after primary anterior shoulder dislocation: a meta-analysis of randomized controlled trials. *American Journal of Sports Medicine* **44** (2), 521–532.

Wilk, K.E., Arrigo, C., 1993. Current concepts in the rehabilitation of the athletic shoulder. *Journal of Orthopaedic and Sports Physical Therapy* **18** (1), 365–378.

Wilk, K.E., Macrina, L.C., Fleisig, G.S. et al., 2011. Correlation of glenohumeral internal rotation deficit and total rotational motion to shoulder injuries in professional baseball pitchers. *American Journal of Sports Medicine* **39** (2), 329–335.

Wolfe, S.W., Wickiewicz, T.L., Cavanaugh, J.T., 1992. Ruptures of the pectoralis major muscle: an anatomic and clinical analysis. *American Journal of Sports Medicine* **20**, 587–593.

Zachazewski, J.E., Magee, D.J., Quillen, W.S., 1996. *Athletic Injuries and Rehabilitation*. W.B. Saunders, Philadelphia.

Zuckerman, J.D. and Rokito, A., 2011. Frozen shoulder: a consensus definition. *J Shoulder Elb Surg* **20**, 322–325.

CHAPTER 13

The elbow

Structure and function

The primary purpose of the shoulder is often described as positioning the arm to facilitate hand action. The elbow, in turn, functions to shorten or lengthen the arm, largely to allow the hand to be brought to the mouth. The elbow complex consists of the humeroulnar and humeroradial articulations and the superior radioulnar joint, all of which share the same capsule (Fig. 13.1).

> ### Definition
> Joints within the elbow are: humeroulnar between the trochlea of the humerus and the trochlea notch of the ulnar; humeroradial between the capitulum of the humerus and the superior surface of the head of the radius; superior radioulnar between the circumference of the head of the radius and the fibro-osseous ring formed by the radial notch of the ulna and the annular ligament.

When viewed from the side, the distal end of the humerus is larger anteriorly and inferiorly, and sits at an angle of 45 degrees to the longitudinal axis of the bone. Similarly, the trochlear notch of the ulna bulges, making a comparable angle to its axis. This structure postpones contact between the humerus

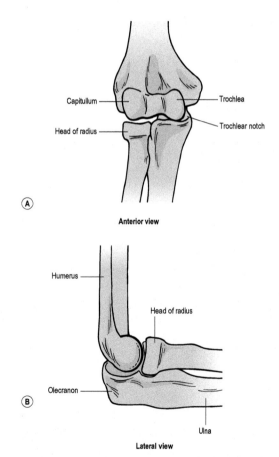

Figure 13.1 Articulations forming the elbow joint. (A) Anterior view. (B) Lateral view.

and ulna on flexion, and allows more space between the bones to accommodate soft tissues. The 'nutcracker effect' is therefore reduced as the bones come together.

Bony alignment and joint contact areas

Viewed from the front, the radius and ulna are slanted laterally to the shaft of the humerus, the angulation forming the carrying angle (Fig. 13.2A). This is approximately 10–15 degrees for men, increasing to 20–25 degrees for women. This bony alignment means that, normally, as the arm is flexed the hand moves towards the shoulder, and the radius and ulna end up in line with the humerus (Fig. 13.2C). Variations in carrying angle between individuals, mainly due to altered configuration of the trochlear groove, may occur and will alter the resting position of the radius and ulnar at full flexion (Fig. 13.2B, D). Changes in bony alignment may also occur after injury – an important factor in rehabilitation following elbow fractures.

The contact area between the joint surfaces of the elbow complex increases throughout flexion. In full extension the lower medial part of the trochlear notch of the ulna is used, with no contact occurring between the radius and ulna. At 90 degrees the contact area is a diagonal (lower medial to upper lateral) across the trochlear surface, with only slight pressure between the humerus and radial head. In full flexion definite contact occurs between the radius and ulna, and the trochlear contact areas increase (Fig. 13.3). Full flexion is thus required to ensure adequate nutrition of the whole articular cartilage, a situation sometimes not possible in obese or heavily muscled individuals due to the approximation of the flexor soft tissues.

Collateral ligaments

The elbow collateral ligaments are positioned on the ulnar (inner) and radial (outer) aspects of the joint. The ulnar or medial collateral ligament (MCL) spreads out from the medial epicondyle to form two thick anterior and posterior bands, joined by a thinner intermediate (oblique) portion, together

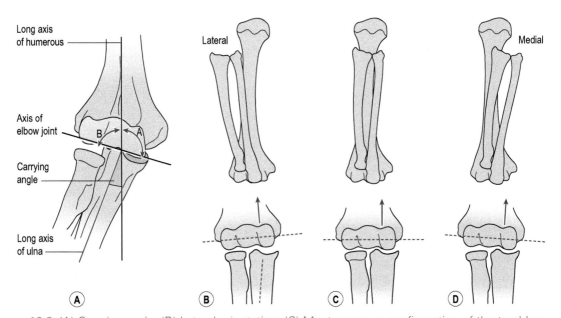

Figure 13.2 (A) Carrying angle. (B) Lateral orientation. (C) Most common configuration of the trochlear groove. (D) Medial orientation. After Norkin and Levangie (1992), with permission.

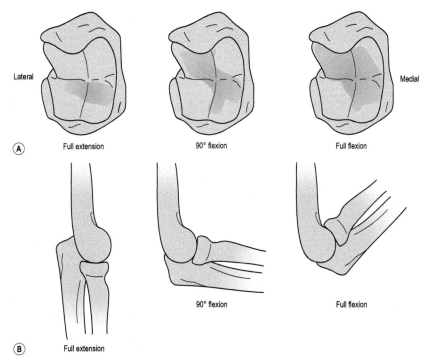

Figure 13.3 Contact areas at different elbow positions. (A) The trochlear notch. (B) The head of the radius. From Palastanga, Field and Soames (2013), with permission.

sometimes being termed the medial collateral ligament complex (MCLC).

> **Key point**
>
> The medial collateral ligament (MCL) has three portions – anterior, posterior and oblique.

The radial or lateral collateral ligament (LCL) is a single triangular structure attaching just below the lateral epicondyle and blending with the annular ligament of the radius. In addition, fibres from the extensor carpi radialis brevis (ECRB) tendon fuse with the LCL, allowing load sharing between the structures (Coombes et al. 2015).

As occurs in the knee, the collateral ligaments of the elbow become taut at different degrees of flexion. The anterior fibres of both the medial and lateral collateral ligaments are taut in extension,

whereas the posterior fibres are taut in flexion. Protection is provided against valgus and varus strains throughout the whole range of joint movement as a result.

Flexion is limited by muscle contact and impingement of the radial head on to the radial fossa. In addition, tension occurs in the triceps and posterior joint capsule, and finally, in lean individuals, the shafts of the radius and humerus themselves come into contact (Fig. 13.4A).

In extension, when the muscles are relaxed, valgus stability is provided by the medial collateral ligament, anterior capsule and bony configuration. As the elbow flexes, the anterior capsule relaxes, and its role is taken on by the medial collateral ligament, which provides 31 per cent of joint stability in extension and 54 per cent at 90-degrees flexion (Table 13.1). In contrast, varus stress is resisted in the main by bone contact supplemented by the anterior capsule. The lateral collateral

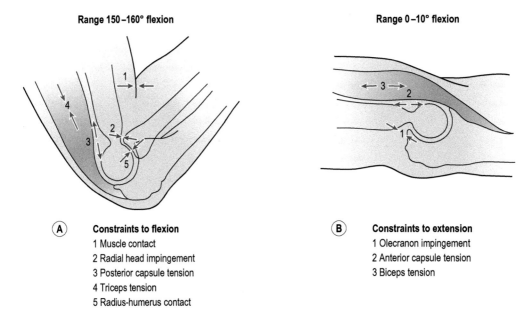

Figure 13.4 Constraints to (A) flexion and (B) extension. From Reid (1992), with permission.

Table 13.1 Percentage contribution of elbow structures to stability of the joint

Limiting structure	Valgus %		Varus %		Distribution %	
	0°	90°	0°	90°	0°	90°
Medial collateral ligament	31	54	—	—	6	78
Lateral collateral ligament	—	—	14	9	5	10
Joint capsule	38	10	31	13	85	8
Bone contact	31	33	55	75	—	—

After Morrey and Kai-Nan (1983).

ligament only contributes 14 per cent of the total stability of the joint with the elbow in full extension, and 9 per cent with it flexed to 90 degrees (Morrey and Kai-Nan 1983). With joint distraction, the main limiting factor in extension is the joint capsule, and with the joint flexed to 90 degrees, the medial collateral ligament. End-range is limited by a combination of the olecranon impinging into the olecranon fossa, and tension in the anterior capsule and biceps (Fig. 13.4B).

Pronation and supination of the forearm involve not just the superior and inferior radioulnar joints, but also the ulnohumeral, radiohumeral and radiocarpal joints. With pronation, the head of the radius twists on the capitulum and swings on the radial notch of the ulna, tightening the quadrate ligament. The radial head tilts, and is pulled into the capitulotrochlear groove, and the ulna moves into slight extension and abduction at the ulnohumeral joint. Consequent to this, at the inferior radioulnar joint the ulnar notch of the radius swings medially over the ulnar head. A traumatic injury to the elbow is therefore likely to affect the wrist, and, to be complete, clinical examination should include both joints.

Screening examination

Prior to objective examination, a full subjective history is taken. Key points with elbow injury are a history of falling onto the outstretched arm or of the elbow being pulled and feeling as though it 'came out' when hanging from a bar or throwing. This would suggest the need for imaging. Altered sensation or skin discoloration may imply neurological involvement, and any change in grip or finger movement should be investigated further.

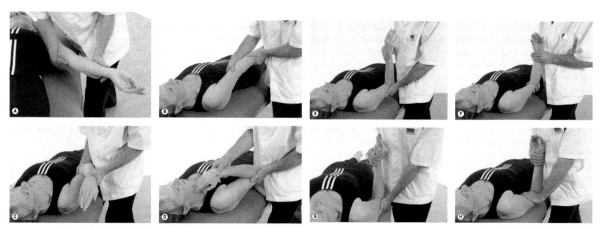

Figure 13.5 (A) Abduction; (B) adduction; (C) flexion–abduction; (D) flexion–adduction; (E) pronation; (F) supination; (G) compression; (H) distraction.

Objective examination begins with observation of the body region followed by active and then passive movements. Flexion and extension are each performed to full range, noting the joint end-feel. The normal end-feel to extension is hard while that to flexion is soft. Pronation and supination are performed with the elbow held to the side of the body and the arm flexed to 90 degrees. The end-feel should be springy. Further differentiation may be obtained by combining flexion and extension with abduction and adduction (valgus/varus) stresses, and by assessing gliding motions of the individual component joints of the elbow complex (Fig. 13.5). The capsular pattern is of flexion more limited than extension, and rotations relatively free.

The inferior radioulnar joint is stressed by pronation and supination, and may require further examination if pain is produced. Screening examinations of the neck and shoulder are performed if referred pain is suspected, and full neurological examination may be required. The front of the elbow lies within the C5 and C6 dermatomes, while the back of the elbow is in the C7 dermatome. Pain may therefore be referred to the elbow from the cervical nerve roots or the shoulder region.

The contractile structures are examined by resisted movements, performed first with the elbow flexed to 90 degrees. One of the therapist's hands supports the elbow to restrict shoulder movement and the other applies resistance to flexion and extension. For pronation and supination, the lower forearm (not the hand) is gripped. The grip must be tight and positioned over the radial styloid to avoid a friction burn to the patient's skin. Resisted wrist flexion and extension are performed with the elbow locked.

Ligamentous instability may be assessed by combining movement of the forearm and upper arm. The MCL is assessed by applying an abduction force to the forearm with the elbow unlocked. At the same time the humerus is laterally rotated. For the LCL the technique is reversed, an adduction force being imposed on the forearm and the humerus pulled into medial rotation. In each case, both excessive movement and reproduction of the patient's symptoms indicate a positive test result.

Lateral pain

The term 'tennis elbow' is often used colloquially as a blanket description for any soft tissue pain between the shoulder and wrist, and there has been little agreement in the past as to the exact site of the lesion. The condition was first

Table 13.2 General causes of tennis elbow

Radiohumeral bursitis
Periostitis of the common extensor tendon
Tendinitis: extensor carpi radialis brevis, supinator
Microtendinous tears of the common extensor tendon with subtendinous granulation and fibrosis
Myofascitis
Radial head fibrillation/chondromalacia
Calcification
Radial nerve entrapment and subsequent fibrosis
Stenosis of the orbicular ligament
Hyperaemic synovial fringe
Inflammation of the annular ligament
Cervical radiculopathy

From Lee, D.G. (1986), with permission.

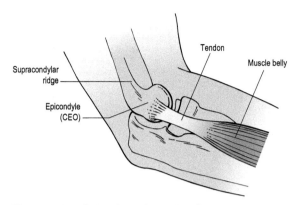

Figure 13.6 Palpation of tennis elbow.

documented in the late 1800s, when it was described as 'lawn tennis arm'. Cyriax (1936) described 26 different lesions to which the condition had been attributed, while Lee (1986) cited 12 more general causes, as shown in Table 13.2. The terms 'lateral' and 'medial tennis elbow' have been used (Nirschl 1988), but in this book the name tennis elbow is used to describe lateral epicondylitis while 'golfer's elbow' refers to medial epicondylitis. The ratio of lateral to medial epicondylitis encountered clinically has been shown to be 7:1 (Leach and Miller 1987).

Tennis elbow (lateral epicondylalgia) is a lesion to the common extensor origin (CEO), with the primary site being the tendon of extensor carpi radialis brevis (ECRB) and/or the extensor carpi radialis longus (ECRL). ECRL attaches to the *lateral supracondylar ridge* (lower third) and travels to the base of the *second metacarpal*, while ECRB attaches more distally to the *lateral epicondyle* itself via the common extensor tendon where it spreads onto the lateral ligament of the elbow. From here the muscle inserts into the base of the *third metacarpal*. When testing for tennis elbow (see below) the muscles may be differentiated by placing resistance over the second and third metacarpals. Pain with rested middle finger extension (third metacarpal) suggests ECRB. Most commonly, the injury is at the tenoperiosteal junction of the tendons, but scar tissue may

form onto the tendons themselves or the musculotendinous junction (Fig. 13.6).

> **Key point**
>
> Tennis elbow affects: (i) the tendon of extensor carpi radialis brevis at the epicondyle; (ii) tendon of extensor carpi radialis longus onto the supracondylar ridge.

Pathophysiology

The pathological features of tendinopathy have been covered in previous chapters for the Achilles (Chapter 6), patellar tendon (Chapter 4) and rotator cuff (Chapter 12). In the case of tennis elbow local tendon pathology is that of immature and dysfunctional healing called *angiofibroblastic hyperplasia*. This process has four key elements: (i) collagen cell numbers and the amount of ground substance increase, (ii) vascular hyperplasia (neovascularization) is seen, (iii) there is an increase in the concentration of local neurochemicals and (iv) collagen is both disorganized and immature (Coombes, Bissel and Vicenzino 2009). In line with other types of tendinopathy, standard inflammatory markers are not present, although neurogenic inflammation has been identified (Fredberg and Stengaard-Pedersen 2008).

Definition

Neurogenic inflammation occurs when there is a local release of inflammatory chemicals from sensory (afferent) nerves. Chemicals involved include Substance P, calcitonin gene-related peptide (CGRP) and glutamate.

Stress imposed on the affected tissues is not uniform, with the deeper tendon regions being placed under a lesser load (stress shielding). These areas may be open to overload, and in the case of ECRB the deep and anterior fibres have been highlighted as potentially problematic.

In addition to tendon pathology, both *pain system change* and *motor impairment* have been proposed as important for a multimodal treatment approach (Coombes, Bissel and Vicenzino 2009). As with many painful conditions, tennis elbow is characterized by an exaggerated response to noxious stimuli (hyperalgesia). Testing local pain response using pressure, tennis elbow sufferers have been shown to have a lower pain threshold (66 per cent) on the injured side compared to the uninjured side (Pienimäki et al. 2002). This change in pain threshold is often bilateral, implying an alteration in central sensitization. In addition, tennis elbow sufferers often have positive cervical joint signs and/or positive radial nerve bias upper limb tension test (ULTT), suggesting that neural involvement is not restricted to the local tissues.

Morphological changes in the muscles affected by tennis elbow include fibre necrosis, increased fast twitch fibre ratio and muscle fibre regeneration (Coombes, Bissel and Vicenzino 2009), consistent with the finding that grip strength is reduced in tennis elbow patients. In addition, motor control changes occur with wrist position changing during standard grip task, with less extension being present. Normal grip requires the wrist extensors to stabilize the wrist against the strong pull of the long finger flexors, which tend to flex the wrist. In a group of 40 subjects, Bisset et al. (2006) showed wrist postures that were less extended (mean value 11 degrees) and upper-limb reaction times which were significantly altered.

Key point

Tennis elbow patients show a combination of altered tissue pathology, pain system change and upper limb motor impairment. These changes require a multimodal treatment approach.

Clinical presentation

Tennis elbow usually presents as pain over the region of the lateral epicondyle, extending distally. The pain may build up slowly (overuse) or be the result of a single incident (trauma). Pain is usually increased with resisted wrist extension. Depending on the site of the lesion, pain can be made worse by adding forearm supination (but see radial tunnel syndrome, below), and radial deviation of the wrist (Halle, Franklin and Karalfa 1986). Performing resisted wrist extension with the elbow fully extended will usually elicit pain, even in mild cases. Resisting the third metacarpal places the emphasis on ECRB rather than ECRL, which attaches to the base of the second metacarpal (Maudsley's test).

The condition is most common with athletes over 30 years of age, and occurs normally when repeated wrist extension is combined with forearm supination. Racquet sports involve this action, but several occupational stresses can also be causal factors. Hammering, painting and using heavy spanners will all exacerbate the problem, so any training modification which is prescribed must also take into account an athlete's job. Pain usually increases when small objects are gripped, as this hand position places additional stretch on the forearm extensors.

Key point

Tennis elbow is exacerbated by activities involving repeated wrist extension while gripping a thin object.

As with most overuse syndromes, the ache may initially subside when the stressful activity is discontinued, but as the condition progresses pain even occurs at rest. Patients complain of a weak grip, and wasting of the affected muscles may be seen in long-standing cases. Close inspection will often reveal slight swelling over the affected area, but this is rarely obvious to the patient.

Treatment

Acute phase

Treatment aims initially to reduce pain and swelling. The POLICE protocol is used, and reducing the stress applied to the tendon is important. Active rest from exacerbating activities and the use of counterforce bracing can be effective. A wait-and-see approach (load reduction, self-administered medication, ice or heat usage) has been recommended for those subjects at low risk (Coombes et al. 2015). Low risk may be assessed using outcome measures such as the Patient Related Tennis Elbow Evaluation (PRTEE), which is a reliable and valuable questionnaire (Vincent and MacDermid 2014). It consists of 15 questions (5 related to pain and 10 to function) which give a total score of 100 (worse pain and disability). Scores greater than 54 represent a severe condition, those less than 33 a mild one. The PRTEE score may be downloaded from this site: http://srs-mcmaster.ca/wp-content/uploads/2015/05/English-PRTEE.pdf.

Taping and bracing may be useful to modulate pain. The counterforce brace consists of a tight strap which is placed around the upper forearm to create a lateral pressure when an object is gripped. The aim is to redirect and disperse overload to healthy tissue or to the band itself, and in so doing reduce painful inhibition and permit a more forceful contraction. Using this technique, grip strength has been shown to improve (Wadsworth et al. 1989), and a positive effect has been shown using biomechanical analysis and technique correction of tennis serves and backhand strokes (Groppel and Nirschl 1986).

Deload taping may also be used (Fig. 13.7). The tape aims to offload pain at its site on the common extensor origin (CEO). Rigid tape is applied under traction, with four pieces forming a diamond shape,

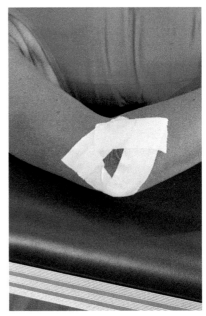

Figure 13.7 Deload taping.

in each case drawing the skin towards the CEO to give a puckered (orange peel) skin effect. Pain-free grip strength has been shown to reduce by 24 per cent from baseline in a small study (n=16), with a 19 per cent reduction in pressure pain threshold (Vicenzino 2003).

The use of nitric oxide given in a transdermal patch as glyceryl trinitrate (GTN) has been described in the treatment of tennis elbow. When compared to placebo, patients in the glyceryl trinitrate group had significantly reduced pain with activity, reduced epicondylar tenderness and increased wrist extensor force. A concentration of 1.25 mg per 24 hours is traditionally used, cutting a 0.5 mg patch into four and applying this quarter of a patch each day. However, a more recent study (Paoloni et al. 2009) did not support these earlier results, showing a significant decrease in elbow pain with activity using GTN at a concentration of 0.72 mg/day compared to placebo, but not with 1.25, 1.44 or 3.6 mg/day. In addition, GTN patches can give complications including headache, weakness, dizziness and skin irritation, causing 12 per cent of patients to discontinue treatment as a result of these side effects (Coombes, Bissel and Vicenzino 2009).

Exercise

As the local swelling adheres and shrinks, inelastic scar tissue can be formed. Stretching exercises can therefore be of value. A useful forearm extensor stretch may be performed with the athlete facing a wall (Fig. 13.8A). The dorsum of the hand is placed flat onto the wall, and the elbow remains locked. By leaning forwards, the wrist is forced into 90-degree flexion, stretching the posterior forearm tissues. Wrist flexion may be combined with a pronation stretch (Fig. 13.8B). Keeping the elbow locked, the forearm is maximally pronated and the wrist flexed. Overpressure is applied with the

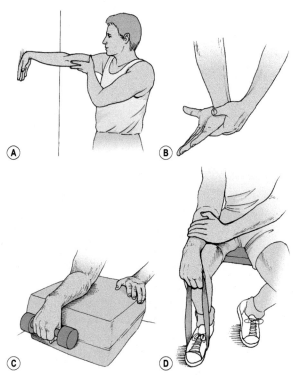

(A)   (B)

(C)   (D)

Figure 13.8 Exercise therapy for tennis elbow. (A) Forearm extensor stretch against wall. (B) Combined flexion–pronation of wrist. (C) Resisted forearm extension (dumb-bell). (D) Resisted extension (band).

other hand and a static stretch performed. The scar tissue is more pliable when warm so the athlete is advised to practise stretching after a hot bath or shower.

Resistance exercises (weight or powerband) are used to re-strengthen the forearm extensors. Wrist extension may be performed holding a small (2 kg) dumb-bell. The forearm is supported on a block or over the couch side and full range movement is attempted (Fig. 13.8C). Initially this is performed with the elbow flexed to reduce pain on the affected muscle (ECRL), and as pain allows the elbow is extended. Powerband extension is performed with the athlete sitting. One end of the band is placed beneath the foot and the other end gripped. The forearm is supported along the athlete's thigh (Fig. 13.8D). Initially, eccentric contractions are likely to be less painful than concentric, and the use of ice massage to produce a temporary anaesthesia before exercise (cryokinetics) is often used.

One word of caution: negative transfer effects have been described when using high-weight, low-repetition training following tennis elbow. To avoid this, Nirschl (1988) recommended the use of high-speed skill training as part of the total rehabilitation programme.

Use of an eight-week programme of stretching and strengthening involving a progression of slow wrist and forearm stretching, muscle conditioning and occupational exercises (Pienimäki et al. 1996) has been shown to result in significantly less pain, both at rest and under strain, and an improved subjective ability to work when compared to a group using ultrasound alone. Comparing supervised exercise, Cyriax treatment (manual therapy and friction massage) and light therapy (Bioptron) given three times per week over a four-week period, Stasinopoulos and Stasinopoulos (2006) found that the supervised exercise programme produced the largest effect in terms of pain reduction and improvement of function.

Key point

Exercise therapy has been shown to produce statistically significant results in the treatment of tennis elbow, and should be considered in all cases of this condition.

Manual therapy

Manual therapy, including local massage to reduce swelling and produce hyperaemia, and transverse frictions to modulate pain and mobilize soft tissue, can be of use. It is important to locate the exact site of injury for transverse frictions to be effective. The forearm should be pronated and supinated while the area is palpated to find the exact site of the CEO. The lateral epicondyle should be identified, as should the supracondylar ridge, and each considered as a possible source of pain. The teno-osseous junction is best frictioned with the forearm in mid-position to let the CEO relax slightly and allow the palpating finger to get right onto the bony surface. The tendon itself is treated on stretch with the elbow and wrist flexed, and forearm pronated (Fig. 13.9A).

Mills manipulation (Mills 1928), although originally designed to stress the annular ligament, can be performed to stretch the CEO. The patient's arm is held in extension at the shoulder, with the elbow comfortably flexed and wrist and forearm fully flexed and pronated (Fig. 13.9B). A high-velocity, low-amplitude thrust is applied to the elbow to fully extend it. Cyriax and Cyriax (1983) claimed this procedure would pull apart the tissue surfaces joined by a painful scar, the fresh tear being replaced by new fibrous tissue under no tension.

Mobilization with movement has been shown to be an effective treatment for this condition (Vicenzino and Wright 1995). In this technique, a sustained mobilization is applied to a joint, normally at 90 degrees to the plane of movement, to correct joint tracking (Mulligan 1989). The mobilization is applied at the same time as the patient performs a painful action with the affected joint. In the case of tennis elbow, this action is normally extension of the wrist or fingers (especially the third finger).

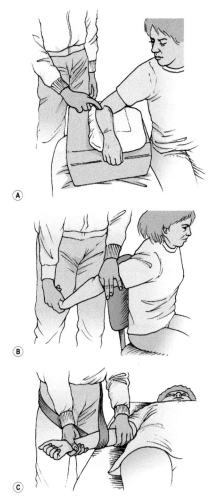

Figure 13.9 Manual therapy for tennis elbow. (A) Deep transverse friction to the common extensor origin. (B) Mills manipulation. (C) Mobilization with movement using belt.

This technique has been shown to be effective in the treatment of tennis elbow. In a study of 25 subjects, Abbott, Patla and Jensen (2001) used a single mobilization with movement (MWM) treatment and found less pain with active motion, greater pain-free grip strength and improved maximum grip in 92 per cent of subjects.

With the patient in a supine position, the therapist wraps a belt around his or her own hips and the athlete's forearm. The proximal edge of the belt is level with the elbow joint. The humerus and forearm are stabilized by the therapist's hands. The mobilization (lateral glide of the ulna) is carried out by the therapist gently leaning back (Fig. 13.9C). The aim is to reduce the pain of the finger extension action, initially while the mobilization is applied and eventually during free movement. MWM using a posteroanterior (PA) glide on the radial head may also be used (see below).

Key point
Research supports the use of mobilization with movement (MWM) in the treatment of tennis elbow.

Where general elbow stiffness is present as a result of previous inflammation, joint mobilization may be required. Overpressure to either flexion or extension may be combined with adduction and abduction to regain accessory movement. Mobilization of the radial head may also be useful in cases of tennis elbow, and end-range pronation and supination with overpressure may be performed. Direct palpation may be given to the radial head using the therapist's thumbs. For a PA (posteroanterior) glide, the patient's elbow is flexed and the bony contour of the radial head is easily palpable. AP (anteroposterior) glides are performed with the patient's arm extended, and the radial head is palpated through the anterior soft tissues.

Radial head PA glides may also be used as an MWM. The subject grips maximally and relaxes to assess grip strength (dynamometry) and pain (NRS). The PA glide is applied and sustained as the subject repeatedly grips and relaxes. Where grip strength increases and/or pain is reduced, the MWM is repeated several times.

Neurodynamic treatment in tennis elbow pain

Manual therapy to the cervical or thoracic spine may also be useful where elbow symptoms are reproduced using cervical spine movement to neurodynamic testing. Local joint mobilization may be used to assess for reproduction of the subject's familiar pain, and the radial nerve neurodynamic test may be performed. For this procedure the subject is supine and shoulder girdle depression, elbow extension, shoulder adduction and internal rotation, forearm pronation, and wrist and finger flexion are combined. Mechanosensitivity is present where the subject's symptoms (caused by the arm/hand wind-up) are reduced using ipsilateral lateral flexion of the cervical spine or scapular elevation. Where mechanosensitivity is present, slider or tensioning actions may be used with the radial nerve test.

For the radial nerve stretch, (Fig. 13.10A) the subject begins standing with the shoulder depressed. The action is to adduct the affected shoulder, rotating it inwards to place it behind the small of the back. The wrist is flexed and the forearm pronated. The stretch can be increased by flexing the neck, while shrugging the shoulders (scapular elevation) reduces the stretch.

The radial nerve slider (Fig. 13.10B) begins with the subject sitting on a stool or gym bench. The right arm is bent at the elbow and the forearm supinated. At the same time the head is tilted away from the arm (cervical lateral flexion). Using a single smooth action, the arm is straightened and medially rotated, bending the wrist and fingers to bring the palm upwards. The head is then laterally flexed and rotated to look at the hand. The aim is to slide the radial nerve but maintain its overall length. As the arm straightens, the radial nerve is lengthened in the arm, but as the head looks towards the arm the nerve is shortened in the neck.

Biomechanics

The extensor carpi radialis brevis is under maximum tension when it contracts in a position of forearm pronation, wrist flexion and ulna deviation (Briggs and Elliott 1985). This is a typical position for a backhand shot in racquet sports, and elements of this anatomical alignment are seen in many repetitive actions in sport and daily living. Repeated practice will cause hypertrophy of this muscle and

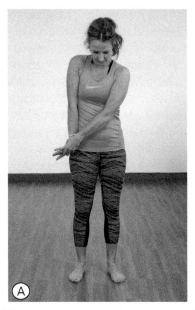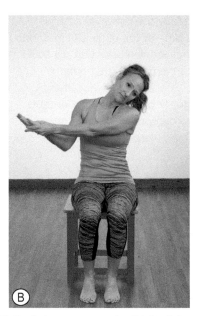

Figure 13.10 Radial nerve neurodynamic treatment. (A) Radial nerve stretch. (B) Radial nerve slider.

often a resultant loss of flexibility. In addition, an imbalance may exist between the forearm flexors and extensors. Normally, the wrist extensors should be at least 50 per cent of the flexors, but in many recreational sports an individual may have considerably weaker wrist extensors in proportion to flexors. The combination of weaker and less flexible wrist extensors placed in a demanding situation of the backhand stroke (or similar occupational action) exceeds the load capacity of the tissues. One action an athlete may take as part of a preventive programme for this condition, therefore, is to maintain the flexibility of the wrist musculature, and build up the strength of the wrist extensors to as much as 75 per cent of the flexor strength.

Ergonomics can play an important part in the management of this condition. Enlarging the grip of any object being held, be it a racquet or a spanner, is important in most cases. The correct grip size can be calculated by measuring from the tip of the ring finger to the bottom lateral crease of the palm, directly below (Fig. 13.12). The figure obtained represents the circumference of the racquet handle. Placing a thick piece of sponge

around a handle is also useful to enlarge the grip and reduce shock travelling from the handle to the hand. In some cases a grip which is too large may also be a problem, so to assess if grip size is a relevant feature, ask the patient to grip a thin object (a pencil) and a large one (a bottle) and find which gives less pain. In general terms, when prolonged grip is applied, the therapist should be able to place one finger between the tips of the athlete's fingers and thumb.

In tennis, higher impact and torsion forces are produced by a wet, heavy ball or a racquet which is too tightly strung. The closer the ball is to the centre of percussion (the mathematical point on the racquet face where no torsion will occur on impact), the less strain on the elbow tissues.

Key point

One factor in prevention of tennis elbow is to increase forearm extensor strength and flexibility. In addition, the circumference of the object being gripped should be increased, so that one finger width can be placed between the athlete's fingers and thumb.

Treatment note 13.1 Trigger points and acupuncture points in the treatment of tennis elbow

Both classical acupuncture points and trigger points (TrPs) may be useful in the treatment of tennis elbow, and have been shown to be superior to sham points (Molsberger and Hille 1994, Fink et al. 2002). TrPs in the extensor carpi radialis longus and brevis may be palpated with the elbow flexed and hand unsupported. Begin over the common extensor origin and palpate distally. Central points are located on the ulnar side of the brachioradialis muscle 4–5 cm distal to the elbow crease (at the approximate point of the classical points LI-10, LI-9 and LI-8) while attachment TrPs are located at the common extensor origin.

The TrP may be treated with either dry needling or deep massage. For massage, the therapist's thumbs are used beginning over the patient's supracondylar ridge and epicondyle, extending into the muscle belly. The whole of the area may be treated using a muscle stripping technique, pressing in a line from the epicondyle to the thumb. Ischaemic compression may be used over a single active point using a plunger and the patient may be taught self-palpation (Fig. 13.11).

Dry needling uses either an intramuscular technique to a depth of 0.5–1.5 cm depending on muscle bulk, or needling close to the epicondyle with the intention of striking the bone using a periosteal technique. Here, the aim is to stimulate the richly innervated periosteum to give pain relief (Mann 1992).

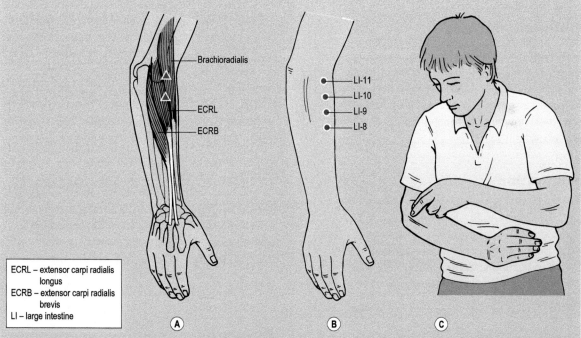

Brachioradialis

ECRL

ECRB

LI-11
LI-10
LI-9
LI-8

ECRL – extensor carpi radialis
longus
ECRB – extensor carpi radialis
brevis
LI – large intestine

(A)　　　(B)　　　(C)

Figure 13.11 Tennis elbow treatment. (A) Trigger points. (B) Classical acupuncture points. (C) Self-treatment.

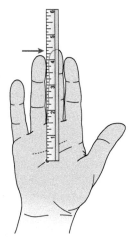

Figure 13.12 Hand measurement to determine proper grip handle size. The distance from the proximal palmar crease to the tip of the middle finger determines the proper size. From Nirschl (1988), with permission.

Osteochondrosis

The most common site for osteochondrosis in the elbow is the anterolateral surface of the capitulum. In younger children (under 11) this may represent Panner's disease, and the two are often described together; however, osteochondrosis occurs in adolescents.

> **Definition**
>
> *Osteochondrosis* is an interruption of the blood supply to the epiphyses (growth region) of a bone. *Osteochondritis* is inflammation of the bone or cartilage within a joint which may lead to cartilage fragmentation. *Osteonecrosis* is death of a portion of bone due to disruption of its blood flow.

The aetiology is generally either traumatic or vascular, although some familial tendency may be present. The condition is most commonly related to throwing or racquet sports. In throwing, the angular velocity experienced at the joint may exceed 300°/s. This, coupled with a valgus force and an extension stress, causes the radial head to impinge against the capitulum. Ultimately, a breakdown can occur in the capitulum surface and the radial head may hypertrophy.

The vascular supply to the area can be disrupted by this repeated trauma. Up until the age of five years the capitulum has a good blood supply, but later the nucleus of the capitulum receives only one or two vessels. These pass into the area posteriorly through soft, compressible cartilage – a possible site of damage. Early stages of osteochondrosis (see Chapter 1) show as a radiolucent (more transparent) area with an open capitellar growth plate. Later stages show as a closed growth plate. Normally X-rays are taken with the elbow flexed to 45 degrees to visualize the capitulum changes.

The typical subject is an active individual in early adolescence (usually male) who shows limitation of elbow extension with local swelling. Onset is often insidious and the patient may have been experiencing difficulties over a protracted period. If the osteochondrotic fragment is free within the joint, locking or catching may be experienced with certain movements. Radiographs may show blunting of the capitulum with enlargement of the radial head. Often an island of bone is seen surrounded by an area of rarefaction. Premature epiphyseal closure may also be noted to either the humerus or the proximal radius.

In the initial stages of the condition with a young subject, rest is all that is required, splinting being indicated if the patient fails to heed this advice. If stress has been allowed to continue and bony degeneration has occurred, drilling or grafting of the attached fragment may be required. In late-stage conditions loose bodies may need to be removed, and unfortunately the prognosis is sometimes poor.

> **Key point**
>
> With Osteochondrosis of the elbow: (i) the patient is typically a male, involved in a throwing sport, and in early adolescence, (ii) pain comes on gradually, (iii) extension is reduced and (iv) there may be local swelling.

Conservative management consists of avoidance of heavy usage of the elbow, usually for a six-month period. In a study of 176 competitive baseball players, Matsuura et al. (2008) showed healing in 90.5 per cent of Stage I patients and 52.9 per cent of Stage II, patients with the mean healing period being 14.9 and 12.3 months, respectively. Mihara et al. (2009) showed spontaneous healing of the capitellar growth plate in 25 out of 30 early-stage lesions, but only 1 out of 9 advanced-stage lesions. These authors recommended surgery to achieve healing in advanced cases.

Medial pain

Lesions to the medial side of the joint occur most often with throwing actions. Although different sports demand different throwing techniques, similarities still exist. Initially, the shoulder is abducted and taken into extreme external rotation and extension, while the elbow remains flexed (cocking phase). Then, the shoulder and trunk rapidly move forward, leaving the arm behind (acceleration phase). This action imposes a valgus stress on the joint and stretches the ulnar collateral ligament in particular. The shoulder flexors and internal rotators contract powerfully, flinging the arm forward and resulting in stress to the olecranon as the arm extends rapidly to full range (deceleration phase and follow-through).

The throwing action imposes a number of stresses on the elbow (Fig. 13.13). The lateral joint line is subjected to compression forces, in the olecranon fossa there are shearing forces, while the medial joint line experiences tensile forces. These forces, if repeated, can give rise to specific injuries and general degeneration reflecting the stress imposed on the elbow structures (Table 13.3).

Medial epicondylitis

This is a lesion of the common flexor origin (CFO) on the medial epicondyle, and is commonly called golfer's elbow. The primary site is the origin of pronator teres and flexor carpi radialis on the medial epicondyle, hence the term *flexor/*

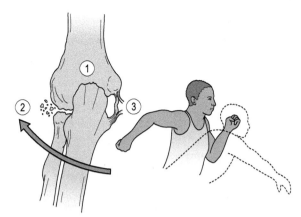

Figure 13.13 Forces on the elbow during throwing. 1. Hypertension – olecranon shear. 2. Valgus – compresses laterally, radial head damage. 3. Valgus – distracts medially, collateral ligament damage.

Table 13.3 Throwing injuries to the elbow

Medial tension	Lateral compression	Posterior shear
Muscular overuse	Osteochondrosis	Muscular strain
Ligamentous injury	Fractured capitulum	Impingement
Capsular injury	Lateral epicondylitis	Olecranon fracture
Ulnar traction spur		Bony hypertrophy
Medial epicondylitis		Loose bodies

pronator tendinopathy. The flexor carpi ulnaris may occasionally be affected. Golfer's elbow is less common than tennis elbow, occurring at a ratio of about 1:15. The injury can be complicated by ulnar nerve involvement, the nerve being compressed at a point distal to the medial epicondyle.

> **Key point**
> Golfer's elbow (medial epicondylitis) mainly affects the pronator teres and flexor carpi radialis muscle. Flexor carpi ulnaris is affected less often, and ulnar nerve involvement may also occur.

585

Sensory symptoms are often present and Tinel's sign (tapping the ulnar nerve at the elbow to produce pain or tingling in the ulnar portion of the hand) is positive. Chronic conditions may see calcium deposits developing within the tendon itself.

Pain is felt more locally than with tennis elbow, and is increased on resisted wrist flexion and sometimes forearm pronation. The condition may be differentiated from chronic medial ligament sprain by applying the valgus stress test, which should not give pain or laxity in epicondylitis.

The treatment is for the most part like that for tennis elbow, including soft tissue manipulation and biomechanical changes to ease pain in the reactive phase of the condition, followed by progressive tissue loading in the recovery stage. Transverse frictions are now performed with the elbow and wrist in extension, with the forearm supinated. Counterforce bracing is again used, but this time the brace extends up to the medial epicondyle to avoid interfering with elbow flexion.

Medial collateral ligament (thrower's elbow)

Repetitive stresses to this ligament are common in throwing athletes, particularly in events such as the javelin. Pain is generally quite localized over the medial joint line, and exacerbated by applying an elbow abduction stress test, forcing a valgus strain on the joint in 20-degree flexion. With severe injuries, gapping of the joint may be apparent.

> **Key point**
>
> Pain in the MCL of the elbow is reproduced using the passive elbow abduction test. For this a valgus (inner opening) strain is placed on the joint in slight flexion.

Initial treatment is to remove the causal stress and rest from throwing, followed by progressive re-strengthening. Operative repair of a ruptured medial collateral ligament is sometimes

recommended for athletes and those involved in heavy manual labour where conservative management has failed. MCL reconstruction typically involves use of an autograft tendon (often palmaris longus) which is placed into ulnar and humeral tunnels. Systematic review (8 studies) has shown excellent results in 83 per cent of patients, with a 10 per cent complication rate. The most common complication (6 per cent) was ulnar neuropathy (Vitale and Ahmad 2008).

Posterior elbow pain

Pain at the back of the elbow is common in activities which rapidly extend or hyperextend the joint. These include the throwing sports, punching in martial arts and pressing actions in weight training. Structures involved, either individually or in combination, include the insertion of the triceps, the olecranon bursa and the olecranon itself (Fig. 13.14).

Olecranon bursitis

The olecranon bursa is placed at the bony point of the elbow, over the olecranon process subcutaneously. A deeper bursa is sometimes

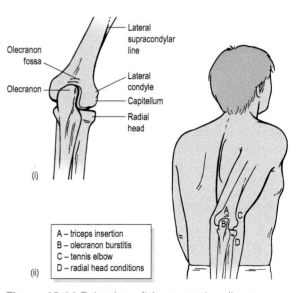

Figure 13.14 Palpation of the posterior elbow.

present between the capsule and triceps. When the elbow is extended, the margins of the olecranon bursa cause a circular ridge of skin about 1.5–2 cm in diameter to be pulled up on the posterior aspect of the elbow.

The bursa can become inflamed by leaning on the elbow for a prolonged period (student's elbow), or from a direct fall onto the point of the elbow. This latter case may induce haemorrhage into the bursal sac itself. Examination of the joint reveals no abnormality, but pain and thickening occur to direct palpation over the bursa. Treatment is to remove the cause, pad the point of the elbow and aspirate the fluid.

Where the bursa becomes infected (septic bursitis), immediate drainage (aspiration) and/or surgical washout may be required, followed by immobilization and oral antibiotics. Signs of bursal infection include local erythema and warmth, marked swelling and sudden symptom exacerbation. General fever and cellulitis of the surrounding skin may also be present.

> **Key point**
> Septic bursitis requires immediate hospital referral for aspiration and antibiotic administration.

Triceps insertion

Triceps tendinopathy may occur in throwing athletes, weight-lifters, and others performing rapid ballistic extension movements. Pathology is usually limited to the olecranon insertion of the muscle. Damage can be to the musculotendinous or teno-osseous junctions, and cessation of activity and correction of technique, coupled with modalities to reduce local inflammation and pain, are usually curative. Treatment is for standard tendinopathy (Chapter 1), with tissue unloading and protection in the reactive phase, and graduated loading in the recovery phase.

Unusually, the medial head of the triceps may sublux over the medial epicondyle during flexion causing a snapping sensation ('snapping elbow syndrome'; Dreyfuss and Kessler 1978). This must be distinguished from subluxation of the ulnar nerve from its groove, which may occur in up to 16 per cent of the population (Reid 1992). Subluxation is normally due to laxity of the ulnar collateral ligament and/or a shallow ulnar groove.

> **Key point**
> Laxity of the ulnar collateral ligament and a shallow ulnar groove can allow the ulnar nerve to sublux and causes neurological symptoms into the fourth and fifth fingers.

Rupture of the triceps tendon, either partial or complete, is unusual, and the muscle belly itself is even less frequently injured. When rupture does occur, there is usually a palpable defect in the musculotendinous junction of the muscle, with scarring in the chronic injury. Active extension is lost, and a large haematoma, later developing into bruising, is noted locally. The majority of patients are in their 30s or 40s, and the injury almost always occurs either following a fall onto the outstretched hand or from a 'chopping' action. In either case, the stress is one of deceleration imposed on an already contracting muscle.

A small fragment of the olecranon may be avulsed and shows up on a lateral radiograph of the elbow, and occasionally radial head fractures are associated with the condition. Conservative management is reserved for partial ruptures (Bach, Warren and Wickiewicz 1987) distinguished by an ability to partially extend the arm against gravity. Surgical management for avulsion injuries involves drilling the olecranon and suturing the muscle. Post-operatively, the patient is immobilized for three to four weeks in a cast or long arm splint at 30–45-degree elbow flexion. Early controlled motion is begun 10–14 days post-operatively, aiming at full elbow extension and limited flexion. The latter is progressed at a timescale dependent on the surgical procedure used.

Posterior impingement

Posterior impingement of the olecranon into its fossa is common in sports where the elbow is 'snapped back'. This is especially the case with rapid weight (circuit) training, and martial arts, where subjects reach upwards as if 'punching the air' while performing Kata (exercise sequences). Throwing events will tend to cause impingement of the medial aspect of the olecranon on the follow-through movement due to the hyperextended valgus angle of the action.

Examination usually reveals point tenderness over the posterior or posteromedial aspect of the olecranon. This is made worse by forced extension, and extension/abduction. Chronic injuries may show osteophyte formation posteromedially. Cortical thickening is also usually seen on radiograph, but this is thought to represent adaptation of the bone to repetitive stress (Garrick and Webb 1990).

Treatment is initially to limit extension and valgus stress by strapping, or if this fails, to rest the elbow completely. The elbow flexors are strengthened (especially eccentrically) to enhance their action as decelerators of elbow extension, and to shorten them and therefore limit hyperextension.

Stress fracture of the olecranon is a rare but often overlooked outcome of posterior impingement, and has been described in javelin throwers and baseball pitchers. Pain usually follows the pattern typical of a stress fracture, eventually limiting performance. Many lesions will respond to rest and splinting, but some require surgery, including excision of the olecranon tip and inlaid bone block graft (Torg 1993). Traumatic fracture of the olecranon may occur through a fall onto the point of the elbow. Where the fragment is undisplaced, immobilization in a posterior splint is normally the treatment of choice. Displaced olecranon fractures require open reduction and internal fixation.

Muscular injury

The biceps, triceps and brachialis may all be injured in sport. The most common injury for the biceps is to its long head (see Chapter 12), but its lower insertion may also be injured occasionally. Pain is reproduced to resisted elbow flexion and supination, and passive pronation, resisted shoulder flexion may also be added. If resisted flexion is painful but supination is not, the brachialis is indicated. The site of pain is the centre of the front of the arm, often radiating as far as the wrist in severe cases.

The usual site for injury to the *triceps* is the musculotendinous junction, but the belly may be injured. Pain on resisted elbow (and shoulder) extension is the clinical sign, but when this test gives pain in the upper arm felt nearer to the shoulder, referred pain from impingement of a shoulder structure should be considered. In this case the triceps contraction pulls the humerus up into the acromion approximating the joint.

Myositis ossificans traumatica

Injury to the *brachialis* should always be treated with caution, because this muscle shares with the quadriceps the potential for myositis development (see Chapter 1).

The history is usually that of a direct blow, for example from a knee or head in rugby or a foot in martial arts. Most commonly, a second blow has been experienced to the same area. The typical findings are tenderness persisting for two to three weeks after injury, and difficulty in regaining full-range motion. On examination, a fibrous mass is often palpable within the muscle over the anterior aspect of the arm.

Key point

The possibility of myositis in the brachialis muscle exists when: (i) there is a history of a number of direct blows to the same area; (ii) tenderness has persisted for two to three weeks after injury; (iii) full range of motion cannot be regained; (iv) there is a palpable mass over the anterior aspect of the arm when compared to the uninjured side.

Where these findings are present, X-ray is required. Often heterotrophic bone formation is seen, showing a diffuse fluffy callus. As the callus matures it will shrink and its margins become better defined. Bone scan will reveal whether the condition is still active.

Management aims initially to minimize the damage. Local swelling is reduced where possible, and activity limited. Mobility exercise is begun with caution when radiographic evidence shows that the condition is no longer active. Resisted work is the last exercise to be started, and when sport is resumed, the area is protected with padding. Rehabilitation of this type, emphasizing joint mobilization and eccentric strengthening especially, has been shown to give full range of motion at the elbow after nine weeks. Follow-up (nine months) showed nearly complete bone maturation and a full return to competitive sport (De Carlo et al. 1992).

Elbow dislocations

Posterior or posterolateral dislocation of the elbow is seen following a fall onto the outstretched arm, sometimes associated with a fracture to the olecranon, coronoid process, or radial head. Mild (Grade I) injuries present as subluxation only, while moderate (Grade II) injuries dislocate with the coronoid process ending up on top of the trochlea. In a severe injury (Grade III) the joint moves further with the coronoid passing behind the trochlea, and the medial collateral ligament (MCL) may rupture.

The injury is more common when falling from a horse or bicycle, and from gymnastic accidents. Roller-skating and skateboarding are also prime causes, as the athlete usually falls backwards onto an abducted straight arm. There is often a snap or crack at the time of injury, with immediate swelling. On examination, the arm is held flexed, and a gross deformity is apparent on the posterior aspect of the elbow. The normal triangular alignment of the olecranon and two epicondyles is lost (Fig. 13.15). Radiographic examination is required to assess bony damage, and on no account should reduction

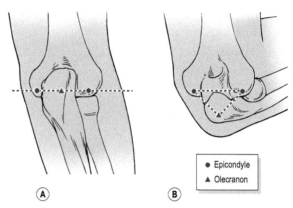

● Epicondyle
▲ Olecranon

Ⓐ Ⓑ

Figure 13.15 Triangular relation of epicondyles and olecranon with elbow flexion.

on the field be attempted because of the risk of neural complications, or interruption to the vascular supply to the forearm. Reduction is achieved by downward pressure on the forearm initially to disengage the coronoid from the olecranon fossa and then the forearm is brought forwards. As with the shoulder, reduction, unless immediate, will usually require analgesia.

Conservative management is usually sufficient following subluxation or dislocation with no bony injury. Bracing is used in a pronated resting position to shorten the lateral ligament. If the arm is immobilized for more than a week, the resting position is generally in as much extension as possible. This is important because reduced flexion is far easier to regain during rehabilitation than is extension. With an uncomplicated injury, gentle isometric exercise is begun as pain and swelling settles. After two to three days, active mobility exercise is started with caution in the pain-free range, the athlete remaining in a sling between exercise periods for protection.

Early mobilization of this injury is importantly. Mehlhoff et al. (1988) described 52 adults with elbow dislocation. Those immobilized for less than 18 days showed significantly better results than those inactive for longer periods, and patients immobilized for more than 4 weeks all showed only fair or poor results. None of the patients redislocated.

Following this injury, there is normally a slight loss of extension. If the elbow has previously hyperextended, this is not usually a problem. However, where the arm remains slightly flexed, weightbearing activities, such as handstands and cartwheels, will tend to push the arm into flexion. To stabilize the arm and obtain some degree of functional locking, the triceps must be built up extensively.

> **Key point**
>
> Early mobilization following elbow dislocation gives better results than prolonged inactivity.

Radial head

Compression fracture of the radial head may occur with a vertical fall onto the outstretched arm, but more commonly the injury which affects the radial head is a *dislocation*. This is usually seen in children, where the radial head is pulled through the annular ligament, limiting extension. The peak incidence of injury occurs between the ages of two and three years, this being the age when the annular ligament is thinner and more easily disrupted. The injury is twice as common in girls as in boys, and the left elbow is affected more often than the right. The mechanism of injury is a sudden traction applied to an extended and pronated arm as an adult lifts the child while gripping the child's hand.

Reduction, if carried out before muscle spasm sets in, may be performed by holding the elbow flexed to 90 degrees and lightly rotating the forearm. The therapist holds the child's elbow in his or her cupped hand and places the thumb over the radial head. The other hand holds the child's hand, and the manipulation is produced with a high velocity supination of the patient's forearm while maintaining thumb pressure over the radial head. At the same time, the radius and humerus are gently pulled together and the radial head is felt to click back beneath the annular ligament on full supination. Often this condition reduces spontaneously.

Nerve involvement

Ulnar nerve

The ulnar nerve may be involved with medial collateral ligament injuries of the elbow, as outlined above. Friction against this nerve or its sheath may give rise to symptoms, causing cubital tunnel syndrome. Since the sensory fibres of the ulnar nerve are more superficial than the motor fibres, sensory symptoms are more prevalent, with paraesthesia occurring in the fourth and fifth fingers.

The nerve passes through the groove behind the medial epicondyle and is covered by a fibrous sheath, forming the cubital tunnel (Fig. 13.16A). The roof of the tunnel is the aponeurosis of the two heads of flexor carpi ulnaris. This is taut at 90-degree flexion, constricting the tunnel, and slack on extension. The floor of the cubital tunnel is formed from the tip of the trochlea and the medial collateral ligament. The ligament bulges with elbow flexion, an additional factor leading to nerve compression, especially with prolonged periods of end-range flexion.

> **Definition**
>
> Cubital tunnel syndrome occurs when there is friction of the ulnar nerve or its sheath. Altered sensation and tingling (paraesthesia) occurs in the fourth and fifth fingers.

Dislocation of the nerve from the ulnar groove can also occur following fracture and is accompanied by a persistent tingling sensation with certain elbow actions. If motor symptoms are present, wasting may be seen in the hypothenar eminence and the first dorsal interosseous space. Tinel's sign and the elbow flexion test may be positive. This latter test involves maximal flexion of the elbow for five minutes to compress the cubital tunnel. Symptoms produced, including pain, altered sensation and numbness, constitute a positive test.

Management depends very much on the severity of the symptoms. Often rest and elbow padding

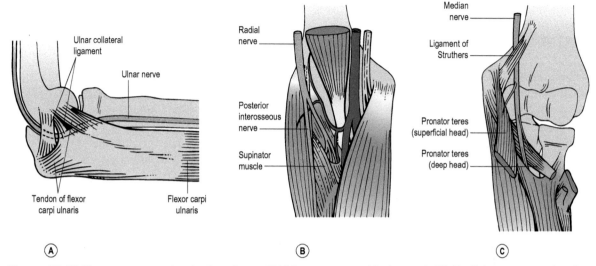

Figure 13.16 Nerve compression in the elbow. (A) Ulnar nerve, cubital tunnel. (B) Radial nerve, arcade of Frohse. (C) Median nerve, pronator teres.

to avoid irritation in contact sports may be all that is required for frictional neuritis. Where adhesions are present following medial joint injury, soft tissue therapy may help. Surgery, if performed early, can be successful in cases of subluxation or bony injury. Nerve transposition combined with excision of a portion of the medial epicondyle and division of the tendinous origin of the flexor carpi ulnaris has been described (Hirsch and Thanki 1985). Neurodynamic testing should be performed, and where positive, neurodynamic treatment (tensioner and/or slider procedures) may be beneficial.

Radial nerve

The radial nerve can be injured in the elbow region. The nerve travels in front of the lateral condyle of the humerus to divide into deep (posterior interosseous) and superficial branches. The superficial branch may be exposed to direct trauma, sometimes being damaged as a complication of fractures to the radial head or neck.

Radial tunnel syndrome occurs when the deep branch of the radial nerve is compressed as it passes under the origin of the extensor carpi radialis brevis and along the fibrous edge of the supinator muscle (arcade of Frohse, Fig. 13.16B). Pain is produced when the arm is fully pronated with the wrist flexed.

Differential diagnosis of radial tunnel syndrome is made by eliciting pain by palpation of the radial head, and pain on resisted supination. True tennis elbow will give pain over the lateral epicondyle (not the radial head), with pain on resisted wrist extension but not supination alone. The condition is seen following repeated contraction of the wrist extensors and forearm supinators against resistance, as in racquet sports in a novice sportsperson.

Most cases respond to activity modification, with neural mobilization being required where symptoms continue. Surgical decompression is reserved for unresolving cases.

Median nerve

In general usage, the medial nerve is most commonly injured by laceration at the wrist, giving an inability to abduct the thumb, a classic 'pointing (index) finger' and sensory loss over the radial digits. In sport, however, medial nerve compression may occur, although it is unusual.

591

At the elbow, the median nerve passes beneath the ligament of Struthers. This is an anomaly found in about 1 per cent of the general population, running from a bony spur on the shaft of the humerus to the medial epicondyle (Fig. 13.16C). Symptoms are generally sensory, with paraesthesia in the forearm and hand. If left untreated, motor symptoms affecting the thumb and forefinger may also occur. Lower down the forearm, the medial nerve passes between the two heads of pronator teres, and it may be compressed here. Resisted pronation may be weak, more noticeably if the movement is maintained for 30–60 seconds, and sensory symptoms may be seen as before. The condition usually responds to an alteration in training, but surgical release may be required.

Testing the elbow following injury

An individual must be able to perform actions relevant to his/her sport or daily living. Maximal functional work of the biceps may be performed by the subject chinning a bar, and for the triceps dipping between two chairs or performing a push-up with the feet on a chair; both of these actions should be slow and controlled until confidence is built. Faster, more demanding actions include press-ups with a clap in between each repetition, and walking hand-to-hand while hanging at arm's length from a horizontal ladder.

Racquet sportspeople should mimic their stroke action with a weighted racquet or heavy club, and can assess their resilience to jarring strains by hitting a club or bat against a firm surface (a medicine ball is ideal). The elbow must be able to take repeated traction and approximation strains, and be pain-free when the arm is locked while holding a weight at arm's length.

References

Abbott, J.H., Patla, C., Jensen, J., 2001. The initial effects of an elbow mobilization with movement technique on grip strength in subjects with lateral epicondylalgia. *Manual Therapy* **6** (3), 163–169.

Bach, B.R., Warren, R.F., Wickiewicz, T.L., 1987. Triceps rupture: a case report and literature review. *American Journal of Sports Medicine* **15** (3), 285–289.

Bisset, L.M., Russell, T., Bradley, S., et al., 2006. Bilateral sensorimotor abnormalities in unilateral lateral epicondylalgia. *Archives of Physical Medicine and Rehabilitation* **87** (4), 490–495.

Briggs, C.A., Elliott, B.G., 1985. Lateral epicondylitis: a review of structures associated with tennis elbow. *Anatomia Clinica* **7**, 149.

Coombes, B.K., Bissel, L., Vicenzino, B., 2009. A new integrative model of lateral epicondylalgia. *British Journal of Sports Medicine* **43**, 252–258.

Coombes, B.K., Bisset, L., Vicenzino, B., 2015. Management of Lateral Elbow Tendinopathy: One Size Does Not Fit All. *Journal of Orthopaedic & Sports Physical Therapy* **45** (11).

Cyriax, J., 1936. Pathology and treatment of tennis elbow. *Journal of Bone and Joint Surgery* **18A**, 921.

Cyriax, J.H., Cyriax, P.J., 1983. *Illustrated Manual of Orthopaedic Medicine*. Butterworth, London.

De Carlo, M.S., Misamore, G.W., Carrell, K.R., Sell, K.E., 1992. Rehabilitation of myositis ossificans in the brachialis muscle. *Journal of Athletic Training* **27** (1), 76–79.

Dreyfuss, U., Kessler, I., 1978. Snapping elbow due to dislocation of the medial head of triceps. *Journal of Bone and Joint Surgery* **60B**, 56.

Fink, M., Wolkenstein, E., Karst, M., Gehrke, A., 2002. Acupuncture in chronic epicondylitis. *Rheumatology* **41** (2), 205–209.

Fredberg, U., Stengaard-Pedersen, K., 2008. Chronic tendinopathy, pain mechanisms, and etiology with a special focus on inflammation. *Scandinavian Journal of Medicine and Science in Sports* **18** (1), 3–15.

Garrick, J.G., Webb, D.R., 1990. *Sports Injuries: Diagnosis and Management*. W.B. Saunders, Philadelphia.

Groppel, J.L., Nirschl, R.P., 1986. A mechanical and electromyographical analysis of the effects of various joint counterforce braces on the tennis player. *American Journal of Sports Medicine* **14**, 195–200.

Halle, J.S., Franklin, R.J., Karalfa, B.L., 1986. Comparison of four treatment approaches for lateral epicondylitis of the elbow. *Journal of Orthopaedic and Sports Physical Therapy* **8** (2), 62–69.

Hirsch, L.F., Thanki, A., 1985. Ulnar nerve entrapment at the elbow: tailoring the treatment to the cause. *Postgraduate Medicine* **77**, 211–215.

Leach, R.E., Miller, J.K., 1987. Lateral and medial epicondylitis of the elbow. *Clinics in Sports Medicine* **6** (2), 259–272.

Lee, D.G., 1986. Tennis elbow: a manual therapist's perspective. *Journal of Orthopaedic and Sports Physical Therapy* **12** (2), 81–87.

Mann, F., 1992. *Reinventing Acupuncture*. Butterworth Heinemann, Oxford.

Matsuura, T., Kashiwaguchi, S., Iwase, T., et al., 2008. Conservative treatment for osteochondrosis of the humeral capitellum. *American Journal of Sports Medicine* **36** (5), 868–872.

Mehlhoff, T.L., Noble, P.C., Bennett, J.B., Tullos, H.S., 1988. Simple dislocation of the elbow in the adult: results after closed treatment. *Journal of Bone and Joint Surgery* **70A**, 244–249.

Mihara, K., Tsutsui, H., Nishinaka, N., Yamaguchi, K., 2009. Nonoperative treatment for osteochondritis dissecans of the capitellum. *American Journal of Sports Medicine* **37** (2), 298–304.

Mills, G.P., 1928. Treatment of tennis elbow. *British Medical Journal* 1 (12).

Molsberger, A., Hille, E., 1994. The analgesic effect of acupuncture in chronic tennis elbow pain. *British Journal of Rheumatology* **33** (12), 1162–1165.

Morrey, B.F., Kai-Nan, A., 1983. Articular and ligamentous contributions to the stability of the elbow joint. *American Journal of Sports Medicine* **11**, 315–318.

Mulligan, B.R., 1989. *Manual Therapy*, Plane View Services, Wellington, New Zealand.

Nirschl, R.P., 1988. Prevention and treatment of elbow and shoulder injuries in the tennis player. *Clinics in Sports Medicine* **7** (2), 289–309.

Paoloni, J.A., Murrell, G.A., Burch, R.M., Ang, R.Y., 2009. Randomised, double-blind, placebo-controlled clinical trial of a new topical glyceryl trinitrate patch for chronic lateral epicondylosis. *British Journal of Sports Medicine* **43** (4), 299–302.

Pienimäki, T., Tarvainen, T., Siira, P., et al., 2002. Associations between pain, grip strength, and manual tests in the treatment evaluation of chronic tennis elbow. *Clinical Journal of Pain* **18** (3), 164–170.

Pienimäki, T.T., Tarvainen, T., Siira, P., Vanharanta, H., 1996. Progressive strengthening and stretching exercises and ultrasound for chronic lateral epicondylitis. *Physiotherapy* **82** (9), 522–530.

Reid, D.C., 1992. *Sports Injury Assessment and Rehabilitation*. Churchill Livingstone, Edinburgh.

Stasinopoulos, D., Stasinopoulos, I., 2006. Comparison of effects of Cyriax physiotherapy, a supervised exercise programme and polarized polychromatic non-coherent light (Bioptron light) for the treatment of lateral epicondylitis. *Clinical Rehabilitation* **20** (1), 12–23.

Torg, J.S., 1993. Comment. *Yearbook of Sports Medicine*. C.V. Mosby, St Louis, p. 72.

Vicenzino, B., 2003. Lateral epicondylalgia: a musculoskeletal physiotherapy perspective. *Manual Therapy* **8**, 66–79.

Vicenzino, B., Wright, A., 1995. Effects of a novel manipulative physiotherapy technique on tennis elbow: a single case study. *Manual Therapy* **1**, 30–35.

Vincent, J., and MacDermid, J.C., 2014. Patient-rated tennis elbow evaluation questionnaire. *Journal of Physiotherapy* **60** (4), 240.

Vitale, M.A., Ahmad, C.S., 2008. The outcome of elbow ulnar collateral ligament reconstruction in overhead athletes: a systematic review. *American Journal of Sports Medicine* **36** (6),1193–1205.

Wadsworth, C.T., Nielsen, D.H., Burns, L.T., Krull, J.D., Thompson, C.G., 1989. Effect of the counterforce armband on wrist extension and grip strength and pain in subjects with tennis elbow. *Journal of Orthopaedic and Sports Physical Therapy* **11**, 192–197.

CHAPTER 14

The wrist and hand

The wrist area has a series of articulations between the distal end of the radius and the carpal bones (radiocarpal joint), and between the individual carpals themselves (intercarpal joints). The radiocarpal joint is formed between the distal end of the radius and the scaphoid, lunate and triquetral, the end of the radius being covered by a concave articular disc. The eight carpal bones are arranged in two rows, the junction between the rows forming the mid-carpal joint. This joint is convex laterally and concave medially, giving it an 'S' shape (Fig. 14.1).

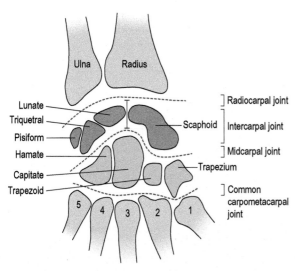

Figure 14.1 The joints of the wrist.

Definition

The radiocarpal joint is formed between the ends of the forearm bones (radius and ulna) and the wrist bones (carpals). The mid-carpal joint is between the two rows of carpal bones themselves.

The wrist is strengthened by collateral, palmar and dorsal ligaments. The ulnar collateral ligament is a rounded cord stretching from the ulnar styloid to the triquetral and pisiform. The radial collateral ligament passes from the radial styloid to the scaphoid and then to the trapezium. The dorsal radiocarpal ligament runs from the lower aspect of the radius to the scaphoid, lunate and triquetral. On the palmar surface, the radiocarpal and ulnocarpal ligaments attach from the lower ends of the radius and ulna to the proximal carpal bones (Fig. 14.2).

The available range of movement at the wrist is a combination of radiocarpal and mid-carpal movement. Flexion occurs more at the mid-carpal joint, while extension is greater at the radiocarpal joint, but the combined movement is about 85 degrees in each direction. Abduction occurs mostly at the mid-carpal joint and has a range of about 15 degrees, whereas adduction involves more movement of the radiocarpal joint and has a range of 45 degrees (Palastanga, Field and Soames

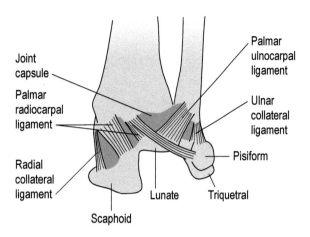

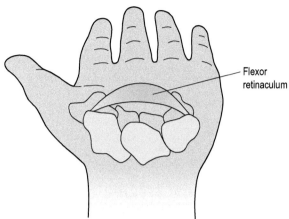

Figure 14.3 Transverse arch of the wrist.

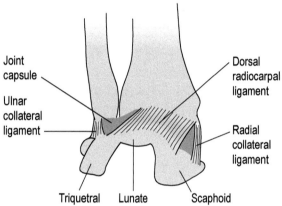

Figure 14.2 The capsular and collateral palmer ligaments of the radiocarpal joint. (A) Anterior. (B) Posterior. After Palastanga, Field and Soames (2013) with permission.

1994). The difference in range occurs because the radial styloid comes down further than the ulnar styloid, and so is more limiting to abduction.

The carpal bones form a transverse arch, concave on their palmar aspect (Fig. 14.3). This arch is maintained by the flexor retinaculum, which attaches medially to the pisiform and the hook of hamate. Laterally, the retinaculum binds to the scaphoid tubercle and to the groove of the trapezium, through which runs the tendon of flexor carpi radialis. The space formed beneath the retinaculum is called the 'carpal tunnel', and the tendons of flexor pollicis longus, flexor digitorum profundus, flexor digitorum superficialis and the median nerve pass through it.

> **Key point**
> The carpel tunnel (i) lies on the palmar (under) side of the wrist, (ii) has a roof formed by the flexor retinaculum, (iii) provides a passage for the flexor tendons and medial nerve.

On the posterior aspect of the wrist the extensor retinaculum stretches from the radius to the hamate and pisiform bones and extends inferiorly to form six longitudinal compartments for the passage of the extensor tendons.

Grip

Prehension (gripping) is an advanced skill in humans, resulting largely from the ability of the thumb to oppose the fingers. Two types of grip may be described – 'precision', involving the thumb and fingers, and 'power', involving the whole hand.

> **Key point**
> Precision grip involves the finger tips; power grip uses the whole hand.

With precision grip, the object is usually small and light. The grip is applied with the nails or fingertips (terminal opposition), pads of the fingers (subterminal opposition), or the pad and side of another finger (subterminal–lateral opposition). This action involves rotation of both the carpometacarpal joints of the thumb and fingers involved in the gripping action. The small finger muscles work in combination with the flexor digitorum profundus and superficialis, as well as the flexor pollicis longus.

In power grips, the long flexors and extensors work to lock the wrist and grip the object. A balance must exist between these two sets of muscles to lock (stabilize) the wrist in its optimal gripping position. Where this balance breaks down, pathology may result. In lateral epicondylalgia, for example, the power of the long extensors is reduced, allowing the flexors to dominate, giving an average of 11 per cent less wrist extension (Bisset et al. 2006). The line of action of the finger flexor muscles (flexor digitorum superficialis and profundus) is at some distance to the axis of the wrist joint. This position creates a significant leverage force, which tends to flex the wrist as well as the fingers. This tendency for wrist flexion is counterbalanced by the extensor carpi radialis muscles to give an optimal gripping position of 35 degree wrist extension and 5 degree ulnar deviation. During light grip, the extensor carpi radialis brevis (ECRB) is most active, but as grip power increases and heavier objects are held, the extensor carpi ulnaris (ECU) and extensor carpi radialis longus (ECRL) are activated (Neumann 2002). Grip force is reduced as wrist flexion increases (Fig. 14.4) due to the shortened position of the finger flexors and the passive extension force created by the finger extensor muscles.

> **Key point**
> Optimal grip force is produced with the wrist in 35-degree extension and 5-degree ulnar deviation. As the wrist is flexed, grip force is reduced.

In the palmar grip, the whole hand surrounds the object, and the thumb works against the fingers. The shape taken up by the hand is largely determined by the size of the object, but the grip is strongest when the thumb can still touch the index finger. This is the type of grip used when holding a racquet or javelin. When the fingers are closed firmly, the fourth and fifth metacarpals move over the hamate bone to further tighten the grip and prevent a smooth object from slipping out of the hand. The hook grip is used when lifting something with a handle, such as a suitcase. Now, the object is held between the flexed fingers and palm, the thumb not being used. Although the grip is quite powerful, the power is in one direction only.

Screening examination

Initial examination of the wrist utilizes a number of movements to cover all the joints involved in wrist articulation. The superior and inferior radioulnar joints are stressed by passive pronation and

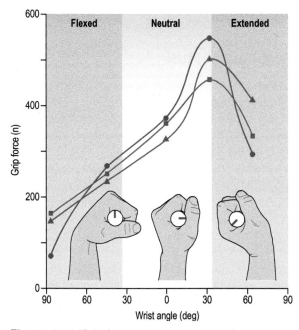

Figure 14.4 Grip force with changing wrist position. Adapted from Neumann (2002).

supination. The wrist itself is assessed by flexion, extension, abduction and adduction, performed both passively and against resistance.

> **Key point**
>
> When the wrist is examined, the superior and inferior radioulnar joints should also be assessed, using passive pronation and supination of the forearm.

At the same time as the wrist is examined, the fingers are also assessed as the two areas are intimately linked. Passive and resisted movements are performed at the thumb and finger joints. Again, flexion, extension, abduction and adduction are used. The capsular pattern for the wrist joint is an equal limitation to passive flexion and extension. Painful resisted movement at the wrist indicates that the lesion is not local but higher up in the muscle bellies, whereas pain to resisted finger movements may give local pain. In addition to pain, crepitus to active movements is an important sign for the long finger tendons.

This examination provides the examiner with enough information to establish whether a lesion is intracapsular or not, and whether contractile tissue is affected. For the therapist, further assessment is usually required to assess and record range of motion and accessory movements. Movements of the individual carpal bones gives more detail about the exact site of the lesion, and the sequence for testing is shown in Table 14.1. In addition, specific tests are used once the initial examination has focused the therapist's attention onto a specific area or series of tissues.

> **Key point**
>
> A screening examination of gross movements allows the examiner to distinguish between pathology at the joint and soft tissues. Examination of individual carpal motion refines the examination and gives an indication of manual therapy required.

Table 14.1 Assessing motion of individual carpal joints

Movements around the capitate
Fixate capitate and move
1. trapezoid
2. scaphoid
3. lunate
Fixate capitate and move
4. hamate
Movements on the radial side
Fixate scaphoid and move
5. the two trapezii
Movements of the radiocarpal joint
Fixate radius and move
6. scaphoid
7. lunate
Fixate ulna (including the disc) and move
8. triquetrum (triquetral)
Movements on the ulnar side
Fixate triquetrum and move
9. hamate
10. pisiform (position the patient's hand in palmar flexion)

From Kaltenborn, F.M. (1993) *The Spine. Basic Examination and Mobilisation Techniques*, 2nd edn. Olaf Norlis Bokhandel, Oslo, Norway. With permission.

Scaphoid fracture

The important feature of this fracture is not the frequency with which it occurs but the number of times it is missed, with pain so often being put down to 'just a sprain'. The usual history is of a fall onto the outstretched arm with the wrist fully extended. When the hand is locked into extension, the athlete is more likely to sustain a scaphoid fracture; this can occur with a vertical fall from gymnastic apparatus, for example. When the hand is more relaxed and the force has some horizontal component, as with a fall when running, the distal radius will usually break (Colles' fracture). The scaphoid fracture is common in the young athlete, while the Colles' fracture is seen more frequently in the elderly. This is partially due to the weakness of the radius with the onset of osteoporosis in the aged.

A further cause of injury to the scaphoid is striking
an object with the heel of the hand, a mechanism
seen in contact sports such as the martial arts,
or in a collision with another player. In addition,
scaphoid fracture can be seen as a punching injury.
Horii et al. (1994) described a series of 125 patients
with fractured scaphoid, 14 per cent of whom had
acquired the injury through punching. Normally it is
a bending force within the scaphoid which creates
the fracture line when falling onto the outstretched
hand. With a punching scaphoid fracture,
however, stress force creates the fracture, making
displacement and delayed union more likely.

Examination

The major symptom of scaphoid fracture is one of
well-localized pain to the base of the thumb, within
the 'anatomical snuffbox'. The athlete's hand is
pronated and gently stressed into ulnar deviation
to make the scaphoid more superficial, as the
snuffbox is palpated. Palpation of the scaphoid
tuberosity with radial deviation of the wrist may
also be painful. In addition, pain is exacerbated
by axial (longitudinal) compression of the first
metacarpal against the scaphoid by pressing the
thumb proximally.

Radiographic examination is helpful, but a negative
X-ray does not rule out fracture, so MRI or CT scan

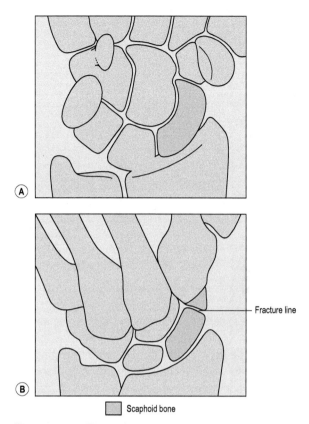

Figure 14.5 The wrist showing the scaphoid bone.
(A) Anteroposterior view. (B) Scaphoid view.

may be better. Non-displaced fractures are often
normal to begin with and only become positive
when some bone reabsorption has occurred, the
fracture line beginning to show up two to four
weeks after injury. Plain AP (anteroposterior) views
of the wrist may easily miss a scaphoid fracture
(Fig. 14.5A), while a specialist scaphoid view
which focuses on the bone itself is more reliable
(Fig. 14.5B).

The scaphoid is 'nut-shaped', with a narrow waist
and two poles (proximal and distal). On the palmar
surface of the distal pole there is a tubercle for
the attachment of the flexor retinaculum and
the tendon of abductor pollicis brevis. The blood
supply to the scaphoid enters through the waist
(centre) of the bone (Fig. 14.6). Smaller arteries
enter from the distal pole and retrograde flow
from these supplies the proximal pole, this pole

599

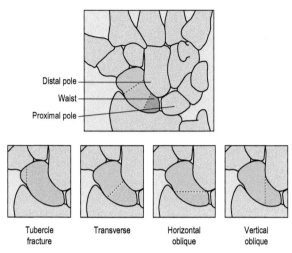

Distal pole
Waist
Proximal pole

| Tubercle fracture | Transverse | Horizontal oblique | Vertical oblique |

Figure 14.6 Classification of scaphoid fracture. From Gutierrez (1996).

having no separate blood supply itself. This has an important clinical bearing, because fractures to the waist of the bone can sever the communicating vessels, starving the proximal segment of blood. This situation makes non-union or malunion more likely.

Classification of injury is important as fractures occurring more proximally tend towards avascular necrosis. In addition, fracture orientation should be noted (see Fig. 14.5) as this will influence stability. Horizontal oblique fractures are generally stable, whereas transverse fractures are inherently unstable.

Management

Scaphoid fracture requires prolonged immobilization of the wrist and thumb. The cast usually extends from the interphalangeal (IP) joint of the thumb to just below the elbow. In some cases, an above elbow splint is used to limit pronation and supination. Uncomplicated fractures of the scaphoid tubercle may heal in as little as four weeks, but fracture to the proximal part of the bone may take as much as twenty weeks. Complications to scaphoid fracture have a poor prognosis. Avascular necrosis may require excision of the avascular fragment, or prosthetic replacement of

the whole bone. Non-union usually demands open reduction and internal fixation (ORIF), percutaneous screw fixation, or bone graft. However, failure rate can be high.

> **Definition**
> (i) Open reduction and internal fixation (ORIF) is surgery where bones are set, consisting of fixation with nails, screws or plates often made from titanium. (ii) Percutaneous procedures are those performed by inserting a needle or other instrument through the skin rather than cutting the skin open with a scalpel.

Successful union has been shown in 90 per cent of patients treated with a differential pitch screw (which is completely buried in the bone) combined with bone grafting (Bunker, McNamee and Scott 1987). This type of fixation significantly reduces the time to return to active sport. With fixation, return in some athletes is immediate, but on average occurs after 4.3 weeks. Athletes treated non-operatively with a playing cast return on average in 11 weeks (Rettig, Weidenbener and Gloyeske 1994). In a systematic review (12 studies met the inclusion criteria out of 112 initially considered), Modi et al. (2009) found percutaneous fixation to give faster rates of union and an earlier return to sport (mean 7 weeks) compared with cast immobilization. A meta-analysis of 14 studies (2,219 patients) showed that displaced scaphoid fractures were four times more likely to progress to non-union that un-displaced fractures, where both were treated in a standard cast. The risk was significantly reduced when displaced fractures were surgically fixated (Singh et al. 2012).

Rehabilitation

Immobilization of the wrist can lead to gross movement loss. It is important, therefore, that subjects perform a range of motion exercise of the shoulder and elbow and free fingers while the cast is still on. Once the cast has been removed, wrist mobilization exercise is essential to regain flexion/extension, abduction/adduction and pronation/supination (see below). In addition, individual carpal joint mobilization (glides) will also be required, moving the whole lateral side of the wrist and hand, but particularly focusing on the thumb. Both open- and closed-chain re-strengthening is needed. Grip and both approximation (push-up) and traction (pull-up on bar) are important if wrist function for sport is not to be limited.

Wrist pain

Sprains

A 'sprained wrist' is a common diagnosis, but really only indicates the area of pain, and the fact that soft tissue is the likely structure affected. The most common tissues affected are the *intercarpal ligaments*, with or without subluxation of a carpal bone. Pain is reproduced to passive wrist flexion and is generally well localized to the particular tissue injured. Common ligaments affected include the lunate-capitate and scapho-lunate. Deep tissue mobilization (massage and transverse frictions) to the ligament with the wrist flexed can be effective at modulating pain prior to exercise therapy.

Sprain to the ulnar or radial collateral ligaments is rare, but if present gives pain to end-range passive abduction and adduction.

Carpal dislocation

Subluxation or dislocation of a carpal bone, rather than a scaphoid fracture, may occur from a fall onto the outstretched hand. The bone most commonly affected is the lunate, although the capitate may also sublux. Movement is generally limited in one direction only (contrast the capsular pattern). Pain is localized by palpating in a line along the third finger to reach the third metacarpal. In the normal hand the capitate lies in a hollow just proximal to the base of the third metacarpal and the lunate is felt proximal to this, and slightly towards the ulna.

> **Key point**
>
> When palpating the dorsum of the wrist, the capitate bone lies in a hollow just proximal to the base of the third (centre) metacarpal and the lunate is felt proximal to this, and slightly towards the ulna (see Fig. 14.1).

When the capitate subluxes, the wrist is held in flexion, and a prominent bump is seen over the dorsum of the wrist as the capitate stands proud of its neighbours. Reduction of a minor subluxation is often spontaneous, but if not, may be achieved during traction by a repeated anterior and posterior glide, with the wrist positioned over the edge of the treatment couch. The wrist is immobilized in a splint until the acute pain subsides, when rehabilitation is begun.

Full dislocation of the lunate may occur with a fall onto the extended wrist. The shape and position of the lunate lying between the lower radius and capitate make it prone to dislocation. On forced wrist extension, the wedge-shaped lunate is squeezed out from between the two bones to lie on the palmar surface of the carpal region (Fig. 14.7) as an apparent 'swelling'. If the athlete

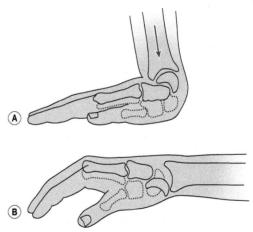

Figure 14.7 Lunate dislocation injury occurs when the radius forces the lunate in a palmar direction, (B) resulting in dislocation. From Hertling and Kessler (1990), with permission.

is asked to form a fist, the third metacarpal head should normally project above the second and fourth. Where the lunate has dislocated, however, all three metacarpal heads may appear in line (Magee 2002).

During lunate dislocation, the scaphoid-lunate ligament usually ruptures and the lunate rotates. Radiographs taken with the forearm fully supinated show a separation of the scaphoid-lunate joint of more than 2 mm. The dislocated lunate may impinge on the median nerve, and the flexor tendons may be compressed within the carpal tunnel.

Reduction under anaesthesia is possible if the condition is diagnosed early, with the wrist being immobilized in some degree of flexion initially, and then protected from forced extension when sport is resumed. If left, damage to the median nerve is more likely and open reduction is usually required.

Occasionally, the lunate may stay in place against the radius, and the carpal bones surrounding it dislocate posteriorly to give a perilunar dislocation. This normally occurs in association with a scaphoid fracture, part of the fractured bone remaining with the radius and lunate. Specialist referral to a hand surgeon is required.

Forced extension injury

Repetitive forced extension causes compression and impaction forces on the wrist. This type of movement is common in gymnastics, and in exercises such as the 'press-up with clap'. In addition, heavy bench press exercises used in training or powerlifting force extension at the wrist. When this occurs, the athlete may experience pain over the dorsum of the wrist, and end-range flexion and extension are painfully limited. The main fault initially may be an impingement of the dorsal wrist structures, resulting in capsular inflammation. If impact forces continue, however, carpal subluxation or fracture may occur in the adult, and epiphyseal damage in the adolescent.

Key point

Repetitive forced extension (gymnastics, push-ups, rapid bench press) may cause impingement, inflammation, carpal bone subluxation and, in children, growth plate injury.

Triangular fibrocartilage

The distal end of the ulna has a triangular fibrocartilage complex (TFCC) which separates it from the lunate. The complex consists of the triangular fibrocartilage itself, the ulnar meniscus, the ulnar collateral ligament, and the extensor carpi ulnaris (ECU). The TFCC prevents ulnocarpal abutment by cushioning forces between the ulna and lunate. Trauma may cause thinning of the meniscus, and a reduction in shock-absorbing capacity. Cadaver studies have shown that the radius takes 60 per cent of axial loading to the wrist when the meniscus is intact, but this is increased to 95 per cent when the disc is excised (Palmer and Werner 1981).

Testing is to load the area by passive wrist extension and ulnar deviation such as pushing up from a chair when sitting (press test). Initial treatment is conservative to protect the area by taping or splinting to avoid wrist extension and ulnar deviation. As pain settles, first isometric and then limited-range strengthening is begun. Progression is to full motion range and strength. For those injuries which do not respond to activity modification, an MRI scan may be required to image the injury, and arthroscopy excision can be required in extreme cases.

Children

Forced extension is of particular concern in the child. Normally, closure of the distal ulnar growth plate should precede that of the radius. However, the structure and function of the distal radial growth plate can be altered by repetitive loading from gymnastics or other sports, and may fuse prematurely, giving radial shortening with respect to the normal ulna. On posterior–anterior radiographs, the position of the ulna may be compared to that of the radius. If the ulnar is longer, positive ulnar variance exists; if shorter, negative variance is present. As the radial growth plate closes after that of the ulna, negative ulnar variance is the norm. However, gymnasts have been shown to have significant positive ulnar variance when compared to controls (Mandelbaum et al. 1989).

Key point

Normally the ulna should be shorter than the radius (negative ulna variance). If the radial growth plate closes prematurely, radial bone growth will stop and ulna growth will continue. Positive ulna variance has been created.

With positive variance, in addition to bone changes, the articular disc between the ulna and lunate may be thinner and less stable. The combination of reduced shock absorption and stability may lead to a chronic degenerative condition.

In the adolescent, rest from activities involving extension and loading of the wrist is essential, with significant healing expected within three months following cessation of gymnastics.

Kienbock's disease

Keinbock's disease (also called lunatomalacia) is an avascular necrosis (osteochondritis) of the lunate, and must be differentiated from a stress reaction of the lunate. The condition may result from direct trauma, such as a compression fracture, or following repeated microtrauma from impact stresses. Industrial stresses, such as hammering, and impact forces in sports, such as tennis, karate, volleyball and golf, can also be factors. Although the progress of the condition is similar in both sporting and non-sporting populations, athletes develop symptoms more quickly.

The condition is seen from adolescence up to the mid-thirties. The lunate atrophies, becomes sclerosed, and later decalcifies, showing flattening and fragmentation on X-ray. The main symptom is wrist pain, with range of motion and grip strength reducing.

Marked deformity of the bone occurs, unless the condition is identified early enough, when pressure on the wrist during sport should be eliminated. If the condition is too advanced to respond to conservative management (normally reserved for stress reaction), surgery is required. As the patients are young, and remodelling of the lunate can be expected, osteotomy is frequently performed rather than carpectomy.

Key point

Kienbock's disease is osteochondrosis of the lunate bone in the wrist. There is pain, reduced motion and weaker grip strength.

Wrist mobilization

Mobilization of the various joints of the wrist is useful both for pain reduction and movement enhancement.

▶ The *inferior radioulnar* joint is mobilized by gripping the lower ends of the radius and ulna and working the hands forwards and backwards against each other (Fig. 14.8A).
▶ The *radiocarpal* joint may be mobilized by gripping the athlete's wrist in one hand and their hand in the other. The edge of the therapist's hands are aligned with the radiocarpal joint line. Again, the hands are worked against each other to perform both transverse mobilizations and anteroposterior movements. Greater purchase may be gained by supporting the athlete's forearm on a low block or on the couch edge (Fig. 14.8B).
▶ *Pronation* and *supination* at the radiocarpal joint is performed using a 'wringing' action (Fig. 14.8C).

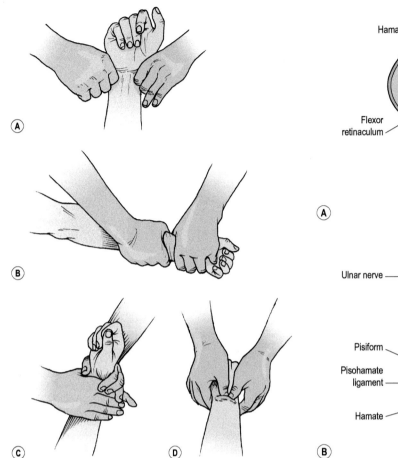

Figure 14.8 Examples of wrist mobilization. From Corrigan and Maitland (1983), with permission.

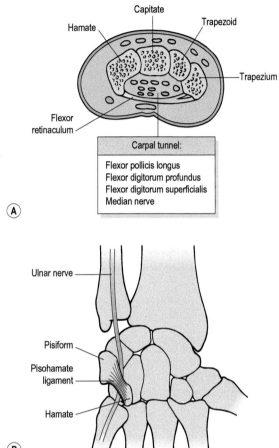

Figure 14.9 Nerve compression in the wrist. (A) Carpal tunnel, (B) Guyon's canal.

▶ *Intercarpal* movements (see Table 14.1) are performed using the thumb pads (Fig. 14.8D).

Compression neuropathies

Carpal tunnel syndrome

Carpal tunnel syndrome (CTS) is a compression neuropathy of the median nerve as it passes beneath the flexor retinaculum and into the carpal tunnel (Fig. 14.9A). It is more common in women than men, and occurs typically later in life (40–60 years), although it is seen in younger individuals secondary to trauma. Paraesthesia (numbness, burning, tingling) is felt over the first three fingers

and the radial half of the fourth. Pain is made worse with repeated movements, and prolonged (1 minute) wrist flexion can reproduce the symptoms (*Phalen's test*). Percussion of the medial nerve (*Tinel's sign*) within the centre of the carpal tunnel with the wrist extended may also be positive.

> **Key point**
>
> With carpal tunnel syndrome, numbness, burning and/or tingling are produced with prolonged wrist flexion (Phalen's test) and tapping over the middle of the wrist (Tinel's sign).

A number of factors may contribute to the condition, and these generally fall into one of two categories. First, factors which increase the size of the structures within the carpal tunnel. This could be through swelling of the flexor tendon sheaths (tenosynovitis) as a result of repeated or sustained flexor activity (gymnasts, cyclists, weight-lifters). Secondly, factors which reduce the size of the carpal tunnel itself, such as arthritic changes secondary to a Colles' fracture, fluid retention during pregnancy and obesity. Interestingly up to 50% of women suffer from CTS in late pregnancy, but the condition is transient. CTS must be differentiated from vascular insufficiency which usually gives a glove-like distribution of symptoms, and entrapment of the C6/C7 nerve root, which does not give increased pain to repeated wrist movements.

Management of the condition is initially to rest the wrist in a splint (day and night), as in the neutral position there is less pressure within the carpal tunnel. In addition, the flexor retinaculum may be mobilized by separating the pisiform and hamate from the trapezium and scaphoid. In severe cases, especially when the median nerve is degenerating, surgery is performed to cut the transverse carpal ligament to relieve tension (Carpal tunnel release). Surgery may be performed through an incision at the wrist (open technique), or using a keyhole (endoscopic technique) which can also be called stitch-less endoscopic carpal tunnel release or SECTR. This technique is carried out through a tiny hole at the wrist or palm. Open surgery gives a better view of tissue damage, but requires an incision through the skin and tissue above the transverse carpal ligament and the cut is larger. Arthroscopic technique uses a smaller cut and passes a tube below the ligament to cut from there. Open surgery will require more recovery (3 months) than arthroscopic (1 month). A period of rehabilitation will be required after surgery to get the hand and fingers moving again and prevent complications.

Electroacupuncture treatment using local points on the pericardium meridian (PC6 and PC7) can be useful clinically to reduce pain. An RCT of acupuncture versus sham used the above points (8 sessions of 60 minutes) and assessed both nerve conduction velocity and global symptom score (GSS) rating. The control group (sham) went from a GSS of 23.7 (mean value) prior to treatment to 22.5 four weeks after treatment, while the acupuncture group went from 24.1 down to 14.6 (Khosrawi et al. 2012). Acupuncture (twice a week for 4 weeks) has also been compared to anti-inflammatory medication (Ibuprofen 400 mg three times daily for 10 days). Outcome was assessed on visual analogue scale (VAS) score, Boston Carpal Tunnel Questionnaire and electrodiagnostic findings following treatment and at 1 month follow-up. Both groups showed significant improvements, with results tending to favour acupuncture (Hadianfard et al. 2015). Although positive results have been produced, a systematic review of 6 RCT's found 5 of the 6 to show acupuncture to be effective for CTS, but with methodological limitations (Sim et al. 2011).

Manual therapy (MT) has also been compared to surgery in the treatment of CTS, when looking at pain severity and functional status. Desensitizing movements of the nerve were used for 30 minutes once a week for 3 treatment sessions. In the short term (1 & 3 months) MT gave greater relief than surgery, but over a period of 1 year the results were the same, indicating that in many cases MT may replace the need for surgery as it has fewer risks (Fernández-de-las Peñas et al. 2015)

Ulnar nerve compression

Ulnar nerve compression (cyclist's palsy) is an unusual condition. The ulnar nerve and artery passes into the hand through Guyon's canal, a shallow trough formed between the pisiform and the hook of hamate, running beneath the pisohamate ligament (Fig. 14.9B). During cycling, the nerve is stretched by hyperextension and ulnar deviation of the wrist. Stresses taken by the hand in cycling can be greater than the athlete's bodyweight, and altered conduction velocity of the distal ulnar nerve has been shown in long-distance cyclists. The condition may also be seen in martial arts where an open hand palm strike is used. In addition to nerve changes, restriction of the ulnar arterial blood flow may occur.

Motor and sensory symptoms may be caused, affecting the fourth and fifth fingers. Weakness and clumsiness of fine finger movements may be seen with a reduction in pinch grip strength. The latter is tested by asking the athlete to pinch a piece of paper between the thumb and radial side of the second finger.

Initial management is by ensuring a correct cycle frame size to prevent the athlete overstretching. Extra padding on the handlebars or in cycling gloves will reduce compression stress, but if symptoms persist, the athlete should refrain from cycling for as long as 4 months to allow recovery of motor function.

Key point

Cylist's palsy is: (i) a compression neuropathy of the ulnar nerve as it passes through the wrist and into the hand; (ii) brought on by prolonged hyperextension and ulnar deviation of the wrist; (iii) fine finger movements are eroded, and there is a loss of pinch grip power between the thumb and index finger.

Thumb

Ulnar collateral ligament rupture

Injury to the ulnar collateral ligament (UCL) of the metacarpophalangeal (MCP) joint of the thumb is common in any sport where the thumb is forced into excessive abduction. This may occur in alpine skiing, where the strap of the ski pole pulls the thumb. It has been estimated that around 10 per cent of all alpine skiing injuries involve this ligament, giving a total of between 50,000 and 200,000 injuries per year (Peterson and Renstrom 1986). The injury also occurs less commonly in contact sports, when the thumb becomes trapped as a player falls.

Chronic insufficiency of the ligament (gamekeeper's thumb) is distinct from complete rupture (skier's thumb). Complete rupture usually occurs from the distal attachment at the base of the proximal phalanx, and in about 30 per cent of cases an avulsion fracture occurs. The UCL lies beneath the adductor pollicis, and with complete rupture the aponeurosis of this muscle (adductor aponeurosis) may be trapped between the pieces of torn ligament which retracts proximally – a so-called 'Stener lesion' (Stener 1962). When the ligament is completely ruptured, contraction of the adductor pollicis will tend to sublux the joint rather than give true adduction, and so grip is weakened.

Definition

A Stener lesion exists when the ulnar collateral ligament of the thumb retracts proximal to the adductor aponeurosis

Symptoms are reproduced by passive extension and abduction of the thumb, and the pain is usually well localized to the ulnar side of the joint. A valgus stress to the MCP joint will stretch the ligament and again gives pain, and this force may also be used to test for ligamentous instability. If the valgus stress is applied with the joint in complete extension (close pack) the joint may appear stable. Unlocking the joint, however, reveals the instability when compared to the non-injured side. In complete rupture, the end-feel of the joint is limp, and a dorsal haematoma may be visible over the thumb interphalangeal joint, indicating that blood has diffused along the extensor pollicis longus.

Key point

Gamekeeper's or skier's thumb is an injury to the ulnar collateral ligament of the MCP joint of the thumb. Extension and abduction of the thumb causes pain, and ligamentous instability may be noted when a valgus stress is imposed on the joint.

Treatment

Treatment of a Grade I injury is initially by rest and ice in the acute phase and then the joint is actively mobilized as pain and swelling settle. Grade II injuries require immobilization for as much as four weeks in a strapping or splint to limit abduction, and in severe cases a cast may be required. Complete ligamentous ruptures generally require surgery, and about a quarter may be expected to have displaced bone fragments (Moutet et al. 1989), which will require fixation.

Following surgical repair, the thumb is immobilized in a cast for four to six weeks, and later a full rehabilitation programme is begun. Movement and strength of the thumb are trained, with an emphasis on thumb opposition and functional gripping actions.

De Quervain's tenovaginitis

De Quervain's syndrome (also called Hoffman's disease) is an inflammation and thickening of the synovial lining of the common sheath of the abductor pollicis longus and extensor pollicis brevis tendons (Fig. 14.10). The thickening occurs particularly at the point where the tendons pass over the distal aspect of the radius (radial styloid or Lister's tubercle). The incidence is higher in females due to the greater angulation of the styloid process. The history is usually of overuse and the condition represents a common occupational injury, but is also seen in rock climbers. There is pain to resisted thumb extension and abduction. In addition, pain is caused by passively ulnar deviating the wrist while keeping the thumb fully flexed (Finkelstein's test), a movement which stretches the tendon and sheath. Local tenderness is found to palpation, again with the tendon on stretch. Crepitus is often present to repeated movements. The condition must be differentiated from arthritis of the carpometacarpal joint of the thumb, which will not give pain on resisted movements, or tendon stretch, but will give pain in roughly the same area.

> **Key point**
>
> Finkelstein's test is used to identify De Quervain's tenovaginitis. It consists of passive ulnar deviation of the wrist while keeping the thumb fully flexed. Pain in the tendon sheath must be differentiated from pain in the carpometacarpal joint of the thumb.

Frictional massage with the tendon on stretch may modulate pain, but immobilization of the thumb in a splint to reduce loading is the key treatment. Corticosteroid injection into the tendon sheath is reserved for persistent cases. In cases of failed conservative management, endoscopic or open surgical release may be required. A comparison of the two techniques (Kang et al. 2013) showed that endoscopic release provided earlier improvement, fewer superficial radial nerve complications and greater scar satisfaction.

Importantly, the stressor causing this injury must be identified and removed. Often, the type of grip and repetition of movement are the two deciding factors. Experimenting with alternative grip types and size of grip is useful to increase the variety of stress imposed on the affected tissues.

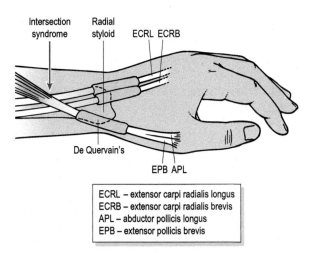

ECRL – extensor carpi radialis longus
ECRB – extensor carpi radialis brevis
APL – abductor pollicis longus
EPB – extensor pollicis brevis

Figure 14.10 Thumb tendinitis.

Intersection syndrome

Intersection syndrome (oarsman's wrist) is a tendinitis between the abductor pollicis longus and extensor pollicis brevis (first dorsal compartment of wrist) on one side and the extensor carpi radialis longus and brevis (second compartment) on the other (see Fig. 14.10). The two sets of tendons are in separate sheaths which cross each other at a 60-degree angle about two to three finger breadths proximal to the wrist crease, and proximal to the radial styloid (the site of De Quervain's syndrome). The condition may also coincide with a compartment syndrome of the thumb extensors. The condition is common in rowing and skiing, and in any activity involving repeated wrist extension and radial deviation. This is often visible swelling along the tendon sheaths and palpable crepitus. Management is by reduction of activity and wrist splinting initially. Steroid injection into the tendon sheath may be required for persistent cases.

Key point

Differentiation of De Quervain's syndrome and intersection syndrome is by palpation. De Quervain's gives pain directly over the radial styloid, while intersection syndrome gives pain 2–3 cm proximal and medial to this point.

Arthrosis

The carpometacarpal (CMC) joint which forms the thumb base, or the STT joint, may all develop arthrosis and give pain on thumb movement.

Definition

The STT (scapho-trapezo-trapezoidal) joint is formed between the three wrist bones connecting to the thumb: the scaphoid, trapezium and trapezoid.

The capsular pattern at the carpometacarpal joint is a limitation of abduction only. The condition is more usual in women and is frequently bilateral, but can also occur secondarily to Bennett's fracture (see below). The typical patient seen by the sports physiotherapist is a mature woman who plays casual racquet sports. The pain is made worse with increasing frequency of play, particularly with a sustained grip. Pain is well localized to the base of the thumb and must be distinguished from De Quervain's (see above). Sudden shooting pains may cause the patient to drop an object in extreme cases, and accessory movements are limited and painful, particularly axial rotations. Pinch grip power is reduced.

Splinting the joint may allow the acute inflammation to subside. Joint mobilization, including longitudinal oscillations, and abduction/adduction while stabilizing the trapezium are effective for pain relief or increasing motion.

Fracture

The base of the first metacarpal is often fractured from a longitudinally applied force, as occurs from a punch in sports such as boxing and karate. Transverse or oblique fracture lines may occur, and if the fracture line affects the joint surface (Bennett's fracture), secondary osteoarthritis may occur in later years. Oblique fractures are often displaced, with the abductor pollicis longus pulling the shaft of the metacarpal proximally (Fig. 14.11). These injuries require manipulation under anaesthetic to reduce them. Maintenance of reduction is by casting the thumb, wrist and forearm, keeping the first metacarpal in extension. Fixation may be required where the joint surface is involved to improve the alignment of the bone fragments.

Immobilization is usually for a period of about three weeks. Active mobility exercises are begun immediately the cast is removed, as stiffness is a severe impairment to normal hand function. Following restoration of joint mobility and strength, functional actions and confidence may be regained using force application along the bone shaft. Exercises include pressing the end of the locked

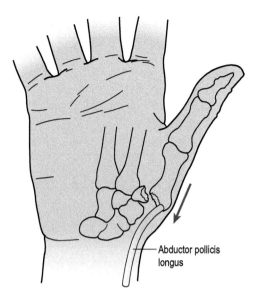

Figure 14.11 Bennett's fracture displaced proximally by the pull of the abductor pollicis longus. From Reid (1992), with permission.

thumb into firstly a foam cushion and then a gym mat.

> **Definition**
> Bennett's fracture is a fracture to the base of the first metacarpal which extends onto the joint surface.

The fingers

The fingers are commonly injured in sport by being 'pulled back' when hit by a ball or opponent (Fig. 14.12). In addition, sports which place great strain on the fingers themselves, such as rock climbing and certain martial arts techniques, may also give problems.

Dislocation

Dislocations of the proximal interphalangeal (PIP) joints, especially that of the fifth finger, are the most commonly seen types. These result from a hyperextension force, with posterior dislocation being more common. Radiographic

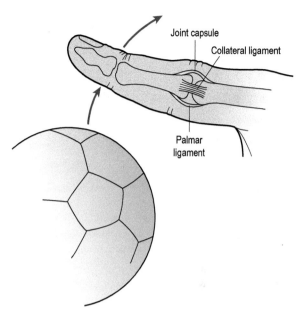

Figure 14.12 Hyperextension injury of the finger. Hyperextension injury (ball hitting finger) may damage the joint capsule and palmar ligament. Greater force creates a dislocation.

appearance is of the middle phalanx overriding the proximal, a condition which is often associated with detachment of the palmar ligament (volar plate) from the base of the middle phalanx. Once reduced, these injuries should be protected in a splint which prevents hyperextension, but allows early flexion.

Where the force is less severe, dislocation may be avoided, but the palmar ligament and joint capsule may still be disrupted. The anterior aspect of the joint is tender to palpation, and the joint is splinted as for a dislocation.

Fracture dislocation can result when an axially directed force is imposed on a semi-flexed finger. The middle phalanx shears and hits onto the condyle of the proximal phalanx, dislodging a bony fragment. When the fragment involves less than a third of the articular line (Fig. 14.13), the collateral ligament usually remains intact and ensures joint stability. Closed reduction is used, with splinting to prevent the last 15 per cent of extension. Where the joint surface is fragmented the collateral

609

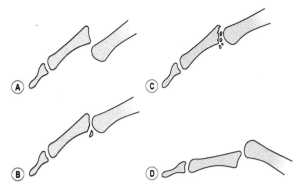

Figure 14.13 Dislocations of the proximal interphalangeal joint. (A) Reducible dislocation. (B) Fracture-dislocation involving less than one third of the articular base. (C) Articular fragmentation involving more than one third of the articular base. (D) Anterior (volar) dislocation.

ligament will usually be disrupted, and repeated subluxation is likely to occur. Open reduction with internal fixation may therefore required.

It is often tempting to reduce finger dislocations straight away, and this is certainly easier than when muscle spasm has set in. As the joint capsule is intact the procedure is usually quite successful. However, the danger of fracture dislocation or the imposition of soft tissue between the bone ends makes it necessary to err on the side of caution. Close examination is needed, and longitudinal traction should be gently applied. The joint may reduce easily, but this should be checked by X-ray.

> **Key point**
>
> Only put back (reduce) a dislocated finger joint after close examination. Do not force the joint, but apply longitudinal traction until the joint reduces spontaneously.

Collateral ligament injuries

The MCP and IP joints have loose capsules which are lax in extension. Each joint has obliquely placed collateral ligaments which become increasingly tight with flexion. In addition, the palmar ligaments are fibrocartilage structures attached loosely to the metacarpals but firmly to the bases of the proximal phalanges. Proximally, the palmar ligament thins out to become membranous. During flexion, this thin portion folds like a bellows, but with hyperextension it is stretched and provides the support lacking from the joint capsule (Fig. 14.14). The fibrous flexor sheaths (containing the tendons of flexor digitorum superficialis and flexor digitorum profundus) in turn attach to the palmar ligaments.

Valgus and varus forces directed against the PIP joints will usually result in partial tearing of the collateral ligaments but leave the joint stable. The injuries respond to strapping to the adjacent finger (buddy splinting) to protect the joint and at the same time facilitate early mobility.

Complete ligamentous disruption may warrant surgical intervention, especially where the radial collateral ligament of the index or little finger is

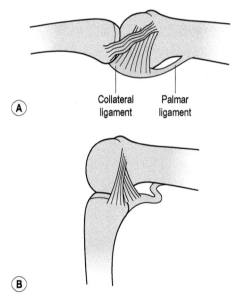

Figure 14.14 Interphalangeal joint of the finger. (A) Extension – collateral ligament lax, palmar ligament tight. (B) Flexion – collateral ligament tight, palmar ligament lax. From Hertling and Kessler (1990), with permission.

affected, as these are subjected to greater stress in normal gripping activities. The ligament normally ruptures at the level of the joint line, possibly with avulsion. After suture repair the finger is maintained in 60-degree flexion for approximately three weeks.

Muscles

The muscles most commonly injured within the hand are the interossei, usually by overstretching the fingers. Pain is highly localized, and increased to abduction (dorsal interossei) or adduction (plantar interossei). As the muscle fibres travel parallel to the finger, transverse friction massage is given by the therapist placing his or her finger between those of the athlete and using a rotation action by pronating and supinating his or her own forearm. Hand rehabilitation exercise is required once pain has begun to subside.

Tendon injury

Prolonged gripping with the tips of the fingers, such as may occur in rock climbing, can cause injury to the flexor tendons. The distal IP joint is extended, while the proximal IP is flexed, stressing flexor digitorum profundus. Long-term exposure to this type of stress may also damage the flexor sheath, increasing the bowstringing effect to resisted finger flexion (Bollen 1988).

Hyperflexion may disrupt the extensor tendon and avulse it from the base of the distal phalanx (mallet finger) or cause the middle section of the tendon to rupture (boutonniere or 'buttonhole' deformity) (Fig. 14.15). This can occur when the end of the terminal phalanx is struck by a ball, for example. When the extensor mechanism is disrupted in this way, the athlete can flex the finger, and while elastic recoil enables the joint to extend slightly, normal extension is impossible.

With mallet finger, tenderness occurs at a point between the nail and the distal IP joint, and the fingertip is held slightly flexed when resting. In a buttonhole deformity, tenderness is more proximal, and the finger is hyperextended at the

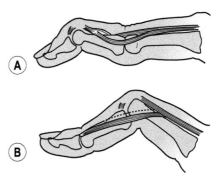

Figure 14.15 Results of injury to the extensor tendon mechanism. (A) Mallet deformity. (B) Buttonhole deformity. From Reilly (1981), with permission.

distal interphalangeal joint. Radiographs reveal the avulsed fragment. Treatment is by immobilization in a splint which maintains hyperextension of the distal IP joint, or occasionally by surgical intervention. Conservative management has been shown to give a very high satisfaction level. In an evaluation of 26 outcome studies, Geyman, Fink and Sullivan (1998) showed an 83.4 per cent satisfaction level with conservative management and recommended that surgical treatment should be reserved for chronic or recurrent injuries only.

> ### Key point
>
> With mallet finger, the fingertip is held slightly flexed when resting. In a buttonhole deformity, the finger is hyperextended at the distal interphalangeal joint.

Inflammation of the extensor tendons (tendinitis), or tendon sheaths (tenosynovitis) may occur with repetitive finger movements. Although more common as an occupational injury (keyboard operators), the condition can occur through excessive training activities. Pain and crepitus occur to repeated movements, with pain localized to the extensor tendon sheaths. Treatment is to remove the stressor and reduce the inflammation with ice and modalities.

Finger pulley injuries

The long flexor tendons of the fingers, flexor digitorum profundus (FDP) and flexor digitorum superficialis (FDS), intertwine with the FDP travelling to the distal phalanx and passing through the FDS, which travels to the middle phalanx. To prevent the tendons from bowstringing as the fingers bend, a system of pulleys exists, making up the flexor sheath. The pulley system consists of fibrous bands of various thicknesses described as five annular pulleys travelling at 90 degrees to the flexor tendons and three cruciform pulleys which criss-cross the tendons (Fig. 14.16). The annular (A) pulleys are named A1–A5 and the cruciform (C) pulleys C1–C3. They are arranged as follows:

▶ The A1 pulley overlies the transverse metacarpal ligament at the *head of the metacarpal* level of the metacarpal phalangeal (MCP) joint and is 8 mm wide.
▶ The A2 pulley is 17 mm wide and originates at the *midshaft of the proximal phalanx*.
▶ The A3 pulley lies at the *distal part of the proximal phalanx* level with the proximal interphalangeal (PIP) joint and is 3 mm wide.
▶ The A4 pulley is located *central to the middle phalanx* and is 6.7 mm wide. It is considered the most important for separate movement of interphalangeal joints.
▶ The A5 pulley lies at the *base of the distal phalanx*, level with the distal interphalangeal (DIP) joint, and is 4 mm wide.
▶ Each of the cruciform (C) pulleys lies in relation to the annular (A) pulleys: C1 distal to A2, C2 between A3 and A4, and C3 distal to A4.

The base of the annular pulleys lies close to the bone and is wider than its palmar surface. This triangular cross-section allows them to come together as the fist is closed to form a continuous tunnel.

One of the most common finger pulley injuries in sport is an A2 pulley injury in rock climbers (Bollen 1988, Logan et al. 2004). The A2 pulley is usually injured during a crimp (cling) grip where the fingertips grip the rock surface, giving DIP hyperextension and proximal interphalangeal joint (PIP) flexion (Fig. 14.17). In this position the A2

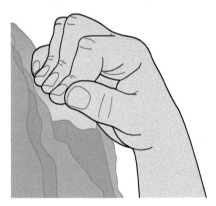

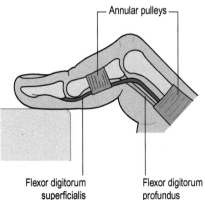

Figure 14.17 Effect of crimp (cling) grip on finger tendons. Adapted from Bollen (1988).

Figure 14.16 Finger pulleys.

pulley sustains 40 per cent more tension than the tendon itself (Logan et al. 2004). Tenderness is usually at the base of the middle phalanx over the FDS insertion of the ring and middle fingers. The crimp hold places the FDP at a mechanical disadvantage, and damage to the A2 pulley has been claimed to increase bowstringing on examination (Bollen 1988).

Treatment is rest from the painful activity and a gradual return to sport. The increased tension taken by the A2 pulley makes taping to support the area important. The finger is taped in flexion with a single stirrup surrounding the pad of the distal phalanx (Fig. 14.18). A rein is laid beneath the finger and secured by a second stirrup around the proximal phalanx. The tape is held firm by a third and final stirrup around the middle phalanx. Each stirrup avoids the joint line, and is placed without excess tension to allow unimpeded circulation. To test tightness, the nail bed is compressed to turn it white and then released; the normal pink colour of the nail bed should return within ten to twenty seconds. On no account should an athlete use taping to cover up an injury. A2 pulley damage requires rest from the stress which caused it. Taping should be used once the injury has recovered.

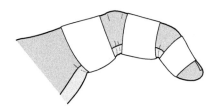

Figure 14.18 Finger taping for the prevention of 'rock climber's finger'.

> ### Key point
> Fingers should be taped to support the distal interphalangeal (DIP) joint and limit hyperextension during rock climbing activities.

Rehabilitation of wrist and hand injuries

Hand injuries occur in both sport and daily living, and there is often a tendency for subjects to play the injury down, especially in cases of contact sport or manual work where heavy hand usage is involved. Subjects may often be found some years later to still have a lack of movement or strength when compared to the uninjured side. This leads to alteration in technique in actions where the hand is used extensively, and can lay the foundation for arthrosis in later years. Hand rehabilitation is no less important than that of, say, a hamstring or injured collateral ligament of the knee, and this must be stressed from the outset.

For soft tissue injuries, especially those affecting the fingers, mobility following injury is an all-important factor. Where splinting is required, this should be in the 'protective position', which prevents capsular and ligamentous contracture while protecting the joint from further injury. The IP joints are immobilized in extension, the MCP joints in flexion, and the thumb in abduction. Movement must be begun as soon as possible after injury. Gentle isometrics and mobility exercise within the pain-free range can usually be begun one or two days after injury.

Following this, exercise progresses as hand function returns. For convenience, wrist and finger exercises will be dealt with separately, although many of the exercises will be used together.

> ### Key point
> Early mobilization of finger injuries is vital to prevent long-term stiffness.

Wrist exercises

Three exercises can be used to form a basis for regaining wrist mobility. The first two are performed with the hand flat on a table top.

▶ Initially, the hand is placed palm down on the table surface, with the wrist crease at the table edge. The contralateral hand is placed on top of the injured one, and the elbow is moved up and down to produce flexion and extension of the wrist. The leverage of the forearm and bodyweight may be used to actively assist movement at end-range (Fig. 14.19A).

▶ The hand is then moved into the centre of the table, so that the whole forearm is supported; again the contralateral hand holds the injured one flat against the table surface, stopping it moving. The elbow on the injured side is moved from side to side, sliding over the table surface to perform abduction and adduction of the injured wrist (Fig. 14.19B).

▶ Finally, the arm is held at 90-degree flexion, with the elbow held close into the side of the body, the injured forearm supported by the cupped contralateral hand. A stick is held in the hand, and pronation and supination performed,

aiming to move the stick into a horizontal position (Fig. 14.19C). Range of motion is measured regularly, and realistic targets are set for the athlete to achieve.

Strength of the wrist is regained by performing movements against the resistance of a powerband or small weight. Flexion/extension may be performed holding a light dumb-bell, with the forearm supported. The other movements are performed with one weight of the dumb-bell removed (hammerbell), or using a hammer. The forearm is positioned with the side supported, and the hand holds the free end of the dumb-bell. Abduction is performed with the dumb-bell weight above the hand, and adduction with it below; in each case a 'chopping' action is used (Fig. 14.20). Pronation and supination are again executed using the hammerbell. The forearm is supported, and pronated and supinated to perform an arc with the hammerbell weight.

In addition to mobility and strength, compression, distraction and combined movements using functional activities are important. The ability of the wrist to take weight (press-up, bench press), to lock (straight arm actions holding a dumb-

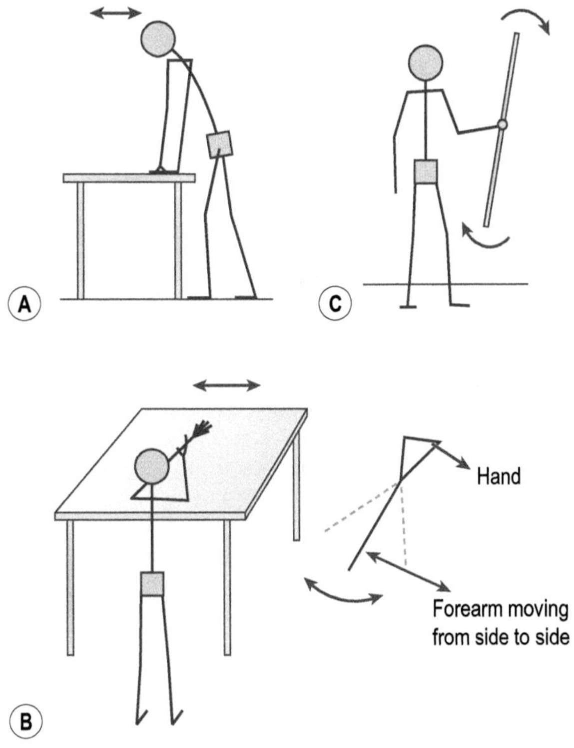

Hand

Forearm moving from side to side

Figure 14.19 Autotherapy wrist mobilizations. (A) Flexion/ extension. (B) Abduction/adduction. (C) Pronation/supination with a broom handle.

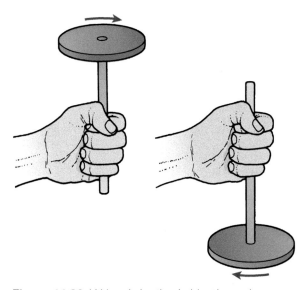

Figure 14.20 Wrist abduction/adduction using a modified dumb-bell.

bell), and to take tension (chinning a bar) must be redeveloped. Rapid actions such as punching, catching and throwing all form part of the late-stage rehabilitation programme.

> **Key point**
>
> Functional wrist exercise includes taking weight (compression) through the wrist, tensioning (traction) the wrist and locking the wrist at various angles.

Finger exercise

Many finger exercises may be begun using simple pinch grip and power grip actions. Grip and release movements, holding and lifting may be performed using small objects with two fingers (pinch) or larger objects and all the fingers (power). Mobility may be performed by isolating the movement to the affected joint and simply teaching the athlete to perform autotherapy activities with the other hand. These are easier when the joint is warm and any tight skin is made more flexible, so hot soaking and the use of oil or cream is encouraged.

Isolation exercises for strength may be accomplished using therapeutic putty, rubber bands of varying sizes and small weights. Again, functional activities, the ability to push, pull and lock, and rapid grip and release actions are important. Simple actions such as screwing and unscrewing varying sized nuts and bolts improve dexterity. Pushing with the finger straight into a thick piece of foam rubber and pulling using pinch, ring, power and key grips help to restore tension and compression ability. Rapid throwing and catching actions with objects of varying sizes and weight rehabilitate grip and release.

> **Key point**
>
> Functional activities for the fingers are vital. Pushing and pulling with the fingers, using the fingers locked (stable) and rapidly gripping and releasing should all be practised.

References

Bisset, L.M., Russell, T., Bradley, S., Ha, B., Vicenzino, B.T., 2006. Bilateral sensorimotor abnormalities in unilateral lateral epicondylalgia. *Archives of Physical Medicine and Rehabilitation* **87** (4), 490–495.

Bollen, S.R., 1988. Soft tissue injury in extreme rock climbers. *British Journal of Sports Medicine* **22** (4), 145–147.

Bunker, T.D., McNamee, P.B., Scott, T.D., 1987. The Herbert screw for scaphoid fractures: a multicentre study. *Journal of Bone and Joint Surgery* **69B**, 631–634.

Fernández-de-las Peñas, C. et al., 2015. Manual physical therapy versus surgery for carpal tunnel syndrome: a randomized parallel-group trial. *Journal of Pain* **16** (11), 1087–1094.

Geyman, J.P., Fink, K., Sullivan, S.D., 1998. Conservative versus surgical treatment of mallet finger. *Journal of the American Board of Family Practitioners* **11**, 382–390.

Hadianfard, M., Bazrafshan, E., Momeninejad, H., Jahani, N., 2015. Efficacies of acupuncture and anti-inflammatory treatment for carpal tunnel syndrome. *J Acupunct Meridian Stud* **8** (5), 229–235.

Horii, E., Nakamura, R., Watanabe, K., Tsunoda, K., 1994. Scaphoid fracture as a 'Puncher's fracture'. *Journal of Orthopaedic Trauma* **8**, 107–110.

Kang, H.J., Koh, I.H., Jang, J.W., Choi, Y.R., 2013. Endoscopic versus open release in patients with De Quervain's tenosynovitis: a randomised trial. *Bone Joint Journal* **95-B** (7), 947–951.

Khosrawi, S., Moghtaderi, A., and Haghighat, S., 2012. Acupuncture in treatment of carpal tunnel syndrome: A randomized controlled trial study. *J Res Med Sci* **17** (1), 1–7.

Logan A.J., Makwana N., Mason G., Dias J., 2004. Acute hand and wrist injuries in experienced rock climbers. *British Journal of Sports Medicine* **38**, 545–548.

Magee, D.J., 2002. *Orthopedic Physical Assessment*, 4th ed. Saunders, Philadelphia.

Mandelbaum, B.R., Bartolozzi, A.R., Davis, C.A., Teurlings, L., Bragonier, B., 1989. Wrist pain syndrome in the gymnast: pathogenetic, diagnostic and therapeutic considerations. *American Journal of Sports Medicine* **17** (3), 305–317.

Modi, C.S., Nancoo, T., Powers, D., et al., 2009. Operative versus nonoperative treatment of acute undisplaced and minimally displaced scaphoid waist fractures – a systematic review. *Injury* **40** (3), 268–273.

Moutet, F., Guinard, D., Lebrun, C., Bello-Champel, P., Massart, P., 1989. Metacarpo-phalangeal thumb sprains: based on experience with more than 1000 cases. *Annales de Chirugie de la Main* **8**, 99–109.

Neumann, D.A., 2002. *Kinesiology of the Musculoskeletal System*. Mosby / Elsevier, St Louis, MO.

Palastanga, N., Field, D., Soames, R., 1994. *Anatomy and Human Movement*. 2nd ed. Butterworth-Heinemann, Oxford.

Palmer, A.K., Werner, F.W., 1981. The triangular fibrocartilage complex of the wrist: anatomy and function. *Journal of Hand Surgery* **6**, 153–162.

Peterson, L., Renstrom, P., 1986. *Sports Injuries*, Martin Dunitz, London.

Rettig, A.C., Weidenbener, E.J., Gloyeske, R., 1994. Alternative management of midthird scaphoid fractures in the athlete. *American Journal of Sports Medicine* **22**, 711–714.

Sim, H., Shin, B.C., Lee, M.S., Jung, A., Lee, H., Ernst, E., 2011. Acupuncture for carpal tunnel syndrome: a systematic review of randomized controlled trials. *J Pain* **12** (3), 307–314.

Singh, H.P., Taub, N., Dias, J.J., 2012. Management of displaced fractures of the waist of the scaphoid: meta-analyses of comparative studies. *Injury* **43** (6), 933–939.

Stener, B., 1962. Displacement of the ruptured ulnar collateral ligament of the metacarpophalangeal joint of the thumb: a clinical and anatomical study. *Journal of Bone and Joint Surgery* **44B**, 869.

Figure and table acknowledgements

Permission given by the following copyright holders is gratefully acknowledged. These figures and tables were reproduced with kind permission. Every effort has been made to contact copyright-holders. Please advise the publisher of any errors or omissions, and these will be corrected in subsequent editions.

Figures

1.1 Reprinted from Oakes, B.W. (1992) The classification of injuries and mechanisms of injury, repair and healing, in *Textbook of Science and Medicine in Sports* (eds Bloomfield, P.A., Fricker, P.A., and Fitch, K.D.). Used with permission from John Wiley and Sons.

1.3 Reprinted from Evans, D.M.D. (1990) Inflammation and healing, in *Cash's Textbook of General Medical and Surgical Conditions for Physiotherapists*, 2nd Edition, (ed. P.A. Downie). Used with permission from Faber and Faber.

1.5 Reprinted from Petty, N.J., Moore, A.P. (2001) *Neuromusculoskeletal Examination and Assessment*, 2nd Edition. Used with permission from Elsevier.

1.6 Reprinted from Low, J. and Reed, A. (1990) *Electrotherapy Explained: Principle and Practice*. Used with permission from Elsevier.

1.10 Reprinted from Oakes, B.W. (1992) The classification of injuries and mechanisms of injury, repair and healing, in *Textbook of Science and Medicine in Sport* (eds J. Bloomfield, P.A. Fricker and K.D. Fitch). Used with permission from John Wiley and Sons.

1.12 Reprinted from Hunter, G. (1998) Specific soft tissue mobilization in the management of soft tissue function, in *Manual Therapy*, 3 (1), 2–11. Used with permission from Elsevier.

1.14 Reprinted from Salter, R.B. and Harris, W.R. (1963) Injuries involved in the epiphyseal plate, in *Journal of Bone and Joint Surgery*: American Volume, 45A, 587. Used with permission from Wolters Kluwer Health.

1.15 Reprinted from Gartland, J.J. (1987) *Fundamentals of Orthopaedics*, 4th Edition. Used with permission from Elsevier.

1.16 Reprinted from Apley, A.G. and Solomon, L. (1998) *Concise System of Orthopaedics and Fractures, 1st Edition*. Used with permission from Elsevier.

1.17 Reprinted from Wolman, R.L. and Reeve, J. (1994) Exercise and the Skeleton, in *Oxford Textbook of Sports Medicine* (eds Harries, M. et al). Used with permission from Oxford University Press.

1.18 Reprinted from Wolman, R.L. and Reeve, J. (1994) Exercise and the Skeleton, in *Oxford Textbook of Sports Medicine* (eds Harries, M. et al). Used with permission from Oxford University Press.

1.19 Reprinted from Bennell, K., Khan, K., McKay, H. (2000) The role of physiotherapy in the prevention and treatment of osteoporosis, in *Manual Therapy* 5 (4), 198–213. Used with permission from Elsevier.

Figure and table acknowledgements

1.20 Reprinted from Gould, J.A. (1990) *Orthopaedic and Sports Physical Therapy*, 2nd Edition. Used with permission from Elsevier.

1.21 Reprinted from Hertling, D. and Kessler, R.M. (1990) *Management of Common Musculoskeletal Disorders*. Used with permission from Wolters Kluwer Health.

1.22 Reprinted from Butler, D.S. (1991) *Mobilisation of the Nervous System*. Used with permission from Elsevier.

2.1 Reprinted from Norris, C.M. (2013) *The Complete Guide to Exercise Therapy*. Used with permission of Bloomsbury Sport, an imprint from Bloomsbury Publishing PLC.

2.3 Reprinted from Enoka, R.M. (2001) *Neuromechanical Basis of Kinesiology*, 3rd Edition, Human Kinetics, Champaign, Illinois. Used with permission from Human Kinetics.

2.5 Reprinted from Safran, M.R., Garrett, W.E., Seaber, A.V., Glisson, R.R, Ribbecsk, B.M. (1988) The role of warmup in muscular injury prevention, in *American Journal of Sports Medicine*, 16 (2), 123–129. Used with permission from SAGE Publications, Inc. Journals.

2.12 Reprinted from Sale, D.G. (1988) Neural adaptation to resistance training, in *Medicine and Science in Sports and Exercise*, 20 (5), 135–145. Used with permission from Wolters Kluwer Health.

2.13 Reprinted from Norris, C.M. (2013) *The Complete Guide to Exercise Therapy*. Used with permission from Bloomsbury Sport, an imprint of Bloomsbury Publishing PLC.

2.18 Reprinted from Jull, G.A. (1994) Headaches of cervical origin, in *Physical Therapy of the Cervical and Thoracic Spine*, 3rd Edition (Grant, R ed.). Used with permission from Elsevier.

2.19 Reprinted from Richardson, C.A., Bullock, M.I. (1986) Changes in muscle activity during fast, alternating flexion-extension movements of the knee, in *Scandinavian Journal of Rehabilitation Medicine*, 18, 51–58. Used with permission from Taylor and Francis.

2.21 Reprinted from Gossmann, M.R., Sahrmann, S.A., Rose, S.J. (1982) Review of length associated changes in muscle, in *Physical Therapy*, 62 (12), 1799–1808. Used with permission from Oxford University Press – Journals.

2.22 Reprinted from Petty, N.J., Moore, A.P. (2001) *Neuromusculoskeletal Examination and Assessment*, 2nd Edition. Used with permission from Elsevier.

3.3 Reprinted from Norkin, C.C. and Levaigne, P.K. (1992) *Joint Structure and Function*, 2nd Edition. Used with permission from F.A. Davis Company.

3.4 Reprinted from Palastanga, N., Field, D., Soames, R. (2013) *Anatomy and Human Movement*, 2nd Edition. Used with permission from Elsevier.

3.5 Reprinted from Magee, D.J. (2002) *Orthopedic Physical Assessment*, 4th Edition. Used with permission from Elsevier.

3.7 Reprinted from Reid, D.C. (1992) *Sports Injury Assessment and Rehabilitation*. Used with permission from Elsevier.

3.21 Reprinted from Magee, D.J. (2002) *Orthopedic Physical Assessment*, 4th Edition. Used with permission from Elsevier.

3.25 Reprinted from Read, M.T. (2000) *A Practical Guide to Sports Injuries*. Used with permission from Elsevier.

3.33 Reprinted from Borley, N.R. (1997) *Clinical Surface Anatomy*, Manson Publishing, London.

4.3 Reprinted from Cox, A.J. (1990) Biomechanics of the Patello-femoral Joint, in *Clinical Biomechanics*, 5, 123–130. Used with permission from Elsevier.

4.6 Reprinted from Magee, D.J. (2002) *Orthopedic Physical Assessment*, 4th Edition. Used with permission from Elsevier.

4.10 Reprinted from Arno, S. (1990) The A angle: a quantitative measurement of patella alignment and realignment, in *Journal of Orthopaedic and Sports Physical Therapy*, 12 (6), 237–242.

4.14 Reprinted from Apley, A.G. and Solomon, L. (1993) *Apley's System of Orthopaedics and Fractures*, 7th Edition. Used with permission from Elsevier.

4.15 Reprinted from Magee, D.J. (2002) *Orthopedic Physical Assessment*, 4th Edition. Used with permission from Elsevier.

4.20 Reprinted from Reid, D.C. (1992) *Sports Injury Assessment and Rehabilitation*. Used with permission from Elsevier.

4.24 Reprinted from Reid, D.C. (1992) *Sports Injury Assessment and Rehabilitation*. Used with permission from Elsevier.

4.25 Reprinted from Magee, D.J. (2002) *Orthopedic Physical Assessment*, 4th Edition. Used with permission from Elsevier.

4.28 Reprinted from Baratta, R., Solomonow, M., Zhou, B.H., et al. (1988) Muscular coactivation: the role of the antagonist musculature in maintaining knee stability. in *American Journal of Sports Medicine*. Used with permission from Sage Publications Ltd.

4.29 Reprinted from Beard, D.J., Kyberd, P.J., O'Connor, J.J., et al. (1994) Reflex hamstring contraction latency in anterior cruciate ligament deficiency, in *Journal of Orthopaedic Research*, 12 (2), 219–227. Used with permission of John Wiley and Sons.

4.31 Reprinted from Henning, C.E. (1988) Semilunar cartilage of the knee: function and pathology, in *Exercise and Sports Sciences Review*, 16, 67–75. Used with permission from Wolters Kluwer Health.

4.41 Reprinted from Reid, D.C. (1992) *Sports Injury Assessment and Rehabilitation*. Used with permission from Elsevier.

4.44 Reprinted from Zuluaga, M., Briggs, C., Carlisle, J. (1995) *Sports Physiotherapy*. Used with permission from Elsevier.

4.57 Reprinted from Reid, D.C. (1992) *Sports Injury Assessment and Rehabilitation*. Used with permission from Elsevier.

4.59 Reprinted from Reilly, B.M. (1991) *Practical Strategies in Outpatient Medicine*.

5.3 Reprinted from Detmer, D.E. (1986) Chronic shin splints: classification and management of medial tibial stress syndrome, in *Sports Medicine*, 3, 436–446. Used with permission from Springer.

5.13 Reprinted from McBryde, A.M. (1985) Stress fractures in runners, in *Clinics in Sports Medicine*, 4 (4), 737–752. Used with permission from Elsevier Science and Technology Journals.

5.14 Reprinted from Read, M.T. (2000) *A Practical Guide to Sports Injuries*. Used with permission from Elsevier.

5.16 Reprinted from Pillai, J. (2008) A current interpretation of popliteal vascular entrapment, in *Journal of Vascular Surgery*, 48 (6), 61–65. Used with permission from Elsevier.

6.1 Reprinted from Burdett, R.G. (1982) Forces predicted at the ankle during running, in *Medicine and Science in Sports and Exercise*, 14 (4), 308–316. Used with permission from Wolters Kluwer Health.

6.10 Reprinted from Eechate, C., Vaes, P., Duquet, W. (2008) The chronic ankle instability scale: Clinimetric properties of a multidimensional, patient-assessed instrument, in *Physical Therapy in Sport*, 9, 57–66. Used with permission from Elsevier.

6.11 Reprinted from Brodsky, A.E. and Khalil, M.A. (1987) Talar compression syndrome, in *Foot and Ankle*, 7, 338–344. Used with permission from Elsevier.

6.16 Reprinted from Magee, D.J. (2002) *Orthopedic Physical Assessment*, 4th Edition. Used with permission from Elsevier.

7.1 Reprinted from Gould, J.A. (1990) *Orthopaedic and Sports Physical Therapy*, 2nd Edition. Used with permission from Elsevier.

7.2 Reprinted from Subotnick, S.I. (1989) *Sports Medicine of the Lower Extremity*, Churchill

Livingstone. Used with permission from Elsevier.

7.3 Reprinted from Reid, D.C. (1992) *Sports Injury Assessment and Rehabilitation*. Used with permission from Elsevier.

7.4 Reprinted from McGlamry, J.G. (1987) *Fundamentals of Foot Surgery*, Williams and Watkins, Baltimore.

7.5 Reprinted from Reid, D.C. (1992) *Sports Injury Assessment and Rehabilitation*. Used with permission from Elsevier.

7.6 Reprinted from Subotnick, S.I. (1989) *Sports Medicine of the Lower Extremity*, Churchill Livingstone. Used with permission from Elsevier.

7.11 Reprinted from Rodgers, M.M. and Cavanagh, P.R. (1989) Pressure distribution in Morton's foot structure, in *Medicine and Science in Sports and Exercise*, 21, 23–28. Used with permission from Wolters Kluwer Health.

7.12 Reprinted from Magee, D.J. (2002) *Orthopedic Physical Assessment*, 4th Edition. Used with permission from Elsevier.

7.14 Reprinted from Hutchison, J.. (2015) Functional atlas of the human fascial system, in *International Journal of Osteopathic Medicine*, 18 (4), 319–320. Used with permission from Elsevier.

7.21 Reprinted from Dandy D. and Edwards, D. (2009) *Essential Orthopaedics and Trauma*, Churchill Livingston. Used with permission from Elsevier.

7.28 Reprinted from Sesseger, B. et al. (1989) *The Shoe in Sport*. Used with permission from Elsevier.

7.29 Reprinted from Sesseger, B. et al. (1989) *The Shoe in Sport*. Used with permission from Elsevier.

7.30 Reprinted from Neale, D., Adams, I.M. (1989) *Common Foot Disorders*, Churchill Livingstone. Used with permission from Elsevier.

7.31 Reprinted from Neale, D., Adams, I.M. (1989) *Common Foot Disorders*, Churchill

Livingstone. Used with permission from Elsevier.

7.33 Reprinted from Subotnick, S.I. (1989) *Sports Medicine of the Lower Extremity*, Churchill Livingstone. Used with permission from Elsevier.

7.34 Reprinted from Sesseger, B. et al. (1989) *The Shoe in Sport*. Used with permission from Elsevier.

7.35 Reprinted from Robbins, S.E. and Gouw, G.J. (1978) Athletic footwear and chronic overloading, in *Sports Medicine*, 9 (2), 76–85. Used with permission from John Wiley and Sons.

8.1 Reprinted from Middleditch, A. et al. (2005) *Functional Anatomy of the Spine*, 2nd Edition. Used with permission from Elsevier.

8.2 Reprinted from Bogduk, N. et al. (1991) *Clinical Anatomy of the Lumbar Spine*. Used with permission from Elsevier.

8.3 Reprinted from Adams, M. et al. (2002) *The Biomechanics of Back Pain*, Churchill Livingstone. Used with permission from Elsevier.

8.4 Reprinted from Adams, M. et al. (2002) *The Biomechanics of Back Pain*, Churchill Livingstone. Used with permission from Elsevier.

8.5 Reprinted from Nachemson, A. (1976) The lumbar spine: an orthopaedic challenge, in *Spine*, 1, 59–71. Used with permission from Wolters Kluwer Health.

8.6 Reprinted from Bogduk, N. et al. (1991) *Clinical Anatomy of the Lumbar Spine*. Used with permission from Elsevier.

8.7 Reprinted from Bogduk, N. et al. (1991) *Clinical Anatomy of the Lumbar Spine*. Used with permission from Elsevier.

8.8 Reprinted from O'Sullivan, P.B. (2000) Masterclass. Lumbar segmental 'instability': clinical presentation and specific stabilizing exercise management, in *Manual Therapy*, 5 (1), 2–12. Used with permission from Elsevier.

8.10 Reprinted from Norris, C. (2008) *Back Stability*, 2nd Edition, Human Kinetics,

Champaign, Illinois, USA. Used with permission from Human Kinetics.

8.11 Reprinted from Kapandji, I. (1974) The physiology of joints, in *Spine*, 3. Used with permission of Editions Maloine (an imprint of V.O.G.).

8.12 Reprinted from Middleditch, A. et al. (2005) *Functional Anatomy of the Spine*, 2nd Edition. Used with permission from Elsevier.

8.19 Reprinted from Herzog, W. (2010) The biomechanics of spinal manipulation, in *Journal of Bodywork and Movement Therapies*, 14 (3), 280–286. Used with permission from Elsevier.

8.21 Reprinted from Twomey, L.T. et al. (1994) *Physical Therapy of the Lower Back*, 2nd Edition. Used with permission from Elsevier.

8.22 Reprinted from Magee, D.J. (2002) *Orthopedic Physical Assessment*, 4th Edition. Used with permission from Elsevier.

8.24 Reprinted from Magee, D.J. (2002) *Orthopedic Physical Assessment*, 4th Edition. Used with permission from Elsevier.

8.30 Reprinted from Gould, J.A. (1990) *Orthopaedic and Sports Physical Therapy*, 2nd Edition. Used with permission from Elsevier.

8.31 Reprinted from Corrigan, B. and Maitland, G.D. (1983) *Practical Orthopaedic Medicine*. Used with permission from Elsevier.

8.32 Reprinted from Magee, D.J. (2002) *Orthopedic Physical Assessment*, 4th Edition. Used with permission from Elsevier.

8.34 Reprinted from Panjabi, M. (1992) The stabilizing system of the spine. Part I. Function, dysfunction, adaptation, and enhancement, in *Clinical Spine Surgery*, 5 (4). Used with permission from Wolters Kluwer Health.

8.35 Reprinted from Norris, C. and Matthews, M. (2008) The role of an integrated back stability program in patients with chronic low back pain, in *Complementary Therapies in Clinical Practice*, 14 (4), 255–263. Used with permission from Elsevier.

8.37 Reprinted from Norris, C. (2008) *Back Stability*, 2nd Edition, Human Kinetics, Champaign, Illinois, USA. Used with permission from Human Kinetics.

9.4 Reprinted from Butler, D.S. (1991) *Mobilisation of the Nervous System*. Used with permission from Elsevier.

9.15 Reprinted from Norris, C. (2015) *The Complete Guide to Back Rehabilitation*. Used with permission from Bloomsbury Publishing PLC.

9.16 Reprinted from Palastanga, N., Field, D., Soames, R. (2013) *Anatomy and Human Movement*, 2nd Edition. Used with permission from Elsevier.

9.21 Reprinted from Read, M.T. (2000) *A Practical Guide to Sports Injuries*. Used with permission from Elsevier.

10.3 Reprinted from Drake, R.L. et al. (2010) *Gray's Anatomy for Students*.

10.4 Reprinted from Grant, R. (1994) Vertebral artery concerns: pre-manipulative testing of the cervical spine, in *Physical Therapy of the Cervical and Thoracic Spine*, 3rd Edition (Grant, R. ed.). Used with permission from Elsevier.

10.7 Reprinted from Butler, D.S. (1991) *Mobilisation of the Nervous System*. Used with permission from Elsevier.

11.1 Reprinted from Drake, R.L. et al. (2010) *Gray's Anatomy for Students*.

11.2 Reprinted from Drake, R.L. et al. (2010) *Gray's Anatomy for Students*.

11.3 Reprinted from Reid, D.C. (1992) *Sports Injury Assessment and Rehabilitation*. Used with permission from Elsevier.

11.5 Reprinted from Magee, D.J. (2002) *Orthopedic Physical Assessment*, 4th Edition. Used with permission from Elsevier.

12.3 Reprinted from Reid, D.C. (1992) *Sports Injury Assessment and Rehabilitation*. Used with permission from Elsevier.

12.4 Reprinted from Palastanga, N., Field, D., Soames, R. (2013) *Anatomy and Human Movement*, 2nd Edition. Used with permission from Elsevier.

Figure and table acknowledgements

12.6 Reprinted from Fleisig, G.S., Dillman, C.J., Andrews, J.R. (1994) Biomechanics of the shoulder during throwing, in *The Athlete's Shoulder* (ed. J.R. Andrews and K.E. Wilks).

12.8 Reprinted from Garrick, J.G, Webb, D.R. (1990) *Sports Injuries: Diagnosis and Management*. Used with permission from Elsevier.

12.15 Reprinted from Kamkar, A., Irrang, J.J., Whitney, S.L. (1993) Nonoperative management of secondary shoulder impingement syndrome, in *Journal of Orthopaedic and Sports Physical Therapy*, 17 (5), 212–224. Used with permission from Journal of Orthopaedic and Sports Physical Therapy.

12.32 Reprinted from Cyriax, J.H. and Cyriax, P.J. (1989) *Illustrated Manual of Orthopaedic Medicine*. Used with permission from Elsevier.

12.33 Reprinted from Keirns, M.A. (1994) Conservative management of shoulder impingement, in *The Athlete's Shoulder* (ed. J.R. Andrews and K.E. Wilks).

12.39 Reprinted from Reid, D.C. (1992) *Sports Injury Assessment and Rehabilitation*. Used with permission from Elsevier.

12.40 Reprinted from Reid, D.C. (1992) *Sports Injury Assessment and Rehabilitation*. Used with permission from Elsevier.

12.53 Reprinted from Palastanga, N., Field, D., Soames, R. (2013) *Anatomy and Human Movement*, 2nd Edition. Used with permission from Elsevier.

12.58 Reprinted from Norris, C. (1996) *Weight Training*, CD-ROM Package.

13.2 Reprinted from Norkin, C.C. and Levangie, P.K. (1992) *Joint Structure and Function*, 2nd Edition. Used with permission from F.A. Davis Company.

13.3 Reprinted from Palastanga, N., Field, D., Soames, R. (2013) *Anatomy and Human Movement*, 2nd Edition. Used with permission from Elsevier.

13.4 Reprinted from Reid, D.C. (1992) *Sports Injury Assessment and Rehabilitation*. Used with permission from Elsevier.

13.12 Reprinted from Nirschl, R.P. (1988) Prevention and treatment of elbow and shoulder injuries in the tennis player, in *Clinics in sports medicine*, 7 (2), 289–309. Used with permission from Elsevier.

14.2 Reprinted from Palastanga, N., Field, D., Soames, R. (2013) *Anatomy and Human Movement*, 2nd Edition. Used with permission from Elsevier.

14.4 Reprinted from Neumann, D.A. (2002) *Kinesiology of the Musculoskeletal System*. Used with permission from Elsevier.

14.6 Reprinted from Gutierrez, G. (1996) Office management of scaphoid fractures, in *Physician and Sports Medicine*, 24 (8), 1–8. Used with permission from Taylor and Francis.

14.7 Reprinted from Hertling, D. and Kessler, R.M. (1990) *Management of Common Musculoskeletal Disorders*. Used with permission from Wolters Kluwer Health.

14.8 Reprinted from Corrigan, B. and Maitland, G.D. (1983) *Practical Orthopaedic Medicine*. Used with permission from Elsevier.

14.11 Reprinted from Reid, D.C. (1992) *Sports Injury Assessment and Rehabilitation*. Used with permission from Elsevier.

14.14 Reprinted from Hertling, D. and Kessler, R.M. (1990) *Management of Common Musculoskeletal Disorders*. Used with permission from Wolters Kluwer Health.

14.15 Reprinted from Reilly, T. (1981) The concept, measurement and development of flexibility, in *Sports Fitness and Sports Injuries* (ed. T. Reilly). Used with permission from Faber.

14.17 Reprinted from Bollen, S.R. (1988) Soft tissue injury in extreme rock climbers, in *British Journal of Sports Medicine*, 22 (4). Used with permission from BMJ Publishing Group Ltd.

Tables

1.1 Reprinted from Magee, D.J. (2002) *Orthopedic Physical Assessment*, 4th Edition. Used with permission from Elsevier.

1.2 Reprinted from Magee, D.J. et al. (2002) Systematic reviews of bed rest and advice to stay active for acute low back pain, in *British Journal of General Practice*, 47, 647–652. Used with permission from the Royal College of General Practitioners.

1.5 Reprinted from Watson, T. (2016) Soft tissue repair and healing review, www.electrotherapy.org. Used with permission from Tim Watson.

1.6 Modified from Magee, D.J. (2008) *Orthopedic Physical Assessment*, 5th Edition. Saunders (Elsevier), St Louis, Missouri. Table 1.35, p.58. Used with permission from Elsevier.

1.8 Reprinted from World Health Organization (1994) Assessment of Fracture Risk and its Application to Screening for Osteoporosis, in Report of the WHO study group, Geneva.

1.10 Reprinted from Jones, M. and Amendola, A. (2007) Acute treatment of inversion ankle sprains: immobilization versus functional treatment, in *Current Orthopaedic Practice*. Used with permission from Wolters Kluwer Health.

1.12 Reprinted from Reid, D.C. (1992) *Sports Injury Assessment and Rehabilitation*. Used with permission from Elsevier.

1.13 Reprinted from Mueller-Wolfhart, H.W. et al. (2013) Terminology and classification of muscle injuries in sport: The Munich consent statement, in *British Journal of Sports Medicine*, 47 (6). Used with permission from BMJ Publishing Group Ltd.

1.15 Reprinted from Cook, J.L. and Purdam, C.R. (2009) Is tendon pathology a continuum? A pathology model to explain the clinical presentation of load-induced tendinopathy, in *British Journal of Sports Medicine*, 43 (6). Used with permission from BMJ Publishing Group Ltd.

1.17 Reprinted from Kesson, M. and Atkins, E. (1998) *Orthopaedic Medicine*. Used with permission from Elsevier.

1.18 Reprinted from Kesson, M. and Atkins, E. (1998) *Orthopaedic Medicine*. Used with permission from Elsevier.

2.2 Reprinted from Kreher, J.B. and Schwartz, J.B. (2012) Overtraining Syndrome, in *Sports Health*, 4 (2), 128–138. Used with permission from Sage Publications, Inc. Journals.

2.3 Reprinted from American College of Sports Medicine (ACSM), (1978) The recommended quality and quantity of exercise for developing and maintaining fitness in healthy adults, in *Medicine and Science in Sports and Exercise*, 10, 7–10. Used with permission from Wolters Kluwer Health.

2.5 Reprinted from American College of Sports Medicine (ACSM), (1990) The recommended quality and quantity of exercise for developing and maintaining fitness in healthy adults, in *Medicine and Science in Sports and Exercise*, 22, 265–274. Used with permission from Wolters Kluwer Health.

2.6 Reprinted from US Department of Health and Human Sciences, (1999) Physical Activity and Health, Report of the Surgeon General, www.cdc.gov.

2.8 Reprinted from Anshel, M.H. (1991) A psycho-behavioral analysis of addicted versus non-addicted male and female exercisers, in *Journal of Sport Behavior*, 14 (2), 145–154. Used with permission from Journal of Sport Behavior.

2.10 Reprinted from McArdle, W.D., Katch, F.I. and Katch, V.L. (1996) *Exercise Psychology, Energy, Nutrition, and Human Performance*, 4th Edition. Used with permission from Wolters Kluwer Health.

2.14 Reprinted from McArdle, W.D., Katch, F.I. and Katch, V.L. (1996) *Exercise Psychology, Energy, Nutrition, and Human Performance*, 4th Edition. Used with permission from Wolters Kluwer Health.

Figure and table acknowledgements

2.16 Reprinted from Potteiger, J.A. (1999) Muscle power and fiber characteristics following 8 weeks of plyometric training, in *Journal of Strength and Conditioning Research*, 13 (3), 275–279. Used with permission from Wolters Kluwer Health.

2.22 Reprinted from Röijezon, U., Clark, N.C., Treleaven, J. (2015) Proprioception in musculoskeletal rehabilitation. Part 1: Basic science and principles of assessment and clinical interventions, in *Manual Therapy*, 20 (3), 368–377. Used with permission from Elsevier.

2.23 Reprinted from Norris, C. (1995) Spinal stabilisation 2. Limiting factors to end-range motion in the lumbar spine, in *Physiotherapy*, 81 (2), 64–72. Used with permission from Elsevier.

3.2 Brukner, P., Nealon, A., Morgan, C. et al. (2014) Recurrent hamstring muscle injury: applying the limited evidence in the professional football setting with a seven-point programme, in *British Journal of Sports Medicine*, 48, 929–938. Used with permission from BMJ Publishing Group Ltd.

3.3 Reprinted from Reid, D.C. (1992) *Sports Injury Assessment and Rehabilitation*. Used with permission from Elsevier.

3.5 Reprinted from Askling, C.M., Tengvar, M., Tarassova, O. et al. (2014) Acute hamstring injuries in Swedish elite sprinters and jumpers: a prospective randomised controlled clinical trial comparing two rehabilitation protocols, in *British Journal of Sports Medicine,* 48 (7), 532–539. Used with permission from BMJ Publishing Group Ltd.

3.6 Reprinted from Wollin, M., Lovell, G. (2006) Oseitis pubis in four young football players: a case series demonstrating successful rehabilitation, in *Physical Therapy in Sport*, 153–160. Used with permission from Elsevier.

3.8 Reprinted from Wollin, M., Lovell, G. (2006) Oseitis pubis in four young football players: a case series demonstrating successful rehabilitation, in *Physical Therapy in Sport*, 153–160. Used with permission from Elsevier.

3.9 Reprinted from Grimaldi, A. (2011) Assessing lateral stability of the hip and pelvis, *Manual Therapy*, 16, 26–32. Used with permission from Elsevier.

3.10 Reprinted from Wall, P.D., Dickenson, E.J., Robinson, D. et al. (2016) Personalised hip therapy: development of a non-operative protocol to treat femoroacetabular impingement syndrome in the FASHIoN randomised controlled trial, in *British Journal of Sports Medicine*, 50, 1217–1223. Used with permission from BMJ Publishing Group Ltd.

3.12 Reprinted from Sahrmann, A. (2002) *Diagnosis and treatment of movement impairment syndromes*. Used with permission from Elsevier.

4.2 Reprinted from Crossley, K. et al. (2007) Anterior knee pain, in *Clinical Sports Medicine*, 3rd Edition (ed. P. Brukner and K. Khan). Used with permission from McGraw Hill.

4.4 Reprinted from Reid, D.C. (1992) *Sports Injury Assessment and Rehabilitation*. Used with permission from Elsevier.

4.5 Reprinted from Jensen, K. (1990) Manual laxity tests for anterior cruciate ligament injuries, in *Journal of Orthopaedic and Sports Physical Therapy*, 11 (10), 474–481.

4.7 Reprinted from Herrington, L., Myer, G., and Horsley, I. (2013) Task based rehabilitation protocol for elite athletes following anterior cruciate ligament reconstruction: a clinical commentary, in *Physical Therapy in Sport*, 14, 188–198. Used with permission from Elsevier.

4.8 Reprinted from Herrington, L., Myer, G., and Horsley, I. (2013) Task based rehabilitation protocol for elite athletes following anterior cruciate ligament reconstruction: a clinical commentary, in *Physical Therapy in Sport*, 14, 188–198. Used with permission from Elsevier.

4.9 Reprinted from Caraffa, A., Cerulli, G.,

Projetti, M., Aisa, G. (1992) Prevention of anterior cruciate ligament injuries in soccer, in *Knee Surgery, Sports Traumatology, Arthroscopy: Official Journal of the ESSKA*, 4, 19–21. Used with permission from Springer Science and Bus Media B V.

4.10 Reprinted from Pasanen, K. et al. (2008) Neuromuscular training and the risk of leg injuries in female floorball players: cluster randomised controlled study, in *The British Medical Journal*, 337. Used with permission from BMJ Publishing Group Ltd.

4.11 Reprinted from Norris, C. (2003) *Bodytoning*, A&C Black. Used with permission from John Wiley and Sons.

4.12 Reprinted from Jorgensen, U., Sonne-Holm, S., Lauridsen, E. (1987) Long term follow up of meniscectomy in athletes: a prospective longitudinal study, in *Journal of Bone and Joint Surgery*, 69, 80. Used with permission from Wolters Kluwer Health.

4.14 Reprinted from Cook, J., Khan, K., Purdam, C. (2001) Conservative treatment of patellar tendinopathy, in *Physical Therapy in Sport*, 2, 54–65. Used with permission from Elsevier.

5.4 Reprinted from Puffer, J.C., Zachazewski, J.E. (1988) Management of overuse injuries, in *American Family Physician*, 38 (3), 225–232.

5.6 Reprinted from Cook, J.L. and Purdum, C.R. (2009), Is tendon pathology a continuum? A pathology model to explain the clinical presentation of load-induced tendinopathy, in *British Journal of Sports Medicine*, 43 (6). Used with permission from BMJ Publishing Group Ltd.

6.1 Reprinted from Palastanga, N., Field, D., Soames, R. (2013) *Anatomy and Human Movement*, 2nd Edition. Used with permission from Elsevier.

6.4 Reprinted from Kosik, K.B., McCann, R.S., Terada, M., Gribble, P.A. (2017) Therapeutic interventions for improving self-reported function in patients with chronic ankle instability: a systematic review, in *British*

Journal of Sports Medicine, 51 (2). Used with permission from BMJ Publishing Group Ltd.

7.3 Reprinted from Irving, D.B., Cook, J.L., Menz, H.B. (2006) Factors associated with chronic plantar heel pain: a systematic review, in *Journal of Science and Medicine in Sport*, 9 (1), 11–22. Used with permission from Elsevier.

7.4 Reprinted from Rathleff, M.S., Molgaard, C.M., Fredberg, U., et al. (2014) High-load strength training improves outcomes in patients with plantar faciitis: a randomized controlled trial with 12-month follow-up, in *Scandinavian Journal of Medicine*. Used with permission from John Wiley and Sons.

8.1 Reprinted from Airaksinen, O., Brox, J.J., Cedraschi. (2005) European Guidelines for the Management of Chronic Non-Specific Low Back Pain, European Commission Publications, Brussels.

8.2 Reprinted from Thompson, B. (2002) How should athletes with chronic low back pain be managed in primary care?, in *Evidence-Based Sports Medicine*. Used with permission from John Wiley and Sons.

8.4 Reprinted from Darlow, B. and O'Sullivan, P.B. (2016) Why are back pain guidelines left on the sidelines? Three myths appear to be guiding management of back pain in sport, in *British Journal of Sports Medicine*, 50 (21). Used with permission from BMJ Publishing Group Ltd.

8.5 Reprinted from Norris, C. (2000) *Back Stability*, 2nd Edition, Human Kinetics, Champaign, Illinois, USA. Used with permission from Human Kinetics.

8.6 Reprinted from Norris, C. (2008) *Back Stability*, 2nd Edition, Human Kinetics, Champaign, Illinois, USA. Used with permission from Human Kinetics.

8.7 Reprinted from Norris, C. (2008) *Back Stability*, 2nd Edition, Human Kinetics, Champaign, Illinois, USA. Used with permission from Human Kinetics.

8.8 Reprinted from Norris, C. (2008) *Back*

Stability, 2nd Edition, Human Kinetics, Champaign, Illinois, USA. Used with permission from Human Kinetics.

8.9 Reprinted from Hodges, P. and Falla, D. (2015) Interaction between pain and sensorimotor control, in *Grieve's Modern Musculoskeletal Physiotherapy*, 53–67. Used with permission from Elsevier.

8.10 Reprinted from Hodges, P. (2015) The role of motor control training, in *Grieve's Modern Musculoskeletal Physiotherapy*, 482–487. Used with permission from Elsevier.

8.11 Reprinted from O'Keefe, M. et al. (2015) Individualised cognitive functional therapy compared with a combined exercise and pain education class for patients with non-specific chronic low back pain: study protocol for a multicentre randomised controlled trial, in *BMJ Open*, 5 (6). Used with permission from BMJ Publishing Group Ltd.

8.13 Reprinted from Norris, C. (2015) *The Complete Guide to Back Rehabilitation*. Used with permission from Bloomsbury Publishing PLC.

8.14 Reprinted from Nijs, J. and Meeus, M. (2014) A modern neuroscience approach to chronic spinal pain: combining pain neuroscience education with cognition-targeted motor control training, in *Physical Therapy*, 94 (5). Used with permission from Oxford University Press.

9.4 Reprinted from Boulding, R., Stacey, R., Niven, R. and Fowler, S.J. (2016) Dysfunctional breathing: a review of the literature and proposal for classification. Reproduced with permission from the © ERS 2016. *European Respiratory Review Sep 2016*, 25 (141), 287–294; DOI: 10.1183/16000617.0088-2015.

9.5 Reprinted from Unverzagt, C., Schuemann, T., Mathisen, J. (2008) Differential diagnosis of a sports hernia in a high school athlete, in *Journal of Orthopaedic and Sports Physical Therapy*, 38, 63–70.

9.7 Reprinted from Sheen, A.J. et al. (2014) 'Treatment of the sportsman's groin': British Hernia Society's 2014 position statement based on the Manchester Consensus Conference, in *British Journal of Sports Medicine*, 48 (14). Used with permission from BMJ Publishing Group Ltd.

9.8 Reprinted from Grieve, G.P. (1986) *Modern Manual Therapy of the Vertebral Column*. Used with permission from Elsevier.

10.1 Reprinted from Grant, R. (1994) Vertebral artery insufficiency: a clinical protocol for pre-manipulative testing of the cervical spine, in *Grieve's Modern Manual Therapy*, 2nd Edition (ed. J.D. Boyling and N. Palastanga). Used with permission from Elsevier.

10.2 Reprinted from Rushton, A., Rivett, D., Carlesso, L., Flynn, T., Hing, W. and Kerry, R. (2014) International framework for examination of the cervical region for potential of cervical arterial dysfunction prior to orthopaedic manual therapy intervention, in *Manual Therapy*, 19 (3), 222–228. Used with permission from Elsevier.

10.3 Reprinted from Wainner, R., Fritz, J., Irrang, J. et al. (2003) Reliability and diagnostic accuracy of the clinical examination and patient self-report measures for cervical radiculopathy, in *Spine*, 28 (1). Used with permission from Wolters Kluwer Health.

10.4 Reprinted from Gunn, C.C. (1996) *Treatment of Chronic Pain*, 2nd Edition. Used with permission from Elsevier.

10.5 Reprinted from Jull, G., Sterling, M., Falla, D., Treleaven, J. (2008) *Whiplash, Headache and Neck Pain: Research Based Directions for Physical Therapies*. Used with permission from Elsevier.

11.1 Reprinted from French, R., St. George, G., Needleman, I. et al. (2017) Face, eyes and teeth, in *Clinical Sports Medicine*, 5th Edition (ed. P. Brukner, B. Clarsen and J. Cook et al). Used with permission from McGraw Hill.

11.2 Reprinted from Magee, D.J. (2002) *Orthopedic Physical Assessment*, 4th Edition. Used with permission from Elsevier.

11.3 Reprinted from McCrory, P. et al. (2017) Consensus statement on concussion in sport – the 5th international conference on concussion in sport held in Berlin, October 2016, in *British Journal of Sports Medicine*, 51 (11). Used with permission from BMJ Publishing Group Ltd.

11.4 Reprinted from McCrory, P. et al. (2017) Consensus statement on concussion in sport – the 5th international conference on concussion in sport held in Berlin, October 2016, in *British Journal of Sports Medicine*, 51 (11). Used with permission from BMJ Publishing Group Ltd.

12.2 Reprinted from McClure, P.W., Michener, L.A. (2015) Staged approach for rehabilitation classification: shoulder disorders (STAR-shoulder), in *Physical Therapy*, 95 (5). Used with permission from Oxford University Press.

12.8 Reprinted from Jaggi, A., Lambert, S. (2010) Rehabilitation for shoulder instability, in *British Journal of Sports Medicine*, 44 (5). Used with permission from BMJ Publishing Group Ltd.

12.9 Reprinted from Peat, M., Culham, E. (1994) Functional anatomy of the shoulder complex, in Andrews J.R. and Wilks, K.E. (eds) *The Athlete's Shoulder*. Used with permission from Elsevier.

12.11 Reprinted from Reid, D.C. (1992) *Sports Injury Assessment and Rehabilitation*. Used with permission from Elsevier.

12.14 Reprinted from Sheridan, M.A. and Hannafin, J.A. (2006) Upper extremity: emphasis on frozen shoulder, in *Orthopedic Clinics of North America*, 37 (4), 531–539. Used with permission from Elsevier.

12.15 Reprinted from Lewis, J. (2015) Frozen shoulder contracture syndrome – aetiology, diagnosis and management, in *Manual Therapy*, 20 (1), 2–9. Used with permission from Elsevier.

13.1 Reprinted from Morrey, B.F. and Kai-Nan, A. (1983) Articular and ligamentous contributions to the stability of the elbow joint, in *American Journal of Sports Medicine*, 11, 315–318. Used with permission from Sage Publications Inc., Journals.

13.2 Reprinted from Lee, D.G. (1986) Tennis elbow: a manual therapist's perspective, in *Journal of Orthopaedic and Sports Physical Therapy*, 12 (2), 81–87. Used with permission from Journal of Orthopaedic and Sports Physical Therapy.

14.1 Reprinted from Kaltenborn, F.M. (1993) *The Spine. Basic Examination and Mobilisation Techniques*, 2nd Edition, Olaf Norlis Bokhandel, Oslo, Norway.

Index

Note: Page numbers in *italics* represent figures and those in **bold** represent tables.